PROCEDURES

D0150802

KINN'S
THE ADMINISTRATIVE MEDICAL ASSISTANT

AN APPLIED LEARNING APPROACH

Brigitte Niedzwiecki, MSN, RN, RMA
Medical Assistant Program Director & Instructor
Chippewa Valley Technical College
Eau Claire, Wisconsin

Julie Pepper, BS, CMA (AAMA)
Medical Assistant Instructor
Health Navigator Program Director
Chippewa Valley Technical College
Eau Claire, Wisconsin

P. Ann Weaver, MSEd, MT (ASCP)
Medical Assistant Instructor
Chippewa Valley Technical College
Eau Claire, Wisconsin

14th EDITION

ELSEVIER

Elsevier
3251 Riverport Lane
St. Louis, Missouri 63043

KINN'S THE ADMINISTRATIVE MEDICAL ASSISTANT: AN APPLIED
LEARNING APPROACH, FOURTEENTH EDITION

ISBN: 978-0-323-61365-1

Notices

International Standard Book Number: 978-0-323-61365-1

Publishing Director: Kristin Wilhelm
Content Development Manager: Ellen Wurm-Cutter
Senior Content Development Specialist: Becky Leenhouts
Publishing Services Manager: Julie Eddy
Senior Project Manager: Richard Barber
Design Direction: Ryan Cook

Printed in Canada

Last digit is the print number: 9 8 7 6 5 4 3 2 1

Working together
to grow libraries in
developing countries

www.elsevier.com • www.bookaid.org

REVIEWERS

Kristi Bertrand, MPH, CMA (AAMA)
Owner/Founder, Chief Academic Officer
Medical Career & Technical College
Richmond, Kentucky

Michelle Buchman, MA, BSN
Michel Assisting Chair and Assistant Professor
Medical Assisting
Cox College
Springfield, Missouri

Candace S. Dailey, MSN, RN, CMA (AAMA)
Dean Health Occupations
Medical Assistant Program Director
Health Occupations
Nicolet College
Rhinelander, Wisconsin

Amy Eady, MT (ASCP), MS, RMA
Medical Assistant Program Director
Dean of Occupations & Program Assessment
Montcalm Community College
Sidney, Michigan

Michael Freeman, CMA
Roseville, Ohio

Tracie Fuqua, BS, CMA (AAMA)
Program Director
Medical Assistant Program
Wallace State Community College
Hanceville, Alabama

Pamela Harvey, RN, MSNED, CPR
Medical Assistant Instructor
North Florida Technical College
Santa Fe College
Gainesville, Florida
Starke, Florida

Angela Kortemeier, MS, RHIA, CHTS-TR, CCMA
Instructor
Business – Medical Coding and Billing
Gogebic Community College
Ironwood, Michigan

Brandi Lippincott, BS, MOS Master
Director
Merit Training Institute
Mount Laurel, New Jersey

LaToya N. Mason, CMA (AAMA), MBA, MHA
Director, Health Sciences
Health Sciences
Lake Michigan College
Benton Harbor, Michigan

Penny Mints, MSB, CCMA, RDMS (AB,OB/GYN), MT (ASCP)
Faculty
Allied Health Department
Northern Maine Community College
Presque Isle, Maine

Norma Moore, BS, MSHA, MT (ASCP), CCMA
Medical Assistant Program Director
Health Sciences Division
Laredo Community College
Laredo, Texas

Robert W. Mun
Program Coordinator of the General Sciences
Department of Education
Hawaii Medical College
Honolulu, Hawaii

PREFACE

Medical assisting as a profession has changed dramatically since *The Office Assistant in Medical and Dental Practice,* by Portia Frederick and Carol Towner, was first published in 1956. Each subsequent edition of this textbook has reflected the age in which it was published. Now, *Kinn's The Medical Assistant: An Applied Learning Approach,* fourteenth edition, continues to represent a long-standing commitment to high-quality medical assisting education with its engaging, straightforward writing style and demonstrated positive outcomes. Hundreds of instructors in classrooms across the country have used this text to teach thousands of students over the years. Many of these students have gone on to teach students of their own with this very same trusted resource. To continue the use and growth of this text and its features, the fourteenth edition continues to offer the most comprehensive, up-to-date, and innovative approach to teaching this subject today.

This textbook has endured throughout the years because it has been able to keep pace with an ever-changing profession while producing students who are well trained and qualified to enter medical practices across the country. This dependability is the reason the market continues to rely on this text, edition after edition. Underlying this dependability is a foundation of pedagogic features that has stood the test of time and that has been expanded and improved upon yet again in this latest edition. Such features include the following:

- An easy-to-read, highly interactive writing style that engages students through practical applications of medical assistant competencies
- An emphasis on skill development, with procedural steps outlining each skill, supported by rationales that provide meaning to each step
- A pedagogic framework based on the use of learning objectives, vocabulary terms, and supportive student supplements
- A package of supportive materials to accommodate a wide variety of student learning types and instructor teaching styles

NEW TO THIS EDITION

- **New chapter** on medical terminology, anatomy, and pathology
- **Reorganized and expanded content** on medical office accounts, law and ethics, math skills, behavioral health, and disease processes
- **New artwork** focused on the workings of a modern medical office, with updated illustrations and photographs of office procedures and medical records
- **Streamlined presentation** with combined chapters and an easier-to-read format
- **New Patient Coaching** section addresses providing information to patients in a supportive environment that allows them to grow, change, or improve their situation
- **More certification practice** with expanded and updated sample exams

EVOLVE

The Evolve site features a variety of student resources, including Chapter Review Quizzes, new Procedure Videos, Medical Terminology Audio Glossary, practice certification exams, and much more! The instructors' Evolve Resources site consists of TEACH Instructor Resources, including Lesson Plans, PowerPoint Presentations, Answer Keys for Chapter Review Quizzes, and a retooled Test Bank with more than 5000 questions.

STUDY GUIDE AND PROCEDURE CHECKLIST MANUAL

The Study Guide provides students with the opportunity to review and build on information they have learned in the text through vocabulary reviews, case studies, workplace applications, and more. The updated Procedure Checklists include CAAHEP and ABHES competencies that can be traced to the online correlation grid.

FEATURES

A Scenario is presented at the beginning of each chapter so the student can envision a real-world situation when reading the chapter content.

Scenario questions provide a way for students to apply the concepts they are learning and think about decisions they would make in real situations.

Learning Objectives emphasize the cognitive and performance objectives presented in the chapter.

Each chapter contains a vocabulary list with definitions so students can first familiarize themselves with the important terms associated with each chapter.

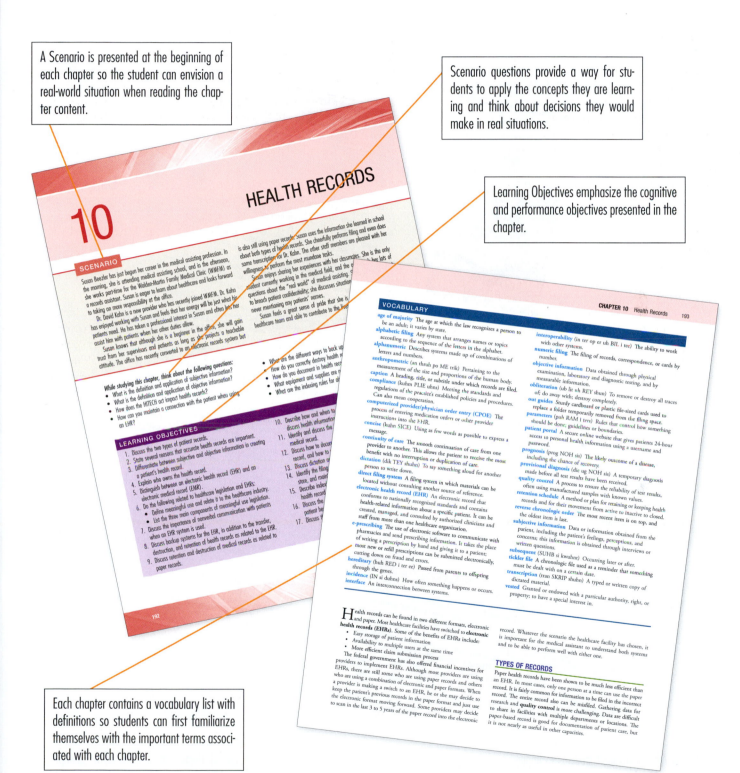

FIGURE 19.5 *Personal Protective Equipment.*

shoe covers, laboratory coats, masks and respirators, protective eyewear, and face shields (Fig. 19.5).

Gloves are the most commonly used PPE in a healthcare facility. Gloves must be worn if the medical assistant is at all likely to be involved in any of the following activities (see Procedure 19.1, p. 425):

- Touching a patient's blood, body fluids, mucous membranes, or skin that is not intact.
- Handling items and surfaces contaminated with blood and body fluids.
- Performing venipuncture, fingerstick/capillary puncture, injections, and other vascular procedures. If a glove is torn during the procedure, the glove should be removed, the hands washed carefully, and new gloves put on as soon as possible.
- Assisting with any surgical procedure.
- Handling, processing, and disposing of all blood and body fluid specimens.
- Cleaning and decontaminating spills of blood or other body fluids.

The same pair of gloves cannot be worn for the care of more than one patient; new disposable gloves must be used for each individual patient.

Safety Alert

Protective equipment contaminated with body fluids of any kind must be removed and placed in a designated area or biohazard waste container. The hands or any other exposed areas must be washed or flushed as soon as possible. Face shields that cover the mouth, nose, and eyes must be worn whenever splashes, sprays, or droplets are possible. Utility gloves may be reused if they are intact (i.e., have no cracks, tears, or punctures). All PPE must be removed before the medical assistant leaves the medical facility (Fig. 19.6).

CRITICAL THINKING APPLICATION   **19.4**

Rosa is caring for an injured 3-year-old child with an open wound on his right knee. She puts on disposable gloves to clean the wound, and the mother demands to know why. How can she explain her actions?

Environmental Protection

Environmental protection refers to minimizing the risk of injury by isolating or removing any physical or mechanical health hazard in the workplace. Every medical assistant must adhere to these safety rules:

- Read warning labels on biohazard waste containers and equipment.
- Minimize splashing or spraying of OPIM. Blood that splatters onto exposed areas of the skin or mucous membranes is a proven mode of HBV transmission.
- Bandage any breaks or lesions on your hands before gloving.
- If any body surface is exposed to potentially infectious material, scrub the area with soap and warm, running water as soon as possible after the exposure.
- If your eyes come in contact with body fluids, continuously flush them with water as soon as possible for a minimum of 15 minutes using an eye wash unit. A stationary unit connected to warm, running water is the best method for properly flushing potentially infectious material out of the eyes.
- Contaminated needles and other sharps should never be recapped, bent, broken, or resheathed; needle units must have protective safety devices to cover the contaminated needle after injection.
- Contaminated sharp instruments, such as operating scissors, should not be processed in a way that requires employees to reach into containers to grasp them.
- Immediately after use, dispose of syringes and needles, scalpel blades, and other disposable sharp items in a labeled, leakproof, puncture-resistant biohazard container. The container must be located as close as possible to the area where the item is used.
- All specimens must be placed in a container that prevents leakage during collection, handling, processing, storage, transport, and shipping. Avoid contaminating the outside of the container or the label with the specimen substance. The container must have a biohazard label to alert others that it holds potentially infectious material. Gloves should be worn throughout this procedure.
- Equipment requiring repair that has been contaminated with blood or body fluids should be decontaminated before being repaired in the office or transported for repair. There is no documented evidence of HIV transmission from contaminated environmental surfaces, but surface contamination is a proven mode of transmission of HBV.
- Smoking, eating, drinking, applying cosmetics or lip balm, and handling contact lenses are prohibited in work areas where there is a reasonable likelihood of contamination by pathogens.
- Food and beverages cannot be kept in refrigerators, freezers, or cabinets or on countertops where infectious materials could be present.

Safety Alert boxes alert students to important safety information and reinforce the importance of safety in the profession.

Critical Thinking Application boxes prompt students to apply what they have learned as they read and study the chapter.

PROCEDURE 20.4   Obtain a Temperature Using a Tympanic Thermometer

Task: Accurately determine and record a patient's temperature using a tympanic thermometer.

EQUIPMENT and SUPPLIES

- Patient's record
- Tympanic thermometer
- Disposable probe covers
- Alcohol wipes
- Waste container

PROCEDURAL STEPS

1. Wash hands or use hand sanitizer.
   PURPOSE: To ensure infection control.
2. Gather the necessary equipment and supplies.
3. Greet the patient. Identify yourself. Verify the patient's identity with full name and date of birth. Explain the procedure to be performed in a manner that the patient understands. Answer any questions the patient may have about the procedure.
   PURPOSE: Identification of the patient prevents errors, and explanations are a means of gaining implied consent and patient cooperation.
4. Clean the probe with an alcohol wipe if indicated. Place a disposable cover on the probe (see the following figure).
   PURPOSE: To ensure a clean surface and prevent cross-contamination.

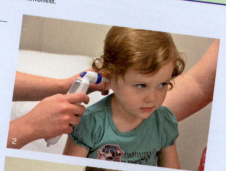

1

5. Insert the probe into the ear canal far enough to seal the opening. Do not apply pressure. For children younger than age 3, gently pull the earlobe down and back (see the first of the following figures); for patients older than age 3, gently pull the top of the ear (pinna) up and back (see the second of the following figures).
   PURPOSE: The external ear must be pulled gently to open the external auditory canal and expose the tympanic membrane for an accurate reading.

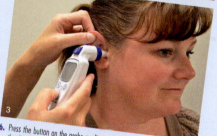

2

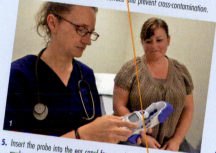

3

6. Press the button on the probe as directed. The temperature will appear on the display screen in 1 to 2 seconds.
7. Remove the probe, note the reading, and discard the probe cover into a waste container without touching it.
   PURPOSE: The probe cover is contaminated and must be discarded in a waste container.
8. Wash hands or use hand sanitizer and disinfect the equipment if indicated. See the manufacturer's manual for cleaning the probe tip. Many recommend cleaning the probe lens with alcohol wipes.
   PURPOSE: To ensure infection control.
9. Document the reading in the patient's medical record (e.g., T: 98.6°F [T]).
   PURPOSE: Procedures that are not recorded are considered not done.

7/11/20xx 2:20 p.m. T: 101.2°F (T) --------------------------------------
-- C. Ricci, CMA (AAMA)

Step-by-step Procedure boxes demonstrate how to perform and document procedures encountered in the healthcare setting.

the anger or become argumentative. Medical assistants must use good listening skills with angry people and must be empathetic. Notify the facility's administrator of all difficult patients or ask for help from co-workers.

There should be a policy in place for dealing with potentially dangerous individuals. Policies can include:

- Making sure that you can reach the exit if you take the patient to another room
- Having another employee close by
- Knowing under what circumstances you should contact the police or building security for assistance

Patient Checkout

When patients return to the front office for checkout, greet them with a friendly smile and call the individual by name. Check the health record to determine when the provider wants the patient to return. Most providers note this information on the encounter form. Make the return appointment. Remember to give the patient an appointment reminder card. If the copayment was not collected prior to the visit it may be collected during checkout.

The medical assistant can convey a sense of caring by terminating the visit cordially. Thank the patient for coming. If the patient will return for another visit, the assistant can say something such as, "We'll see you next week." If the patient will not be returning soon, a pleasant "I hope you'll be feeling better soon" is appropriate. In addition, tell patients to call the facility if they have any questions or if they need additional care. Whatever words of goodbye are chosen, all patients should leave the facility feeling that they have received top-quality care and were treated with friendliness, respect, and courtesy.

CLOSING COMMENTS

Patient Coaching

Providing patients with an information booklet about the healthcare facility can familiarize them with policies and procedures. Many providers compile an extensive booklet that even provides tips as to when the provider should be called immediately, listing symptoms and signs of emergencies.

Educating the patient about the healthcare facility's policies helps the facility run smoothly from day to day. All patients should be familiar with the policies about appointments. This leads to fewer misunderstandings and conflicts over bills that might include a charge for a missed appointment.

If the facility offers internet-based appointment scheduling or forms completion, patients must be taught how to use the system. A printed pamphlet or information sheet is helpful for providing instructions to the patient. A wise option is to have a special phone number that patients can call if they have problems with the system. For best results, choose a program that is simple to use, easy to understand, and does not breach patient confidentiality.

Legal and Ethical Issues

As mentioned earlier, the appointment schedule may be used as a legal record and could be brought by subpoena into a court of law.

Make sure all handwriting in the book is completely legible and that information is routinely collected in a consistent manner for each entry. Do not fail to note a no-show both in the patient's health record and the appointment schedule. This often is helpful when a provider must prove that the patient did not follow medical advice or that the patient contributed to his or her poor condition by missing appointments. Old appointment schedules should be kept for a time equal to that of the statute of limitations in the state where the practice is located.

A medical assistant must never offer medical advice to a patient. The patient sees the medical assistant as an extension of the provider and tends to weigh advice and comments by the medical assistant with the same validity as if they came from the provider. Provide only information the provider has approved or that is included in the healthcare facility's policies and procedures manual.

When a patient complains, listen carefully and try to resolve the problem or assure the patient that the issue will be discussed with the appropriate staff member to find a solution. If someone other than the patient asks for information about the patient, refrain from discussion unless the patient or provider has authorized the release of information.

Patient-Centered Care

Going to a healthcare facility can be intimidating and uncomfortable for many patients. It is important that the medical assistant try to put everyone at ease. Cultivate the habit of greeting each patient immediately in a friendly, self-assured manner. Establish eye contact and smile while introducing yourself to the patient.

Small talk can help put a patient at ease. Talking about the weather or an uncontroversial topic may make the patient more comfortable. Asking personalized questions can also help. Providers and staff members sometimes make brief notes in the health record about the current events in the patient's life. On the next visit, the staff or provider can use this information to start a conversation with the patient. For instance, the patient may state she is going to Florida for a vacation. During the next visit, the provider may start off the visit by asking how her Florida trip was. Asking personalized questions will solidify the personal connection with patients. They may feel important, less intimidated, and more comfortable. It is a great way to provide excellent customer service.

Professional Behaviors

When working in scheduling and helping patients move through the healthcare facility, medical assistants have many opportunities to demonstrate professionalism. It is important to remember that we are often seeing patients when they are not at their best, so we must learn not to take all of the responses personally. When an angry patient approaches the reception desk, you should smile politely, ask how you can help the person, and respond in a soothing tone of voice. When a patient calls for an appointment and demands a day and time when the provider is not available, you should remain calm and explain why that day and time are not an option. As a medical assistant in the front office, you have the opportunity to make an amazing first impression on patients. Remember to always behave professionally.

Patient Coaching sections address how the MA can provide information to patients in a supportive environment that allows them to grow, change, or improve their situation.

NEW! Professional Behaviors boxes provide tips on professional behavior that are specific to each chapter's content.

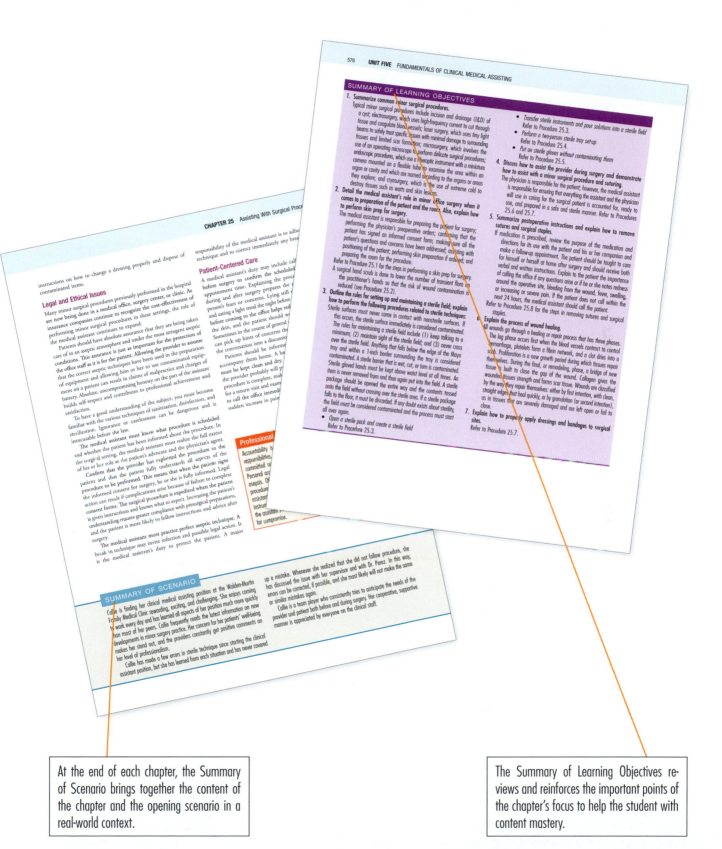

576 **UNIT FIVE** FUNDAMENTALS OF CLINICAL MEDICAL ASSISTING

SUMMARY OF LEARNING OBJECTIVES

1. **Summarize common minor surgical procedures.**
Typical minor surgical procedures include incision and drainage (I&D) of a cyst; electrosurgery, which uses high-frequency current to cut through tissue and coagulate blood vessels; laser surgery, which uses tiny light beams to safely treat specific issues with minimal damage to surrounding tissues and limited scar formation; microsurgery, which involves the use of an operating microscope to perform delicate surgical procedures; endoscopic procedures, which use a fiberoptic instrument with a miniature camera mounted on a flexible tube to examine the area within an organ or cavity and which are named according to the organs or areas they explore; and cryosurgery, which is the use of extreme cold to destroy tissues such as warts and skin lesions.

2. **Detail the medical assistant's role in minor office surgery when it comes to preparation of the patient and the room. Also, explain how to perform skin prep for surgery.**
The medical assistant is responsible for preparing the patient for surgery; performing the physician's preoperative orders; confirming that the patient has signed an informed consent form; making sure all the patient's questions and concerns have been addressed; assisting with positioning of the patient; performing skin preparation if ordered; and preparing the room for the procedure.
Refer to Procedure 25.1 for the steps in performing a skin prep for surgery.
A surgical hand scrub is done to lower the number of transient flora on the practitioner's hands so that the risk of wound contamination is reduced (see Procedure 25.2).

3. **Outline the rules for setting up and maintaining a sterile field; explain how to perform the following procedures related to sterile techniques:**
Sterile surfaces must never come in contact with nonsterile surfaces. If this occurs, the sterile surface immediately is considered contaminated. The rules for maintaining a sterile field include (1) keep talking to a minimum; (2) maintain sight of the sterile field; and (3) never cross over the sterile field. Anything that falls below the edge of the Mayo tray and within a 1-inch border surrounding the tray is considered contaminated. A sterile barrier that is wet, cut, or torn is contaminated. Sterile gloved hands must be kept above waist level at all times. An item is never removed from and then again put into the field. A sterile package should be opened the entire way and the contents tossed onto the field without crossing over the sterile area. If a sterile package falls to the floor, it must be discarded. If any doubt exists about sterility, the field must be considered contaminated and the process must start all over again.
   - *Open a sterile pack and create a sterile field*
     Refer to Procedure 25.3.

   - *Transfer sterile instruments and pour solutions into a sterile field*
     Refer to Procedure 25.3.
   - *Perform a two-person sterile tray set-up*
     Refer to Procedure 25.4.
   - *Put on sterile gloves without contaminating them*
     Refer to Procedure 25.5.

4. **Discuss how to assist the provider during surgery and demonstrate how to assist with a minor surgical procedure and suturing.**
The physician is responsible for the patient; however, the medical assistant is responsible for ensuring that everything the assistant and the physician will use in caring for the surgical patient is accounted for, ready to use, and prepared in a safe and sterile manner. Refer to Procedures 25.6 and 25.7.

5. **Summarize postoperative instructions and explain how to remove sutures and surgical staples.**
If medication is prescribed, review the purpose of the medication and directions for its use with the patient and his or her companion and make a follow-up appointment. The patient should be taught to care for himself or herself at home after surgery and should receive both verbal and written instructions. Explain to the patient the importance of calling the office if any questions arise or if he or she notes redness around the operative site, bleeding from the wound, fever, swelling, or increasing or severe pain. If the patient does not call within the next 24 hours, the medical assistant should call the patient. Refer to Procedure 25.8 for the steps in removing sutures and surgical staples.

6. **Explain the process of wound healing.**
All wounds go through a healing or repair process that has three phases. The lag phase occurs first when the blood vessels contract to control hemorrhage, platelets form a fibrin network, and a clot dries into a scab. Proliferation is a new growth period during which tissues repair themselves. During the final, or remodeling, phase, a bridge of new tissue is built to close the gap of the wound. Collagen gives the wounded tissues strength and forms scar tissue. Wounds are classified by the way they repair themselves: either by first intention, with clean, straight edges, that heal quickly, or by granulation (or second intention), as in tissues that are severely damaged and are left open or fail to close.

7. **Explain how to properly apply dressings and bandages to surgical sites.**
Refer to Procedure 25.7.

CHAPTER 25 Assisting With Surgical Proce...

instructions on how to change a dressing properly and dispose of contaminated items.

Legal and Ethical Issues
Many minor surgical procedures previously performed in the hospital are now being done in a medical office, surgery center, or clinic. As insurance companies continue to recognize the cost-effectiveness of performing minor surgical procedures in these settings, the role of the medical assistant continues to expand.

Patients should have absolute assurance that they are being taken care of in an aseptic atmosphere and under the most stringent aseptic conditions. This assurance is just as important for the protection of the office staff as it is for the patient. Allowing the provider to assume that the correct aseptic techniques have been used in the preparation of equipment and allowing him or her to use contaminated equipment on a patient can result in claims of malpractice and charges of battery. Absolute, uncompromising honesty on the part of the assistant builds self-respect and contributes to professional achievement and satisfaction.

To have a good understanding of the subject, you must become familiar with the various techniques of sanitization, disinfection, and sterilization before you act. Ignorance or carelessness can be dangerous and is inexcusable before the law.

The medical assistant must know what procedure is scheduled and whether the patient has been informed about the procedure. In the surgical setting, the medical assistant must realize the full extent of his or her role as the patient's advocate and the physician's agent.

Confirm that the provider has explained the procedure to the patient and that the patient fully understands all aspects of the procedure to be performed. This means that when the patient signs the informed consent for surgery, he or she is fully informed. Legal action can result if complications arise because of failure to complete consent forms. The surgical procedure is expedited when the patient is given instructions and knows what to expect. Increasing the patient's understanding ensures greater compliance with presurgical preparations, and the patient is more likely to follow instructions and advice after surgery.

The medical assistant must practice perfect aseptic technique. A break in technique may invite infection and possible legal action. It is the medical assistant's duty to protect the patient. A major

responsibility of the medical assistant is to adhe... technique and to correct immediately any brea...

Patient-Centered Care
A medical assistant's duty may include call... before surgery to confirm the scheduled ... appointment time. Explaining the proce... during and after surgery prepares the ... person's fears or concerns. Lying still ... and eating a light meal the night before ... before coming to the office helps red... the skin, and the patient should w... Sometimes in the course of general ... can pick up hints of concerns th... the conversation into a discussio...

Patients should be informe... accompany them home. A ba... must be kept clean and dry... the provider probably will p... procedure is complete, mak... for a return visit and exam... to call the office immedia... sudden increase in pain...

SUMMARY OF SCENARIO

Callie is finding her clinical medical assisting position at the Walden-Martin Family Medical Clinic rewarding, exciting, and challenging. She enjoys coming to work every day and has learned all aspects of her position much more quickly than most of her peers. Callie frequently reads the latest information on new developments in minor surgery practice. Her concern for her patients' well-being makes her stand out, and the providers constantly get positive comments on her level of professionalism.

Callie has made a few errors in sterile technique since starting the clinical assistant position, but she has learned from each situation and has never covered

up a mistake. Whenever she realized that she did not follow procedure, she has discussed the issue with her supervisor and with Dr. Perez. In this way, errors can be corrected, if possible, and she most likely will not make the same or similar mistakes again.

Callie is a team player who consistently tries to anticipate the needs of the provider and patient both before and during surgery. Her cooperative, supportive manner is appreciated by everyone on the clinical staff.

At the end of each chapter, the Summary of Scenario brings together the content of the chapter and the opening scenario in a real-world context.

The Summary of Learning Objectives reviews and reinforces the important points of the chapter's focus to help the student with content mastery.

CONTENTS

THE PROFESSIONAL MEDICAL ASSISTANT AND THE HEALTHCARE TEAM

SCENARIO

Carmen Angelos is a new student in a medical assisting program accredited by the Commission on Accreditation of Allied Health Education Programs (CAAHEP) at Butler County Community College. Carmen is returning to school after working at a local pharmacy for 5 years, where she became very interested in pursuing a career in medical assisting. She has been out of high school for a few years but is very excited about her new career choice.

While studying this chapter, think about the following questions:

- Why is professionalism an important attribute in the field of medical assisting?
- What is a typical job description for an entry-level medical assistant?
- How will scope of practice and standards of care determine your role as a medical assistant?
- Why is it important to learn about professional medical assisting organizations?
- Studying may be a challenge for Carmen. What skills can she use to help her learn new material and prepare for examinations?
- Why is it important for medical assisting students to learn about the various healthcare facilities and medical specialties?
- How can Carmen show professional behavior toward all patients in the healthcare setting?
- How can time management strategies help Carmen prioritize her responsibilities as a member of the healthcare team?

LEARNING OBJECTIVES

1. Discuss the typical responsibilities of a medical assistant and describe the role of the medical assistant as a patient navigator.
2. Discuss the attributes of a professional medical assistant, project a professional image in the ambulatory care setting, and describe how to show respect for individual diversity.
3. Differentiate between scope of practice and standards of care for medical assistants.
4. List and discuss professional medical assisting organizations.
5. Examine your learning preferences and interpret how your learning style affects your success as a student.
6. Integrate effective study skills into your daily activities, design test-taking strategies that help you take charge of your success, and incorporate critical thinking skills and reflection to help you make mental connections as you learn material.
7. Summarize the history of medicine and its significance to the medical assisting profession.
8. Summarize the various types of medical professionals, allied health professionals, and healthcare facilities.
9. Define a patient-centered medical home (PCMH) and discuss its five core functions and attributes.
10. Explain the reasons professionalism is important in the medical field, describe work ethics, and stress the importance of cooperation.
11. Apply time management strategies to prioritize the medical assistant's responsibilities as a member of the healthcare team.
12. Respond to criticism, problem-solve, identify obstacles to professional behaviors, and define the principles of self-boundaries.

VOCABULARY

allopathic (al uh PATH ik) A system of medical practice that treats disease by the use of remedies, such as medications and surgery, to produce effects different from those caused by the disease under treatment; medical doctors (MDs) and osteopaths (DOs) practice allopathic medicine; also called conventional medicine.

complementary and alternative medicine (CAM) A group of diverse medical and healthcare systems, practices, and products that are not generally considered part of conventional medicine. Complementary medicine is used in combination with conventional medicine (allopathic or osteopathic); alternative medicine is used instead of conventional medicine.

conscientious (kon shee EN shuhs) Meticulous, careful.

contamination (kun tam i NAY shun) The process by which something becomes harmful or unusable through contact with something unclean.

critical thinking The constant practice of considering all aspects of a situation when deciding what to believe or what to do.

demeanor (dih MEE ner) Behavior toward others; outward manner.

detrimental (de truh MEN tl) Harmful.

holistic (hoh LIS tik) A form of healing that considers the whole person (i.e., body, mind, spirit, and emotions) in individual treatment plans.

hospice (HOS pis) A concept of care that involves health professionals and volunteers who provide medical, psychological, and spiritual support to terminally ill patients and their loved ones.

indicator (IN di kay ter) An important point or group of statistical values that, when evaluated, indicates the quality of care provided in a healthcare facility.

initiative (i NISH eh tive) The ability to determine what needs to be done and to take action on your own.

integrity (in TEG ri tee) Adhering to ethical standards or right conduct standards.

learning style The way an individual perceives and processes information to learn new material.

mnemonic (ni MON ik) A learning device (e.g., an image, a rhyme, or a figure of speech) that a person uses to help him or her remember information.

morale (muh RAL) Emotional or mental condition with respect to cheerfulness or confidence.

negligence (NEG li jens) Failure to act as a reasonably prudent person would under similar circumstances; such conduct falls below the standards of behavior established by law for the protection of others against unreasonable risk of harm.

overlearn To learn or memorize beyond the point of proficiency or immediate recall.

patient navigator A person who identifies patients' needs and barriers; then assists by coordinating care and identifying community and healthcare resources to meet the needs. May also be called *care coordinator*.

perceiving (per SEEV ing) How an individual looks at information and sees it as real.

processing (prah CES ing) How an individual internalizes new information and makes it his or her own.

reflection (ree FLEK shun) The process of thinking about new information so as to create new ways of learning.

reliable (ree LIE ah bul) Dependable, able to be trusted.

triage (tree AHZH) The process of sorting patients to determine medical need and the priority of care.

What an exciting and challenging career you have chosen! Medical assistants are multiskilled healthcare workers who function under the direction of a licensed provider and are primarily employed in outpatient or ambulatory care facilities, such as medical offices and clinics. According to the U.S. Bureau of Labor Statistics, medical assisting is one of the nation's fastest growing careers, and employment opportunities are projected to grow 29% through 2026.

This growth in job opportunities for medical assistants is due to multiple factors, including a steady increase in the aging population as baby boomers spur demand for preventive health services from physician offices and ambulatory care centers. Since medical assistants are trained in both administrative and clinical skills, they are the perfect employees to meet the needs of this increasing population. In addition, the switch to electronic health records (EHRs) in ambulatory care centers will also open up employment opportunities for medical assistants who are trained in EHR computer software.

RESPONSIBILITIES OF THE MEDICAL ASSISTANT

Medical assistants are the only allied health professionals specifically trained to work in ambulatory care settings, such as physicians' offices, clinics, and group practices. That training includes both clinical and administrative skills, covering a multitude of medical practice needs. The skills performed by an entry-level medical assistant depend on his or her place of employment, but all graduates of accredited programs are taught a similar skill set.

Clinical skills include:

- Assisting during physical examinations
- Performing patient screening procedures
- Assisting with minor surgical procedures, including sterilization procedures
- Performing electrocardiograms (ECGs)
- Obtaining and recording vital signs and medical histories
- Performing phlebotomy
- Performing tests permitted by the Clinical Laboratory Improvement Amendments (i.e., CLIA-waived tests)
- Collecting and managing laboratory specimens
- Following Occupational Safety and Health Administration (OSHA) regulations on infection control
- Administering vaccinations and medications as ordered by the provider
- Performing patient education and coaching initiatives within the scope of practice
- Documenting accurately in a paper record or an EHR
- Performing first aid procedures as needed
- Performing infection control procedures
- Applying therapeutic communication techniques
- Adapting to the special needs of a patient based on his or her developmental life stage, cultural diversity, and individual communication barriers

- Acting as a patient advocate or navigator, including referring patients to community resources
- Acting within legal and ethical boundaries

Administrative skills include:

- Answering telephones
- Managing patient scheduling
- Creating and maintaining patient health records
- Documenting accurately in a paper record and an EHR
- Performing routine maintenance of facility equipment
- Performing basic practice finance procedures
- Coordinating third-party reimbursement
- Performing procedural and diagnostic coding
- Communicating professionally with patients, family members, practitioners, peers, and the public
- Managing facility correspondence
- Performing patient education and coaching initiatives within the scope of practice
- Following legal and ethical principles
- Complying with facility safety practices

These lengthy lists of capabilities that make up the basic skill set are not all that is expected of entry-level medical assistants; they also play a significant role as the patient's advocate. Current research describes this role as being a **patient navigator** (Fig. 1.1). If you have ever had a loved one who was very ill and required medical attention from a number of different practitioners and allied health specialty groups, you understand what a complex and overwhelming task it can be to make decisions and coordinate a loved one's care. Care coordination originated from the patient navigator program. This program was established at the Harlem Hospital Center in 1990. The goal was to assist cancer patients in accessing quality healthcare. Many patient navigator positions were funded with the assistance of the Patient Navigator, Outreach and Chronic Disease Prevention Act of 2005. Today, patient navigator positions are commonly called *care coordinators*. These positions can be found in ambulatory care settings and hospitals. In hospitals, the care coordinators help manage the acute care services and also help patients transition home or to other healthcare settings.

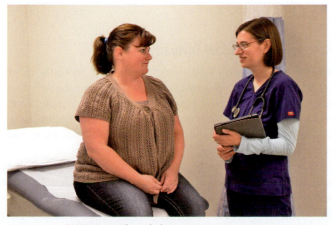

FIGURE 1.1 The medical assistant as a patient navigator.

CRITICAL THINKING APPLICATION 1.1

Medical assistants have long been encouraged to act as patient advocates in the ambulatory care setting. Given their multilevel training, medical assistants can help patients navigate through a wide variety of confusing issues. Let's think about how you could help a patient and family navigate the following scenario:

Mrs. Jana Green is an 82-year-old patient at Walden-Martin Family Medical Clinic. Mrs. Green recently suffered a mild cerebrovascular accident (CVA), and her son is trying to help coordinate her care. Mrs. Green does not understand when or how to take her new medications; she is concerned about whether her health insurance will cover the cost of frequent clinic appointments and assistive devices; she doesn't understand how to prepare for an MRI the provider ordered; and she dislikes having to have blood drawn every week.

Based on what you have learned about the job description of a medical assistant, how can you help Mrs. Green and her family navigate through this complex and challenging medical regimen? What specific actions could help Mrs. Green and her son manage her care?

Customer Service

Another aspect of being a medical assistant is providing excellent customer service. Customer service closely relates to professional behaviors. One must be professional to provide exceptional customer service. In healthcare today, many of our patients have the ability to choose where they go to seek care. The ambulatory care facility needs to attract and retain patients to remain open and for you to have a job. Two of the quickest ways to lose patients are to treat them poorly and to act in an unprofessional manner. Happy patients will tend to tell others about their experiences. Great customer service leads to a successful healthcare facility and allows growth.

To understand customer service, we first need to know who our customers are. A *customer* is one who purchases goods or services. A customer can also be a person whom you deal with in the work environment. By that definition, we can see that patients are our customers. They choose our ambulatory care facility to seek healthcare services. They (or their insurance company) pay for the services provided. Patients are considered *external customers,* or people we do business with who are "outside" (i.e., not employed by) the healthcare facility. Other external customers include medical equipment and supply vendors and pharmaceutical representatives.

The second part of the customer definition relates to *internal customers,* or people whom you deal with in the work environment. These are individuals we interact with inside the facility. They include our co-workers, employees in other departments, and the administrative staff. Both internal and external customers are important for the success of the healthcare facility.

Customer service is whatever we do for our customers to improve their experience at our healthcare facility. People may have different ideas about how they should be treated during their interactions. Our goal is to provide *customer satisfaction,* or a sense of contentment with the interaction. Typically, the more we get to know the customer, the better we can provide customer service. This might not always be possible. For instance, a new patient comes for an appointment.

If you are at the reception desk, you do not have a lot of time to get to know the patient. The most important things for you to do are:

- Be considerate and treat the patient as you would want to be treated
- Look and act professional

CRITICAL THINKING APPLICATION   **1.2**

During Carmen's orientation, she learned about customer service and customer satisfaction. In your own words, how would you define both of these phrases?

CHARACTERISTICS OF PROFESSIONAL MEDICAL ASSISTANTS

Medical assistants must have professional *characteristics*, or distinguishing traits. You will start developing these traits while in school. You will put them into practice during practicum. They will follow you into your first job. If a student is unprofessional during practicum, it will be difficult to get a job. That behavior may be **detrimental** to the medical assistant's professional career.

Professionalism

As a healthcare professional, medical assistants represent the healthcare facility. They are viewed as an extension of the provider and the facility. A healthcare professional:

- has high ethical standards.
- displays **integrity**.
- completes work accurately and in a timely fashion.

It is important for successful professionals to show *professionalism*; that is, having courteous, **conscientious**, and respectful behaviors. This approach is used during all interactions and situations in the workplace. Our patients and co-workers expect professional behavior. Patients base much of their trust and confidence in those who show professionalism. How health professionals act is a direct reflection on the facility and provider. If a medical assistant is rude to a patient, the patient may think that the provider is rude. The perceived quality of care will be negative. Medical assistants must always display professionalism. This includes their attitude, appearance, and behavior. Regardless of the situation, they must always act professionally.

Courtesy and Respect

Courtesy, respect, and dignity often come together when discussing professionalism. *Courtesy* is having good manners or being polite. Courteous behavior is polite, open, and welcoming. *Respect* means to show consideration or appreciation for another person. *Dignity* is the state or quality of being worthy of respect.

We show our patients dignity by treating all patients the way we would want to be treated. It does not matter if the patient has bad body odor or is dressed in tattered clothes. The patient is a person worthy of respect. Patients expect to be treated as individuals who matter. They want to be respected and not to be treated as an annoyance or a medical condition. How can the medical assistant treat others with courtesy and respect?

- Make patients feel welcome and respected. A pleasant greeting and eye contact should be the first things patients experience. Thanking patients at the end of the visit is also important.
- Display positive nonverbal behaviors. Use a calm tone of voice, eye contact when appropriate, and provide privacy for patients. Maintain patient confidentiality.

- Learn about other cultures in your area. When working with patients from those cultures, make sure to avoid gestures, words, and behaviors that could be perceived as disrespectful.
- Always use proper grammar, without slang words. Explain medical treatments and conditions in simple lay language. If you need to use a medical term, explain it to the patient.

Empathy and Compassion

It is important that professional medical assistants demonstrate empathy and compassion to their patients. Empathy, sympathy, and compassion can easily be confused. *Empathy* is the ability to understand another's perspective, experiences, or motivations. We can share another's emotional state. Empathy differs from sympathy. *Sympathy* is feeling sorrow, concern or pity for what the other person has gone through. *Compassion* means we have a deep awareness of the suffering of another and wish to ease it. These characteristics will help to build our positive relationship with our patients.

Tact and Diplomacy

Tact and diplomacy are extremely valuable traits in healthcare professionals. Being *tactful* means being acutely sensitive to what is proper and appropriate when interacting with others. A tactful person has the ability to speak or act without offending others. Being *diplomatic* means using tact and sensitivity when interacting with others. The medical assistant must be sensitive to the needs of others. How can a medical assistant use these traits when communicating with others?

- Consistently be polite and honest during your communication. Show sensitivity to others through your communication and behaviors.
- Recognize the needs and rights of others. Attempt to reach a mutually beneficial resolution to the problem.
- Assess your personal response to the situation. Your personal beliefs and biases should not prevent you from interacting diplomatically and tactfully with others.

CRITICAL THINKING APPLICATION   **1.3**

During Carmen's orientation, she learned about the importance of courtesy, respect, empathy, compassion, tact, and diplomacy. Select three of these words and share with a peer examples of how a medical assistant could display these traits.

Respect for Individual Diversity

Medical assistants work with diverse populations. Your patients will come from different backgrounds. *Diversity* describes the differences and similarities in identity, perspective, and points of view among people. When talking about diversity people usually think of things such as nationality or race, but diversity can also include things such as age and economic status.

It is important to be open and nonjudgmental when working with patients and workers who are different than ourselves. Be aware and accepting of other cultural differences. Be aware of your own cultural values. What preconceived ideas do you have of other diverse groups? How might your biases affect the care you provide to those in different groups?

It is important to educate yourself about other groups. Get to know their customs and practices. Culture can affect healthcare. It can influence how people describe their symptoms, when healthcare is sought, and how treatment plans are followed. For instance, people in some cultures eat traditional foods high in sodium. This could be an issue if a person has high blood pressure or kidney disease. Understanding and accepting the differences represented by your patients will help you provide the best care possible for them.

Honesty, Dependability, and Responsibility

Honest means to be sincere and upright. *Dependable* is the same as trustworthy. *Responsible* is defined as being trusted or depended upon. These are three traits that employers value in their employees. Professional medical assistants should be honest, dependable, and responsible. When given a task, they should complete it accurately, on time, and to the best of their ability. If they make an error, they should be upfront about it. Patient safety is the number one priority. Any mistake in patient care needs to be reported immediately to the provider and to the supervisor. Dependability and honesty are critical components in earning the trust and respect of others. How can medical assistants perform their duties using these three characteristics?

- Be honest and straightforward when interacting with others.
- Accept responsibility for your mistakes. Determine how to prevent them in the future.
- Follow through on your promises.
- Complete your work to the best of your abilities. Complete it on time.
- Be self-motivated. Don't wait to be asked to complete a task.
- Embrace change.

Professional Appearance

Most ambulatory healthcare facilities have dress codes for employees. Medical assistants are usually required to wear scrubs, along with the facility's nametag (and a photo) clearly visible (Fig. 1.2). Table 1.1 provides a typical dress code. Dress codes will vary by facility. Some communities are more conservative, and thus the dress codes reflect this.

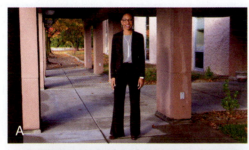
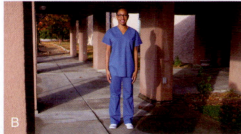

FIGURE 1.2 A professional appearance is important for a medical assistant. **(A)** Business attire. **(B)** Scrubs.

Typically, healthcare facilities include terms such as "modest" and "business attire" in describing their dress codes. The rule of thumb is to make sure the employee does not expose too much at the neckline, the abdomen, and below the waist when bending and raising the arms. Business attire is not casual clothing. Casual clothes include jeans, T-shirts, shorts, exercise/sports clothing, and so on. Business attire is considered dressier, more professional, than casual clothes. Dress pants and a dress shirt would be considered business attire for men. Dress pants, a dress shirt, modest dresses, and modest skirts and blouses would be considered business attire for women.

> **CRITICAL THINKING** APPLICATION   **1.4**
> Rosie, a business office employee at Walden-Martin Family Medical Clinic, is allowed to dress in business attire. She interacts with patients who have questions about their bill. Describe how Rosie should dress.

SCOPE OF PRACTICE AND STANDARDS OF CARE FOR MEDICAL ASSISTANTS

Scope of practice is defined as the range of responsibilities and practice guidelines that determine the boundaries within which a healthcare worker practices. What is the scope of practice of a medical assistant? There is no single definition of the scope of practice for medical assistants throughout the United States, but some states have enacted scope of practice laws covering medical assistant practice. These states include Alaska, Arizona, California, Florida, Georgia, Illinois, Maine, Maryland, Montana, Nevada, New Jersey, New York, Ohio, South Dakota, Virginia, Washington, and West Virginia. Medical assistants working in those states must refer to the identified roles specified in the law. However, for those employed in states without scope of practice laws, medical assistant practice is guided by the norms of that particular location, facility policies and procedures, and individual physician-employers. In some states, medical assistants are overseen by the board of nursing, whereas in others, the board of medicine oversees medical assistants. Make sure you are aware of your state's rules governing medical assistant scope of practice.

One fact is absolutely true about all practicing medical assistants – they are not independent practitioners. Whether certified or not, regardless of length of training or experience, every medical assistant must practice under the direct supervision of a physician or other licensed provider (e.g., nurse practitioner or physician assistant).

Earlier in this chapter we discussed the typical tasks performed by a medical assistant, so you already know generally what duties medical assistants perform in ambulatory care centers; however, some specific tasks are beyond the scope of practice of medical assistants, including the following:

- Performing telephone or in-person **triage**; medical assistants are not legally authorized to assess or diagnose symptoms
- Prescribing medications or making recommendations about over-the-counter drugs and remedies
- Giving out drug samples without provider permission
- Automatically submitting refill prescription requests without provider orders
- Administering intravenous (IV) medications and starting, flushing, or removing IV lines unless permitted by state law
- Analyzing or interpreting test results

TABLE 1.1   Typical Dress Code for Medical Assistants

DRESS CODE	PROFESSIONAL	UNPROFESSIONAL	COMMENTS
Uniform: scrubs and white shoes	• Scrubs must be clean, pressed (ironed), and fit properly. • Scrub pants must be hemmed to the appropriate length. • Closed-toed shoes must be white and clean.	• Dirty, wrinkled, ripped scrubs • Scrub pants dragging on the floor • Scruffy, dirty shoes • Open shoes (sandals), fabric shoes	• Shoes need to protect your feet. Cloth and open-toed shoes provide very little protection. • Pants dragging on floors pick up and transfer bacteria.
Hair	• Natural colors; clean and styled • Long hair must be tied back	• Unnatural colors; dirty, messy hair • Hair in face or hanging down	• Hair hanging in front can interfere with patient care, spread bacteria, and get caught in equipment.
Fingernails	• Cut short, unpolished	• Long, polished, artificial nails	• Bacteria can multiply and grow under long, artificial, and/or polished nails.
Cosmetics and body odors	• Professional makeup • No odors on the body	• Overuse of makeup • Wearing perfume, cologne, etc. • Using scented lotions • Smelling like a cigarette • Body odor (from not bathing)	• Too much makeup can look unprofessional. • Smells like perfumes, colognes, or cigarettes can trigger allergies in others. • Offensive body odor is unprofessional because we are in patients' intimate/personal space.
Jewelry	• Wedding band (no stones) • One pair of earrings (studs) • Watch	• Rings with stones • Multiple earrings on each ear • Necklaces, bracelets • Lanyards	• Bacteria can accumulate in rings and bracelets. • Necklaces and lanyards can be choking hazards if grabbed by a patient.
Tattoos and body piercings	• Tattoos and body piercings must follow the healthcare facility's policy	• Not following the healthcare facility's policy	• In conservative communities, body piercings and tattoos may be perceived as unprofessional.
Professional dress (street clothes) for special events	• Blouse, top, or sweater • Dress pants • Dress or skirt (to the top of the knee) • Dress shoes	• Low-cut tops; sheer tops • Jeans, ripped pants, exercise clothes • Flip-flops, tennis shoes • Mini skirts	• Clothes should look professional; should not be ripped or casual in appearance.

- Operating laser equipment
- Performing laboratory tests that are not CLIA-waived
- Ordering diagnostic or radiographic tests/procedures

What is the difference between scope of practice and standards of care? The scope of practice for a medical assistant is what has been established by law in some states or by practice norms, institutions, or physician-employers in states without scope of practice laws. *Standards of care*, however, is a legal term that refers to whether the level and quality of patient service provided is the same as what another healthcare worker with similar training and experience in a similar situation would provide. Standards of care set minimum guidelines for job performance. They define what the expected quality of care is and provide specific guidelines on whether the care standard has been met. Medical assistants not meeting the expected standard of care may be charged with professional **negligence** (discussed in greater detail in Chapter 3).

The following are examples of breaks in the standards of care in medical assisting.

- A patient calls reporting a persistent headache for 3 days. You tell the patient to get some rest and take ibuprofen, without referring the call to a provider. What standard of care has been broken?
- A patient asks you to explain his lab report. You do your best to explain what his blood count levels mean. What is the problem here?
- An elderly patient tells you she cannot afford to get her prescriptions filled. The provider is busy, but you know there are samples of the prescribed drug in the medication cupboard, so you give her several packets. Does this follow standard of care?
- A patient tells you her son fell on the playground yesterday, and he is complaining that his arm hurts. You tell the mother

it is probably just a strain and suggest she wrap the arm with an elastic bandage. Why is this a problem?

- You overhear a patient calling one of the other medical assistants "nurse." Should your co-worker correct the patient? Why?

Hopefully you are beginning to see that the practice of medical assisting is limited not only by individual state laws or norms, but also by the standards and scope of practice established by the supervising providers where the medical assistant is employed. Remember, the scope of practice and expected standards of care for licensed medical professionals are quite different from those for medical assisting practice. The medical assistant must refer to the provider for orders and guidance on what behaviors are expected for medical assistants in that facility. The medical assistant can *never* independently diagnose, prescribe, or treat patients. She or he must *always* have the written order of a provider or follow established policies and procedures when performing clinical skills.

PROFESSIONAL MEDICAL ASSISTING ORGANIZATIONS, CREDENTIALS, AND CONTINUING EDUCATION

Becoming a member of a professional organization, obtaining credentials, and participating in continuing education are all part of being a professional medical assistant. In this next section you will find information about professional organizations, how to obtain a medical assistant credential, and continuing education.

Professional Organizations for Medical Assistants

Most healthcare occupations have a professional organization that sets high standards for quality and performance. A code of ethics is also developed by the organization to help guide the actions of those in that particular profession. Professional organizations provide many benefits to their members, including opportunities for continuing education, national and regional conventions, and networking opportunities. Medical assisting is no different. Becoming a member of a professional organization will also show your employer that you are committed to being the best possible medical assistant. The following sections provide descriptions of three of the professional medical assisting organizations available.

American Association of Medical Assistants

The American Association of Medical Assistants (AAMA) was created in 1956 and remains the only association devoted exclusively to the medical assisting profession. According to the AAMA's website (*www.aama-ntl.org*), becoming a member includes the following benefits:

- AAMA legal counsel represents medical assistants across the United States to fight for the rights of medical assistant practice; in addition, the counsel stays abreast of federal and state laws regarding medical assisting.
- Members receive a complimentary subscription to *CMA Today*, an informative magazine devoted entirely to the medical assistant profession; each issue (six per year) offers continuing education unit (CEU) articles, medical assisting news, and healthcare information.

More information about the AAMA is available on the organization's website: *www.aama-ntl.org*.

American Medical Technologists (AMT)

The American Medical Technologists (AMT) was founded in 1939 as a nationally recognized certification agency for multiple allied health professionals, including Medical Assistant (RMA), Medical Laboratory Technician (MLT), Phlebotomy Technician (RPT), Medical Administrative Specialist (CMAS), and Dental Assistant (RDA).

According to the AMT's website (*www.americanmedtech.org*), becoming a member includes the following benefits:

- Professional publications
- Annual convention
- State society meeting and seminars
- Continuing education
- Career services
- Awards and scholarships

Additional information on the AMT is available on the organization's website: *www.americanmedtech.org*.

The National Healthcareer Association (NHA)

The National Healthcareer Association (NHA) was established in 1990 to offer certification examinations in a number of allied health programs; for example, certification is granted for pharmacy, phlebotomy, and electrocardiography (ECG) technicians. The NHA also offers two different medical assisting certifications: Certified Clinical Medical Assistant (CCMA) and Certified Medical Administrative Assistant (CMAA). The NHA is not involved in program curriculum standards or program accreditation. It simply offers certification if the applicant can successfully pass the NHA examination developed for each particular medical discipline. You can find out more about the certifications offered through the NHA at the association's website: *www.nhanow.com/*.

Achieving a Credential

Medical assistants have several options if they choose to become credentialed. Being a credentialed medical assistant has certain benefits:

- Credentialed medical assistants have had to pass a national standardized exam. Passing the exam indicates that they have the knowledge to perform the medical assistant's duties.
- Some employers require the credential prior to hiring or within a few months after hiring.
- Some employers will pay more if a person has achieved a medical assistant credential.

There are several national agencies that will provide credentials to medical assistants upon successful completion of their exam. Table 1.2 presents some of the more common medical assistant credentials. It is important for graduating medical assistants to research whether credentials are preferred or required by local employers. It is also important to identify which credential is most wanted by local employers. Your instructors are also excellent resources if you have additional questions on credentials for medical assistants.

Continuing Education

For a professional medical assistant, it is important to stay current (up-to-date) with the newest medications, treatments, and diagnostic tests. Education beyond your medical assistant degree is considered continuing education. Most healthcare professionals need to do continuing education to renew their certification or license. There are many opportunities for continuing education. These include:

TABLE 1.2   Credentialing Agencies for Medical Assistants

AGENCY/WEBSITE	CREDENTIAL	RECERTIFICATION METHODS
American Association of Medical Assistants (AAMA) http://www.aama-ntl.org	Certified Medical Assistant (CMA [AAMA])	Recertify every 5 years either by exam or by earning 60 continuing education points. Specific points must be achieved in the three content areas. At least 30 points must be from AAMA-approved continuing education units (CEUs).
American Medical Technologists (AMT) https://www.americanmedtech.org	Registered Medical Assistant (RMA)	Recertify every 3 years either by exam or by completing specific activities.
National Healthcareer Association (NHA) https://www.nhanow.com	Clinical Medical Assistant (CCMA) Medical Administrative Assistant (CMAA)	Recertify every 2 years either by exam or by earning 10 continuing education credits.
National Center for Competency Testing (NCCT) https://www.ncctinc.com	Medical Assistant (NCMA)	Recertify every year either by exam or by completing 14 contact hours of continuing education.

- Reading professional journals and reputable health websites
- On-the-job educational conferences
- Local, state, and national medical assistant conferences

Typically, additional continuing education opportunities exist if a medical assistant is a member of an organization.

HOW TO SUCCEED AS A MEDICAL ASSISTANT STUDENT

Who You Are as a Learner: How Do You Learn Best?

You have taken the first step toward becoming a successful student by choosing your profession and field of study. Becoming a medical assistant opens the doors to a wide variety of opportunities in both administrative and clinical practice at ambulatory or institutional healthcare facilities. To become a successful medical assistant, you first must become a successful student. This section will help you discover the way you learn best, and it provides multiple strategies to assist you in your journey toward success.

Think about what you do when you are faced with something new to learn. How do you go about understanding and learning the new material? Over time you have developed a method for **perceiving** and **processing** information. This pattern of behavior is called your **learning style**. Learning styles can be examined in many different ways, but most professionals agree that a student's success depends more on whether the person can "make sense" of the information than on whether the individual is "smart." Determining your individual learning style and understanding how it applies to your ability to learn new material are the first steps toward becoming a successful student.

Learning Style Inventory

For you to learn new material, two things must happen. First, you must perceive the information. This is the method you have developed over time that helps you examine new information and recognize it as real. Once you have developed a method for learning about the new material, you must process the information. Processing the information is how you internalize it and make it your own. Researchers

believe that each of us has a preferred method for learning new material. By investigating your learning style, you can figure out how to combine different approaches to perceiving and processing information that will lead to greater success as a student.

The first step in learning new material is determining how you perceive it, or as some experts explain, what methods you use to learn the new material. Some learners opt to watch, observe, and use **reflection** to think about and learn the new material. These students are *abstract perceivers,* who learn by analyzing new material, building theories about it, and using a step-by-step approach to learning. Other students need to perform some activity, such as rewriting notes from class, making flash cards, and outlining chapters, to learn new information. Students who learn by "doing" are called *concrete perceivers.* Concrete learners prefer to learn things that have a personal meaning or that they believe are relevant to their lives. So, which type of perceiver do you think you are? Before you actually learn new material, do you need time to think about it, or do you prefer to "do" something to help you learn the material?

The second step in learning new material is information processing, which is the way learners internalize the new information and make it their own. New material can be processed by two methods. *Active processors* prefer to jump in and start doing things immediately. They make sense of the new material by using it *now.* They look for practical ways to apply the new material and learn best with practice and hands-on activities. *Reflective processors* have to think about the information before they can internalize it. They prefer to observe and consider what is going on. The only way they can make sense of new material is to spend time thinking and learning a great deal about it before acting. Which type of information processor do you think you are? Do you prefer to jump in and start doing things to help you learn, or do you need to analyze and consider the material before you can actually learn it?

Using Your Learning Profile to Be a Successful Student: Where Do I Go From Here?

No one falls completely into one or the other of the categories just discussed. However, by being aware of how we generally prefer first to perceive information and then to process it, we can be more sensitive to our learning style and can approach new learning situations with a plan for learning the material in a way that best suits our learning preferences.

Your preferred perceiving and processing learning profile will fall into one of the following four stages of the Learning Style Inventory, which was created by David Kolb of Case Western Reserve University.

- *Stage 1* learners have a *concrete reflective* style. These students want to know the purpose of the information and have a personal connection to the content. They like to consider a situation from many points of view, observe others, and plan before taking action. They feel most comfortable watching rather than doing, and their strengths include sensitivity toward others, brainstorming, and recognizing and creatively solving problems. If you fall into this stage, you enjoy small-group activities and learn well in study groups.

- *Stage 2* learners have an *abstract reflective* style. These students are eager to learn just for the sheer pleasure of learning, rather than because the material relates to their personal lives. They like to learn lots of facts and arrange new material in a clear, logical manner. Stage 2 learners plan studying and like to create ways of thinking about the material, but they do not always make the connection with its practical application. If you are a stage 2 learner, you prefer organized, logical presentations of material and therefore enjoy lectures and readings and generally dislike group work. You also need time to process and think about new material before applying it.

- *Stage 3* learners have an *abstract active* style. Learners with this combination learning style want to experiment and test the information they are learning. If you are a stage 3 learner, you want to know how techniques or ideas work, and you also want to practice what you are learning. Your strengths are in problem solving and decision making, but you may lack focus and may be hasty in making decisions. You learn best with hands-on practice by doing experiments, projects, and laboratory activities. You enjoy working alone or in small groups.

CRITICAL THINKING APPLICATION   **1.5**
- Consider the two ways to perceive new material. Are you a concrete perceiver, who ties the information to a personal experience, or are you an abstract perceiver, who likes to analyze or reflect on the meaning of the material? Choose the type you think most accurately describes your method of learning.
- Now, think about the way you process learning. Are you an active processor, who always looks for the practical applications of what you learn, or are you a reflective processor, who has to think about new material before internalizing it?
- After completing this activity, write down the combination of your perceiving and processing learning styles and share it with your instructor.

- *Stage 4* learners are *concrete active* learners. These students are concerned about how they can use what they learn to make a difference in their lives. If you fall into this stage, you like to relate new material to other areas of your life. You have leadership capabilities, can create on your feet, and usually are vocal in a group, but you may have difficulty completing your work on time. Stage 4 learners enjoy teaching others and working in groups and learn best when they can apply new information to real-world problems.

To get the most out of knowing your learning profile, you need to apply this knowledge to how you approach learning. Each of the learning stages has pluses and minuses. When faced with a learning situation that does not match your learning preference, see how you can adapt your individual learning profile to make the best of the information. For example, if you are bored by lectures, look for an opportunity to apply the information being presented to a real problem you are facing in the classroom or at home. If you are an abstract perceiver, take time outside of class to think about new information so that you are ready to process it into your learning system. If you benefit from learning in a group, make the effort to organize review sessions and study groups. If you learn best by teaching others, offer to assist your peers with their learning. By taking the time now to investigate your preferred method of learning, you will perceive and process information more effectively throughout your school career.

CRITICAL THINKING APPLICATION   **1.6**
Take a few minutes to reflect on a time when you really enjoyed learning about something new. How was the material presented, and what did you do to "make it your own"? What do you need to do to become a more effective learner?

Study Skills: Tricks for Becoming a Successful Student

Let's investigate some ideas that are useful for learning new material. These study skills include memory techniques, active learning, brain tricks, reading methods, and note-taking strategies.

Several techniques can help you store and remember information. The first of these involves organizing information into recognizable groups so that the brain can find it easily. You can organize information by getting the big picture first before trying to learn the details. One way to implement this strategy is to skim a reading assignment before actually reading and taking notes on the material, thus getting a general impression of what you need to learn before tackling the details. Depending on your learning style, it may also help to find a way of making the new information meaningful. Think about your educational goals and how the new material will help you achieve those goals.

Another way of remembering material is to create an association with something you already know. If new material is grouped with already stored material, the brain remembers it much more easily. For example, maybe you took a biology class in high school and learned the basics about human anatomy and physiology. Try to create a link between what you previously learned and the details of the new information you are expected to learn now. Or maybe you have a family member who suffers from a particular disease. Think about that individual's signs and symptoms while learning more details about the disease so that you can apply your learning to his or her situation.

A useful study skill for some learners is to be physically active while learning. Some students learn best if they walk or talk out loud while studying. Besides encouraging learning, moving and talking while studying relieve boredom and keep you awake. Another way to be actively involved in learning is to use pictures or diagrams to represent the material you are studying. Some people are visual learners, and creating pictures of the material is the easiest method for them to retain the information. Other students find that rewriting notes, making lists of information, creating flash cards, color-coding notes, or highlighting important material in a textbook helps them retain the material. Writing also helps students who need to "do" something to learn.

Studying goes much more smoothly if you work with your brain rather than against it. If you tend to get anxious and worried while studying, you may be acting as your own worst enemy. One way of dealing with a topic you are anxious about is to **overlearn** it. If material is overlearned, you are much less likely to experience test anxiety. Another method for remembering material is to review it quickly after class. This mini-review helps the new information become part of your long-term memory system.

Many students find creating songs, dances, or word associations an effective way to learn and remember new material. Putting details into a familiar song and moving to it can help trick the brain into remembering the information. This is especially helpful when trying to learn anatomy and physiology. For example, think about one of your favorite songs and "dance" your way through the blood flow through the heart. Or, if you are finding the organization of the body especially tricky to remember, such as the movement of food through the gastrointestinal (GI) system, create a **mnemonic** that helps you remember the information. The most common one suggested for the parts of the intestines is: **D**ow **J**ones **I**ndustrial **C**limbing **A**verage **C**losing **S**tock **R**eport. The first letter of each word stands for an anatomic part of the intestines – *d*uodenum, *j*ejunum, *i*leum, *c*ecum, *a*ppendix, *c*olon, *s*igmoid, and *r*ectum. You can make up your own mnemonics or memory tricks to help you learn complicated material.

Another excellent way of learning information is to actually teach it to someone else. Teaching requires you to have a good understanding of the material and the ability to describe it for others. It can be an effective reinforcement of complicated material.

A great deal of the learning process is expected to take place from assigned readings. You can use several methods to make reading assignments more meaningful. If you find a reading assignment challenging or difficult to understand, the first step is to take the time to read it again. Sometimes the first time through the material is not enough to gain understanding. As you read, highlight important words or thoughts and stop periodically to summarize the material. Some students find outlining new material helpful. This is another way to use active learning to help you make the information "your own."

If you get bored while reading, use your body; walk or talk your way through the assignment. Take the time to look up words or terms you do not understand or ask your instructor or tutor for help. The best way to determine whether you have learned anything from your reading is to try to explain the material to someone else. For example, you can meet with other students and explain to them what you learned. If you can do that effectively, you know you have acquired the knowledge needed from the reading assignment.

Many students find effective note taking a challenge. The big question is, "How much of what the instructor says do I actually need to write down?" The first step in effective note taking is to come to class prepared. The more familiar you are with the material, the easier it will be to determine the important parts of the instructor's lecture. Pay attention to the instructor and look for clues to what he or she thinks is important. Ask questions about the material if you do not understand it, rather than writing down information that makes no sense to you. Think critically about what you hear before you write it down, so you can start to build relationships among the things you want or need to know.

If your instructor uses PowerPoint presentations to teach a lesson, request copies of the slides before the lecture so you have an opportunity to review them as you are doing your reading. Many courses have an online website where PowerPoints or other lecture materials are available for review. Take advantage of these added materials to be prepared for each class so that you can ask questions about anything you don't understand. In addition, this textbook has an extensive online site that you can access for learning resources. Investigate the site and see whether something there can help you reach your learning goals.

When it comes to actual note taking, some strategies can make the process of recording notes an active learning tool. Organize the information as much as possible while you are writing or typing, either in an outline or a paragraph format. If you take notes on a laptop or tablet, make sure your keyboarding skills are good enough for you to keep up with the flow of information and that you review your notes shortly after class to fill in any missing details. If you take notes on paper, use only one side of the page (for easier reading) and leave blank spaces where needed to fill in details later. Use key words to help you remember the material and create pictures or diagrams to help visualize it. If permitted, record the lecture and make sure you have copies of any handouts or notes distributed by your instructor that cover material written on the board or provided in a PowerPoint presentation. If your instructor refers the class to a YouTube video or other website, transcribe the site address correctly to refer to it at a later time. Another helpful tool is to develop your own system of abbreviations to help simplify the note-taking process.

The most effective way to use your notes is to review them shortly after class and then find a time to review them every day. This is the time to add details, clarify information, or make notes about asking the instructor for explanations during the next class. You could even exchange notes with students you trust to compare information. Some students find it beneficial to create an electronic copy of their notes (if they wrote them out on paper) or to rewrite them. This gives you an opportunity to learn the material as you transcribe it. As you are reviewing your notes, you also can draw mind maps of the information or diagram outlines to help you better understand and remember the material.

Creating mind maps is a way of representing the main idea of a topic and supporting important details with a figure or picture. Healthcare textbooks present complicated concepts with multiple main ideas, each with its own important details. Mind maps are a way of combining complex details and organizing them into a format that is easier to remember. The *spider map* (Fig. 1.3) presents a method for including several main ideas with details in one study guide. The *fishbone map* (Fig. 1.4) can be used to learn complicated causes of disease. The *chain-of-events map* (Fig. 1.5) displays the cause and effect of events, such as infection control or the history of medicine. The *cycle map* (Fig. 1.6) shows the connection between factors, such

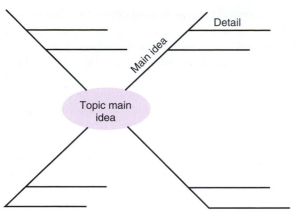

FIGURE 1.3 Spider map showing multiple main ideas with supporting details.

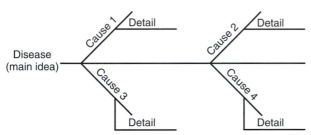

FIGURE 1.4 Fishbone map used to describe cause of disease.

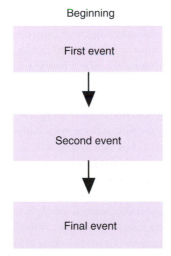

FIGURE 1.5 Chain-of-events map showing the cause and effect of events.

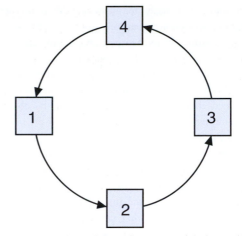

FIGURE 1.6 Cycle map illustrating the way one action leads to another.

Test-Taking Strategies: Taking Charge of Your Success

What happens when you do not know the answer to the first question on a test? What if you do not know the next one? Are you able to go on without panicking? Many people find taking tests the most challenging part of being a successful student. Multiple approaches are available that you can use to take charge of your success and improve your ability to take tests. These include such strategies as adequate preparation, controlling negative thoughts during test time, and understanding ways to manage various types of questions.

The first step is to go into a test adequately prepared. Use the time management skills discussed later in this chapter to prepare for the big day. Recognize and use your preferred learning style to overlearn the material and increase your confidence. Use memory tools (e.g., flash cards, checklists, and mind maps) to help you visualize the material. Form a study group if you are the type of learner who benefits from studying in groups. Schedule and plan study time and reward yourself for your hard work. It also is important to go into the test rested and relaxed; therefore, you should eat, exercise to relieve stress, and sleep before the test so that you are as alert as possible.

Before you start the test, make sure you read the directions carefully. If possible, begin with the easiest or shortest questions to build your confidence. Be aware of the amount of time allotted for the examination, and pace yourself accordingly. As you go through the test, look for clues to answers in other questions. During test time, remember to use positive self-talk at the first indication of panic. Repeatedly remind yourself that you are well prepared; relax and think about the material before you get worried. You need to stop negative thoughts as soon as they arise and instead visualize yourself being successful. Use slow, deep breathing to relax and, if helpful, close your eyes for a minute and visualize a relaxing place before you go on with the test.

as in the chain of infection. Creating your own mind maps is a way of making the information more meaningful and easier for you to understand and remember.

Although many techniques can help you study, perhaps the most important one is your attitude toward learning. Some students fall into the "I can't possibly learn this material" trap. That type of attitude only leads to self-defeat. The way to overcome barriers is first to recognize that they exist. Once you know your weak spots, use the suggested study skills to improve in those areas. Do not be afraid to ask questions or to ask for help if you do not understand the material. Use as many different strategies as necessary to become a successful student.

Certain strategies are useful for answering different types of questions. With multiple choice questions, try to identify key words or clues in each question. Read the question carefully and answer it in your head before you review the provided answers. If you are not absolutely sure of the answer, make an educated guess or follow your instincts in choosing an answer. If there are answers that you know are not correct, that can eliminate the "all of the above" answer choice. By eliminating the answers that you know are incorrect, you can focus on the other answer choices.

"True or false" questions give you a 50/50 chance of being correct. Remember that if any part of the question is not true, then the statement is false. Again, check the statements for key words that help indicate the direction of the answer. Look for qualifying terms (e.g., *always, never, sometimes*) that are the key to understanding the meaning of the true or false statement.

CRITICAL THINKING APPLICATION   **1.8**

Think about a time you experienced test anxiety. Write down the details of the situation and how you felt. Choose four test-taking strategies you think would be beneficial for handling similar situations in the future.

Becoming a Critical Thinker: Making Mental Connections

The ability to process information and arrive at reasonable conclusions is crucial to all healthcare workers. The process of **critical thinking** involves (1) sorting out conflicting information, (2) weighing your knowledge about that information, (3) ignoring or letting go of personal biases, and (4) deciding on a reasonable belief or action. Critical thinking is actually an active search for the truth.

Critical thinking could be described as thorough thinking because it requires learners to keep an open mind to all possibilities. Successful students are thorough thinkers because they must determine the facts about a topic and come to logical conclusions about the material. Critical thinkers also are inquisitive learners; they constantly analyze and sort out conflicting information to reach conclusions.

A crucial step in critical thinking is evaluating the results of your learning. Reflection is the key to critical thinking. "How did I learn what I learned?" and "What does it mean in my life?" are questions that must be asked consistently to continue to learn. Becoming a successful student, and ultimately a successful member of the allied health team, requires critical thinking skills.

Using these tools to become the best possible medical assistant student will also help you become the best possible professional medical assistant.

THE HISTORY OF MEDICINE

Although religious and mythologic beliefs were the basis for care for the sick in ancient times, evidence suggests that drugs, surgery, and other treatments based on theories about the body were used as early as 5000 BC. Moses presented rules of health to the Hebrews in approximately 1205 BC. He was the first advocate of preventive medicine and is considered the first public health officer. Moses knew that some animal diseases could be passed to humans and that **contamination** existed; therefore, a religious law was developed forbidding humans to eat or drink from dirty dishes. The people of

that era believed that doing so would defile their bodies, and they would lose their souls.

Hippocrates, known as the Father of Medicine, is the most famous of the ancient Greek physicians. He was born in 450 BC on the island of Cos in Greece. He is best remembered for the Hippocratic Oath, which has been administered to physicians for more than 2000 years. To this day, most graduating medical school students swear to some form of the oath (Fig. 1.7).

Hippocrates is credited with taking mysticism out of medicine and giving it a scientific basis. During this period of history, most believed that illness was caused by demonic possession; to cure the illness, the demon had to be removed from the body. Hippocrates' clinical descriptions of diseases and his volumes on epidemics, fevers, epilepsy, fractures, and instruments were studied for centuries. He believed that the body had the capacity to heal itself and that the physician's role was to help nature. It is also interesting to see that Hippocrates addressed confidentiality and understood that it was important to maintain patient privacy.

Medical knowledge developed slowly, and distribution of such knowledge was poor. In the 17th century, European academies or societies were established, consisting of small groups of men who met to discuss subjects of mutual interest. One of the earliest academies was the Royal Society of London, formed in 1662. In the United States, medical education was greatly influenced by the Johns Hopkins University School of Medicine in Baltimore, Maryland, established in the early 1890s. The school admitted only college graduates with at least one year's training in the natural sciences. The clinical education at Johns Hopkins was superior because the school partnered with Johns Hopkins Hospital, which had been created expressly for teaching and research by members of the medical faculty. Table 1.3 presents selected medical pioneers and their achievements.

The History of Medical Assisting

As physicians made the switch from going to patients' homes for treatment to having the patient come to their office, some physicians hired nurses to help in their practices. Gradually, the administrative part of running a practice became increasingly complicated and time-consuming, and physicians realized that they needed an assistant with both administrative and clinical training. Nurses were likely to have training only in clinical skills; therefore, many physicians began training individuals – medical assistants – to assist with all the office duties.

The first medical assistants started working in individual physicians' offices with on-the-job training to help out when an extra pair of hands was needed. Today medical assisting is one of the most respected allied health fields in the industry, and training is readily available through community colleges, junior colleges, and private educational institutions throughout the United States.

CRITICAL THINKING APPLICATION   **1.9**

- In Table 1.3, review the list of individuals who have made significant contributions to medicine. Which one do you believe had the greatest impact on modern healthcare?
- Consider how the medical assisting profession began. How do you think advances in medicine throughout history have affected the current practice of medical assisting?

I swear to fulfill, to the best of my ability and judgment, this covenant:

I will respect the hard-won scientific gains of those physicians in whose steps I walk, and gladly share such knowledge as is mine with those who are to follow.

I will apply, for the benefit of the sick, all measures [that] are required, avoiding those twin traps of overtreatment and therapeutic nihilism.

I will remember that there is art to medicine as well as science, and that warmth, sympathy, and understanding may outweigh the surgeon's knife or the chemist's drug.

I will not be ashamed to say "I know not," nor will I fail to call in my colleagues when the skills of another are needed for a patient's recovery.

I will respect the privacy of my patients, for their problems are not disclosed to me that the world may know. Most especially must I tread with care in matters of life and death. If it is given me to save a life, all thanks. But it may also be within my power to take a life; this awesome responsibility must be faced with great humbleness and awareness of my own frailty. Above all, I must not play at God.

I will remember that I do not treat a fever chart, a cancerous growth, but a sick human being, whose illness may affect the person's family and economic stability. My responsibility includes these related problems, if I am to care adequately for the sick.

I will prevent disease whenever I can, for prevention is preferable to cure.

I will remember that I remain a member of society, with special obligations to all my fellow human beings, those sound of mind and body as well as the infirm.

If I do not violate this oath, may I enjoy life and art, respected while I live and remembered with affection thereafter. May I always act so as to preserve the finest traditions of my calling and may I long experience the joy of healing those who seek my help.

Written in 1964 by Louis Lasagna, Academic Dean of the School of Medicine at Tufts University, and used in many medical schools today.

FIGURE 1.7 Modern version of the Hippocratic Oath.

MEDICAL PROFESSIONALS

Now that you have an understanding of the medical assistant profession, let's take a look at other areas in healthcare. Physicians and providers (e.g., nurse practitioners and physician assistants) are portals of entry or first contacts for patients seeking medical care. *Primary care providers* (PCPs) are healthcare practitioners who monitor a patient's overall health. Family medicine, internal medicine, and pediatrics are generally considered primary care specialties. After the initial assessment or with the diagnosis of a more complex health issue, patients may be referred to a medical specialist for further examination and treatment.

Doctors of Medicine

Medical doctors (Doctor of Medicine [MD]) are considered **allopathic** physicians. They are the most widely recognized type of physician. They diagnose illness and disease and prescribe treatment for their patients. MDs have a wide variety of rights, including writing prescriptions, performing surgery, offering wellness advice, and performing preventive medicine procedures. Becoming an MD requires 4 years of undergraduate university training (premed) and 4 years of medical school. Regardless of where premed students attend college, a national standard of course work is required to apply to medical school. They must take entry and advanced levels of biology, physics, organic and inorganic chemistry, mathematics, English, humanities, and social sciences. The United States has approximately 125 allopathic medical schools. After medical school, the student faces 3 to 8 years of residency programs, depending on the medical specialty he or she pursues. After completion of a residency program, a physician can obtain board certification in one or more of 37 different specialty areas recognized by the American Board of Medical Specialties (Table 1.4). An MD must have a state license to practice, and continuing education is required to maintain the license. Graduates of foreign medical schools usually can obtain a license in the United States after passing an examination and completing a residency program in this country.

Doctors of Osteopathy

Osteopathic physicians (Doctor of Osteopathy [DO]) complete requirements similar to those of MDs to graduate and practice medicine. Osteopaths use medicine and surgery, in addition to osteopathic manipulative therapy (OMT), in treating their patients. Andrew Taylor Still is considered the father of osteopathic medicine, which he established in 1874. He believed in a more **holistic** approach to medicine, and although he was an MD, he founded the American School of Osteopathy in Kirksville, Missouri. The school originally was chartered to offer an MD degree but later focused more on the osteopathic approach. DOs stress preventive medicine and holistic patient care, in addition to a special focus on the musculoskeletal system and OMT. Premed students moving toward osteopathic medicine complete the same undergraduate course work as allopathic candidates and 4 years of medical studies at a school for osteopathic medicine. Over the years there have become fewer differences between allopathic and osteopathic programs, with many DO physicians earning residency programs in the same institutions as MDs.

TABLE 1.3   Medical Pioneers and Their Achievements

NAME	ACHIEVEMENT	NAME	ACHIEVEMENT
Andreas Vesalius (1514–1564)	Father of modern anatomy; wrote first anatomy book	Robert Koch (1843–1910)	Developed Koch's postulates, a theory of causative agents for disease; discovered the cause of cholera
William Harvey (1578–1657)	Discovered the circulatory system	William Roentgen (1845–1923)	Discovered the x-ray
Anton van Leeuwenhoek (1632–1723)	First to observe microbes through a lens; developed the first microscope	Walter Reed (1851–1902)	Proved that yellow fever was transmitted by mosquito bites while in the U.S. Army serving in Cuba
John Hunter (1728–1793)	Founder of scientific surgery	Paul Ehrlich (1854–1915)	Injected chemicals for the first time to treat disease (syphilis)
Edward Jenner (1749–1823)	Developed smallpox vaccine	Marie Curie (1867–1934)	Discovered radium and polonium
Ignaz Semmelweis (1818–1865)	First physician to recommend hand washing to prevent puerperal fever; believed there was a connection between performing autopsies and then delivering babies that caused puerperal fever in new mothers	Alexander Fleming (1881–1955)	Discovered penicillin
		Albert Sabin (1906–1993)	Developed the oral live-virus vaccine for polio 10 years after Salk developed the first injected vaccine
Florence Nightingale (1820–1910)	Founder of nursing	Virginia Apgar (1909–1974)	Founded neonatology; developed the Apgar score, which assesses the status of newborns
Clara Barton (1821–1912)	Established the American Red Cross	Jonas Salk (1914–1955)	Developed the first safe and effective injectable vaccine for polio
Elizabeth Blackwell (1821–1910)	First woman in the United States to earn a Doctor of Medicine degree	Christiaan Barnard (1922–2001)	Performed the first human heart transplant
Louis Pasteur (1822–1895)	Father of bacteriology and preventive medicine; developed pasteurization and established the connection between germs and disease	Edwin Carl Wood (1929–2011)	Pioneered the technique of in vitro fertilization (IVF)
Joseph Lister (1827–1912)	Father of sterile surgery; developed antiseptic methods for surgery	David Ho (1952–)	Research pioneer in acquired immunodeficiency syndrome (AIDS)

TABLE 1.4   Examples of Medical Specialties

SPECIALTY	PRACTITIONER'S TITLE	DESCRIPTION
Allergy and immunology	Allergist/ immunologist	Allergists/immunologists are trained to evaluate disorders and diseases of the immune system. This includes conditions such as adverse reactions to drugs and food, anaphylaxis, and problems related to autoimmune diseases, asthma, and insect stings.
Anesthesiology	Anesthesiologist	Anesthesiologists provide pain relief and pain management during surgical procedures and also for patients with long-standing conditions accompanied by pain.
Colon and rectal surgery	Colorectal surgeon	Colorectal surgeons diagnose and treat conditions affecting the intestines, rectum, and anal area, in addition to organs affected by intestinal disease.
Dermatology	Dermatologist	Dermatologists work with adult and pediatric patients in treating disorders and diseases of the skin, hair, nails, and related tissues. Dermatologists are specially trained to manage conditions such as skin cancers, cosmetic disorders of the skin, scars, allergies, and other disorders, both malignant and benign.

TABLE 1.4   Examples of Medical Specialties—*continued*

SPECIALTY	PRACTITIONER'S TITLE	DESCRIPTION
Emergency medicine	Emergency physician	Emergency physicians are experts in assessing and treating a patient to prevent death or serious disability. They provide immediate care to stabilize the patient's condition, and then refer the patient to the appropriate professional for further care.
Family medicine	Primary care provider (PCP)	PCPs offer care to the whole family, from newborns to elderly adults. They are familiar with a wide range of disorders and diseases, and preventive care is their primary concern.
General surgery	Surgeon	General surgeons correct deformities and defects and treat diseases or injured parts of the body by means of operative treatment.
Genetics	Medical geneticist	Geneticists are physicians trained to diagnose and treat patients with conditions related to genetically linked diseases. They provide genetic counseling when indicated.
Internal medicine	Internist	Internists are concerned with comprehensive care, often diagnosing and treating those with chronic, long-term conditions. They must have a broad understanding of the body and its ailments.
Neurologic surgery	Neurosurgeon	Neurosurgeons provide surgical care for patients with conditions of the central, autonomic, and peripheral nervous systems.
Neurology/ psychiatry	Neurologist/ psychiatrist	Neurologists diagnose and treat disorders of the nervous system. Psychiatrists are physicians who specialize in the diagnosis and treatment of people with mental, emotional, or behavioral disorders. A psychiatrist is qualified to conduct psychotherapy and to prescribe medications.
Nuclear medicine	Nuclear medicine specialist	These specialists use radioactive substances to diagnose, treat, and detect disease.
Obstetrics and gynecology	Obstetrician/ gynecologist	Obstetricians provide care to women of childbearing age and monitor the progress of the developing child. Gynecologists are concerned with the diagnosis and treatment of the female reproductive system.
Ophthalmology	Ophthalmologist	Ophthalmologists diagnose, treat, and provide comprehensive care for the eye and its supporting structures. These physicians also offer vision services, including corrective lenses.
Otolaryngology	Otolaryngologist	Otolaryngologists treat diseases and conditions that affect the ear, nose, and throat and structures related to the head and neck. Problems that affect the voice and hearing are also referred to this specialist.
Pathology	Pathologist	Pathologists study the causes of diseases. They study tissues and cells, body fluids, and organs themselves to aid in the process of diagnosis.
Pediatrics	Pediatrician	Pediatricians promote preventive medicine and treat diseases that affect children and adolescents. They monitor the child's growth and development and provide a wide range of health services.
Physical medicine and rehabilitation	Physiatrist	Physiatrists assist patients who have physical disabilities. This may include rehabilitation, patients with musculoskeletal disorders, and patients suffering from pain as a result of injury or trauma.
Plastic surgery	Plastic surgeon	Plastic surgeons work with patients who have a physical defect as a result of some type of injury or condition. They perform reconstructive cosmetic enhancements and elective procedures.
Preventive medicine	Preventive medicine specialist	Preventive medicine specialists are concerned with preventing mental and physical illness and disability. They also analyze current health services and plan for future medical needs.
Radiology	Radiologist	Radiology is a specialty in which x-rays are used to diagnose and treat disease. A diagnostic radiologist specializes in using x-rays, ultrasound, nuclear medicine, computed tomography, and magnetic resonance imaging to detect abnormalities throughout the body.
Thoracic surgery	Thoracic surgeon	Thoracic surgeons are concerned with the operative treatment of the chest and chest wall, lungs, heart, heart valves, and respiratory passages.
Urology	Urologist	Urologists are concerned with the treatment of diseases and disorders of the urinary tract. They diagnose and manage problems with the genitourinary system and practice endoscopic procedures related to these structures.

Doctors of Chiropractic

Chiropractors (Doctor of Chiropractic [DC]) focus on the relationship between the spine and the function of the body. The goal is to correct alignment problems and thereby alleviate pain, improve function, and support the body's natural ability to heal itself. Spinal manipulation has been shown to be beneficial for low back pain, headaches, neck pain, whiplash-associated disorders, and upper and lower extremity joint conditions. Chiropractic care is one of the most common fields of **complementary and alternative medicine (CAM)**. Examples of complementary and alternative medicine can be found in the following box.

Complementary and Alternative Medicine Therapies

- Chiropractic
- Massage therapy
- Acupuncture
- Biofeedback
- Meditation
- Guided imagery
- Healing touch
- Natural products
- Yoga, Tai Chi, or Qi Gong
- Homeopathy
- Naturopathy
- Progressive relaxation
- Hypnotherapy
- Ayurvedic medicine

Chiropractic doctors have at least 4 years of additional training beyond a bachelor's degree. The training includes both classroom and direct patient care. The doctors must pass the national licensing exam. State law regulates their practice, and many state boards require continuing education to maintain the license.

Hospitalists

Hospitalists are physicians whose primary professional focus is the general medical care of hospitalized patients. Most hospitalists are employed by the healthcare facility instead of having individual freestanding offices in which patients are seen and treated. Perhaps the most attractive benefit of becoming a hospitalist is the quality of life for the physician and his or her family. Hospitalists work a specific, set number of hours each week and receive a set salary from their employers. In addition, most institutions that employ hospitalists cover these physicians with blanket malpractice insurance, saving the practitioner the expense of costly premiums. Although the hospitalist is in charge of the patient while the person is in the hospital, if the patient has a PCP, he or she may still visit the patient. The hospitalist would still refer the patient to medical specialists as needed for more advanced care.

Nurse Practitioners

Nurse practitioners (NPs) provide basic patient care services, including diagnosing and prescribing medications for common illnesses, or they may have additional training and expertise in a specialty area of medicine. These professionals must have advanced academic training beyond the registered nurse (RN) degree and also vast clinical experience. An NP is licensed by individual states and can practice independently or as part of a team of healthcare professionals.

Physician Assistants

A physician assistant (PA) is a certified healthcare professional who provides diagnostic, therapeutic, and preventive healthcare services under the supervision of a medical doctor. Physician assistants must be licensed, which requires completion of a physician assistant program that is typically at the master's degree level. Physician assistants must pass the Physician Assistant National Certifying Examination to practice in any state. They may also complete advanced training to focus on a particular specialty practice.

ALLIED HEALTH PROFESSIONALS

In addition to doctors, nurse practitioners, and physician assistants the healthcare team includes allied health professionals. The definition of an allied health professional can vary, but it loosely refers to those who can act only under the authority of a licensed medical practitioner (e.g., MD, DO, optometrist, dentist, pharmacist, podiatrist, or chiropractor). Allied health professionals include respiratory therapists, radiation therapists, occupational therapists, physical therapists, technologists of various types, dental hygienists, medical assistants, phlebotomists, pharmacy technicians, and other professionals who do not independently diagnose and prescribe treatment, but perform diagnostic procedures, therapeutic services, and provide care.

The allied health professions fall into two broad categories: technicians (assistants) and therapists. Technicians are trained to perform procedures, and their education lasts 2 years or less. They are required to work under the supervision of medical providers or licensed therapists. This part of the allied health field includes, among others, physical therapy assistants, medical laboratory technicians, radiology technicians, occupational therapy assistants, recreational therapy assistants, respiratory therapy technicians, and medical assistants (Table 1.5).

The educational process for nurses and therapists is more intensive. These professions require a state-issued license and an advanced degree, showing that the individual is trained to evaluate patients, diagnose conditions, develop treatment plans, and understand the rationale behind various treatments (Table 1.6).

Allied health professionals typically work as part of a healthcare team, which is what you will do as a professional medical assistant.

As a new medical assistant, you will enter the ranks of an ever-growing group of allied health professionals who provide services for patients in a variety of settings in today's healthcare system. Allied health professionals comprise nearly 60% of the healthcare workforce. The term "allied health" is used to identify a cluster of health professions, encompassing as many as 200 careers. In the United States, about 5 million allied health professionals work in more than 80 different professions; they represent approximately 60% of all healthcare providers.

TYPES OF HEALTHCARE FACILITIES

Hospitals

Hospitals are classified according to the type of care and services they provide to patients and by the type of ownership. There are three different levels of hospitalized care, which are interconnected.

TABLE 1.5   Allied Health Occupations Recognized by the American Medical Association

TITLE	CREDENTIAL	JOB DESCRIPTION
Anesthesiology assistant	AA	Functions as a specialty physician assistant under the direction of a licensed and qualified anesthesiologist; assists in developing and implementing the anesthesia care plan.
Art therapist	ATR	Uses drawings and other art and media forms to assess, treat, and rehabilitate patients with mental, emotional, physical, and/or developmental disorders.
Athletic trainer	ATC	Provides a variety of services, including injury prevention, assessment, immediate care, treatment, and rehabilitation after physical injury or trauma.
Audiologist	CCC-A	Identifies individuals with symptoms of hearing loss and other auditory, balance, and related neural problems; assesses the nature of those problems and helps individuals manage them.
Blood bank technology specialist	SBB	Performs routine and specialized tests in blood center and transfusion services, using methods that conform to the accepted standards in the blood bank industry.
Diagnostic cardiovascular sonographer/ technologist	RDCS, RVT	Using invasive or noninvasive techniques (or both), performs diagnostic examinations and therapeutic interventions for the heart and blood vessels at the request of a physician.
Clinical laboratory science/medical technologist	MT, MLT	In conjunction with pathologists, performs tests to diagnose the causes and nature of disease; also develops data on blood, tissues, and fluids of the human body using a variety of methodologies.
Counseling-related professional	LPC, LMHC	Deals with human development through support, therapeutic approaches, consultation, evaluation, teaching, and research; practices the art of helping people to grow.
Cytotechnologist	CT	Works with pathologists to evaluate cellular material from all body sites, primarily through use of the microscope; examines specimens for normal and abnormal cytologic changes, including malignancies.
Dance therapist	DTR, ADTR	Uses the psychotherapeutic properties of movement as a process that furthers the emotional, cognitive, social, and physical integration of the patient as a tool for healing.
Dental assistant, dental hygienist, dental laboratory technician	CDA, RDH, CDT	Performs a wide range of tasks, from assisting the dentist to teaching patients how to prevent oral disease and maintain oral health.
Diagnostic medical sonographer	RDMS	Uses medical ultrasound to gather sonographic data, which can aid the diagnosis of a variety of conditions and diseases; also monitors fetal development.
Dietitian, dietetic technician	DTR	Integrates and applies the principles of food science, nutrition, biochemistry, physiology, food management, and behavior to achieve and maintain good health.
Electroneurodiagnostic technologist	REEG-T	Records and studies the electrical activity of the brain and nervous system; obtains interpretable recordings of patients' nervous system function.
Genetics counselor	IGC	Provides genetic services to individuals and families seeking information about the occurrence or risk of a genetic condition or birth defect.
Health information management professional	RHIA, RHIT	Provides expert assistance in the systems and processes for health information management, including planning, engineering, administration, application, and policy making.
Kinesiotherapist	RKT	Provides rehabilitation exercise and education designed to reverse or minimize debilitation and enhance the functional capacity of medically stable patients.
Massage therapist	MT	Applies manual techniques, and may apply adjunctive techniques, with the intention of positively affecting the health and well-being of a patient or client.

Continued

TABLE 1.5   Allied Health Occupations Recognized by the American Medical Association—*continued*

TITLE	CREDENTIAL	JOB DESCRIPTION
Medical assistant	CMA, RMA, CCMA, CMAA	Functions as a member of the healthcare delivery team and performs both administrative and clinical procedures and duties; a multiskilled health professional.
Medical illustrator	MI	Specializes in the visual display and communication of scientific information; creates visuals and designs communication tools for teaching both medical professionals and the public.
Music therapist	MT-BC	Uses music in a therapeutic relationship to address the physical, emotional, cognitive, and social needs of individuals of all ages; assesses the strengths and needs of clients and patients.
Nuclear medicine technologist	RT	Uses the nuclear properties of radioactive and stable nuclides to make diagnostic evaluations of anatomic or physiologic conditions of the body; also provides therapy with unsealed radioactive sources.
Ophthalmic laboratory technician, medical technician/technologist	COT, COMT	Collects data and performs clinical evaluations; performs tests and protocols required by ophthalmologists; assists in the treatment of patients.
Orthoptist	CO	Performs a series of diagnostic tests and measurements on patients with visual disorders; helps design a treatment plan to correct disorders of vision, eye movements, and alignment.
Orthotist/prosthetist	RTO, RTP, RTPO	Designs and fits devices (orthoses) to patients who have disabling conditions of the limbs and spine and/or partial or total absence of a limb.
Perfusionist	CCP	Operates extracorporeal circulation and autotransfusion equipment during any medical situation in which the patient's respiratory or circulatory function must be supported or temporarily replaced.
Pharmacy technician	CPhT	Assists pharmacists with duties that do not require the expertise or judgment of a licensed pharmacist.
Radiation therapist, radiographer	RRTD	Delivers prescribed dosages of radiation to patients for therapeutic purposes; provides appropriate patient care and maintains accurate records of the treatment provided.
Rehabilitation counselor	CRC	Determines and coordinates services to assist people with disabilities in moving from psychological and economic dependence to independence.
Respiratory therapist, respiratory therapy technician	RRT, CRT, RPFT, CPFT	Evaluates, treats, and manages patients of all ages with respiratory illnesses and other cardiopulmonary disorders. Advanced respiratory therapists exercise considerable independent judgment.
Surgical assistant	CSA	Assists in exposure, hemostasis, closure, and other intraoperative technical functions that help surgeons carry out a safe operation with optimal results for the patient.
Surgical technologist	ST, CST	Helps prepare patients for surgery and maintain the sterile field in the surgical suite, making sure all members of the surgical team follow sterile technique.
Therapeutic recreation specialist	CTRS	Uses treatment, education, and recreation services to help people with illnesses, disabilities, and other conditions develop and use their leisure in ways that enhance their health.

- Primary level of care
  - Smaller city or community hospitals
  - Usually serve as the first level of contact between the community members and the hospital setting
- Secondary level of care
  - Both PCPs and specialists provide care
  - Larger municipal or district hospitals that provide a wider variety of specialty care and departments

- Tertiary level of care
  - Referral system for primary or secondary care facilities
  - Provide care for complicated cases and trauma
  - Medical centers, regional and specialty hospitals

Private hospitals are run by a corporation or other organization and usually are designed to produce a profit for the owners or stockholders. *Nonprofit* hospitals exist to serve the community in which they are located and are normally run by a board of directors.

TABLE 1.6   Licensed Healthcare Professions

TITLE	CREDENTIAL	JOB DESCRIPTION
Certified nurse midwife	CNM	Registered nurse (RN) with additional training and certification; performs physical exams; prescribes medications, including contraceptive methods; orders laboratory tests as needed; provides prenatal care, gynecologic care, labor and birth care, and health education and counseling to women of all ages.
Diagnostic cardiac sonographer or vascular technologist	DCS or DVT	Assists in the diagnosis and treatment of cardiac and vascular diseases and disorders; performs noninvasive tests, including echocardiographs and electrocardiographs.
Emergency medical technician	EMT	Progresses through several levels of training, each providing more advanced skills. EMTs' medical education encompasses managing respiratory, cardiac, and trauma cases and often emergency childbirth. Some states also recognize specialties in the EMT field, such as EMT-Cardiac, which includes training in cardiac arrhythmias, and EMT-Shock Trauma, which includes starting intravenous fluids and administering specific medications.
Licensed practical or vocational nurse	LPN or LVN	Provides bedside care, assisting with the day-to-day personal care of inpatients; assesses patients, documents their progress, and administers medications and intravenous fluids when allowed by law; often works in hospitals or skilled nursing facilities and in physicians' offices.
Medical technologist	MT	Performs diagnostic testing on blood, body fluids, and other types of specimens to assist the provider in arriving at a diagnosis.
Nurse anesthetist	NA	RN who administers anesthetics to patients during care provided by surgeons, physicians, dentists, or other qualified health professionals.
Nurse practitioner	NP	Provides basic patient care services, including diagnosing and prescribing medications for common illnesses; must have advanced academic training, beyond the registered nurse (RN) degree, and also must have extensive clinical experience.
Occupational therapist	OT	Assists in helping patients compensate for loss of function.
Paramedic	Paramedic	Specially trained in advanced emergency skills to aid patients in life-threatening situations.
Physical therapist	PT	Assists patients in regaining their mobility and improving their strength and range of motion. Devises treatment plans in conjunction with the patient's physician.
Physician assistant	PA	Provides direct patient care services under the supervision of a licensed physician; trained to diagnose and treat patients as directed by the physician. In most states is allowed to write prescriptions; take patient histories, order and interpret tests, perform physical examinations, and make diagnostic decisions.
Radiology technician	RT	Uses various machines to help the provider diagnose and treat certain diseases; machines may include x-ray equipment, ultrasonographic machines, and magnetic resonance imaging (MRI) scanners.
Registered dietitian	RD	Thoroughly trained in nutrition and the different types of diets patients require to improve or maintain their condition. Designs healthy diets for patients during hospital stays and can help plan menus for home use. Also teaches patients about their recommended diet.
Registered nurse	RN	Provides direct patient care, assesses patients, and determines care plans; has many career options.
Respiratory therapist	RT	Commonly uses oxygen therapy to assist with breathing; also performs diagnostic tests that measure lung capacity. Most work in hospitals. All types of patients receive respiratory care, including newborns and geriatric patients.

The term *nonprofit* sometimes is misleading, because "profit" is different from "making money." A nonprofit hospital or organization may make money in a campaign or fundraiser, but all of the money is returned to the organization. Nonprofit hospitals and organizations must follow strict guidelines in the area of finance and must account to the government for the money brought in and the purposes for which it is used.

A *hospital system* is a group of facilities that are affiliated and work toward a common goal. Hospital systems may include a hospital and a cancer center in a small community or may consist of a group of separate hospitals in a specific geographic region. Many hospital systems are designed as integrated delivery systems. An integrated delivery system (IDS) is a network of healthcare providers and organizations that provides or arranges to provide a coordinated continuum of services to a defined population and is willing to be held clinically and fiscally accountable for the clinical outcomes and health status of the population served. An IDS may own or could be closely aligned with an insurance product, such as a type of insurance policy. Services provided by an IDS can include a fully equipped community and/or tertiary hospital, home healthcare and **hospice** services, primary and specialty outpatient care and surgery, social services, rehabilitation, preventive care, health education and financing, and community provider offices. An IDS can also be a training location for health professional students, including physicians, nurses, and allied health professionals.

Accreditation is considered the highest form of recognition for the quality of care a facility or an organization provides. Not only does it indicate to the public that the facility is concerned with providing high-quality care, it also provides professional liability insurance benefits and plays a role in regulatory agency relicensure and certification efforts. Hospitals and other healthcare facilities are accredited by The Joint Commission, an organization that promotes and evaluates the quality of care in healthcare facilities. Standards or **indicators** have been developed that help determine when patients are receiving high-quality care. The term "quality" refers to much more than whether the patient liked the food served or had to wait to have a procedure or test performed. Categories of compliance include:

- Assessment and care of patients
- Use of medication
- Plant, technology, and safety management
- Orientation, education, and training of staff
- Medical staff qualifications
- Patients' rights

Accreditation by The Joint Commission is required to obtain reimbursement from Medicare, managed care organizations, and insurance companies. Besides accrediting healthcare facilities, The Joint Commission carefully evaluates patient safety. It has established the National Patient Safety Goals, which must be addressed by member facilities. The 2018 safety goals for ambulatory organizations took effect January 1, 2018. They included:

- Identifying patients correctly
- Using medicines safely
- Preventing infection
- Preventing mistakes in safety

All these safety factors are addressed in future chapters.

Ambulatory Care

Ambulatory care centers include a wide range of facilities that offer healthcare services to patients who seek outpatient health services. Physicians' offices, group practices, and multispecialty group practices are common types of ambulatory care facilities, and medical assistants can be employed in all of these practices. Group practices may involve a single specialty, such as pediatrics, or may be a multispecialty. A multispecialty practice might consist of an internal medicine physician, an oncologist, a cardiologist, and an endocrinologist.

Usually the providers in the practice refer patients to each other when indicated. This is not only more convenient for the patients, but also more profitable for the members in the practice. A patient seeing a provider for the first time is considered a *new* patient, whereas a patient who has seen the provider on previous occasions is called an *established* patient. Most providers charge new patients more than established patients because the levels of decision making, the extent of the physical examination, and the complexity of the medical history require that more time be directed toward the new patient.

Occupational health centers are concerned with helping patients return to work and productive activity. Often, physical therapy is used in conjunction with rehabilitation services to assist the patient in regaining as much of his or her previous level of ability as possible. Also, freestanding rehabilitation centers can assist patients with a wide range of services. Pain management centers help patients deal with discomfort associated with their condition. Sleep centers diagnose and treat people with sleep problems. Freestanding urgent or emergency care centers provide patients with an alternative to hospital emergency departments (EDs) and are typically open when traditional provider offices are closed.

Surgery has become more convenient because of the number of ambulatory surgical centers that exist today. Many insurance companies now prefer day surgery because it is more cost-effective. A wide variety of outpatient surgical facilities is available, offering procedures in ophthalmology, plastic surgery, and gastrointestinal concerns, including colonoscopies.

Dialysis centers offer services to patients with severe kidney disorders, and many of the larger cities across the country have cancer centers for patients who need treatment by oncologists. Among the many other types of ambulatory care facilities are centers that provide magnetic resonance imaging (MRI), student health clinics, dental clinics, community health centers, and women's health centers.

Other Healthcare Facilities

Several other types of healthcare facilities deserve attention in the broad overview of the healthcare industry. Diagnostic laboratories offer testing services for patients referred by their providers. The enactment of CLIA in 1967 and its amendment in 1988 established that the only laboratory tests that can be performed in a physician's office lab are those designated as *CLIA-waived*. You will learn how to perform many CLIA-waived tests in your medical assistant program. Larger ambulatory care centers may contain an on-site advanced diagnostic laboratory where all studies can be completed. Smaller or independent practices typically have to send non-CLIA-waived tests to an outside diagnostic facility.

Home health agencies or hospital-affiliated home healthcare organizations provide crucial services to patients who require medical

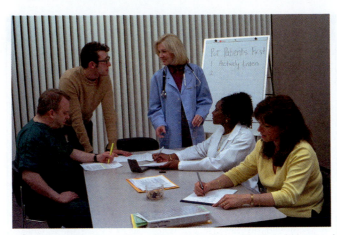

FIGURE 1.8 Teamwork is a vital part of the medical profession. All staff members must work together to care for the patient and perform required duties in the healthcare facility.

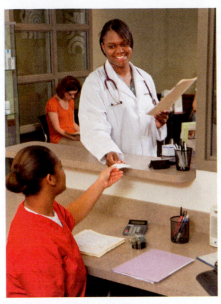

FIGURE 1.9 Knowing which employee to call when help is needed promotes goodwill among employees and often gets a task done more efficiently.

follow-up but are not in a hospital setting. Home healthcare includes therapy services, administration of and assistance with medications, wound care, and other services so that the patient can remain at home, yet still obtain consistent medical attention. Hospice care is a type of home health service that provides medical care and support for patients facing end-of-life issues and their families. The goal of hospice is to provide peace, comfort, and dignity while controlling pain and promoting the best possible quality of life for the patient. Some communities have inpatient hospice services available either in a special unit in a hospital or in an independent hospice center.

THE HEALTHCARE TEAM

To deliver comprehensive quality care, everyone who interacts with patients, from the time they enter the facility to the time they leave, must work as a cooperative member of the healthcare team. If managers were asked to name the most important attributes for medical professionals, teamwork would be high on the list (Fig. 1.8). Staff members must work together for the good of the patients. They must be willing to perform duties outside a formal job description if they are needed in other areas of the office. Many supervisors frown on employees who state, "That's not in my job description." A professional medical assistant should perform the duty and later discuss with the supervisor any valid reasons that the task should have been assigned to someone else. However, if the task is illegal, unethical, or places the patient or anyone else in danger, it should not be done. If you are ever concerned about patient safety, you should discuss the situation with your supervisor before performing the task.

Although we all would enjoy working in an office where everyone gets along and likes every other employee, this does not always happen. Personal feelings must be set aside at work, and all employees must cooperate with others to get the job done efficiently. If a medical assistant has an issue with another employee, the first move would be to discuss it privately with the other person. If the situation does not improve, perhaps a supervisor (office or practice manager) should be involved for further discussions. Do not bring the provider into the discussion unless there is no choice because the facility manager is expected to deal with personnel issues (Fig. 1.9).

Patient-Centered Medical Home

The Patient Centered Medical Home (PCMH) is a model of patient care. In this model, patient care is looked at from a holistic approach. The healthcare team wants to be able to assist that patient with any issues that come up about his or her care. This means having multiple team members available. The provider and the medical assistant would provide the primary care. There would also be a nurse who coordinates all of the care for the patient, including issues about home healthcare, financial issues, transportation issues, and so on. Many models include a clinical pharmacist who is available to discuss medication questions and concerns with the patient.

Research indicates that PCMHs are saving money by reducing hospital and ED visits while at the same time improving patient outcomes. The Agency for Healthcare Research and Quality (AHRQ), which is part of the Department of Health and Human Services (HHS), believes that improving our primary care system is the key to achieving high-quality, accessible, efficient healthcare for all Americans. The agency recognizes that health information technology (IT) plays a central role in the successful implementation of the key features of the primary care medical home. According to the AHRQ, the PCMH has five core functions and attributes:

1. *Comprehensive care:* The primary care practice has the potential to provide physical and mental healthcare, prevention and wellness, acute care, and chronic care to all patients in the practice. However, comprehensive care cannot be provided by only the practicing physician. It requires a team of care providers. The healthcare team for a PCMH includes physicians, nurse practitioners, physician assistants, nurses, pharmacists, nutritionists, social workers, educators, and medical assistants. If these specialty individuals are not readily available to smaller physician practices, virtual teams can be created online to link providers and patients to services in their communities.
2. *Patient-centered care:* The PCMH provides primary healthcare that is holistic and relationship based, always considering the

individual patient and all facets of his or her life. However, establishing a partnership with patients and their families requires understanding and respect of each patient's unique needs, culture, values, and preferences. Medical assistants are trained to provide respectful patient care regardless of individual patient factors. The goal of the PCMH is to encourage and support patients in learning how to manage and organize their own care. Patients and families are recognized as core members of the care team.

3. *Coordinated care:* The PCMH coordinates care across all parts of the healthcare system, including specialty care, hospitals, home healthcare, and community services. Coordination is especially important when patients are transitioning from one site of care to another, such as from hospital to home. The PCMH works at creating and maintaining open communication among patients and families, the medical home, and members of the broader healthcare team.

4. *Accessible services:* The PCMH is designed to deliver accessible care. This is achieved by establishing policies that create shorter wait times for urgent needs, expanded office hours, around-the-clock telephone or electronic access to a member of the care team, and alternative methods of communication, such as email and telephone care.

5. *Quality and safety:* The PCMH is committed to delivering quality healthcare by providing evidence-based medicine and shared decision making with patients and families; assessing practice performance and working on improvements; collecting safety data; and measuring and responding to patients' experiences and satisfaction. All of this information is made public to allow an open assessment of the practice and suggestions for possible methods of improvement.

The goal of the PCMH is to improve patient outcomes and reduce costs. There are accreditation processes that must be completed for a healthcare facility to be recognized as a PCMH. For further information about the PCMH model, refer to the Patient Centered Medical Home Resource Center, Department of Health and Human Services: http://pcmh.ahrq.gov.

PRACTICING PROFESSIONALISM AS A TEAM MEMBER

A *team* is a group of people organized for work or a specific purpose. In the healthcare setting, usually the team consists of the employees working in the same department. A broader definition could include all the employees at the facility. A *team member* is loyal to the group and works well with the other people in the group. As a member, the medical assistant must help the team function. To do this, it is important to know the roles of the different team members. Tables 1.5 and 1.6 describe various healthcare professionals found in ambulatory care facilities.

To be a valuable team member, it is important to have several qualities. Work ethic, punctuality, cooperation, and the willingness to help are important traits in a team member. It takes all members working together to make an effective and productive team. When a member "drops the ball," others must step in and do extra work.

Exceptional Customer Service

To provide exceptional customer service, medical assistants need to:
- Remember that patients, family members, and co-workers are all customers.
- Be professional in behavior and appearance.
- Consider cultural differences when using nonverbal communication.
- Prepare clear, concise verbal communication (written and oral).
- Use therapeutic communication, including active listening.

To help promote professionalism when you first meet a patient, it is important to GIVE:
- **G**reet the patient.
- **I**dentify yourself.
- **V**erify the patient's identity by asking for the person's full name and date of birth.
- **E**xplain the procedure to be performed in a manner that is understood by the patient.

The Meaning of Professionalism

Professionalism is defined as having a courteous, conscientious, and respectful approach to all interactions and situations in the workplace. It is characterized by or conforms to the recognized standard of care for the profession. Conducting themselves in a professional manner is essential for successful medical assistants. The attitude of those in the medical profession generally is more conservative than that seen in other career fields. Patients expect professional behavior and base much of their trust and confidence in those who show this type of **demeanor** in the healthcare facility (Fig. 1.10).

Work Ethic and Punctuality

A *work ethic* is composed of sets of values based on hard work and diligence. The medical assistant should always display **initiative** and be **reliable**. People with a good work ethic arrive on time, are rarely absent, and always perform to the best of their ability. Co-workers become frustrated if another employee consistently arrives late or is absent. This forces others to take on additional duties, and it may prevent them from completing their own work. One missing employee

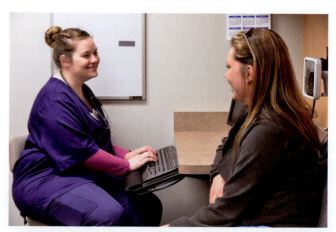

FIGURE 1.10 The professional medical assistant is an asset to the healthcare facility.

can disrupt the entire day. Phones may not be answered promptly. Patients may have to wait longer for appointments. Lunch breaks may be shortened to allow all the work to be done. All employees should know and follow the attendance policies of the facility as outlined in the policies and procedures manual.

Most new hires have a probationary period that may last 30 to 90 days. Excessive absences or *tardiness* (being late) will negatively affect the employee. It may be grounds for *termination* (job loss). If the medical assistant must be absent or tardy, the supervisor must be notified prior to the start time. Make sure to follow the office policy. All employees must be *punctual* (on time) every day. Providers and patients alike expect this reliability.

CRITICAL THINKING APPLICATION   **1.10**

Carmen tends to arrive at the clinic with about 1 minute to spare. She realizes that she needs to change her habits and arrive about 10 minutes before her start time. This would give her a little "cushion" if traffic is slow. If you were Carmen, what strategies could you use to make sure to get to the healthcare facility 10 minutes before the start time?

Cooperation and Willingness to Help

Each team member must be willing to cooperate and help others on the team. It is not uncommon that one team member might be very busy or handling an emergency. Other team members must be willing to step up and lend a helping hand. For instance, a medical assistant may be tied up caring for a very sick patient. Other patients who have appointments are waiting to be seen. One of the other team members needs to help room the patients (e.g., take their vital signs and histories for the provider). This is how the department can provide exceptional customer service. Team members watch out for each other. If someone is getting behind, others help out.

Through cooperation, the team is more productive. Team members have greater job satisfaction. When members cooperate and work together, there is a great sense of communication and understanding in a team. Most importantly, the patients are cared for, and great customer service is provided.

Prioritizing and Time Management Skills

Prioritizing duties and using time management skills are critical for the success of medical assistants. *Prioritizing* means to arrange and complete duties in the order of most importance. *Time management strategies* are methods that maximize personal efficiencies and prioritize tasks. This means that we are to use our time efficiently and concentrate on the most important duties first. To do this, we must first prioritize our duties. We must arrange our schedules to ensure that these duties can be performed. The first way to improve time management is to plan the tasks that need to be done that day. Take 10 minutes to write down the tasks for the day. This helps ensure the tasks get done. Make sure to reference the list throughout the day to keep on track. Don't schedule too much to do each day, so that it is impossible to get everything done. Keep the list manageable. You need to build in some extra time in case of emergencies or urgent issues that come up. The key to managing time is prioritizing.

Time Management Strategies

- Organize and review your daily "to do" list. If you honestly believe you can't possibly get everything that is a priority done, ask for help. It is better to admit you can't do it all than to ignore a task that is important.
- Brainstorm with your peers about ways to achieve all the tasks facing everyone each day. Maybe someone can come up with a unique way to solve a problem; but if not, at least all of you will be on the same page.
- Make a master list of important tasks so nothing is forgotten.
- Try to accomplish like tasks in the same block of time. If you have phone calls to return or insurance referrals to complete, do both at the same time to be more efficient.
- At the end of each day, create a new "to do" list for the next day so that nothing important is forgotten.

When prioritizing your tasks, use a code system to indicate when they need to be done. For instance:

- Use an "M" for tasks that *must* be done that day.
- Use an "S" for tasks that *should* be done that day.
- Use a "C" for tasks that *could* be done if time permits.

Once the tasks have been divided into these categories, they can be further classified in each section. For instance, if category *M* has six tasks, they can be numbered in the order they should be performed. The same process is completed with the tasks in categories *S* and *C*. As the tasks are completed, they are checked off. At the end of each day, create a new "to do" list for the next day so that nothing important is forgotten.

CRITICAL THINKING APPLICATION   **1.11**

Carmen needs to practice her time management skills. Using the system described, make your "to do" list. Use M, S, and C to categorize your activities.

Responding to Criticism

As we work, we are evaluated by others. It may be informal or formal for a job evaluation. We learn from others' feedback on our performance. This criticism can be hard to take. It threatens our confidence and self-esteem. We need to realize the value of the feedback. It will help us improve our skills and refine our professional skills. When a person gives us feedback or criticism, it is important to take it as a professional. Becoming defensive or blaming others is not professional. This type of behavior will be a negative reflection on you.

Problem Solving and Chain of Command

When you are working as part of a team, it is important to understand how to solve differences with other members. Typically, it is best to talk with the person with whom you are having an issue. Try not to use statements that accuse the other person. Refrain from using sentences that start with "You are…" Try to remove the emotion from the situation if you can. Use more "I feel…" statements. If your attempt to resolve the situation is unsuccessful, then it is usually recommended that you talk with the supervisor.

If the issue is related to theft, confidentiality, or harassment, you may need to follow the chain of command in the healthcare facility. Usually, you need to start with your supervisor or the person you report to. Then the next step is the supervisor of your supervisor, and so on. Most employee handbooks discuss the facility's chain of command.

Barriers to Professionalism

At times it is not easy to be a professional. Sometimes patients and co-workers try our patience. It can be difficult to maintain a professional attitude in these cases. Some of the obstructions to professional behavior are discussed in this section.

Attitude

Having a negative attitude can bring down the **morale** of the whole team. Patients can sense when the staff is unhappy, and this makes them wonder why. It is not the patient's responsibility to cheer up the medical assistants. The patients will also be less likely to share personal information with someone who has a negative attitude. Try to find the positive in any given situation.

Complaining can be considered having a negative attitude. If you have a problem you should discuss it, constructively, with someone who can help resolve the situation. Sitting in the break room and complaining to another medical assistant about your schedule will not help to resolve the situation. Talking with your supervisor would be a better solution.

Procrastination

Delaying or putting off tasks can be detrimental to patient care and your relationship with your co-workers. If there is a task that you dread doing, do it quickly and efficiently and you will not have to think about it until the next time. When you are working in healthcare, waiting to do something can put a patient at risk or require that your co-workers do it for you. Either situation can put your job at risk.

Personal Problems and "Baggage"

We all have a personal life. Sometimes things happen in our lives before we go to work. It is important that we push these issues aside and focus on our job. If we carry this "baggage" to work, it can interfere with our ability to do our job. We may be tempted to make personal calls, check emails, and so on. This takes time away from our job, and our focus is not on our job. If the "baggage" is so important and concerning, the medical assistant needs to speak with the supervisor. It might not be appropriate to be working if one cannot concentrate on the job at hand. The patient must be the prime concern of all the employees in the healthcare facility.

Gossip

Gossip is casual or idle chat (rumors) about other people and their business. Many times, the "discussion" is based on someone's opinion and not fact. Most people enjoy working in an environment in which employees cooperate and get along with each other. Rumors and gossip can cause problems with employee morale. They can affect how a team functions. A medical assistant should refuse to participate in the rumor mill (Fig. 1.11). Attempting to be cordial and friendly

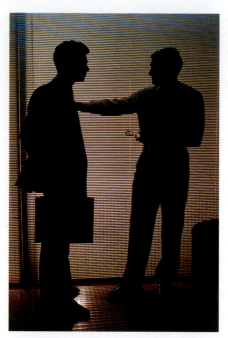

FIGURE 1.11 Gossip and rumors have no place in the medical profession. Avoid employees who participate in this type of activity.

to everyone at work is important. Supervisors regard those who gossip or spread rumors as unprofessional and untrustworthy. You should always avoid passing along work-related rumors to patients and family members.

Personal Communication

The medical assistant should not take unnecessary phone calls from friends and family at the office. The office phone is a business line and must be used as such, except in emergencies. Using personal cell phones during working hours is not acceptable. Use breaks and lunch hours to take care of business on the phone. Never take a personal call or respond to text messages on a cell phone while working with a patient. Many healthcare facilities require cell phones to be silenced and out of sight during the workday. Because most phones have cameras, facility administrators are concerned about unlawful pictures being taken. Many healthcare computer networks block certain nonhealthcare websites (e.g., social media sites). Table 1.7 describes acceptable and unacceptable activities for digital communication devices and online activities.

> **CRITICAL THINKING** APPLICATION **1.12**
>
> Carmen loves her phone. But she learned very quickly that her phone was to be turned off and put away during work hours. Explain why having cell phones out and turned on can create issues in the healthcare facility.

Visitors should not frequent the office, especially the area where the medical assistant is working. If someone must come to the office, always offer the reception area as a waiting room. Visitors should never be allowed to enter patient areas.

Checking personal email also should be avoided in the workplace. Any type of personal business, such as studying, looking up information on the internet for personal use, internet shopping, or using social

TABLE 1.7   Using Digital Communication Devices and Online Activities in Healthcare Facilities

DEVICE/ACTIVITY	ACCEPTABLE, PROFESSIONAL	UNACCEPTABLE, UNPROFESSIONAL
Phone calls/text messages	• Emergency calls only • Turn off or silence ringer • Make personal calls only on break time	• Frequent checking for calls received • Making personal calls • Have phone out and visible when working with patients • Taking pictures
Personal emails and social media	• Do not open, read, or post	• Sending and reading personal emails • Viewing social media postings
Online activities	• Work-related web-related activity	• Shopping, gaming, nonwork websites

media, should be done at home and not in the office. All of these actions distract the medical assistant from the job at hand; the focus should be on serving the patients in the office at all times. Many employees are fired each year for surfing or shopping on the internet for personal reasons or for checking personal email. Make sure all personal business is handled outside of business hours.

Dating Co-Workers

Given the amount of time that we spend with our co-workers, it is not surprising that personal relationships can develop. Dating someone you work with can present professionalism issues. Maintaining a professional demeanor while at work becomes that much harder, especially if you are both on the same team. Other co-workers might think that there is favoritism, especially if one person is the supervisor of another. There can also be issues if the relationship ends badly and both must continue to work together.

Self-Boundaries

When you are working in healthcare, it is important to develop a solid professional relationship with your patients. By establishing realistic self-boundaries, you can protect that relationship.

CLOSING COMMENTS

Medical assisting has developed over the years into a profession that makes considerable contributions to quality patient care in ambulatory care centers. Medical assistants are uniquely trained to manage both the administrative and clinical needs of patients in physicians' offices, clinics, and outpatient facilities. One of the crucial roles of medical assistants is to act as the patient's navigator; that is, to help patients understand and comply with complex care issues. The medical assistant joins a wide range of allied health professionals as part of a healthcare team in which all members work together to best meet the needs of patients. Medical assistants can work in a variety of healthcare facilities and alongside medical specialists to care for patients. They also can act as core members of the PCMH and, along with a variety of community resources, can help provide holistic care to patients in the healthcare system. However, the medical assisting practice must align with the state and regional scope of practice laws and must meet expected standards of care. Medical assistants must always act

under the direction of a physician or provider; they cannot diagnose, prescribe, or treat patients independently.

Patients expect and deserve professional behavior from those who work in medical facilities. Display courtesy and respect toward patients, families, and peers. A diplomatic and tactful person always attempts to interact honestly without giving offense. By displaying these attributes, the medical assistant earns the respect of co-workers and becomes indispensable to his or her employer. Behaving in a professional manner in the medical office helps the medical assistant gain the patient's trust. Trust is one of the most important factors in preventing cases of medical liability. Treating patients with care and not subjecting them to negative behaviors keeps the patient-provider relationship strong and conducive to the health and recovery of the patient. Performing as a cooperative team member goes a long way in promoting a positive healthcare environment for the patient. Incorporating time management strategies into each day not only helps you perform tasks more efficiently, but also ensures that no important tasks are left uncompleted. The entry-level medical assistant can promote professional behavior by joining one of the professional medical assistant organizations and seeking national credentialing.

Patient Coaching

Some patients have very little knowledge about the healthcare industry and may need instruction and explanations about details important to their healthcare. They often call the healthcare facility with questions; therefore, medical assistants must understand the wide variety of healthcare facilities and medical resources available in the community. Become familiar with community resources to make provider-approved referrals for patients who need help from various sources. If a patient seems to have a need, speak with him or her privately and determine whether any agency or organization might help with the issues at hand. The PCMH model relies on all healthcare workers to participate in the care of patients.

Legal and Ethical Issues

Medical assistants are responsible for understanding and following the scope of practice in their communities and for always meeting the expected standards of care. Not meeting these responsibilities can result in serious liability for themselves and their employers.

Remember, the medical assistant must act under the direct supervision of a physician or licensed provider. You must know the limitations placed on your practice by the state in which you live or by the facility or provider who employs you. There is nothing more important than patient safety, so always act within the guidelines of the law and according to the policies and procedures of the facility where you work. Medical assistants are multiskilled healthcare workers who can have a lasting positive effect on patient outcomes. However, never forget that you do not have the authority or education to diagnose, prescribe, or treat patients' clinical problems. Professional credentialing is becoming more important each year.

The workday should be centered around patient care, so never allow personal business to intrude on time that should be spent assisting patients and the provider. Otherwise, the patient may be left with the impression that the medical assistant, or the entire staff, is unprofessional, and this often leads to trust issues with the individuals employed at the facility.

Patient-Centered Care

Patient-centered care involves taking care of the whole patient, not just the physical problems. As a professional medical assistant, you can be instrumental in helping the patient with coordination and integration of care, providing information and education as directed by the provider, involving the family with the patient's care, and above all, respecting the patient's preferences.

Professional Behaviors

Much of this chapter has focused on an introduction to what it means to be a medical assistant and what you will need to learn so you can perform all the skills expected of an entry-level medical assistant. However, working with patients and providing quality care go beyond being able to perform administrative and clinical skills. Each patient must be viewed holistically. This means considering the following patient factors:

- What is the patient's physical condition, and how is it affecting his or her life?
- What is the patient's psychological state; is it preventing the person from following treatment regimens?
- Are any communication barriers preventing the patient from understanding the diagnosis or suggested treatment?
- Is the patient's culture, age, or lifestyle preventing him or her from following the provider's orders?
- Are insurance issues or financial problems preventing the patient from following through with treatment plans?

These are just a few of the factors that can affect patient outcomes. Again, because you will be trained in both administrative and clinical duties, you will be in a unique position to understand all the factors that might affect patient care. It is your responsibility to treat all patients with respect and empathy and to do whatever you can to support them throughout the healthcare experience.

SUMMARY OF SCENARIO

Carmen is a bit overwhelmed but very excited about what she has learned about the role of medical assistants in ambulatory care. She finds it hard to believe that she will become competent in all aspects of the typical medical assistant's job description, but she anticipates learning both administrative and clinical skills. She is looking forward to joining the local AAMA chapter so that she can take advantage of professional development opportunities and networking with other medical assistant professionals and students in her community. Carmen now appreciates the significance of scope of practice and of meeting standards of care, and she is researching the laws affecting medical assistant practice in her state. She can't wait until she is actually able to work with the healthcare team to meet the holistic needs of patients in the practice where she will be employed.

SUMMARY OF LEARNING OBJECTIVES

1. **Discuss the typical responsibilities of a medical assistant and describe the role of the medical assistant as a patient navigator.**
Medical assistants are trained in both clinical and administrative skills that are applicable to ambulatory care settings, such as providers' offices, clinics, and group practices. Graduates of accredited programs are all taught a similar skill set that prepares students for an entry-level position. The actual duties will depend on the place of employment.

Medical assistants have long been encouraged to act as patient advocates in the ambulatory care setting. That role is now described as acting as a patient navigator or care coordinator to help patients manage the complexities of their care. Given their multilevel training, medical assistants can help patients navigate through a wide variety of confusing issues.

2. **Discuss the attributes of a professional medical assistant, project a professional image in the ambulatory care setting, and describe how to show respect for individual diversity.**
Professional medical assistants display courteous, respectful behaviors and communicate with tact and diplomacy. They demonstrate responsible and honest behaviors and always act with integrity. Professional medical assistants view constructive criticism as a way of improving their skill level. Important assumptions are made within seconds of meeting someone based only on how the person looks. Most medical facilities require that medical assistants wear a uniform or scrubs or professional clothing that is not too tight and projects a professional, businesslike appearance. In addition, name badges should be visible; hair should be clean, and longer hair should be tied back; shoes should be clean; nails should be short

and without nail polish (no artificial nails); and no jewelry should be worn.

It is important to recognize that diversity is more than just nationality or race. It can include age, economic status, disabilities, and so on. As professional medical assistants we should learn as much about our patient population as possible, learning about its customs and practices. Being informed will help us to better serve our patients.

3. **Differentiate between scope of practice and standards of care for medical assistants.**

Scope of practice determines the range of responsibilities and practice guidelines for healthcare workers. The scope of practice for a medical assistant is what has been established by law in some states or by practice norms, institutions, or physician-employers in states without scope of practice laws. The standard of care (a legal term) sets the minimum guidelines for job performance. It defines the level and quality of patient service that should be provided by healthcare workers with similar training and experience in a similar situation.

Licensed healthcare professionals have a different scope of practice and expected standard of care than medical assistants. Medical assistants can never diagnose, prescribe, or treat patients. The medical assistant's actions are always done under the supervision of a provider such as a physician, nurse practitioner, or physician assistant. The medical assistant should follow the written order or follow established policies and procedures.

4. **List and discuss professional medical assisting organizations.**

Three professional medical assisting organizations were discussed in this chapter. The American Association of Medical Assistants (AAMA), American Medical Technologists (AMT), and the National Healthcareer Association (NHA). All three organizations offer certification and continuing education.

5. **Examine your learning preferences and interpret how your learning style affects your success as a student.**

Learning preferences are the ways you like to learn and that have proven successful in the past. Your learning style is determined by your individual method of perceiving or examining new material and the way you process it or make it your own. People are either concrete or abstract perceivers and either active or reflective processors.

6. **Integrate effective study skills into your daily activities, design test-taking strategies that help you take charge of your success, and incorporate critical thinking skills and reflection to help you make mental connections as you learn material.**

Study skills, such as memory techniques, active learning, brain tricks, effective reading methods, note-taking strategies, and mind maps, all help students to be more successful.

Test-taking strategies include preparing adequately for the examination, controlling negative thoughts during the examination, and understanding how to deal with different types of questions.

Critical thinking can be defined as thorough thinking because it considers all sides of the information without bias.

Reflection is the process of thinking about or reviewing information before acting.

7. **Summarize the history of medicine and its significance to the medical assisting profession.**

The history of medicine can be traced to ancient practices as far back as 5000 BC. In 1205 BC Moses presented rules of health to the Hebrews, thus becoming the first advocate of preventive medicine. Hippocrates, known as the Father of Medicine, is the most famous of the ancient Greek physicians and is best remembered for the Hippocratic Oath, which has been administered to physicians for more than 2000 years. The medical assisting profession relies on previous medical discoveries to provide patients with safe care in today's healthcare environment. Table 1.3 summarizes medical pioneers and their achievements.

8. **Summarize the various types of medical professionals, allied health professionals, and healthcare facilities.**

Physicians and other providers (e.g., nurse practitioners and physician assistants) are portals of entry or first contacts for patients seeking medical care. Medical professionals include physicians (MDs, DOs), dentists, chiropractors, optometrists, podiatrists, pharmacists, nurse practitioners, and physician assistants. Table 1.4 presents a list of medical specialties.

The definition of an allied health professional can vary, but it loosely refers to those who can act only under the authority of a licensed medical practitioner. Allied health professions fall into two broad categories: technicians (assistants) and therapists. Allied health professionals, including professional medical assistants, typically work as part of a healthcare team. Table 1.5 presents a list of allied health occupations, and Table 1.6 shows a list of licensed healthcare professions.

Healthcare facilities include different levels of hospitals, ambulatory care facilities, and a variety of other institutions that provide specialty care for patients.

9. **Define the Patient-Centered Medical Home (PCMH) and discuss its five core functions and attributes.**

The PCMH is a concept that is transforming the organization and delivery of primary care. The healthcare team looks at patient care from a holistic approach. Improving our primary care system is the key to achieving high-quality, accessible, efficient healthcare for all Americans. The PCMH has five core functions and attributes: (1) comprehensive care, (2) patient-centered care, (3) coordinated care, (4) accessible services, and (5) evidence-based, high-quality, safe care.

10. **Explain the reasons professionalism is important in the medical field, describe work ethics, and stress the importance of cooperation.**

Professionalism is the characteristic of conforming to the technical or ethical standards of a profession. Professionalism is vital in the medical profession because patients expect and deserve to be treated in a professional way. When the medical assistant acts in a professional way, he or she establishes trust with the patient. Patients notice professional behavior, even when it is not directed at them specifically. They notice how others are treated in the reception room and in other areas of the office. Always act in a professional manner while at work.

Continued

SUMMARY OF LEARNING OBJECTIVES—*continued*

Work ethics are sets of values based on the moral virtues of hard work and diligence, involving a whole range of activities, from individual acts to the philosophy of the entire facility.

Each team member must be willing to cooperate and help others on the team. Through cooperation, the team is more productive.

11. **Apply time management strategies to prioritize the medical assistant's responsibilities as a member of the healthcare team.**

Medical assistants need to use time efficiently, prioritize duties, and arrange schedules to ensure that duties can be performed in a timely manner. This can be done by planning tasks that need to be done that day. Most tasks can be prioritized into three general categories: those that must be done that day, those that should be done that day, and those that could be done if time permits.

12. **Respond to criticism, problem-solve, identify obstacles to professional behaviors, and define principles of self-boundaries.**

Criticism can be hard to take, but we need to realize the value of feedback. When you are working as a part of a team, it is important to understand how to resolve differences with other members. If there is an issue related to theft, confidentiality, or harassment, you may need to follow the chain of command in the healthcare facility. Everyone has a life outside the workplace, and sometimes we face challenges and difficult times that are hard to put aside. The professional medical assistant never transfers personal problems or baggage to anyone at the medical facility. The medical assistant should refuse to participate in the office rumor mill and should be cordial and friendly to everyone at work. Avoid personal phone calls and visits unless it is an absolute emergency.

Awareness of personal boundaries helps us determine the actions and behaviors that we find unacceptable. Healthy self-boundaries make it possible to respect our strengths, abilities, and individuality and those of others.

THERAPEUTIC COMMUNICATION 2

SCENARIO

Christi Michelson is a newly hired medical assistant at Walden-Martin Family Medical (WMFM) Clinic. She graduated from the local community college last month. She is currently in her probationary period at WMFM Clinic. Christi has orientation for 1 month, and her probationary period will last for 3 months. Over the next 3 months, she must pass a national certification exam. At the end of 3 months, she will have an evaluation by her supervisor. If the evaluation is positive, she will continue in her position.

Christi is very excited with her first healthcare job. In the past, she has worked as a waitress and a sales clerk. These jobs have helped her learn customer service skills, which she is now using in her current position. Christi is finding that the professionalism at WMFM Clinic is much different than at her previous jobs. Christi is learning the clinic's customer service policies and procedures. She was surprised to learn that her customers include not only the patients, but also her co-workers. Christi is learning new communication skills and is excited to continue learning more skills to help her provide the best patient care possible.

While studying this chapter, think about the following questions:
- What are types of nonverbal communication?
- What are styles and types of verbal communication?
- What are communication barriers and what techniques can help overcome these barriers?
- Why do people behave the way they do?

LEARNING OBJECTIVES

1. Describe the importance of a first impression.
2. Discuss examples of cultural, social, and ethnic diversity, and explain how to demonstrate respect for individual diversity, including gender, race, religion, age, economic status, and appearance.
3. Identify types of nonverbal communication.
4. Discuss the communication cycle, provide tips for composing written communication, and describe the behaviors seen in passive, aggressive, passive-aggressive, manipulative, and assertive communicators.
5. Describe therapeutic communication and active listening, and discuss open and closed questions or statements.
6. Identify barriers to communication, describe techniques for overcoming communication barriers, and discuss how Erikson's psychosocial development stages and Kübler-Ross's stages of grief and dying relate to communication and behavior.
7. Describe personal boundaries with professional verbal communication.
8. Discuss how Maslow's hierarchy of needs relates to communication and behavior.
9. Discuss defense mechanisms and differentiate between adaptive and maladaptive coping mechanisms.

VOCABULARY

adherence The act of sticking to something.
compassion Having a deep awareness of the suffering of another and the wish to ease it.
coping mechanisms Behavioral and psychological strategies used to deal with or minimize stressful events.
defense mechanisms Unconscious mental processes that protect people from anxiety, loss, conflict, or shame.
dignity (DIG ni tee) The inherent worth or state of being worthy of respect.
diversity The differences and similarities in identity, perspective, and points of view among people.

empathy (EM pah thee) The ability to understand another's perspective, experiences, or motivations.
hierarchy (HIE er ar kee) Things arranged in order and rank.
nonverbal communication A type of communication that occurs through body language and expressive behaviors rather than with verbal or written words.
poised (poizd) Having a composed and self-assured manner.
rapport (ra PORE) A relationship of harmony and accord between the patient and the healthcare professional.
respect Showing consideration or appreciation for another person.

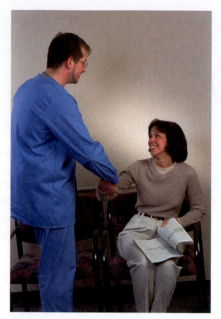

FIGURE 2.1 First impressions are critical in gaining the patient's trust.

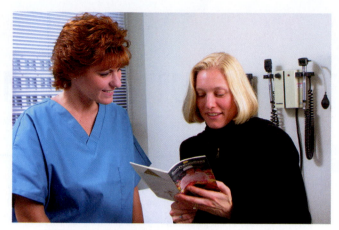

FIGURE 2.2 A bright smile helps to put the patient at ease and to relax.

Communication is the exchange of information, feelings, and thoughts between two or more people using spoken words or other methods. What we say and how we say something directly affects how the other person perceives the message. We need to communicate *effectively*, or in a manner that is clear, concise, and easy to understand. This helps the message to be understood by the other person.

Therapeutic communication is a process of communicating with patients and family members in healthcare. Therapeutic communication requires healthcare professionals to have strong communication skills. It also requires an understanding of how people communicate, the role of diversity in communication, and what impacts behavior. This chapter provides the foundation for therapeutic communication, which will assist as you develop and refine your communication skills.

FIRST IMPRESSIONS

The opinions formed in the early moments of meeting someone remain in our thoughts long after the first words have been spoken. The first impression involves much more than just physical appearance or dress. It includes attitude, **compassion**, and therapeutic communication skills that clearly help the patient and family members realize that the medical assistant is interested in who they are and what they need (Fig. 2.1).

Delivering quality patient care is the primary objective of the professional medical assistant. Patients are the reason the facility exists. Each patient should be welcomed warmly by name and with a polite greeting. The medical assistant should smile and introduce himself or herself to the patient. A smile should show not only on the face, but in the voice and the eyes (Fig. 2.2). This small effort helps put the patient at ease in the healthcare environment.

To provide high-quality patient care, we must communicate effectively with the patient and provide a warm, caring environment.

Positive reactions and interactions with the patient are vital. Because medical care by nature is extremely personal, a medical assistant must always remember that each patient is an individual with certain anxieties. Their anxieties often cause people to act and react in different ways; therefore, effective verbal communication and nonverbal communication with each patient is absolutely essential.

Healthcare professionals accept the responsibility of developing helping relationships with their patients. The interpersonal nature of the patient–medical assistant relationship carries with it a certain amount of responsibility to forget one's self-interest and focus on the patient's needs. A medical assistant can elicit either a positive or a negative response to patient care simply by the way he or she treats and interacts with patients. You usually are the first person with whom the patient communicates; therefore, you play a vital role in initiating therapeutic patient interactions.

DIVERSITY AND COMMUNICATION

Chapter 1 discussed the importance of professionalism and respecting **diversity**. Not only does a medical assistant need to respect diversity, it is also important to understand how it impacts the communication process. Your patients and co-workers will come from backgrounds that are different from your own. Their traditions, customs, beliefs, and values impact how they communicate with others. Knowing more about the diversity around you will help you become a better healthcare professional.

There are several types of diversity, including nationality, race, culture, ethnicity, and social factors. Table 2.1 provides descriptions of the types of diversity. Besides these five types, we also have individual diversity. Factors that relate to individual diversity include language, age, religion, economic status, gender, and appearance. Many times, certain stereotypes, biases, and beliefs are attached to these factors (Table 2.2). Healthcare professionals need to identify personal biases, stereotypes, and beliefs that will prevent effective communication with patients, family, and co-workers. Taking steps to overcome these negative beliefs will help healthcare professionals as they provide respect and dignity to others.

TABLE 2.1 Types of Diversity

TYPE	DESCRIPTION	EXAMPLE
Nationality	Pertains to the country where the person was born and holds citizenship.	John was born in Mexico and moved to the United Stated. He became a U.S. citizen.
Race	A group of people who have the same physical characteristics (e.g., skin color).	Even though John was born in Mexico, his mother is Mongolian, and his father is Caucasian.
Culture	General customs, norms, values, and beliefs held by a group of people.	John has adapted to the U.S. culture. He likes to be on time for appointments. Even though he grew up in a large family (six children), he is comfortable with having two or three children. John values honesty, timeliness, punctuality, and motivation.
Ethnicity	A group of people who share a common ancestry, culture, religion, traditions, nationality, language, and so on.	John states he is Mexican. Growing up he learned his family's Mexican traditions. He plans to share these with his children someday. He values his family and respects his grandparents and parents.
Social factors	All the ways a person is different from others (e.g., lifestyle, religion, tastes, and preferences).	John does not drink alcohol or smoke. He exercises in the gym each day. He likes to visit art museums and learn about history.

TABLE 2.2 Individual Diversity Factors

FACTOR	DISCUSSION
Language	Some people are fluent in more than one language. For others, English is not their primary language. It is important to be sensitive to and respectful of language differences. Using resources (e.g., translated materials, an interpreter) can also show respect to patients.
Age	There are many stereotypes about age. For instance, the older generation may not be college educated, but may have "street smarts." The younger generation may be more comfortable with computers and digital devices. It is important not to stereotype a person because of his or her age. Ask, never assume anything!
Religion	There is a wide range of belief systems in this country. There are also different degrees of religious observations in the workplace. Some patients may refuse certain medical treatments based on their religion. Be sensitive to patients who refuse medical care or want to involve their shaman or healer in their care.
Economic status	Our patients may be from a variety of economic backgrounds. Some patients may be very wealthy and can afford to pay for healthcare without insurance. Other patients may rely on food banks and charities to get by. Be sensitive and respectful if your patient doesn't have the financial means to pay for healthcare services. Help the patient seek resources for medications, transportation, and food.
Gender	There are many stereotypes attributed to gender. We need to make sure we do not stereotype our patients and peers. Some of our patients may identify as a gender other than their birth gender. We need to respect their choices and be sensitive to any issues that arise.
Appearance	Our patients' appearances can greatly vary. If you work in a farming community, patients may come to appointments in their work clothes and smell of the barn. With the popularity of piercings, tattoos, and hair dye, we can see a variety of differences in our patients. We need to move beyond the patient's appearance and provide exceptional patient care.

Demonstrating Respect

Healthcare professionals need to show respect to others. This can be achieved with a smile, a pleasant greeting, and eye contact when first meeting the person. During the interaction, it is important to be courteous, sincere, polite, welcoming, and professional. Using a calm tone of voice, appropriate eye contact, and proper grammar without slang or generational terms also shows respect.

Being respectful also means maintaining the person's dignity, or in other words, treating others as we would want to be treated. People expect to be treated as individuals who matter. By treating others as though they matter, you are also showing them the respect they deserve.

NONVERBAL COMMUNICATION

As mentioned in the opening section, communication occurs by what we say and how we say something. These two forms of communication – verbal and nonverbal – affect how the other person perceives the message. Experts agree that nonverbal communication greatly exceeds verbal communication. In other words, we communicate more by our body language and expressive behaviors than through our words.

Think of a time when you were talking with a person, and that person did something that left a greater impression on you than the verbal message did. Nonverbal communication is powerful. It is important that the verbal message matches the perceived nonverbal message.

With therapeutic communication, we use nonverbal communication to show respect, acceptance, and understanding. We want to appear positive and open with others. We can do this through our nonverbal communication, which involves the following areas:

- *Behaviors*: Include our posture, facial expressions, eye contact, and so on. (Fig. 2.3). Table 2.3 discusses positive and open behaviors that should be used by medical assistants.
- *Communication delivery factors*: Include how we deliver our verbal message, for instance the rate, clarity, and volume of our voice. This helps create the context of the message. Table 2.4 provides a list of delivery factors and the professional expectations that medical assistants should strive for.
- *Other factors*: Include our appearance and spatial distance with another person. How we dress can send a message to others.

For instance, a medical assistant who has a dirty uniform and messy hair may send a negative message to others. Chapter 1 discussed the importance of a professional appearance for medical assistants. *Spatial distance*, or the space between one person and another, will be discussed later in this chapter.

Besides using nonverbal communication to convey acceptance and respect, we also read others' nonverbal communication. This provides us feedback on what is being said and how the person feels (Fig. 2.4). Table 2.3 describes negative and closed nonverbal behaviors.

Examples of how nonverbal behaviors are interpreted include:

- *Self-confident*: The person appears confident and self-assured, has good posture, and makes appropriate eye contact.

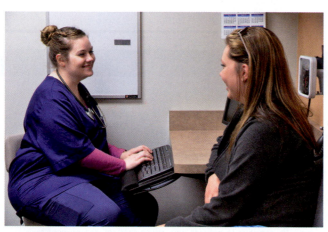

FIGURE 2.3 The medical assistant's position should be at the level of the patient.

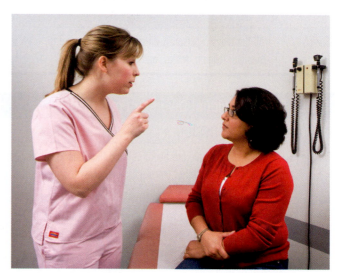

FIGURE 2.4 Pointing often is an accusatory gesture and causes discomfort.

TABLE 2.3	Positive and Negative Nonverbal Behaviors	
NONVERBAL BEHAVIORS	**POSITIVE AND OPEN**	**NEGATIVE AND CLOSED (INTERPRETED AS OR MEANING)**
Position	Be at the level of the other person; angled toward the other person	Being at a higher level (looking down on the person); leaning backward (disinterest); direct face to face (confrontational, intimate)
Arms	Arms at the side	Arms are crossed (discomfort, defensive, disagree); hands behind back (secretive, mistrustful); clenched fists (anger, aggressive); pointing at a person
Posture	**Poised**	Poor or slumped posture (poor self-worth, lack of confidence, unwillingness, lack of interest, less knowledgeable, unreliable); stiff, immobile (uncomfortable)
Facial expression	Smile	Rolling eyes, yawning (boredom); frowning (sadness, disagree, anger)
Gestures	Small gestures	Overuse of hands (nervousness, excitement)
Touch	Light touch on hand, appropriate touch	Inappropriate touching or hugging (makes the person feel uncomfortable or violated)
Eye contact	Movement of eyes, blinking	Staring at the person (makes it awkward); avoiding eye contact (low self-esteem, low confidence, and dishonesty)
Mannerisms	Focus on the person	Fidgeting; looking at a watch, phone, or clock (bored, anxious, impatient)

TABLE 2.4 Nonverbal Communication Delivery Factors

NONVERBAL DELIVERY FACTORS	DEFINITION	PROFESSIONAL EXPECTATIONS
Rate	Refers to the speed at which the speaker talks	Use a moderate rate. If the rate is too fast, the message may be missed. If the rate is too slow, it may be perceived as more negative by the receiver.
Clarity	Refers to the quality of the voice	Use a clear voice when talking with others. Muffled, mumbling, or unclear speech can create inaccuracies with the message.
Volume	Refers to the loudness of the speaker's voice	Use a moderate volume. If too loud, it may be perceived as yelling, and if too soft, the message may be missed. In healthcare, we need to keep information confidential. So, using a loud voice can violate the patient's privacy.
Pitch	Refers to the highness and lowness of the voice	Using a varying pitch, or *inflections*, helps a person to emphasize important points. It is important to have a rhythm in your voice to help the receiver understand what is important.
Tone	Refers to the emotion in the voice	Use an accepting or a neutral tone in healthcare. An angry tone can cause the receiver to misinterpret the message and/or also become angry.
Pauses	Refers to a period of not talking	Using pauses helps the receiver absorb the message. Limit verbalized pauses (e.g., "ah," "umm," and "er").
Intonation	Refers to the melodic pattern or the pitch variation	With statements, we usually use a medium intonation and finish the sentence on a lower pitch. Finishing the statement on a higher pitch usually indicates a question. Using correct intonation will help the correct message to be received.
Vocabulary	Refers to the word choice used	Using precise words helps the message to be correctly received. Incorrect use of words may create a negative impression of the speaker. It is important to use words that the receiver understands. If medical terminology, slang, or generational terms are used, the message may not be understood.
Grammatical structure	Refers to the sentence structure	Using incorrect grammatical sentence structure can create a negative impression of the speaker.
Pronunciation	Refers to how the word is said	Using the correct pronunciation will help ensure the correct message will be received. Incorrect pronunciation of a word (e.g., medication name) may lead to inaccuracies with the message.

- *Insecure*: The person is quiet, courteous, and has good listening skills, but tends to focus more on others than on himself or herself.
- *Arrogant*: The person has increased personal space; appears to bore easily and is a poor listener.
- *Embarrassed*: The person has a nervous giggle; tends to avoid eye contact with others.
- *Fearful*: The person has wide-open eyes, looks around, grasps hands, and has a rigid posture.
- *Resentful*: The person hunches shoulders, crosses his or her arms, and mutters or whispers.

CRITICAL THINKING APPLICATION   **2.1**

While working at the reception desk, Christi needs to demonstrate positive and open nonverbal behaviors. Describe the positive and open nonverbal behaviors she should be demonstrating.

Cultural Differences

The meaning of nonverbal behaviors can greatly vary among cultural groups. What is acceptable to one group may be considered offensive to others. As you work with patients from diverse groups, make sure to learn cultural differences in communication. It will reduce the likelihood of offending the other person. It also will help make the patient's experience a positive one. Table 2.5 provides some examples of cultural differences with nonverbal behaviors.

If you are interacting with a person from another cultural group and you are unfamiliar with it, try following these tips:
- Follow the other person's lead in terms of nonverbal behaviors and personal space.
- Use gestures cautiously.
- Refrain from touching a child's head.
- Remember that facial expressions can be misinterpreted (e.g., grimacing with pain may not be acceptable in some cultures, whereas other cultures "encourage" it).

TABLE 2.5   Cultural Differences in Nonverbal Behaviors

NONVERBAL BEHAVIORS	CULTURAL DIFFERENCES
Eye contact	*Hispanics, Asians, Native Americans, and Middle Easterners:* Eye contact is considered rude and offensive. *Females:* May avoid eye contact with males so it is not perceived as a sign of sexual interest.
Touch	*Asians and Middle Easterners:* The head is a sacred part of the body; it is considered offensive to pat the head. *Middle Easterners:* Left hand is reserved for bodily hygiene; it is inappropriate to use that hand to touch others or transfer objects. *Muslims:* Inappropriate to touch a person of the opposite gender. *Latin Americans and Eastern Europeans:* Very comfortable with touching others, even new acquaintances.
Gestures	*Some cultures:* Using the "come here" finger/hand gesture is used with dogs and considered offensive. Pointing with one finger is considered very rude. *Asians and Indians:* Use the whole hand to point at something or someone. *Venezuelans:* Use their lips to point; finger pointing is impolite.
Winking	*Latin Americans:* Consider winking a romantic or a sexual invitation. *Nigerians:* Wink at children to indicate they should leave the room. *Chinese:* Consider winking rude.
Posture	*Many cultures:* Consider poor posture disrespectful.
Personal space	*Latin Americans and Middle Easterners:* Stand quite close to those they do not know. *Muslim males (even providers):* Cannot be too close to females.

- Lack of eye contact may be related to nervousness or the culture. It is not due to fear or dishonesty.

CRITICAL THINKING APPLICATION   **2.2**

Christi had heard that people from the Hmong and Vietnamese cultures do not likes others commenting on their children. They fear the words might be overheard by a spirit who might try to harm the children. Christi mentions this to a co-worker. The co-worker does not believe in this. Do they need to worry about this belief when working with patients from the Hmong and Vietnamese culture? Explain your answer.

Spatial Distance

As previously mentioned, spatial distance is also considered to be part of nonverbal communication. The distance between ourselves and another person can vary based on our familiarity with that person. There are different types of spaces, including:

- *Intimate or personal space* (distance of 0 to 18 inches): In our personal lives, we allow close family and friends into this space (Fig. 2.5). In healthcare, medical assistants are in the patients' personal space for procedures such as electrocardiograms, wound care, and obtaining vital signs.
- *Casual person space* (distance of 18 inches to 4 feet): In our personal lives, this space is used for conversations with friends. In healthcare, the medical assistant uses this space when talking with the patient. This may include taking a medical history or coaching a patient on home cares.

Spatial Distance in the United States

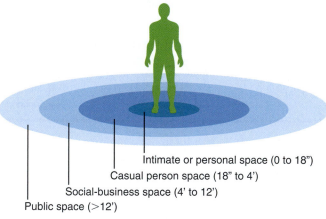

Intimate or personal space (0 to 18")
Casual person space (18" to 4')
Social-business space (4' to 12')
Public space (>12')

FIGURE 2.5 Spatial distance.

- *Social-business space* (distance of 4 to 12 feet): In our personal lives, this is the acceptable space for business transactions and socializing with acquaintances. In healthcare, the medical assistant uses this space when completing business tasks, such as answering billing questions and checking in a patient at the reception desk.
- *Public space* (distance greater than 12 feet): In our personal lives, this space is used for activities in public. In healthcare, this is the acceptable space with group events.

Research has shown that some cultural groups have different acceptable casual person space. For instance, Middle Eastern cultures have about 1 foot, whereas North American and Western European cultures have about 1.5 feet. The Japanese culture is about 3 feet. You may have already experienced this when you are talking with friends. Some friends get closer to you than others. When a person is closer to us than we feel is acceptable for our culture, we may become uncomfortable.

We all have a personal space, or "bubble," around us. We may be uncomfortable and on guard if someone we do not know well gets into our personal space. We may take a step back or move back in a chair to increase the space between us and the other person. If someone is communicating from too far away, we may also feel uncomfortable.

It is important to realize that as healthcare professionals, we move into the personal or intimate space of patients many times while providing care. We need to respect this space. We need to be aware of our grooming, our appearance, and our habits. When working with others, we need to watch for clues regarding the person's comfort level with distance. A person who needs more space may move backward. Leaning, shifting, or moving forward shows the person wants to decrease the distance. It is important to recognize this nonverbal communication.

CRITICAL THINKING APPLICATION   **2.3**

Think about the diverse cultures in your area. What differences have you observed in the nonverbal communication between these groups?

VERBAL COMMUNICATION

Verbal communication can be defined as words used either orally or in written form. Medical assistants use verbal communication all the time. This section will examine the communication process and then discuss the two forms of verbal communication, written and oral communication.

Communication Cycle

The *communication cycle* is a way to describe the communication process (Fig. 2.6). A breakdown of any part of the cycle can lead to a message being misunderstood. The communication cycle proceeds as follows:

- **Sender creates the MESSAGE:** The person with a message is called the *sender*. The sender must organize his or her thoughts and communicate a clear, concise, easy to understand message.
- **Receiver DECODES the message**: The person getting the message is the *receiver*. This person must decode or translate the message based on personal factors and subjective perceptions. If the message was correctly translated within the context of the message sent, then it matches the message the sender sent. If the message was incorrectly translated, then the receiver develops a different perception of the message than what the sender intended.
- **Receiver creates FEEDBACK**: The receiver then provides feedback based on the perceived message.
- **Sender DECODES feedback**: The sender gets the feedback message. Again, the feedback must be decoded correctly for the communication to be accurate

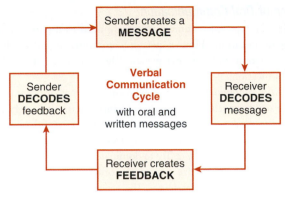

FIGURE 2.6 Verbal communication cycle.

As indicated in Fig. 2.6, the verbal communication cycle exists with written and oral messages. We will examine both types of verbal communication.

Written Communication

Written communication is a type of verbal communication. We create written messages for the receiver. Written communication includes:

- Written messages (e.g., phone messages)
- Letters and emails
- Online information and media (e.g., informational flyer)

It is important that we consider how we state our written message. We want the receiver to get the message we intended on sending. The following box provides tips for composing written communication. Chapter 9 provides additional information on composing professional letters and emails.

Tips for Composing Written Communication

All Forms of Written Communication
- Draft the message and then read what you have written. Make sure the message is clear, concise, easy to understand, and provides the message you intended.
- Check the grammar, spelling, capitalization, punctuation, and sentence structure.
- Make sure to address the message to the correct receiver.

Professional Emails
- Add a few meaningful words in the subject line.
- Start with a courteous greeting.
- Write out all words.
- Write in complete sentences. Capitalize the first letter of the first word and end the statement with the correct punctuation.
- Do not use all-capital letters. It is viewed as shouting at the receiver.

Oral Communication

Oral communication is a type of verbal communication. Oral communication means we talk with others and we listen to others. In the ambulatory care environment, oral communication occurs in person, over the phone, and using remote devices (e.g., webcams).

Styles of Oral Communication

Besides the types of communication, we need to discuss the styles of communication. How a person communicates affects his or her interaction with another person. There are five main styles of communication.

- *Passive communicators*: Avoid expressing feelings or opinions, fail to exert themselves, allow others to infringe on their rights, and tend to speak softly. They may feel depressed, resentful, or anxious because life seems out of their control.
- *Aggressive communicators*: Try to dominate others; have low frustration tolerance, criticize and attack others, have poor listening skills, and use "you" statements. This can cause them to be alienated from or feared by others.
- *Passive-aggressive communicators*: Deny problems; do not confront problems or people, appear to be cooperative, but plan subtle sabotage or disruptions. They may become alienated from others and feel powerless.
- *Manipulative communicators*: Cunning and controlling of others. Use others to get what they want. Can cause others to feel sorry for them or guilty.
- *Assertive communicators*: Clearly state their needs and wants. They use "I" statements and listen without interrupting. They are relaxed, use good eye contact, feel connected with others, and stand up for their rights. They feel in control of their lives and are mature enough to address issues.

It is important that healthcare professionals understand each type. We should also evaluate our own communication style. What style do we use? Identifying how you communicate is an important part of your professionalism journey. A healthcare professional needs to communicate in an assertive manner. This is the healthy form of communication. It leads to better team dynamics.

As you learn about these styles, think about the people you interact with. How do they communicate? How do you feel when you interact with them? Table 2.6 reviews the nonverbal communication behaviors for each communication style. It also identifies common feelings others may have when interacting with such a person.

> **CRITICAL THINKING** APPLICATION   2.4
>
> Of the five communication styles, which one should Christi use at work? Explain your answer.

Therapeutic Communication

As mentioned before, therapeutic communication is a process of communicating with patients and family members in healthcare. It is an interactive relationship that conveys acceptance and respect without judgment or blame. It encourages healthcare professionals to build **rapport** with patients. When that bond develops and grows, patients are more comfortable with expressing their feelings, ideas, and concerns. Thus, therapeutic communication techniques are helpful in building the relationship with the patient. Active listening and other therapeutic communication techniques will be described in the following sections.

TABLE 2.6	Communication Styles		
COMMUNICATION STYLE	NONVERBAL COMMUNICATION BEHAVIORS	OTHERS' FEELINGS WITH THIS BEHAVIOR	HOW TO DEAL WITH THIS STYLE
Passive	Soft voice, head down, fidgets, no eye contact. "Victim mentality." Hesitant, self-conscious, and belittles the person's contribution.	Exasperated and frustrated. Feel they can take advantage of the person.	Be assertive. May need to be firm in your approach, while ensuring you take the time to reassure the person and welcome his or her suggestions and contributions.
Aggressive	Low voice; big, sharp, and fast gestures. Glare and frown. Invade others' personal space intentionally.	Hurt, fearful, afraid, humiliated, and resentful. Loss of respect for the person.	Never become aggressive and always remain calm. Do not take the person's aggression personally. Attempt to see his or her point of view, which will help you communicate yours.
Passive-aggressive	Sugary sweet voice; often looks sweet and innocent. Often in others' personal space and touches others to pretend to be warm and friendly.	Confused, angry, and hurt by the "two-faced" personality of the person.	Try to refrain from drawing negative conclusions immediately. Can use various ways to handle this approach, based on the situation. May use humor and positive discussion.
Manipulative	Patronizing voice; uses high pitch.	Angry, resentful, guilty, and frustrated with being manipulated.	Avoid being manipulated. Respectfully maintain your position.
Assertive	Medium pitch, speed, and volume of voice; good eye contact. Open posture and respectful of others.	Can trust individual. Know the person can handle criticism and accept compliments.	Ideal communication style. Be assertive also!

Active Listening

Active listening is the most important therapeutic communication technique. This skill takes time to master. Active listening means we fully concentrate on what is being said and how it is said. This is different from passively hearing what the speaker is saying and being distracted by our own thoughts.

When a person is actively listening, the speaker can easily see it. The listener shows interest by verbal messages, such as "Yes." The listener also shows interest through nonverbal messages. As discussed earlier, nonverbal messages include eye contact, nodding your head, body position, touch, and facial expressions (Fig. 2.7). The following box lists characteristics of a good listener. Showing interest at this level will encourage the speaker to be more at ease. Communication between the two people will be more open, honest, and clear.

Characteristics of a Good Listener

- Remain nonjudgmental and neutral.
- Refrain from interrupting with a comment or question.
- Allow for periods of silence.
- Smile and nod your head to show you are listening to the message.
- Use appropriate eye contact so the speaker is not intimidated.
- Lean slightly forward or sideways toward the speaker.
- Avoid distractions (e.g., fidgeting, looking at the clock, doodling).

Open and Closed Questions or Statements

When you gather information from a patient, it is helpful to use a combination of open and closed questions or statements. An *open question* or statement asks for general information or states the topic to be discussed, but only in general terms. Use this communication tool to begin a conversation with a patient, to introduce a new section of questions, or whenever the person introduces a new topic. It is a very effective method of gathering more details from the patient about his or her problem. Examples of open questions include:

- "What is the reason for the appointment with Dr. Walden?"
- "How have you been getting along?"

- "You mentioned having problems with your insurance. Can you tell me more about that?"

This type of question or statement encourages patients to respond in a manner they find comfortable. It allows patients to express themselves fully and provide comprehensive information about their chief complaint.

Closed (also called direct) *questions* ask for specific information. In many cases, this form of questioning limits the patient's answer to one or two words, including yes and no. Use this form of question when you need confirmation of specific facts, such as when asking about demographic information. For example:

- "What is the name of your insurance carrier?"
- "What is your birth date?"
- "What pharmacy do you prefer for prescription refills?"

Other Therapeutic Communication Techniques

When you are working with patients and family members, several therapeutic communication techniques can be used. It is critical that we understand the message correctly. We need to make sure patients know we are listening. We also need to check that we understand the message. Assuming what someone means or feels can lead to misunderstanding. Therapeutic communication techniques are detailed in Table 2.7. Procedures 2.1 through 2.3 on pp. 46-49 provide examples of role-playing to practice communicating with patients.

Effective communication is critical for compassionate, quality patient care. Medical assistants must understand barriers that prevent patients from understanding communication or communicating clearly with others. Taking steps to overcome these barriers will help promote effective communication. Table 2.8 discusses common barriers and ways to overcome barriers. The following sections will provide additional information on communication barriers related to anger, age, and disease status.

Anger

As discussed in Table 2.8, anger is a barrier to communication. Medical assistants can encounter angry patients, family members, or co-workers (Fig. 2.8). It is critical to know how to handle and defuse the situation. It is important for the person to feel heard and for the medical assistant to remain safe and follow through on any promises made.

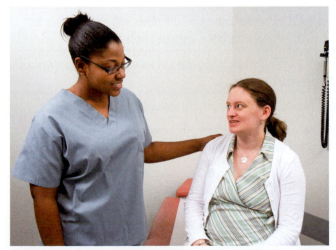

FIGURE 2.7 Touching the patient communicates care and compassion. Careful listening and asking questions help the patient express thoughts and feelings.

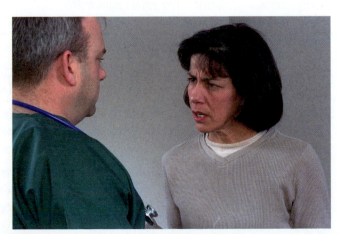

FIGURE 2.8 Remain calm, even if a patient becomes verbally aggressive. Attempt to calm the person by listening and expressing empathy whenever possible.

TABLE 2.7   Therapeutic Communication Techniques

TECHNIQUES	DEFINITION	FEEDBACK TO SPEAKER
Reflection	Putting words to the person's emotional reaction, which acknowledges the person's feelings. Also helps to check what the person is feeling instead of just assuming. Shows **empathy** and helps build **rapport.**	Reflect what you think was said. For example: "It sounds like you are feeling scared…" or "I understand you are having trouble with…" or "You feel that…"
Restatement or paraphrasing	Rewording or rephrasing a statement to check the meaning and interpretation. Also shows you are listening and understanding the speaker.	Do not repeat the person's exact words. Use phrases such as, "What I'm hearing is…" or "It sounds like you are saying…" Refrain from using "I know what you mean."
Neutral	Encourages the speaker to continue and conveys you are interested and listening to the message.	Use phrases such as, "Uh huh," "I see," and "That is very interesting."
Silence	Allows time to gather thoughts and answer questions.	Can be uncomfortable to some people. Allows time to think about what was said.
Clarification	Allows the listener to get additional information.	Using statements such as, "Can you clarify…" and "Do you mean…"
Summarizing	Allows the listener to recap and review what was said.	Using a statement such as, "If I understand how you feel about this situation…"

TABLE 2.8   Barriers to Communication and Ways to Overcome Barriers

TYPE OF BARRIER	PATIENT BARRIERS	WAYS TO OVERCOME BARRIERS
Environmental distractions	Noise, lack of privacy, temperature	Provide privacy for patients. Talk with patients in a quiet room with the door closed. Make sure the room temperature is comfortable.
Internal distractions	Hunger, pain, anger, tiredness	Help make the patient comfortable. Provide food and drink if available. Administer pain medications as ordered.
Visually impaired	Unable to see written communication	Use audio recordings, screen magnifiers, large-print materials, and screen reader software.
Hearing impaired	Unable to hear verbal communication	Use print materials and written instructions. Use videos with captions. Have text telephones (TTYs) available. Use a sign language interpreter.
Intellectual disability	Unable to understand what is being said; may be functioning at a lower age level	Use "functioning age"–appropriate language and materials. Provide information also to the guardian/caregiver.
Illiterate	Unable to read or write	Use pictures and models. Draw pictures and use simple language.
Non-English speaking	English is not the patient's primary language; lack of understanding of medical terminology	Use interpreters and translated materials. Limit medical terminology and define medical terms that must be used. Use culturally appropriate materials and visuals (pictures, graphs, and models).
Emotional distractions (angry, distraught, anxious)	Fear and anxiety related to being judged by the healthcare professional; inability to explain personal feelings; angry or distraught patients may not hear what is said or may not be able to communicate effectively	Provide a warm, caring environment. Make sure your body language (nonverbal behaviors) is consistent with an open, caring manner. Gain the person's trust. Keep your voice at a normal level; raising the voice can increase the person's anger.

If the angry person is in a public area and the medical assistant feels safe, the person should be invited to a more private location. It is important to allow the person to talk out the anger. The medical assistant should present a calm attitude, speak in a low tone of voice, and take notes if needed. The medical assistant should demonstrate empathy by using active listening skills and using therapeutic communication techniques. If the medical assistant responds in anger or becomes argumentative, the situation will intensify, and the person's anger may increase.

Empathy

Healthcare professionals who are empathetic provide better patient care. Showing patients respect and dignity through empathetic care builds trust with patients, which increases their satisfaction and **adherence** to the treatment plan. It is critical when providing patient-centered care. Without empathy, the patients may remain anxious, feel disconnected with their care, lose trust in their healthcare team, and may have less positive health outcomes. Strategies to provide empathetic care include:

- Make sure to listen to your patient and understand his or her experiences, perspective, and concerns.
- Use positive nonverbal behaviors. For instance, position yourself at the same level as the patient. Make good eye contact. Nod your head and lean in as you communicate with the patient.
- Use therapeutic communication techniques (e.g., reflection, paraphrasing, and clarification) as you interact with the patient. Show your support.
- Interpret the patient's nonverbal behaviors and clarify any messages that differ with the verbal message received.
- Be welcoming. Show your patients dignity and respect.

During the interaction with the angry person, the medical assistant must remain safe. There should be a policy in place for dealing with angry individuals. Policies should cover the following:

- Notify the facility's administrator of all difficult patients or ask for help from co-workers.
- Keep yourself at a distance from the person (e.g., try to separate yourself from the person by a desk or another piece of furniture).
- If you are in a room with the angry person, position yourself so you are the closest to the door.
- Have another employee remain close by.
- Know under what circumstances you should contact the police or building security for assistance.

Age

A person's age may be a barrier to communication. Communicating with a 3-year-old child is different than with an 80-year-old adult. A medical assistant must understand the developmental stages to know how to interact with people of different ages.

Erik Erikson, a psychoanalyst, described the emotional, physical, and psychological stages of human development. He stated that a person in each stage had a specific developmental task to complete. Understanding the task or goal of each stage helps healthcare

professionals communicate more effectively with patients. Table 2.9 presents the developmental stages, goals of each stage, and communication tips for healthcare professionals. The following box provides additional suggestions for effective communication with aging patients. Procedure 2.4 on p. 49 provides a role-playing scenario related to an older patient.

Suggestions for Effective Communication With Aging Patients

- Address the patient by Mr., Mrs., Ms., or Miss unless the patient has given you permission to use his or her first name.
- Introduce yourself and explain the purpose of a procedure before performing the procedure.
- Face the aging person and softly touch the individual to get his or her attention before beginning to speak.
- Use expanded speech by lowering the pitch or tone of your voice and speaking firmly, making sure to enunciate each word clearly.
- Use gestures and demonstrations to clarify communication, and print out instructions in block print using a larger font size to be sure aging individuals can read the information.
- If the message must be repeated, paraphrase or find other words to say the same thing.
- Observe the patient's nonverbal behavior for cues indicating whether he or she understands.
- Provide adequate lighting without glare.
- Allow patients time to process information and take care of themselves unless they ask for assistance.
- Conduct communication in a quiet room without distractions.
- Involve family members as needed for continuity of care.
- When leaving a telephone message, remember to speak slowly and clearly and repeat the message in the same manner. It is difficult to interpret a message, and even more difficult to write it down, if the message was delivered in a hurried manner.
- Use referrals and community resources for support.

CRITICAL THINKING APPLICATION   2.5

What communication tips should Christi use when communicating with:
- A 2-year-old child?
- A 13-year-old teen?
- A 30-year-old adult?
- An 80-year-old adult?

Disease Status

A person's disease status also can affect communication. For instance, think about these scenarios:

- Jim was just notified by his provider that he may only have 3 months to live. Jim had been healthy until the last few weeks, when he started to feel very ill.

TABLE 2.9   Erikson's Stages of Psychosocial Development

DEVELOPMENTAL STAGE	GOALS OF STAGE	COMMUNICATION TIPS
Trust versus Mistrust (age range: 0–1.5 years [infancy])	Must develop trust, with the ability to mistrust should the need arise.	Use calm, soothing voice, hold child securely. Loud voices and noises can startle the child.
Autonomy versus Shame and Doubt (age range: 1.5–3 years [toddler])	Must explore and manipulate things in his or her "world" to develop autonomy and self-esteem.	Use simple language. Allow the child to touch and explore objects. Allow the child to play and make choices.
Initiative versus Guilt (age range: 3–6 years [preschool])	Encouraged to try new activities. Must assume responsibilities and learn new skills. Will make the child feel purposeful and increase self-esteem.	Use short, simple sentences. Encourage questions. Use imitation, play, and role-playing.
Industry versus Inferiority (age range: 6–12 years [school age])	Must seek to finish tasks. Recognition for accomplishments is important.	Use engaging simple tools to communicate information (videos, gaming software, pamphlets). Encourage discussion and questions.
Identity versus Role Confusion (age range: 12–18 years [adolescence])	To know who you are as a person and how you fit into the world around you. Creates a meaningful self-image.	Provide privacy and independence. Encourage responsible decision making. Encourage discussion and questions.
Intimacy versus Isolation (age range: 18–25 years [young adult])	Can vary. Develops friendships; takes on commitments.	Identify motivating factors and use them as needed during communication. Realize person may be juggling a lot of obligations.
Generativity versus Stagnation (age range: about 25–60 years [middle adulthood])	Achieve a balance between the concern for the next generation (having a family) and being self-absorbed.	
Ego Integrity versus Despair (age range: 60 and older [late adulthood])	Reflect on one's life and come to terms with it, instead of regretting the past.	Communicate with dignity and respect. Limit slang and "generational" terms. Use simpler language. Speak clearly. Allow the patient time to respond.

- Rose was just informed that she has type 2 diabetes mellitus. She needs to take medication, change her diet, and exercise.

If you were Jim or Rose, how would you feel? Could you understand and remember a lot of new information after hearing the diagnosis? Could you even converse normally with others, or would you be "blown away"? Would you deny the diagnosis?

Elisabeth Kübler-Ross studied people's reactions to dying. She found that people experienced similar stages as they came to terms with the situation. Over the years, these stages have been applied to grief. They can relate to patients who are informed of a chronic or terminal illness. Family and friends of the ill person can also experience these stages. Not everyone progresses through the stages at the same time, nor does everyone get to the final stage. Table 2.10 describes the stages of grief and dying.

When you are communicating with those with a terminal or chronic illness, it is important to understand that they are working through these stages. Remember, the emotions they display may not be related to you. They may be related to the grief the patient is dealing with. For instance, a terminally ill patient yells at the receptionist. He is upset about his wait time, although it was

TABLE 2.10   Stages of Grief and Dying

STAGE	DESCRIPTION
Denial	Refuses to accept the fact (e.g., diagnosis or prognosis). This is a defense mechanism that allows the person to ignore what is happening.
Anger	Can be directed at self or others.
Bargaining	Attempts to bargain with the higher power the person believes in (e.g., God).
Depression	Feels sad, fearful, and uncertain. May not participate in normal activities. Distances self from others.
Acceptance	Has come to terms with situation.

under 5 minutes. His emotions may relate more to his stage of grieving than to his wait time. It is important that we provide a supportive accepting, environment. We should be empathetic to these patients.

Personal Boundaries With Verbal Communication

The previous sections have discussed the types of verbal communication, therapeutic communication, and barriers to communication. The last aspect of verbal communication that needs to be addressed is personal boundaries. Have you ever talked to a person who shared too much personal information? How did you feel? How did that impact your relationship with the other person?

As a healthcare professional, it is important to remember our personal boundaries with verbal communication. When we are talking with family and friends, the topics of our conversations can vary greatly. We can discuss many different things. When we are in the healthcare environment, we need to remember that certain topics are inappropriate. Discussions regarding relationships, politics, religion, and other such topics are not appropriate for the workplace.

Besides what we talk about, we also need to consider the phrases or words we use. Many people swear or use words that are insulting or degrading to others. Some people routinely use religious names (e.g., God) when they are surprised or upset. For some people, religious names have sacred meaning. When you say these names in their presence, it can be offensive. We need to ensure our language is professional.

The relationship between the medical assistant and the patient needs to be professional. It cannot be a dual relationship, in which the medical assistant also becomes a friend to the patient. When working with patients, we need to keep our lives private. It is not appropriate for the medical assistant to:

- Share personal issues, struggles, life stories, or other personal intimate information.
- Contact the patient outside of the work environment.
- Befriend the patient on social media.
- Engage in a flirty or romantic conversation or relationship with the patient.
- Gossip and share what happens in the workplace with patients and others.

These behaviors cross the line between a professional relationship and a personal relationship. It is important for medical assistants to keep a professional relationship with patients and their families.

UNDERSTANDING BEHAVIOR

Throughout this chapter, we have discussed verbal and nonverbal communication. As healthcare professionals, it is important we understand why our patients and peers behave the way they do. Why do they make the choices they make? What is important to them? Many times, their behaviors relate to their needs, **defense mechanisms**, and **coping mechanisms**. By understanding these factors, we can interact more effectively with others.

Maslow's Hierarchy of Needs

In 1943 psychologist Abraham Maslow proposed a **hierarchy** of needs. This is a motivational theory that depicts five levels of needs.

Years later, he expanded the theory to include eight levels of needs. Maslow believed that our human needs can be categorized into these eight levels. Each level must be satisfied before we can move up to the next level. These levels are often depicted as a triangle (Fig. 2.9).

The "*Deficiency*" needs consist of the four bottom levels. They are considered the coping behaviors. We must fulfill these needs to cope with life and survival. We all have similar needs, but when they are not met, it motivates us to get them met. Fulfillment of these needs leads to instant short-term gratification. For example, when we are thirsty, we find water to drink. We are satisfied for the moment but will be thirsty a short time later.

The top four levels are "*Growth*" needs. These levels relate to making ourselves a better person or being all that we can be. Achieving these levels brings long-lasting happiness. The happiness is more meaningful than the gratification achieved from meeting the lower level needs.

Maslow's eight needs, starting at the bottom and working toward the top level, include:

1. **Physiological needs**: These include air, food, drink, shelter, warmth, oxygen, sleep, and so on. We need these things to survive. For instance, when we are hungry, we look for food.
2. **Safety needs**: These include protection from the elements, security, order, law, stability, and so forth. These needs relate to keeping us safe and secure. Unmet safety needs can lead to fear, stress, and anxiety. Some examples of meeting safety needs include:
   - Staying in a job that one really dislikes for the security of the paycheck
   - Staying in an abusive relationship, because it is familiar
   - Getting the brakes on your car fixed
3. **Love and belongingness needs**: These include friendship, intimacy, acceptance in a group, and receiving and giving affection and love. We need to be accepted by others. Unmet needs in this level can lead to feelings of isolation, loneliness, and depression. A person may feel anxious about going out in social situations if this need is not met.
4. **Esteem needs**: These include our self-esteem, achievement, mastery of skills, independence, status, prestige, and so on. Our needs relate to our reputation and what we think of ourselves. It's important to remember the saying, "People who matter do not judge, people who judge do not matter." The only thing we have total control over is what we think of ourselves. Some examples of how people attempt to meet this level include:
   - Buying the latest electronic devices to "show off" to others.
   - Fishing for compliments.
   - Cutting down others to make oneself feel better.
   - Focusing on the positives about yourself.
   - Setting yourself a challenge and meeting it.
5. **Cognitive needs**: These include knowledge, curiosity, understanding, and exploration. We are driven to learn more about something.
6. **Aesthetic needs**: We appreciate and search for beauty, balance, symmetry, form, and so on. Some people find true happiness when they create music, paint a picture, take a picture, or explore nature. Think of how relaxing it is to be at a beach, enjoying the sound of the water and the feeling of nature.

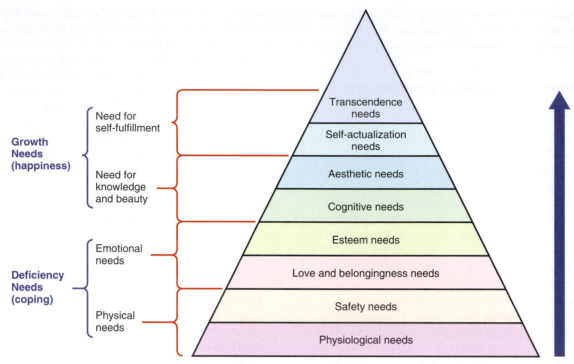

FIGURE 2.9 Maslow's hierarchy of needs.

7. **Self-actualization needs**: We need to realize our potential, seek self-fulfillment, and experience personal growth.
8. **Transcendence needs**: We meet these by helping others achieve their very best, or self-actualization. This requires that we give of our time and talent to help others meet their needs.

Maslow believed that only a few people ever achieve the top levels of the hierarchy. He believed that when people did something bad (e.g., steal, put others down), they were motivated to meet their own needs. The method used to meet needs could be unhealthy or dysfunctional. It is important for medical assistants to realize that people meet their own needs in different ways. Their ways may be different and wrong by our standards. We still need to respect our patients and provide the best possible care.

A medical assistant can help patients meet their deficiency needs in the following ways:
- *Physiological needs*: Provide community resources for basic needs.
- *Safety needs*: Provide domestic abuse hotline numbers and other community resources.
- *Love and belongingness needs*: Be positive and respectful. Have a caring manner when working with patients. Try to make a patient feel important.
- *Esteem needs*: Encourage independence and provide sincere compliments.

Defense Mechanisms

Defense mechanisms are unconscious mental processes that protect people from anxiety, loss, conflict, or shame. We use defense mechanisms and so do our patients and peers. People use defense mechanisms to protect themselves from situations or information they cannot manage psychologically.

Defense mechanisms may hide a variety of thoughts or feelings, including anger, fear, sadness, despair, and helplessness. A patient who uses defense mechanisms can be very difficult to deal with. If medical assistants are aware of a patient's needs for psychological protection, they may be able to find a way to provide excellent care for the patient. There are many types of defense mechanisms. Table 2.11 describes several of the more common behaviors using patient and peer situations.

Coping Mechanisms

Stress is a condition that causes physical and/or emotional tension. Stress can be positive (e.g., learning a new job) or negative (e.g., dealing with a love one's terminal illness). We use coping mechanisms when we are stressed. *Coping mechanisms* are behavioral and psychological strategies used to deal with or minimize stressful events. Two types include:
- *Adaptive* (healthy) *coping mechanisms*: Improve our functioning level and reduce our stress level (Table 2.12).
- *Maladaptive* (nonadaptive or unhealthy) *coping mechanisms*: Reduce the feelings associated with stress for a short time, but do not decrease the actual stressor and can lead to future problems (see Table 2.12).

Understanding the different types of coping mechanisms is important in our own lives and in our role as a healthcare professional. We may have times when we are stressed and tend to use more maladaptive coping mechanisms. It's important for our health

TABLE 2.11   Common Defense Mechanisms

DEFENSE MECHANISM	DESCRIPTION	EXAMPLE
Denial	The person completely rejects the information.	"I couldn't possibly have breast cancer. You must be mistaken."
Repression	The person simply forgets something that is bad or hurtful.	"I wasn't driving the car that killed my best friend."
Regression	The person reverts to an old, usually immature behavior to express her feelings.	Perhaps instead of discussing the diagnosis and the need for treatment, he just storms out of the room and slams the door.
Displacement	The person transfers the emotion toward one person to another person or thing.	After being reprimanded by his supervisor, the person goes home and screams at his children.
Projection	The person accuses someone else of having the feelings that he or she has.	A patient is angry about the diagnosis. She may say, "You do not have to lose your temper about this," even though the medical assistant's demeanor is completely professional.
Suppression	The person is consciously aware of the information or feeling but refuses to admit it.	"I do not think the test is accurate. My mammograms are always normal."
Splitting	The person views another person as all bad or all good and not a mixture of good and bad traits.	An abused patient may say, "He is a good husband and father."
Reaction formation	The person expresses his feelings as the opposite of what he really feels.	A patient is angry at the medical assistant for insisting that a biopsy be scheduled. He expresses the opposite emotion: "I appreciate your trying to help me, but I just can't come to the hospital that day."
Rationalization	The person comes up with various explanations to justify her response.	"I think the results are wrong. I didn't follow the directions for the tests like I should have, and besides, there's no history of breast cancer in my family."

TABLE 2.12   Adaptive and Maladaptive Coping Mechanisms

ADAPTIVE COPING MECHANISMS	MALADAPTIVE COPING MECHANISMS
• Eat healthy, well-balanced meals • Exercise • Drink water • Get plenty of sleep • Take breaks when you feel stressed • Talk and share with others • Get help when you need it	• Hostility, aggression, manipulation • Recognition seeking • Passive-aggressive behavior • Compliance, dependence • Social withdrawal, isolation • Denial, fantasy • Drugs and alcohol use • Gambling, shopping, risk-taking behaviors

CRITICAL THINKING APPLICATION   2.6

Christi is starting to exercise after work each night. She found that it helps her deal with the stress of the day. What coping mechanisms do you use when you are stressed? Are they adaptive or maladaptive coping mechanisms?

CLOSING COMMENTS

Patient Coaching

When coaching patients in the ambulatory care facility, the medical assistant must remember to adapt the teaching for the patient. This means that if the patient has special needs, the medical assistant must attempt to meet those needs. For instance, a patient who has a hearing impairment may struggle to hear the coaching. Writing down the information, speaking slower, and facing the patient may be helpful. When instructing patients from different age groups, the medical assistant will use different techniques. For instance, when coaching young children, the medical assistant would use play techniques and simple words to explain information. Adapting coaching so it works best for the patient is an important role of the medical assistant.

and well-being to use more adaptive strategies. Patients, family members, and co-workers are not immune to stress. They will also be using different coping mechanisms. Our role is to encourage the use of healthy coping mechanisms and provide resources for these strategies.

Legal and Ethical Issues

Overcoming communication barriers is more than just providing great patient care. Healthcare providers are legally required to provide ways to overcome communication barriers. This legal requirement comes from:

- *Civil Rights Act*: All providers who accept federal funds for the healthcare provided must ensure equal access to services.
- *Americans with Disabilities Act (ADA)*: All healthcare providers must provide free effective communication to patients (and companions) with disabilities.
- *Americans with Disabilities Act Amendments Act (ADAAA)*: Expanded the definition of disabilities established in the ADA.

Ways that providers can meet their federal obligations for accommodating patients with communication disabilities include:

- Provide a qualified medical interpreter free of charge to the patient. This can be done by having an interpreter available to the patient or by using online interpretation services during the visit. The interpreter may be present for the visit, available over the phone, or via videoconferencing. Table 2.13 describes types of interpreters used in healthcare.
- Provide informational and educational materials that have been translated into the primary languages of the patients seen in the ambulatory care facility.
- Provide large-print materials.
- Write out instructions.

Patient-Centered Care

Patient-centered care is focused on creating a relationship with the patient and making the patient feel respected, involved, and knowledgeable about the plan of care. The patient has a role in decision making and ultimately the goal is for better health outcomes for the person.

To create this relationship, the healthcare team, which includes the medical assistant, must use therapeutic communication. This process of communication helps build a respectful, empathetic, comfortable, and accepting relationship with the patient. It also gives the patient the self-confidence to express his or her feelings, ideas, questions, and concerns. In turn, the healthcare team members can gather the information, answer questions, and share the patient's concerns and feelings with other members.

TABLE 2.13	Types of Interpreters
TYPE	DESCRIPTION
Sign language interpreter	Uses American Sign Language or Signed English.
Oral interpreter	Silently mouths speech to the hearing-impaired patient. Uses gestures.
Cued-speech interpreter	Does everything an oral interpreter does. Also uses a hand code to stand for each speech sound.
Qualified medical interpreter	Interprets between the healthcare provider and the non-English-speaking or limited English-speaking patient. (Using a family member to interpret can be risky, because the message may be changed. There is no guarantee the family member is translating exactly what the provider states.)

Professional Behaviors

Medical assistants need to be assertive in the healthcare setting. Not every person going into the medical assisting profession is assertive. It is important to learn how to be assertive in school and in your practicum (externship). Practicing assertive skills will help a medical assistant to become more confident and comfortable with that style of communication. Tips for being assertive include:

- Be assertive when you need to; not every situation requires it.
- Use good eye contact.
- Use a medium pitch, speed, and volume of voice.
- Be respectful of others.
- Clearly state your needs; use "I" statements.
- Listen to others.
- Accept compliments graciously and learn to handle criticism professionally.

SUMMARY OF SCENARIO

Christi is enjoying her orientation. She is nervous about her upcoming evaluation, but she knows that she is improving her professionalism. She is now arriving 10 to 15 minutes before her start time. That gives her time to put her things away and wash her hands before the workday begins. She has no issues with the dress code. It is becoming a habit. In addition, she is learning some great communication techniques to use with patients.

Christi feels she is becoming more professional not only with the patients, but also with her team. She really wants to be the best medical assistant she can be. She wants to be dependable and trustworthy. She is already starting to read up on the Hmong and Mexican cultures, because a high percentage of her patients come from those two backgrounds. Christi is also studying to take her CMA (AAMA) exam. She is enjoying working at the clinic.

SUMMARY OF LEARNING OBJECTIVES

1. **Describe the importance of a first impression.**

 First impressions are very important, and they include more than just the first words that are exchanged. We must communicate effectively, both verbally and nonverbally, with the patient and provide a warm, caring environment. The medical assistant plays a vital role in initiating therapeutic patient interactions.

2. **Discuss examples of cultural, social, and ethnic diversity, and explain how to demonstrate respect for individual diversity, including gender, race, religion, age, economic status, and appearance.**

 Cultural diversity includes general customs, norms, values, and beliefs held by a group of people. Examples of cultural diversity may include values like timeliness, punctuality, honesty, and the importance of hard work. Social diversity relates to all the ways a person is different from others. Examples of social diversity include a person's lifestyle, religion, tastes, and preferences. Ethnic diversity relates to a group of people who share a common ancestry, culture, religion, traditions, nationality, and language. Examples of ethnic diversity include family traditions and values.

 Showing respect for individual diversity is important for healthcare professionals. Respect is shown by being courteous, sincere, polite, welcoming, and professional in both verbal and nonverbal communication.

3. **Identify types of nonverbal communication.**

 Communication is the exchange of information, feelings, and thoughts between two or more people using spoken words or other methods. Nonverbal communication includes body language and expressive behaviors. More communication occurs nonverbally than verbally. Nonverbal communication occurs through our position, posture, facial expressions, gestures, touch, eye contact, and mannerisms. Nonverbal communication also occurs through the quality of our vocal expression. For instance, nonverbal communication includes the rate, clarity, volume, pitch, tone, intonation, and vocabulary we use when speaking.

4. **Discuss the communication cycle, provide tips for composing written communication, and describe the behaviors seen in passive, aggressive, passive-aggressive, manipulative, and assertive communicators.**

 The communication cycle is a way to describe the communication process. It involves both a sender and a receiver, in addition to the message and feedback. Oral and written communications are forms of verbal communication. Oral communication means we talk with others and we listen to others. Examples of written communication include written messages, letters, emails, and online information. It is important how we state our written message because we want the receiver to get the message that we are intending to send. Always be courteous, write in complete sentences, and check grammar, spelling, and punctuation.

 Styles of verbal communication include the following communicators: passive, aggressive, passive-aggressive, manipulative, and assertive. The behaviors seen with these styles include:

 • *Passive communicators*: Avoid expressing feelings or opinions, fail to exert themselves, allow others to infringe on their rights, and tend to speak softly.
 • *Aggressive communicators*: Try to dominate others; have low frustration tolerance, criticize and attack others, have poor listening skills, and use "you" statements.
 • *Passive-aggressive communicators*: Deny problems; do not confront problems or people, appear to be cooperative but plan subtle sabotage or disruptions.
 • *Manipulative communicators*: Cunning and controlling of others. Use others to get what they want.
 • *Assertive communicators*: Clearly state their needs and wants. Use "I" statements and listen without interrupting. Are relaxed, use good eye contact, feel connected with others, and stand up for their rights.

 Healthcare professionals should use the assertive communication style.

5. **Describe therapeutic communication and active listening, and discuss open and closed questions or statements.**

 Therapeutic communication is a process of communicating with patients and family members in healthcare. It is an interactive relationship that conveys acceptance and respect without judging or blaming. Active listening is the most important therapeutic communication technique. Active listening means we fully concentrate on what is being said and how it is said.

 When you gather information from a patient, it is helpful to use a combination of open and closed questions or statements. An open question or statement asks for general information or states the topic to be discussed, but only in general terms. It is a very effective method of gathering more details from the patient about his or her problem.

 Closed questions ask for specific information. In many cases, this form of questioning limits the patient's answer to one or two words, including yes and no. Use this form of question when you need confirmation of specific facts, such as when asking about demographic information.

6. **Identify barriers to communication, describe techniques for overcoming communication barriers, and discuss how Erikson's psychosocial development stages and Kübler-Ross's stages of grief and dying relate to communication and behavior.**

 Barriers to communication and ways to overcome the barriers include:
 • Environmental distractions: Provide patients with privacy.
 • Internal distractions: Help make patients comfortable.
 • Visually impaired: Use audio recordings, large-print materials, and screen reader software.
 • Hearing impaired: Use print materials, videos with captions, and sign language interpreters.
 • Non-English speaking: Use interpreters and translated materials.
 • Emotional distractions: Provide a warm, caring environment.

 Erik Erikson described the emotional, physical, and psychological stages of human development. He stated that a person in each stage had a specific developmental task to complete. Understanding the task or goal of each stage helps healthcare professionals communicate more effectively with patients.

 Elisabeth Kübler-Ross studied people's reactions to dying. She found that people went through similar stages: denial, anger, bargaining, depression, and acceptance. These stages have been applied to grief and relate to patients who have a chronic or terminal illness. Not everyone progresses through the stages at the same time, nor does everyone get to the final stage.

Continued

SUMMARY OF LEARNING OBJECTIVES—*continued*

7. Describe personal boundaries with professional verbal communication.

As a healthcare professional, it is important to remember our personal boundaries with verbal communication. When we are in the healthcare environment, we need to remember that certain topics are inappropriate. Discussions regarding relationships, politics, religion, and other such topics are not appropriate for the workplace. We also need to consider the phrases or words we use. Many people swear or use words that are insulting or degrading to others. Some people routinely use religious names when they are surprised or upset. These are not professional.

The relationship between the medical assistant and the patient needs to be professional. It cannot be a dual relationship, where the medical assistant also becomes a friend to the patient. When working with patients, we need to keep our lives personal.

8. Discuss how Maslow's hierarchy of needs relates to communication and behavior.

Maslow described what motivates people. His theory helps describe behaviors of individuals as they cope with the world or strive for happiness. Maslow believed that our human needs can be categorized into eight

levels. Each level must be satisfied before we can move up to the next level. The "Deficiency" needs consist of the four bottom levels and they are considered the coping behaviors. We must fulfill these needs to cope with life and survival, but fulfillment only leads to instant short-term gratification. The top four levels are "Growth" needs, which relate to making ourselves a better person. Achieving these levels brings long-lasting happiness.

9. Discuss defense mechanisms and differentiate between adaptive and maladaptive coping mechanisms.

Defense mechanisms are unconscious mental processes that patients and peers use to protect themselves from situations or information they cannot manage psychologically. Coping mechanisms are behavioral and psychological strategies used to deal with or minimize stressful events. Adaptive (healthy) coping mechanisms improve our functioning level and reduce our stress level. Maladaptive (nonadaptive or unhealthy) coping mechanisms reduce the feelings associated with stress for a short time, but they do not decrease the actual stressor and can lead to future problems.

PROCEDURE 2.1	Use Feedback Techniques and Demonstrate Respect for Individual Diversity: Gender and Appearance

Tasks: Use feedback techniques (e.g., reflection, restatement, and clarification) to obtain patient information. Respond to nonverbal communication. Communicate respectfully with patients with individual diversity related to gender and appearance. Demonstrate empathy, active listening, and nonverbal communication.

Background: When working with a transgender patient, ask the patient privately which pronouns the person prefers. Make sure to add this information into the patient's health record for future reference.

Scenario: You are rooming Crystal Green. You can see that she has expertly applied her makeup, has long red fingernails, long blond hair, and is wearing at least 3-inch heels. You are surprised to see that her birth gender is male. This is the first time you have roomed a transgender patient. You are uncomfortable in this situation because you have strong personal beliefs that birth gender should be maintained throughout a person's life. (Role-play this scenario with a peer, who is the patient.)

EQUIPMENT and SUPPLIES

- Patient health record
- Rooming form (optional)
- Pen

PROCEDURAL STEPS

1. Greet the patient. Identify yourself. Verify the patient's identity with full name and date of birth. Explain the procedure in a manner that is understood by the patient. Answer any questions the patient may have on the procedure.

PURPOSE: It is important to identify the patient in two different ways to ensure that you have the correct patient. Explaining the procedure can make the patient feel more comfortable and helps to reduce anxiety.

2. Demonstrate respect for the patient. Be sincere, courteous, polite, and welcoming. Maintain the patient's dignity. Demonstrate professional, nonjudgmental verbal and nonverbal communication. Ask appropriate questions as information is obtained.

PURPOSE: It is important to provide a respectful and welcoming environment to all patients regardless of individual diversity.

3. Using appropriate closed and open questions and statements, obtain the patient's chief complaint (main reason for the visit), allergies, pregnancy history, and current medications. Document the information in the health record or rooming form.

PURPOSE: Medical assistants need to gather the patient's information prior to the provider seeing the patient.

4. Use feedback techniques, including reflection, restatements, and clarification, as information is obtained.

PROCEDURE 2.1   Use Feedback Techniques and Demonstrate Respect for Individual Diversity: Gender and Appearance—*continued*

PURPOSE: Feedback techniques help to ensure the information is correct.

5. Respond to the patient's nonverbal communication by using feedback techniques (e.g., reflection). If the patient's nonverbal communication is interpreted differently than the patient's oral statements, clarify the information with the patient.
   PURPOSE: Feedback techniques help to ensure the receiver's interpretation of the nonverbal and verbal communication is correct.

6. Use active listening skills. Remain neutral and refrain from interrupting. Allow for periods of silence. Smile and nod your head to show interest. Use appropriate eye contact. Focus on the patient and avoid distractions (e.g., looking at the clock, fidgeting).
   PURPOSE: Demonstrating active listening skills creates a trusting, welcoming environment for the patient. It helps build a trusting, caring relationship with the patient.

7. Use professional, positive nonverbal communication behaviors. Use a clear voice, with a moderate rate and volume. Use a varying pitch and an accepting or a neutral tone. Use words the patient can understand. Correctly pronounce the words. Be at the same eye level as the patient's. Smile and have a poised posture. Use light touch on the hand if appropriate. Maintain proper eye contact.
   PURPOSE: Demonstrating active listening skills and positive nonverbal communication behaviors creates a trusting, welcoming environment for the patient. It helps build a trusting, caring relationship with the patient.

8. Demonstrate empathy by listening to the patient and learning about his or her experiences and concerns. Use therapeutic communication techniques and positive nonverbal behaviors, including good eye contact. Position yourself at the same level as the patient. Show your support and respect.
   PURPOSE: Being empathetic will help build a trusting relationship with the patient.

PROCEDURE 2.2   Use Feedback Techniques and Demonstrate Respect for Individual Diversity: Race

Tasks: Use feedback techniques (e.g., reflection, restatement, and clarification) to obtain patient information. Respond to nonverbal communication. Communicate respectfully with patients with individual diversity related to race. Demonstrate empathy, active listening, and nonverbal communication.

Background: When working with an interpreter, allow time for the person to translate the information to the patient. Also, focus on the patient and do not look at the interpreter when speaking to the patient.

Scenario: You are rooming Maria Hernandez. She is always late for her appointments, and today she was 20 minutes late. She also does not speak English, and you need to use a Spanish interpreter for the visit. You are uncomfortable in this situation because you have not worked with an interpreter before. You are also feeling rushed because she was late for her appointment. (Role-play the scenario with two peers. One peer is the patient, and the other peer is the interpreter.)

EQUIPMENT and SUPPLIES
- Patient health record
- Rooming form (optional)
- Pen

PROCEDURAL STEPS

1. Greet the patient. Identify yourself. Verify the patient's identity with full name and date of birth. Explain the procedure in a manner that is understood by the patient. Answer any questions the patient may have on the procedure.
   PURPOSE: It is important to identify the patient in two different ways to ensure that you have the correct patient. Explaining the procedure can make the patient feel more comfortable and helps to reduce anxiety.

2. Demonstrate respect for the patient. Focus on the patient, not on the interpreter. Pause to give the interpreter and patient time to answer. Be sincere, courteous, polite and welcoming. Maintain the patient's dignity. Demonstrate professional, nonjudgmental verbal and nonverbal communication. Ask appropriate questions as information is obtained.

PURPOSE: It is important to provide a respectful and welcoming environment to all patients regardless of individual diversity.

3. Using appropriate closed and open questions and statements, obtain the patient's chief complaint (main reason for the visit), allergies, pregnancy history, and current medications. Document the information in the health record or rooming form.
   PURPOSE: Medical assistants need to gather the patient's information prior to the provider seeing the patient.

4. Use feedback techniques, including reflection, restatements, and clarification as information is obtained.
   PURPOSE: Feedback techniques help to ensure the information is correct.

5. Respond to the patient's nonverbal communication by using feedback techniques (e.g., reflection). If the patient's nonverbal communication is interpreted differently than the patient's oral statements, clarify the information with the patient.
   PURPOSE: Feedback techniques help to ensure the receiver's interpretation of the nonverbal and verbal communication is correct.

Continued

PROCEDURE 2.2   Use Feedback Techniques and Demonstrate Respect for Individual Diversity: Race—continued

6. Use active listening skills. Remain neutral and refrain from interrupting. Allow for periods of silence. Smile and nod your head to show interest. Use appropriate eye contact. Focus on the patient and avoid distractions (e.g., looking at the clock, fidgeting).
PURPOSE: Demonstrating active listening skills creates a trusting, welcoming environment for the patient. It helps build a trusting, caring relationship with the patient.

7. Use professional, positive nonverbal communication behaviors. Use a clear voice, with a moderate rate and volume. Use a varying pitch and an accepting or a neutral tone. Use words the patient can understand. Correctly pronounce the words. Be at the same position as the patient. Smile and have a poised posture. Use light touch on the hand if appropriate. Maintain proper eye contact.
PURPOSE: Demonstrating active listening skills and positive nonverbal communication behaviors creates a trusting, welcoming environment for the patient. It helps build a trusting, caring relationship with the patient.

8. Demonstrate empathy by listening to the patient and learning about his or her experiences and concerns. Use therapeutic communication techniques and positive nonverbal behaviors, including good eye contact. Position yourself at the same level as the patient. Show your support and respect.
PURPOSE: Being empathetic will help build a trusting relationship with the patient.

PROCEDURE 2.3   Demonstrate Respect for Individual Diversity: Religion and Appearance

Tasks: Respond to nonverbal communication. Communicate respectfully with patients with individual diversity related to religion and appearance. Demonstrate empathy, active listening, and nonverbal communication.

Background: The Sikh religion was founded in northern India. Sikhs believe in one God, the equality of men and women, justice, and community service. Turbans and kachera are worn at all times for religious reasons. Turbans or scarves cover the uncut hair. If the turban or scarf needs to be removed, an alternative head covering should be provided. A turban or scarf should be treated with respect. Placing it on the floor or near shoes would be a sign of disrespect. Kachera are undershorts/undergarments, and at least one leg is to remain in the kachera at all times.

Scenario: You are preparing a patient for an examination. The patient is Sikh. The provider always wants the patient to completely undress, wear a gown, and be seated on the exam table before she comes into the room. You are uncomfortable in this situation because you have never worked with a patient who is Sikh. (Role-play this scenario with a peer, who is the patient.)

EQUIPMENT and SUPPLIES
- Gown and drape sheet (optional)
- Exam table (optional)

PROCEDURAL STEPS

1. Greet the patient. Identify yourself. Verify the patient's identity with full name and date of birth. Explain the procedure (undressing) in a manner that is understood by the patient. Answer any questions the patient may have on the procedure.
PURPOSE: It is important to identify the patient in two different ways to ensure that you have the correct patient. Explaining the procedure can make the patient feel more comfortable and helps to reduce anxiety.

2. Demonstrate respect for the patient. Be sincere, courteous, polite and welcoming. Maintain the patient's dignity. Demonstrate professional, nonjudgmental verbal and nonverbal communication.
PURPOSE: It is important to provide a respectful and welcoming environment to all patients regardless of individual diversity.

3. Respond to the patient's nonverbal communication by using feedback techniques (e.g., reflection). If the patient's nonverbal communication is interpreted differently than the patient's oral statements, clarify the information with the patient.
PURPOSE: Feedback techniques help to ensure the receiver's interpretation of the nonverbal and verbal communication is correct.

4. Use active listening skills. Remain neutral and refrain from interrupting. Smile and nod your head to show interest. Use appropriate eye contact. Focus on the patient and avoid distractions (e.g., looking at the clock, fidgeting).
PURPOSE: Demonstrating active listening skills creates a trusting, welcoming environment for the patient. It helps build a trusting, caring relationship with the patient.

5. Use professional, positive nonverbal communication behaviors. Use a clear voice, with a moderate rate and volume. Use a varying pitch and an accepting or a neutral tone. Use words the patient can understand. Correctly pronounce the words. Be at the same eye level as the patient's. Smile and have a poised posture. Use light touch on the hand if appropriate. Maintain proper eye contact.
PURPOSE: Demonstrating active listening skills and positive nonverbal communication behaviors creates a trusting, welcoming environment for the patient. It helps build a trusting, caring relationship with the patient.

PROCEDURE 2.3	Demonstrate Respect for Individual Diversity: Religion and Appearance—*continued*

6. Demonstrate empathy by listening to the patient and learning about his or her experiences and concerns. Use therapeutic communication techniques and positive nonverbal behaviors including good eye contact. Position yourself at the same level as the patient. Show your support and respect.

PURPOSE: Being empathetic will help build a trusting relationship with the patient.

PROCEDURE 2.4	Use Feedback Techniques and Demonstrate Respect for Individual Diversity: Age, Economic Status, and Appearance

Tasks: Use feedback techniques (e.g., reflection, restatement, and clarification) to obtain patient information. Respond to nonverbal communication. Communicate respectfully with patients with individual diversity related to age, economic status, and appearance. Demonstrate empathy, active listening, and nonverbal communication.

Scenario: You are rooming Mr. Abraham Black (79 years old), who has recently been diagnosed with dementia. He likes to talk about things that happened long before you were born, and you are not interested in those events. He also has a hard time hearing your questions, and you frequently repeat questions. Mr. Black has poor personal hygiene. His clothes are dirty and torn. He has an unpleasant body odor. Mr. Black tells you he can't afford to eat if he buys his medications. He doesn't believe in government programs and refuses to take "handouts." You have worked with Mr. Black in the past and have heard this all before numerous times. You would prefer to work with the younger generation and with patients who have better hygiene. (Role-play this scenario with a peer, who is the patient.)

EQUIPMENT and SUPPLIES

- Patient health record
- Rooming form (optional)
- Pen

PROCEDURAL STEPS

1. Greet the patient. Identify yourself. Verify the patient's identity with full name and date of birth. Explain the procedure in a manner that is understood by the patient. Answer any questions the patient may have on the procedure.
PURPOSE: It is important to identify the patient in two different ways to ensure that you have the correct patient. Explaining the procedure can make the patient feel more comfortable and helps to reduce anxiety.

2. Demonstrate respect for the patient. Be sincere, courteous, polite and welcoming. Maintain the patient's dignity. Demonstrate professional, nonjudgmental verbal and nonverbal communication. Ask appropriate questions as information is obtained.
PURPOSE: It is important to provide a respectful and welcoming environment to all patients regardless of individual diversity.

3. Using appropriate closed and open questions and statements, obtain the patient's chief complaint (main reason for the visit), allergies, and current medications. Document the information in the health record or rooming form.
PURPOSE: Medical assistants need to gather the patient's information prior to the provider seeing the patient.

4. Use feedback techniques including reflection, restatement, and clarification as information is obtained.
PURPOSE: Feedback techniques help to ensure the information is correct.

5. Respond to the patient's nonverbal communication by using feedback techniques (e.g., reflection). If the patient's nonverbal communication is interpreted differently than the patient's oral statements, clarify the information with the patient.
PURPOSE: Feedback techniques help to ensure the receiver's interpretation of the nonverbal and verbal communication is correct.

6. Use active listening skills. Remain neutral and refrain from interrupting. Allow for periods of silence. Smile and nod your head to show interest. Use appropriate eye contact. Focus on the patient and avoid distractions (e.g., looking at the clock, fidgeting).
PURPOSE: Demonstrating active listening skills creates a trusting, welcoming environment for the patient. It helps build a trusting, caring relationship with the patient.

7. Use professional, positive nonverbal communication behaviors. Use a clear voice, with a moderate rate and volume. Use a varying pitch and an accepting or neutral tone. Use words the patient can understand. Correctly pronounce the words. Be at the same eye level as the patient's. Smile and have a poised posture. Use light touch on the hand if appropriate. Maintain proper eye contact.
PURPOSE: Demonstrating active listening skills and positive nonverbal communication behaviors creates a trusting, welcoming environment for the patient. It helps build a trusting, caring relationship with the patient.

8. Demonstrate empathy by listening to the patient and learning about his or her experiences and concerns. Use therapeutic communication techniques and positive nonverbal behaviors, including good eye contact. Position yourself at the same level as the patient. Show your support and respect.
PURPOSE: Being empathetic will help build a trusting relationship with the patient.

3

LEGAL PRINCIPLES

SCENARIO

Daniela Garcia was just hired as a part-time float receptionist at Walden-Martin Family Medical (WMFM) Clinic. As a float receptionist, she will be working with many different co-workers and providers. Besides working, Daniela is enrolled in a medical assistant program at the local community college. She is just starting a law and ethics course. The first part of the course explains legal concepts.

Daniela learned about the government in high school, but she has never been in a courtroom, nor witnessed court proceedings. Learning about law concepts is very different from her other courses. Many of her classmates did not realize that medical assistants need to learn about legal concepts and laws. Daniela hopes that she can relate what she does in the clinic to what she is learning in her course. She finds concepts are easier to remember if she can apply them to real-life situations.

Bella, a newly certified medical assistant (CMA), has offered to help Daniela study for her law course. Bella stated that she enjoyed learning about law and its importance in healthcare. Daniela is considering asking her for help on their breaks. Studying with another person also helps her retain and understand the concepts.

While studying this chapter, think about the following questions:
- What are the different sources of law?
- How do criminal and civil law differ?
- What is the difference between intentional torts and negligent torts?
- What are the requirements for a legal contract?
- How do expressed, implied, and informed consent occur in healthcare?
- What is the difference between the provider's and the medical assistant's scope of practice and practice requirements?

LEARNING OBJECTIVES

1. Discuss the balance of power in the United States and name the four types of laws.
2. Compare criminal and civil law as they apply to the practicing medical assistant.
3. Differentiate between intentional torts and negligent (unintentional) torts.
4. Differentiate between standard of care and scope of practice for a medical assistant, define terms related to a civil lawsuit, and explain the 4 *D*s of negligence.
5. Describe types of professional liability insurance.
6. Explain the five elements required for a contract to be legally binding.
7. Describe the reasons and the steps for terminating the provider-patient relationship.
8. Differentiate between implied consent, expressed consent, and informed consent.
9. List who can give consent and who cannot give consent.
10. Summarize the Patient's Bill of Rights.
11. Describe licensure, certification, registration, and accreditation.

VOCABULARY

arbitration (ahr bi TRAE shuhn) The process in which conflicting parties in a dispute submit their differences to a court-appointed person (arbitrator), who submits a legally binding decision.

common law Unwritten laws that come from judicial decisions based on societal traditions and customs.

damages A monetary settlement the defendant pays the plaintiff in a civil case for loss or injury. Also, one of the 4 *D*s of negligence, meaning the patient suffers a legally recognized injury.

declaratory judgment A court judgment that defines the legal rights of the parties involved.

defendant (dih FEN dant) An individual or a business against whom a lawsuit is filed.

defense (di FENS) A strategy used by the defendant to avoid liability in a lawsuit.

deposition (dep ah ZISH uhn) A sworn testimony made before a court-appointed officer; it is used in the discovery process and may be used in the trial.

emancipated minor (i MANS i pa ted MIE nohr) A minor who has been granted emancipation by the court; the minor can assume the rights and responsibilities of adulthood.

expert witnesses People who are educated and knowledgeable in the area of concern; they testify in court and provide an expert opinion on the topic of concern.

fact witnesses People who observed the situation and testify in court about the facts of the case.

incompetence (in KOM pi tahns) The state of being incompetent or lacking the ability to manage personal affairs due to mental deficiency; an appointed guardian or conservator manages the person's affairs.

injunction (in JUNGK shuhn) A court order by which an individual or institution is required to perform or refrain from performing a certain act.

interrogatory (IN tah rog ah TOOR ee) Written or oral questions that must be answered under oath.

liability (LIE ah bil i tee) The state of being liable or responsible for something.

liable Legally responsible or obligated.

licensure (LIE sen shur) A mandatory process established by state law that ensures a person has met the legal standards for practicing an occupation in that state.

litigious (LI ti jehs) Prone to lawsuits.

locum tenens (LOE kuhm TEE nenz) Latin for "to substitute for"; the term refers to physicians or advanced practice professionals who temporarily contract to provide healthcare services when a facility has a vacancy, vacation, or a leave of absence.

malpractice (mal PRAK tis) A type of negligence in which a licensed professional fails to provide the standard of care, causing harm to a person.

mature minor A person under the age of adulthood who demonstrates the maturity to make a personal healthcare decision and can give informed consent for treatment.

mediation (MEE dee ae shuhn) The process of facilitating conflicting parties to make an agreement, settlement, or compromise.

minor One who has not reached adulthood; usually age 18 or 21, depending on the jurisdiction.

negligence (NEG li juhns) Failure to act as a reasonably prudent person would under similar circumstances; such conduct falls below the standards of behavior established by law for the protection of others against unreasonable risk of harm.

patient abandonment A form of medical malpractice, also called negligent termination; the provider ends the provider-patient relationship without reasonable or adequate notification.

plaintiff (PLAIN tif) An individual or a party who brings a lawsuit to court.

precedent (PRES i dent) A prior court decision that serves as a model for similar legal cases in the future.

res ipsa loquitur (RASE ipsah low kwah tuhr) A Latin term meaning "the thing speaks for itself." A legal concept under which the plaintiff's burden to prove malpractice is minimal, since the jury can clearly understand the details of the injury. For example, a surgical instrument was left in the body during surgery.

res judicata (RASE JOO di kah tah) Latin for "a thing decided." Once a case has been decided by the court, it cannot be litigated again.

respondeat superior (re SPON dee at soo PIR ee ahr) Latin for "let the master answer"; a legal doctrine by which the employer/provider is legally responsible for the wrongful actions or lack of actions of employees if done within the scope of employment.

scope of practice Range of responsibilities and practice guidelines that determine the boundaries within which a healthcare worker practices.

subpoena (suh PEE nuh) A court order requiring a person to appear in court at a specific time to testify in a legal case.

subpoena duces tecum (suh PEE nuh DOO seez TEE kuhm) A legal document commanding a person to bring a piece of evidence (e.g., the plaintiff's health record) to court.

telemedicine (TEL i med i sin) The use of telecommunication technology to provide healthcare services to patients at a distance; it is usually used in rural communities.

tort A civil wrongdoing that causes harm to a person or property, excludes breach of contract.

tortfeasor (TORTE fee zahr) The individual or entity who committed the tort, either intentionally or as a result of negligence.

In the United States, the number of lawsuits has increased over the years. Working in a **litigious** society requires that we know how to protect ourselves against lawsuits. This is the reason that medical assistants need to learn about the law. To avoid the risk of lawsuits, medical assistants need to practice within the guidelines of the law.

SOURCES OF LAW

Law is a custom or practice of a community. It is a rule of conduct or action prescribed or formally recognized as enforceable by a controlling authority. Law is the system by which society gives order to our lives.

The United States has both federal and state laws. The U.S. Constitution is the supreme law of the United States. Each state has a constitution that is the supreme law of that state. State laws cannot conflict with the U.S. Constitution. In the following sections, we will examine the makeup of the federal and state governments and the sources of law.

Balance of Power

The federal government was designed to allow for a balance of power. The three branches of government share power so that no one branch is more powerful than any other. Table 3.1 describes the three branches

TABLE 3.1   Branches of the Federal and State Governments

BRANCH	FEDERAL GOVERNMENT	STATE GOVERNMENT
Legislative	Made up of: • Two houses of Congress (Senate and House of Representatives). Members of the houses are elected by eligible voters from the state they represent. Roles: • Makes new federal laws • Can impeach the President or remove judges from office for misconduct • Must approve: all appointments for judges, budget spending, and treaties • Can override the President's veto of a bill by a ⅔ vote	Made up of: • Most states have two houses, although the names can differ. Officials are elected. Roles: • Introduce legislation to become new state laws • Can impeach state officials for misconduct • Must approve state budget • Can override the governor's veto and amend the state constitution
Executive	Made up of: • President of the United States administers this branch. Roles: • Can issue *executive orders* that become law without the approval of Congress • Creates a budget • Appoints judges • Carries out laws • Makes treaties with other nations • Can veto bills from Congress	Made up of: • Headed by the elected governor; each state has a different executive organizational structure. Roles: • Creates a budget • Carries out laws • Can veto bills from state houses • Issues executive orders • Appoints state court judges (in most states)
Judicial	Made up of: • Supreme Court, which has nine justices Roles: • Interpret laws according to the U.S. Constitution • Determine if laws from Congress and executive actions are constitutional	Made up of: • State supreme court Roles: • Interpret laws according to the state constitution • Hear cases from lower courts • Determine if state laws are constitutional

of the federal government. The states also have three branches of government.

When members of Congress or the state houses want new legislation, a bill is brought forward. After much debate, the bill will either die or be passed and become an *act* or *statute*. The act or statute is now part of the laws for the state or country. (The terms "act" and "statute" are used interchangeably. Most of the time you will hear the word "act" in the name of a specific law; statute is used more to refer to the contents of the actual law.) On the local level, an *ordinance* is a piece of legislation passed by a municipality or local government. A city ordinance to ban smoking from restaurants is an example of local legislation.

Types of Laws

There are four types of laws:
- *Constitutional law*: Derived from the federal and state constitutions, which give power to federal and state governments. Examples of constitutional law include prohibiting slavery (based on an 1865 constitutional amendment) and the power to tax.
- *Case law*: Derived from legal **precedents** and **common law**. Common law originated in England and was used by the

colonists. An example would include the right of criminal defendants to have an attorney even if they cannot afford one, which was a ruling from the Supreme Court (*Gideon v. Wainwright* 372 U.S. 335 [1963]).
- *Regulatory* and *administrative law*: Concerns the procedures, regulations, and rules of federal, state, and local governmental administrative agencies. Examples include: zoning boards, licensing agencies, the Social Security Administration, and unemployment commissions.
- *Statutory law:* Refers to the laws enacted by the state and federal legislatures. An example is the speed limits set by the state legislature.

CRIMINAL AND CIVIL LAW

Laws can be divided into two main categories:
- *Substantive law*: Laws that determine rights and obligations of people derived from common law and statutes. Substantive laws include criminal, civil, military, and international law.
- *Procedural law:* Laws that all parties (courts, officers, and lawyers) must follow when investigating and prosecuting unlawful acts.

TABLE 3.2 Criminal Law Compared to Civil Law

TERM	CRIMINAL LAW	CIVIL LAW
Plaintiff	State or federal government	Victim (individual or institution) of the wrongdoing
Defendant	Person or party accused of the criminal complaint or charge	Wrongdoer (also called **tortfeasor** with tort law); could be a business, individual, or the government
Wrong act against	Wrongful act against the government (state or federal)	Wrongful acts against an individual or an institution (business)
Offense/wrong	Crime	Tort, breach of contract (depends on the type of civil law)
Attorney	Defendant is entitled to an attorney. The state must provide an attorney if the defendant cannot afford one.	Defendant must pay for the attorney or defend himself or herself.
Court	Tried in criminal court system; almost always involves a trial by jury.	Tried in a civil court system; may not involve a jury. Cases are typically decided by the judge.
Standard of proof	Must prove beyond a reasonable doubt.	The preponderance of evidence (more than likely it occurred)
Consequence	Substantial fine and prison time	**Damages**, **injunction**, **declaratory judgment**
Healthcare example	A medical assistant determines a patient should have a specific medication and gives the patient the medication without a provider's order, thus practicing medicine.	A medical assistant changes a sterile dressing per a provider's order but does the procedure incorrectly. The wound develops an infection, and the patient subsequently dies.

With criminal law, procedural law ensures that a person receives due process under the U.S. Constitution.

We will examine criminal and civil law in depth as they relate to healthcare.

Criminal Law

Criminal laws are statutes that define actions or *omissions* (lack of actions) that threaten and/or harm public safety and welfare. These actions or omissions are prohibited by the government and are called *crimes*. Criminal law can be summarized as crimes against the state (or government). When criminal cases are brought to court, the **plaintiff** is the government. The **defendant** is the person or party charged with the offense.

Criminal offenses can vary in severity from traffic violations to murders. In most states criminal offenses are classified as *misdemeanors* and *felonies*, which both appear on a person's criminal record. Misdemeanors are lesser criminal offenses and include: assault, battery, false imprisonment, perjury, shoplifting, and most cases of operating while intoxicated (OWI) and operating under the influence (OUI). A misdemeanor is punishable by a substantial fine and possible jail time under 1 year. (*Jails* are usually operated by local law enforcement and are used for short-term stays.) A felony is a serious criminal offense and is classified by degree, with first degree being the most serious. Examples of felonies include: murder, robbery, rape, sodomy, larceny, manslaughter, kidnapping, embezzlement, arson, mayhem, burglary, and treason. Felonies are punishable by substantial fines and prison time more than 1 year. (*Prisons* are usually operated by the state or federal government and are for long-term stays.) A felony conviction may prevent a person from voting and owning firearms (guns). A felon may have difficulty obtaining a job, especially in healthcare.

Civil Law

Civil laws protect and define private rights. An individual or institution can sue another person, institution (business), or the government in a civil matter (Table 3.2). Civil laws govern disputes related to contracts, property, family law, and personal injury. Common civil disputes involve contract issues, divorce, child custody, product **liability**, and accidents. There are many branches of civil law, including:

- *Tort law:* Applies when one person, business, or the government does a wrongdoing to an individual that causes injury or property damage. Includes intentional tort, negligence, and strict liability (strict duty to ensure safety of manufactured products).
- *Contract law:* Applies to agreements between two or more individuals or parties.
- *Property law:* Applies to personal property (e.g., copyrights, stocks, animals, physical goods) and real property (e.g., land, mineral rights).
- *Family law:* Applies to marriage, divorce, annulment, child custody and support, birth, and adoption.

The following sections will address **tort** law and contract law.

TORT LAW

Tort law enforces rules that we have in our society. If these rules are violated, then an individual can sue another individual, institution (business), or government. There are two types of torts that will be discussed: intentional torts and negligent torts (unintentional torts).

Intentional Torts

With an intentional tort, the plaintiff must prove the defendant had specific intent to perform the action that caused the injury. The focus is not on whether the harm was intended, but if the action was intended. Many intentional torts are also criminal in nature. The defendant may be prosecuted in both a civil court and a criminal court for the action. Common intentional torts include:

- *Assault:* Intentional threat to do harm or acting in a manner that causes another to fear bodily harm. Example: a medical assistant threatens a child to behave by stating "I will give you a 'shot' if you do not behave."
- *Battery:* Intentional harmful or offensive contact with another that was unconsented. This includes unauthorized administration of medical care in a nonemergent situation. Only proof of unconsented contact is required; proof of harm is not required. Example: a medical assistant gives a child a vaccination without consent from the parent or guardian.
- *False imprisonment:* Intentional restraint of another individual without consent or reason. Example: a medical assistant uses restraints to keep a patient in a wheelchair without significant reason.
- *Fraud:* Deceiving (lying to) a person or party for monetary gain. Example: a medical assistant bills an insurance company for services not provided to the patient.
- *Defamation:* Intentionally saying something false about another person, which causes harm. Written defamation is *libel*. Spoken defamation is *slander*. Example: a medical assistant posts lies about a co-worker on a social media site that could cause harm to that person.
- *Invasion of privacy:* Disclosing private facts without the consent of the individual, or intrusion into a person's personal life. Example: a medical assistant tells a family member or friend about a patient who was seen in the department, which is breaching confidentiality.

CRITICAL THINKING APPLICATION   3.2
Bella and Daniela are reviewing civil law concepts after work. Bella asks Daniela how civil law would apply to medical assistants. How might Daniela respond? Discuss your response with a peer.

Negligent Torts

Negligent torts, or unintentional torts, are more common in healthcare because they are unintentional. The harm that is caused by **negligence** is the result of a person's carelessness. Negligence results when a person's conduct falls below the standard of behavior expected of a reasonable person in the same situation.

Legal Example: Defamation Suit

According to the complaint: In 2013 in Fairfax, Virginia, the plaintiff was to have a colonoscopy. He was told he could be groggy afterwards and was concerned about recalling post-procedure instructions. Prior to the procedure, he set his mobile phone to record the post-procedure instructions. His clothing and phone ended up in the operating suite with him during the procedure. His phone recorded the entire procedure. While the plaintiff was unconscious, the doctors and medical assistant joked that he had syphilis and tuberculosis that caused a penile rash. The defendants mocked the patient for a variety of reasons and then discussed how to avoid the patient when he woke up. The medical assistant attempted to mislead the plaintiff. She indicated falsely that the physician spoke to him after surgery, but the patient must not have remembered. The plaintiff and his wife discovered the recording on their way home.

The jury awarded the plaintiff $50,000 in compensatory damages for defamation for the provider's remarks about each disease. He was also awarded $200,000 for overall medical malpractice and $200,000 in punitive damages.

D.B. v Ingham et al., 2013-16811, (2015, Fairfax Circuit Court)

The *reasonable person standard* applies reasonable behavior as an objective test to measure another's actions or lack of actions. The accused person's actions or lack of actions are measured against what a reasonable person would or would not do in the same situation. The accused person is negligent if his or her actions or lack of actions do not measure up to the reasonable person standard. Negligent acts can be classified as:

- *Malfeasance:* Performance of an unlawful, wrongful act. For instance, a medical assistant determines that a patient needs pain medication and gives a large dose without a provider's order. The patient dies from the overdose. (It is illegal for the medical assistant to practice medicine [prescribe the medication], and the dose was incorrect.)
- *Misfeasance:* Improper performance of a lawful act, that causes damage or injury. For instance, a medical assistant gives an injection ordered by the provider. The injection is given in the wrong location, and the patient has lifelong pain.
- *Nonfeasance:* Failure to act when one had a legal duty to act. For instance, after a patient is given an injection, the patient starts to have an adverse reaction. The medical assistant fails to act and notify the provider. The medical assistant sends the patient home, and the patient later dies.

Malpractice is a type of negligence that applies to professionals. Medical malpractice occurs when a healthcare professional's performance falls below the professional minimum standard of care and thus causes harm to the plaintiff. *Standard of care* refers to the level and type of care an ordinary, prudent healthcare professional, having the same training and experience in a similar practice, would have provided under a similar situation.

CRITICAL THINKING APPLICATION   **3.3**

Bella asks Daniela to describe negligence and malpractice in her own words. How might Daniela respond?

The standard of care takes into account the accused person's skills and knowledge. It also considers the environment. For instance, the care provided by Dr. Walden, a family practice doctor practicing in a midsize Midwestern city, would be compared to a family practice doctor who practiced in a similar-sized city in the same geographic location. It would be unfair to compare Dr. Walden's family practice to a large family practice located on the East Coast. The resources available to the providers could be different.

Medical assistants need to be aware of the standard of care. If medical assistants identify themselves as nurses to patients, they may be held to the standard of care (including the educational level) of a nurse. If medical assistants practice beyond their **scope of practice**, they may be held to the higher standard of care. Also, medical assistants who are nationally certified may be held to a higher level than those who are not certified. It is important for credentialed medical assistants to pursue continuing education to keep updated and current in their practice. Scope of practice will be discussed later in the chapter.

CRITICAL THINKING APPLICATION   **3.4**

Daniela asks Bella why medical assistants cannot call themselves nurses. How might Bella address this question? How might scope of practice relate to the question?

Defenses to Liability

When the defendant's attorney accepts a case, a **defense** is planned for the lawsuit. There are three main defenses used for lawsuits: denial, technical, and affirmative. *Denial defense* is used when none of the facts are true. If even just one fact is true, then the denial defense cannot be used. The following sections will describe technical and affirmative defenses.

Technical Defenses. When attorneys review cases, they look for ways to have the cases dismissed based on a legal technicality. Four technical defenses will be discussed: statute of limitations, Good Samaritan law, release of tortfeasor, and res judicata.

The *statute of limitations* is the length of time legal action can be taken after an event has occurred. When the time has expired, the court will reject the claim or lawsuit. The statute of limitations for medical malpractice is usually 2 to 5 years, but it varies from state to state. In most states the "clock" starts when the patient "reasonably should have known" the malpractice occurred. For instance, if a patient awoke after surgery to find that the operation had been performed on the wrong leg, the clock would start then. In some cases, patients do not realize the malpractice occurred for months or years after the event. For instance, something was left in the patient's body during surgery, and it was discovered on an x-ray 3 years later. According to the *Discovery Rule*, the malpractice needs to be discovered (the patient "reasonably should have known") before the "clock starts" on the statute of limitations. The statute of limitations for children greatly varies; some states use age 8, whereas others use age 18.

The *Good Samaritan laws* vary in each state, with some states providing protection if the provider acts "in good faith." For Good Samaritan protection, a person must provide care in a true emergency. The care must be provided outside of a place with necessary medical equipment (e.g., outside of a hospital or ambulatory care facility). The person providing the care cannot bill the patient for the emergency care provided.

The *release of tortfeasor* defense is used when the plaintiff had signed a release and received monetary compensation. The release indicated that the plaintiff would give up all rights to sue the defendant (tortfeasor) in the future, in exchange for a monetary compensation. If this signed release existed and the plaintiff decided to sue the defendant at a later time, the defendant's attorney could use the release of tortfeasor defense.

The final technical defense is **res judicata**, which is Latin for "a thing decided." If a case has already been decided by the court, the plaintiff cannot bring a similar suit against the defendant in the future. The defendant's attorney would use the *res judicata* defense.

Affirmative Defenses. When attorneys review cases, if the denial defense and the technical defense cannot be used, then they attempt to use the affirmative defense. An *affirmative defense* means the defendant admits to wrongdoing, but his or her attorney introduces facts that support the defendant's conduct. If the defense is successful, it will reduce the defendant's legal liability. The following are common affirmative defenses:

- *Contributory negligence*: The plaintiff's actions or lack of actions caused the injury. In other words, had the plaintiff used ordinary care, the injury would not have occurred. The plaintiff's carelessness (e.g., ignoring warnings or safety rules, inattention) caused the injury. (In many states contributory negligence has been replaced by comparative negligence).
- *Comparative negligence*: The plaintiff's action or lack of action caused the injury to a certain percent. The damages to the plaintiff are calculated based on the percent the defendant was responsible.
- *Assumption of risk*: The defendant can show evidence that the plaintiff had actual, subjective knowledge of the risks involved and the plaintiff consented to proceed with the activity. Informed consent is critical for this defense. (Informed consent will be discussed later in the chapter.)
- *Limited or no harm*: The defendant claims the plaintiff suffered no or little harm; much less than what the plaintiff claims.

- *Intervening cause*: The defendant acknowledges the plaintiff suffered injuries due to defendant's negligence, but the injury was made worse by the plaintiff's actions following the situation.

Legal Example: Assumption of Risk

The plaintiff was being treated for bronchitis. Following his clinic visit, a coughing episode caused him to black out and hit his head at home. Upon his return to the clinic a few weeks later for a follow-up visit on the bronchitis, a medical assistant took the plaintiff into the examination room. The medical assistant instructed the plaintiff to sit on the exam table while his vital signs were obtained. The plaintiff mentioned to the medical assistant that he had fainted twice as a result of coughing episodes. After the medical assistant left to get the physician, the plaintiff had a coughing episode, fainted, and fell to the floor. He sustained injuries because of the fall.

The plaintiff sued the clinic and the medical assistant, alleging that the medical assistant was negligent for failing to move him to another location upon learning about his fainting episodes. The defendants moved for a summary judgment. They stated that an assumption of risk defense applied. The plaintiff could have chosen to sit on one of the two chairs present in the room, but he did not. The court agreed. The plaintiff appealed, and the Georgia Court of Appeals unanimously sided with the trial court's ruling. The defendants proved the plaintiff had knowledge of the danger, understood the risks associated with the danger, and exposed himself to the danger. The plaintiff lost the case.

Watson v. Regional First Care, Inc., No. A15A1708, Ga. App. (February 19, 2016).

CRITICAL THINKING APPLICATION   3.5

Daniela is studying affirmative defenses. She asks Bella if she has any study tips for remembering the different affirmative defenses. How might Bella answer? Share your answer with a peer.

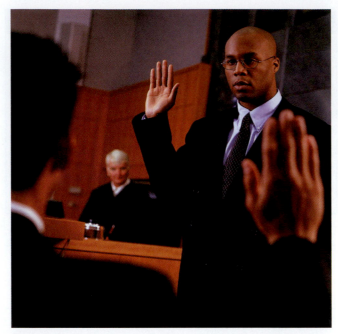

FIGURE 3.1 Witnesses must be credible and must tell the truth on the stand in court to avoid charges of perjury.

If the disputing parties decide to take the lawsuit to court, a specific process must be followed (Fig. 3.1). When a medical negligence suit is brought to court, four elements must be proven for malpractice to be found. These elements are the 4 *D*s of negligence: duty, dereliction, damages, and direct cause. Let's examine the 4 *D*s of negligence.

- *Duty of care*: The healthcare professional has a legal obligation to the patient. Many times, the duty of care comes from the provider-patient relationship. This will be examined in more depth later in the chapter.
- *Dereliction*: The healthcare professional breaches (violates) the duty of care to the patient. In other words, the professional did not follow through with the duty to the patient.
- *Damages*: The patient suffers a legally recognized injury. Examples of such an injury include physical pain, mental anguish, additional medical bills, and loss of work/earning capacity.
- *Direct cause*: The breach of duty of care (the negligent act or lack of action) directly causes the patient's injury.

The plaintiff's attorney is responsible for proving each of these four elements. In many cases, medical experts are hired by attorneys to be expert witnesses. These expert witnesses help establish the standard of care and some of the 4 *D*s. If one of the elements is not proven, malpractice will not be found. For instance, if the provider performed below the standard of care, but the patient did not suffer any harm, malpractice cannot be found.

Proving Malpractice

When a plaintiff sues the defendant, the defendant can attempt to settle outside of court or go to trial. *Alternative dispute resolution* (ADR) is the process of settling disputes outside of litigation. This process is usually cheaper and quicker than going to trial. Two types of alternative dispute resolution are **arbitration** and **mediation.** Both ADR procedures involve a neutral third party who hears both sides. With mediation, the mediator facilitates an agreement that is acceptable to both parties. With arbitration, the arbitrator listens to both sides and makes the final decision, which is *legally binding* (or a legal obligation).

With civil litigation, either party or the judge can move for a summary judgment. A *summary judgment* is a process that can be used if there are no disputes about the facts in the case. This process speeds up cases. It allows a judgment to be made based on the facts. With a summary judgment, there is no trial.

CRITICAL THINKING APPLICATION   3.6

Daniela struggles with remembering the 4 *D*s of negligence. Be creative and work with a peer. How might a person remember the 4 *D*s of negligence?

Stages of a Civil Lawsuit

1. **Pre-filing phase:** The situation occurs, and the patient seeks the advice of a civil attorney. After reviewing the person's story, the medical record, and other documents, the attorney accepts the case.
2. **Initial pleading phase:**
   - The plaintiff's attorney files a complaint with the clerk of the court. The complaint includes the patient's version of the situation and the damages (amount of money) sought from the defendant.
   - The clerk of the court issues a summons to the defendant. The summons outlines the complaint and damages and states a deadline for a response.
   - The defense attorney files an answer or motion with the court. The answer provides the courts with the defendant's version of the situation. (If the deadline is missed, the defendant may be responsible for the damages.)
3. **Discovery phase:**
   - Both sides exchange information and gather evidence to support their side in court.
   - A **subpoena** is issued for the healthcare professionals involved in the case. They may be required to go to court or to attend a **deposition**. They may also be required to complete an **interrogatory.** Failure to comply with a deposition or subpoena will result in a *contempt of court* charge. The person may be fined or imprisoned.
   - A **subpoena duces tecum** may also be issued.
4. **Post discovery phase:**
   - The judge may meet with both attorneys to discuss the case.
   - The plaintiff may drop the case if not enough evidence was available to make the case.
   - The defendant may settle the lawsuit by "making a deal" so it does not move to trial.
5. **Trial phase:** If the case is to be heard by a jury, the jury is selected.. **Expert witnesses** and **fact witnesses** are questioned and cross-examined by the opposing attorney. Closing arguments are made, and the jury retires to make a decision. The verdict is read to the court, and the judge enters the judgment.
6. **Appeals phase:** Post-trial motions are filed. An appeal to a higher court may be made.

CRITICAL THINKING APPLICATION   3.7
Bella is helping Daniela study for a law exam. She asks Daniela to describe the differences between the following sets of terms. How might Daniela respond?
- Subpoena and subpoena duces tecum
- Fact witness and expert witness

In a case in which there was obvious negligence, the doctrine **res ipsa loquitur** may apply. *Res ipsa loquitur* is Latin for "the thing speaks for itself." The *res ipsa loquitur* doctrine may be used for:
- Cases that involve an object being left in the patient's body during a surgery
- Cases that involve an operation on the wrong extremity

The evidence shows that the plaintiff did not cause the injury. The defendant caused the injury as a result of negligence. The defendant breached the duty to the plaintiff.

Damages

The defendant may need to pay **damages** when the plaintiff wins a civil suit. Damages are a monetary settlement. There are several types of damages:
- *Punitive damages*: Very large payment meant to punish the defendant.
- *Nominal damages*: Very small settlement because the plaintiff's injury was slight.
- *Compensatory damages*: A settlement for losses suffered. Losses can be related to loss of income, property damage, and medical care.
- *General damages*: A settlement for emotional pain and anguish, loss of future earning power, and so on. Often sought with compensatory damages.
- *Special damages*: A settlement for a specific dollar amount that directly relates to medical bills.

Professional Liability Insurance

Many people are familiar with car insurance and home owner's insurance. When a person becomes a professional, the risk of being sued increases. Having insurance (to protect oneself in case of civil damages) is important. Providers, nurses, and in some cases medical assistants, purchase annual insurance policies. Ambulatory healthcare facilities also must carry insurance. It is important for medical assistants to understand the types of insurance available.

The person or company purchasing the insurance policy is called the *insured* (*first party*). The insured pays a specific amount of money to the insurance company (*second party*). This payment is called a *premium*. The insurance company is the *insurer*. The insurer agrees to compensate the insured for specific losses covered in the insurance contract or policy. When the insurer (insurance company) pays the plaintiff, the plaintiff is known as the *third party*.

Liability insurance provides protection from claims of injuries or damage to people or property. It can be referred to as third-party coverage because it covers claims from a party other than the insured. Different types of liability insurance include:
- *Professional liability insurance*: A type of liability coverage used by professionals to protect them against liability suits incurred because of errors and omissions while performing their professional services.
  - *Medical malpractice insurance*: A type of professional liability insurance. Protects healthcare professionals, including medical assistants, from liability related to wrongful practices resulting in injury, expense, and property damages. It also covers the cost of defending lawsuits.

- *General liability* or *commercial liability insurance*: A type of liability coverage purchased by companies. It protects businesses from lawsuits for property loss and bodily injury from nonemployees.
- *Personal injury insurance*: A type of liability coverage that protects against claims related to harm other than bodily injury. Coverage can be for invasion of privacy, slander, imprisonment, and so on.

When purchasing a policy, it is important to understand the types of policies.

- *Claims-made policy*: An insurance policy that covers claims made during the policy year. For example: if a provider has a claims-made policy for the current year, any claims that come in this year will be covered.
- *Occurrence policy*: An insurance policy that covers claims for wrongful acts that occurred during the policy year. For example, if a provider has an occurrence policy for the current year, any wrongful acts that occur this year will be covered when the claims are filed in future years.
- *Nose coverage*: A limited-term policy purchased from the new carrier the provider is joining. The policy covers the provider between the end of the prior policy and the start of next policy. Nose coverage can also be referred to as *retroactive* or *prior acts coverage*.
- *Tail coverage*: A limited-term policy purchased from the insurance carrier that the provider is leaving. The policy covers the provider until the new policy starts. A person would need only nose or tail coverage, but not both.

CONTRACTS

Most people are aware of contracts. We sign contracts for cell phone plans, rental properties, and payment plans. We also have contracts in healthcare. The healthcare facility's business manager signs contracts for equipment and building rental, service agreements, and so on. The most common contract is the provider-patient contract.

A *contract* is an agreement between two parties. For a contract to be legally binding, five elements must be present:

- *Offer*: Made by one party. Example: a family practice physician advertises complete physicals for $150.
- *Acceptance*: A second party agrees to the offer. Example: after seeing the advertisement, a patient calls to make an appointment.
- *Consideration*: Each party exchanges something of value. Example: the physician gives a physical exam, and the patient pays $150.
- *Legal subject matter*: The consideration must be legal. Example: the board-certified physician can legally perform physical exams. The payment is legal tender (money).
- *Competency and capacity*: A person entering a contract must have the legal capacity to be held liable for the contract obligation. If one or both parties is underage (a **minor**) or shows signs of **incompetence**, intoxication, or acting under the influence of drugs, this would invalidate a contract. An **emancipated minor** can enter into contracts. Example: both the physician and the patient are adults with the capacity to understand the contract.

Emancipated Minor

Conditions for Emancipation

Must be at least 16 years of age in most states and usually must meet one of the following:

- Married
- In the U.S. military
- Living on his or her own and managing own money

Benefits of Emancipation

- Can be a party in a contract (e.g., rent housing, purchase agreements)
- Can sue
- Can keep earned income and apply for public benefits
- May make all healthcare decisions regarding himself or herself

---

Contracts can either be:

- *Implied contract*: The parties have agreed to the terms of the contract through their actions and behaviors. The provider-patient relationship is an implied contract (Fig. 3.2).
- *Expressed contract:* The parties have specifically stated the terms of the contract in writing, orally, or both. A service contract for office equipment maintenance is an expressed contract.

Specific types of contracts must be in writing to avoid fraud. These types of contracts are outlined in each state's *statute of frauds*. Statutes of fraud vary slightly, but all indicate that contracts need to be in writing and signed by both parties. Contracts that need to be in writing include:

- Contracts that are property related – real estate sales, real estate leases for longer than 1 year, and transfer of property upon the owner's death
- Agreements to pay another's debt
- Contracts that last longer than 1 year or last longer than the life of an individual
- Contracts over a certain amount of money (varies by state)

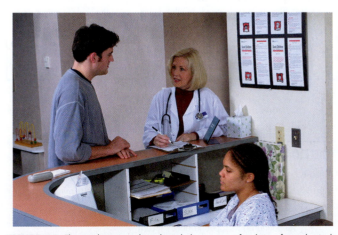

FIGURE 3.2 The provider-patient relationship is built on a strong foundation of trust, but it also is a contractual relationship.

TABLE 3.3 Terminating the Provider-Patient Relationship

REASONS PROVIDERS TERMINATE THE PROVIDER-PATIENT RELATIONSHIP	STEPS TO TERMINATE THE PROVIDER-PATIENT RELATIONSHIP
• Retirement or moving • Patient is not paying for the services provided • Patient is not following or is noncompliant with the provider's treatment plan • Patient's behavior (e.g., rude, abusive, drug seeking, not showing up for appointments)	• Provider must notify the patient in writing of the withdrawal of care. • A date must be indicated for the termination. There must be an adequate period of coverage to allow the patient to find another provider. Fifteen to 30 days is usually recommended. • The termination letter should be sent as a certified letter with return receipt requested. • A copy of the letter and the return receipt need to be placed or scanned into the patient health record. • Scheduling staff should be notified of the termination date, so no appointments are made after that date.

Provider-Patient Relationship

The contract that is established between the provider and the patient is legally binding. The patient accepts the provider's offer when a patient makes an appointment to see the provider. This means the provider has a duty to see, diagnose, and treat the patient. The patient has the responsibility to follow the provider's recommendations and pay the bill.

As indicated earlier, duty to the patient is one of the 4 Ds in proving malpractice. The duty to the patient is established during the initial visit of the patient. From that time onward, the provider has a duty to the patient. Both parties can terminate the contract or relationship. A patient can terminate the contract at any time. The patient may no longer need the provider's services. The patient may decide to use another provider.

The provider must follow the legal process to terminate the contract. Table 3.3 lists reasons providers terminate the patient relationship or contract. A provider can be charged with **patient abandonment** if he or she simply stops providing care to the patient. To prevent abandonment allegations, the provider must follow the correct legal steps to terminate the provider-patient relationship. Table 3.3 lists the steps the provider needs to follow to terminate the contract or relationship with the patient.

There are many situations in which allegations of patient abandonment may occur, including:

- Failing to follow up with the patient. If a patient calls or emails the provider or facility, follow-up with the patient must be made in a reasonable period of time.
- Failing to have another provider cover the practice during vacations or when the facility is closed.
- Discharging a patient without proper instructions.

The medical assistant has an important role in ensuring that the patient is not abandoned. Typically, the medical assistant is responsible for answering patient calls and emails in a timely manner. Documentation in the patient health record must reflect all communication with the patient.

If the medical assistant does not follow up with the patient, allegations of abandonment can be brought against the medical assistant and the provider. *Respondeat superior* is a common law doctrine that means "let the master answer." The doctrine means that the employer/provider is **liable** for actions that the employee did or did not do within the scope of employment. This means that the medical assistant's actions affect the employer and the provider. The medical assistant's actions or lack of actions can lead to malpractice allegations for the provider.

Breach of Contract

A *breach of contract* occurs when the terms of the contract are not fulfilled by one party without a legitimate legal reason. The breach can occur when the terms are not met by the stated deadline. It can also happen when the terms are not met or performed. An allegation of a breach of contract can lead to a lawsuit. The injured party attempts to force the contract terms to be met or to receive compensation for financial loss caused by the breach.

In the healthcare field, a breach of contract can occur with the provider-patient relationship. Breach of contract may occur with improper termination and abandonment situations. Breach of contract may also occur with the business side of the facility, including:

- Business contracts (e.g., leases for equipment)
- Payment contracts with patients

CONSENT

Consent means one party voluntarily agrees with another party's proposition or plan. In healthcare, several types of consent are used.

- *Implied consent*: Consent that is inferred based on signs, actions, or conduct of the patient rather than oral communication (using words). For instance, the medical assistant asks a patient if he can obtain a blood pressure reading. The patient removes her arm from her jacket sleeve and extends it toward the medical assistant.
- *Expressed consent*: Consent that is given either by the spoken or written word. For example, the medical assistant asks the patient's preference for which arm should be used for an injection. The patient states she wants the injection in her upper right arm. The medical assistant gave the patient a choice, and the patient expressed her consent by stating her choice.
- *Informed consent*: A legal process that ensures the patient or guardian understands the treatment and gives consent for the treatment.

With informed consent, the provider must educate the patient on the treatment before the patient signs the consent form. More information on the informed consent doctrine is given in the following section.

Doctrine of Informed Consent

With many medical procedures and treatments, informed consent is required, including:

- Surgical procedures; may include minor surgery done in ambulatory care facilities
- Complex procedures and tests (e.g., endoscopy, biopsy, exercise or nuclear stress test)
- Administration of high-risk medications and most vaccines
- Participation in a research study
- Cancer treatment (e.g., radiation, chemotherapy)
- Some medical laboratory testing

The provider, not the medical assistant, has a duty to provide information to the patient or guardian. The provider must educate the patient on the treatment options. Once the information is given, the patient or guardian makes an informed decision regarding treatment.

Informed consent requirements may vary slightly from state to state. The requirements are usually described in the state's medical practice act. For an informed consent to occur, seven elements must be present:

1. The patient or guardian is competent to understand and decide.
2. The patient or guardian voluntarily decides to agree to or refuse the treatment.
3. The patient or guardian understands the diagnosis and reason for treatment.
4. The patient or guardian understands the proposed treatment and the risks of the treatment.
5. The patient or guardian understands the alternative treatments available and the risks of the treatments.
6. The patient or guardian understands the risks if treatment is delayed or not done.
7. The patient or guardian signs a treatment consent form.

Adults of sound mind can give informed consent. Married minors, minor parents, emancipated minors, and **mature minors** can also give informed consent. Patients who cannot legally give informed consent include:

- Patients under the influence of alcohol or drugs
- Patients medicated with a preoperative medication that may affect their understanding (e.g., a sedative)
- A minor
- A patient who is mentally incompetent
- A patient who speaks little to no English. (An interpreter must be used for the patient to give informed consent. The interpreter will translate the information from the provider, questions from the patient, and the information on the consent form. It is important to document in the health record that an interpreter was used.)

In special situations, such as abortion, sterilization procedures, and human immunodeficiency virus (HIV) testing, each state has specific restrictions. The following box lists possible state restrictions for abortions. Currently, with abortions, the father of the fetus has no rights. No state requires the father to give consent or to be told about the abortion. For sterilization procedures, states may have waiting periods between signing the consent form and the procedure. The patient may have to be an adult (as defined by the state). For HIV testing, the Centers for Disease Control and Prevention (CDC) recommends that a general consent for medical care form be completed prior to HIV testing. Most states have specific language in the statutes regarding consent and counseling for HIV testing.

In many states, the patient's written consent is required to take a video or picture of the patient. Pictures are taken to show before and after images. These pictures are added to the patient electronic health record.

The medical assistant may need to prepare the informed consent form. The following box lists information that should be on the informed consent form. The medical assistant may also need to sign the form as a witness to the signature of the patient. It is important to ask patients before they sign the form if the provider discussed the treatment and if they have any questions. If patients have questions, let the provider know. After all the questions have been answered, then the informed consent form can be signed. Do not have the patient sign if he or she:

- Does not understand the treatment.
- Cannot legally give consent.
- Has questions.

PATIENT'S BILL OF RIGHTS

Congress has attempted to create laws effecting a patient's "bill of rights" related to patient care and services, but none of the proposed bills has passed. The Affordable Care Act's Patient's Bill of Rights focuses on rights related to insurance. With no federal laws to follow, the American Hospital Association created a patient's bill of rights for its members. Since then, many healthcare facilities have created their own patient's bill of rights. Many agencies title theirs as "Patient's Rights and Responsibilities" (Fig. 3.3). The patient's bill of rights

Information on the Informed Consent Forms

- Patient's name, date of birth, and health record number
- Name of hospital or facility
- Name of provider(s) performing treatment(s)
- Risks and benefits of the treatment(s)
- Alternative treatment(s) and risks
- Risk if treatment(s) is delayed or not done
- Statement indicating the treatment was explained to the patient or guardian
- Signature of patient or guardian
- Signature and name of person who explained the treatment options
- Signature of the witness
- Date and time consent form was completed

WALDEN-MARTIN
FAMILY MEDICAL CLINIC
1234 ANYSTREET | ANYTOWN, ANYSTATE 12345
PHONE 123-123-1234 | FAX 123-123-5678

Patient Bill of Rights
RIGHTS

1. **Medical Care and Dental Care.** The right to quality care consistent with available resources and accepted standards. The right to refuse treatment to the extent permitted by law and Government regulations, and to be informed of refusal consequences. When concerned about care received, the right to request review of care adequacy.

2. **Respectful Treatment.** The right to considerate and respectful care, with recognition of personal dignity.

3. **Privacy and Confidentiality.** The right, within law and military regulations, to privacy and confidentiality concerning medical care.

4. **Identity.** The right to know, at all times, the identity, professional status, and professional credentials of health care personnel, as well as the name of the health care provider primarily responsible for his or her care.

5. **Explanation of Care.** The right to an explanation concerning diagnosis, treatment, procedures, and prognosis of illness in terms the patient can understand. When it is not medically advisable to give such information to the patient, information should be provided to appropriate family members or, in their absence, another appropriate person.

6. **Informed Consent.** The right to be advised in non-clinical terms of information (significant complications, risks, benefits, and alternative treatments) needed to make knowledgeable decisions on treatment consent or refusal.

7. **Research Projects.** The right to be advised if the facility proposes to perform research associated with care. The right to refuse to participate in any research projects.

8. **Safe Environment.** The right to care and treatment in a safe environment.

9. **Medical Treatment Facility (MTF) or Dental Treatment Facility (DTF) Rules and Regulations.** The right to be informed of facility conduct rules and regulations. The patient should be informed about smoking rules and should expect compliance with those rules from other individuals. Patients are entitled to information about the MTF or DTF mechanism for the initiation, review, and resolution of patient complaints.

RESPONSIBILITIES

1. **Providing Information.** The responsibility to provide, to the best of his or her knowledge, accurate and complete information about complaints, past illness, hospitalizations, medications, and other matters relating to his or her health. A patient has the responsibility to let his or her primary health care provider know whether he or she understands the treatment and what is expected of him or her.

2. **Respect and Consideration.** The responsibility for being considerate of the rights of other patients and MTF and DTF health care personnel and for assistance in the control of noise, smoking, and the number of visitors. The patient is responsible for being respectful of the property of other persons and of the facility.

3. **Compliance with Medical Care.** The responsibility for complying with medical and nursing treatment plans, including follow-up care, recommended by health care providers. This includes keeping appointments on time and notifying the MTF or DTF when appointments cannot be kept.

4. **Medical Records.** The responsibility for ensuring that medical records are promptly returned to the medical facility for appropriate filing and maintenance when records are transported by the patients for the purpose of medical appointment or consultation, etc. All medical records documenting care provided by any MTF or DTF are the property of the U.S. Government.

5. **MTF and DTF Rules and Regulations.** The responsibility for following the MTF and DTF rules and regulations affecting patient care conduct. Regulations regarding smoking should be followed by all patients.

6. **Reporting of Patient Complaints.** The responsibility for helping the MTF or DTF commander provide the best possible care to all beneficiaries. Patients' recommendations, questions, or complaints should be reported to the patient contact representative.

FIGURE 3.3 Patient's Bill of Rights.

provides patients with information on their rights under federal and state laws. Healthcare professionals must ensure they uphold and respect patients' rights.

A medical assistant is likely to encounter a situation in which a choice of treatments is given to a patient (see Procedure 3.1, p. 67). It is important that the provider discuss the treatment choices with the patient. If the medical assistant is involved, it is important to find out if the patient has any questions. Questions need to be answered before a decision is made. It is important to be respectful and professional during the discussion. Do not attempt to sway the patient in one direction. If the patient selects the treatment that was not the provider's top choice, it is important to respect the patient's decision. The medical assistant should relay the information to the provider.

A medical assistant should know how to handle the situation if a patient refuses a procedure or treatment (see Procedure 3.1). It is important to follow the facility's policy and procedure in such a situation. Most times the following applies when a patient refuses treatment or procedures:

- Show sensitivity to the patient's rights by being respectful and professional. Remember, it is the right of the patient to refuse.
- Ask the patient if he or she has questions regarding the procedure. If so, let the provider know.
- Notify the provider of the refusal.
- Document the refusal in the health record. Make sure to include which provider was notified.

CRITICAL THINKING APPLICATION   **3.10**

Bella is working with Daniela on the Patient's Bill of Rights. Bella asks Daniela to summarize these rights. What might Daniela say?

CRITICAL THINKING APPLICATION   **3.11**

Daniela asks Bella how much a medical assistant really uses the Patient's Bill of Rights. Bella provides this scenario for Daniela: Mrs. Ella Jones, a new patient to the practice, comes in for her 28-week pregnancy check. After the provider examines her, he comes out and gives you an order for the patient. You are to give the patient RhoGAM, because she has Rh-negative blood. This is a standard practice with mothers who have Rh-negative blood. You prepare the medication and go to the exam room. You explain to Mrs. Jones what the provider ordered. She asks, " Is RhoGAM a blood product?" and you reply that it is. She refuses it, explaining that she is a Jehovah's Witness and cannot accept blood products. Bella asks Daniela, "Keeping in mind the Patient's Bill of Rights, how might a medical assistant demonstrate sensitivity to Mrs. Jones' rights in this situation?" How might Daniela answer? Discuss your answer with a peer.

PRACTICE REQUIREMENTS

Many healthcare professionals are required to complete an educational program before they can work in healthcare. Upon completion, they usually must pass an exam before practicing. This section will

discuss the practice requirements and scope of practice of physicians, advanced practice professionals, and other healthcare professionals (Table 3.4).

Practice Acts and State Boards

The Tenth Amendment of the U.S. Constitution empowers each state to establish laws that protect the health and safety of that state's citizens. Each state has passed laws and regulations that govern the practice of medicine. These laws and regulations are in a state statute called the *Medical Practice Act*. The Medical Practice Act also outlines the responsibility of the state medical board.

Each state's medical board issues licenses to practice medicine. The board also investigates complaints and disciplines members who violate the law. The state medical board creates policies related to the practice of medicine. Other healthcare professionals (i.e., nurses) have Practice Acts and state boards with similar roles.

Licensure

Many healthcare professionals must have a state license before they begin their practice. The **licensure** process allows the state board to ensure that the healthcare professional meets the educational and training requirements. Passing the state licensing exam is a requirement for the license. Once a person gets a license, it needs to be renewed, about every 1 to 2 years. Besides the renewal fee, many state boards require evidence of continuing education.

If a healthcare professional is already licensed in one state, there are different methods of obtaining a license in additional states, including:

- *Licensing exam*: Passing the state's licensing exam and meeting the requirements.
- *Endorsement*: A state board grants a license to a person who is currently licensed in another state that has the same or stricter standards.
- *Reciprocity*: A state has a written agreement with another state to recognize licenses issued by that state without additional review of the person's credentials.

In 2015 the Interstate Medical Licensure Compact was created. This compact helped create a streamlined pathway for physicians to get licensure in multiple states. With the changes in healthcare, more rural care is provided by **telemedicine**, and more physicians are becoming *locum tenens*. With these changes, the need for licensure from multiple states has increased. To be eligible for licensure through the compact's process, physicians need to meet several requirements. Eligible physicians can select the compact member states where they would like to practice. Once the verification process has been completed, the physician will get a full, unrestricted license to practice medicine in those states.

Scope of Practice

The *scope of practice* for an occupation defines the procedures, actions, and processes that individuals are permitted to perform. A state board determines the scope of practice for that state's specific occupations. In some cases, the medical state board oversees the scope of practice of other healthcare occupations. If healthcare professionals practice beyond their scope of practice, they risk being sued for malpractice.

TABLE 3.4   Physicians, Advanced Practice Professionals, and Other Healthcare Professionals

TITLE	SCOPE OF PRACTICE	EDUCATION	CREDENTIAL AND LICENSE
Physicians			
Doctor of Medicine (MD)	Trained in all areas of medicine to diagnose and treat illness and prescribe medications; more focus on symptoms experienced by patient.	Beyond a bachelor's degree, must complete 4 years of medical school and 2–4 years of residency. Additional years of training may be required for specialties.	Must pass all three parts of the United States Medical Licensing Examination (USMLE). Must obtain state license to practice.
Doctor of Osteopathy (DO)	Trained in all areas of medicine, as is an MD. Specially trained in the nervous and musculoskeletal systems and their influence on health and disease.		
Advanced Practice Professionals			
Physician Assistant (PA)	Diagnoses and treats illness and prescribes medication; may specialize. Supervised by physician.	Must complete a 3-year PA program beyond a bachelor's degree.	Physician Assistant–Certified (PA-C) after passing the national exam. Must obtain state license to practice.
Advanced Practice Registered Nurse (APRN)		Must complete a master's degree beyond Registered Nurse (RN) training.	Must pass the national certification exam. Must obtain state license to practice.
Clinical Nurse Specialist (CNS)	Diagnoses and treats patients. Many work in hospital and community settings.		
Nurse Practitioner (NP)	Diagnoses and treats patients and prescribes medication; may specialize. Depending on state law, can be more independent than a PA.		
Certified Nurse Midwife (CNM)	Provides prenatal and postpartum care; delivers babies.		
Certified Registered Nurse Anesthetist (CRNA)	Gives anesthesia and related care to patients in surgery and for outpatient procedures.		
Other Healthcare Professionals			
Registered Nurse (RN)	Works in a wide range of positions, including clinical and administrative; performs more advanced assessments, patient care, and treatments than LPNs.	Has 2–4 years of education.	Must pass a licensure exam to practice.
Licensed Practical Nurse (LPN)	Works in long-term care, ambulatory care, and hospital settings; performs basic patient assessments, patient care, and treatments.	Has 1 year of education.	Must pass a licensure exam to practice.
Medical Assistant (MA)	Primarily works in ambulatory care settings. Performs administrative, clinical, and CLIA-waived laboratory testing under the supervision of a provider.	Varies from about 8 to 24 months; may get a diploma or an associate degree.	National certification exam is optional.

Legal Example: Scope of Practice

An obstetrician-gynecologist performed a procedure on a patient in her office. A few days after the procedure, the patient had increased pain that radiated along her side to her back. The patient called the office and spoke to a medical assistant. She mentioned the increase in pain, bleeding, and changes in her bowel movement. The medical assistant thought she had a urinary tract infection, so she asked the patient if she had any of the typical symptoms. The medical assistant did not talk to the provider about the patient's pain or bleeding because she did not think the complaints were serious enough. The medical assistant did not ask more questions about the pain or bleeding. The medical assistant told the patient her symptoms could be normal and advised her to take 800 mg of ibuprofen. (The medical assistant had been instructed by the providers to advise patients to take ibuprofen, 800 mg, every 8 hours as needed, for any sort of abdominal or back pain.) Later the patient was admitted to the intensive care unit, had to undergo a hysterectomy, and later died. Two months after the procedure, the patient's antibiotic prescription was found at the front desk. (The front desk staff had failed to give the patient the prescription after the procedure.)

The plaintiff sued for damages for the doctor's professional negligence (malpractice) and the clinic for the medical assistant's and front desk staff's negligence. After a 16-day trial, the jury returned a verdict for the defense. The plaintiff appealed. The appeals court ruled that the complaint was ordinary negligence and not medical malpractice. The appeals court also stated that the plaintiff could sue the clinic and medical assistant. The jury would have to decide if the medical assistant had practiced medicine without a license.

Wong v. Chappell, No. 333 Ga. App. 422 (2015).

Typical Duties of a Medical Assistant

- Obtain and record the patient's history and personal information
- Obtain and record vital signs (blood pressure, pulse, respiration rate), height, and weight
- Assist the provider during physical exams
- Administer oral, injectable, and inhaled medications as directed by provider and as permitted by state law
- Obtain blood samples for laboratory tests
- Perform CLIA-waived laboratory tests
- Schedule patients for appointments
- Perform receptionist duties
- Bill patients for services

- *License suspended*: Person cannot practice in that occupation for a specific period of time.
- *License surrendered*: Person voluntarily gives up license.
- *Probation*: Person's license is monitored for a specific period of time.
- *Reprimand*: Person is sent a warning or letter of concern.

Examples of Unprofessional Conduct by Physicians

- Substance and alcohol abuse
- Neglect of a patient
- Sexual misconduct
- Not meeting the accepted standard of care
- Dishonesty when obtaining a license or failing to meet the continuing education requirement
- Convicted of a felony or fraud
- Inadequate record keeping
- Delegating others to practice medicine

The scope of practice for physicians is similar across the states. Physicians diagnose, treat, prevent, or monitor disease conditions. The scope of practice differs between specialties. For instance, a family practice physician cannot perform heart surgery.

For medical assistants, the scope of practice laws vary by state. The following box provides a list of common medical assistant duties. Some states allow medical assistants to perform injections. Some states do not allow medical assistants to give certain types of injectable medications or to calculate the medication amount. It is important for you to know the legal scope of practice in your state (see Procedure 3.2, p. 70).

Disciplinary Action

The state boards have an obligation to the public to protect consumers. To do this, state boards take disciplinary action against licensed professionals for felony convictions and unprofessional, improper, or incompetent practice. The following box lists examples of unprofessional conduct for physicians. The following are some of the disciplinary actions state boards can take against healthcare professionals:

- *License revoked*: License is terminated, and the person can no longer practice in that occupation in the state.

Certification and Registration

For some healthcare professional occupations, certification or registry is available. *Certification* is a voluntary process indicating that a person has met predetermined criteria. The certification is granted by a nongovernmental agency, such as a national association. Most certifications require educational preparation and passing the certification exam. Medical assistants can obtain a certification. For advanced practice professionals, many state boards require certification before the professional can apply for a license. Ongoing certification requirements vary by state. In many states, the ongoing certification is voluntary.

Some healthcare occupations have *registration*. People working in a specific occupation have their name entered into an official registry. To become registered, a person must meet requirements. These may include educational training, passing a registry exam, participating in continuing education, and conditions of that registry.

Accreditation

Accreditation differs from licensure and certification. *Accreditation* is a recognition granted by a specific organization to educational, health-care, or managed care organizations that have demonstrated compliance with standards. Common accreditation organizations include:

- *The Joint Commission*: Accredits ambulatory care facilities, hospitals, behavioral healthcare facilities, home healthcare agencies, and laboratory services.
- *National Committee for Quality Assurance (NCQA)*: Accredits health plans (i.e., managed care plans).
- *College of American Pathologists (CAP) Laboratory Accreditation Program*: Accredits medical laboratories.
- *Commission on Accreditation of Allied Health Education Programs (CAAHEP)*: Accredits specific allied health programs, including medical assisting.
- *Accrediting Bureau of Health Education Schools (ABHES)*: Accredits both schools and specific allied health programs, including medical assisting.

There are advantages to being accredited. Students from accredited medical assisting programs can take specific certification examinations. Agencies that have Joint Commission accreditation gain the community's confidence in the quality and safety of the care provided. The accreditation is recognized by insurance companies and may reduce liability insurance costs.

CLOSING COMMENTS

Patient Coaching

As stated in Chapter 1 with GIVE (*g*reet, *i*ntroduce, *v*erify, and *e*xplain), it is important for the medical assistant to explain the procedure or treatment to the patient before it begins. As part of the Patient's Bill of Rights, patients need to be coached on what is going to occur. The medical assistant must use words that the patient understands and answer any patient questions. If the medical assistant does not know the answer, it is important to talk with the provider and then make sure the patient's question gets answered.

Legal and Ethical Issues

Learning about concepts of law is important for all healthcare professionals. The medical assistant is trained to perform administrative, patient care, and laboratory skills that are CLIA-waived (i.e., permitted for medical assistants by the Clinical Laboratory Improvement Amendments). With this wide range of duties, it is critical that the

medical assistant always remember to work within the boundaries of the law and his or her scope of practice.

Areas that can be problematic for medical assistants and may lead to lawsuits include:

- Not following up with patients who call the ambulatory care facility
- Not getting consent before giving a child a vaccination
- Not documenting phone calls, procedures, and treatments
- Identifying oneself as another type of healthcare professional (e.g., a nurse)
- Giving advice to patients without the permission of healthcare providers

With the increase in lawsuits through the years, healthcare professionals must practice within their scope of practice and ensure that patients have no grounds for lawsuits.

Patient-Centered Care

One of the elements of patient-centered care is respect for patients' preferences. The medical assistant may not understand why a patient refuses a test, procedure, or treatment. Some patients do not share their thoughts on such matters. Other patients may cite a personal belief or a religious belief. As a medical assistant, you might not agree with the patient's ideas or beliefs. To provide exceptional customer service, a medical assistant must be sensitive to the patient's rights. This means the medical assistant must be respectful of the patient's right to refuse and must notify the provider. It is not appropriate for the medical assistant to:

- Pressure the patient into changing the refusal.
- Gossip with peers about the patient's refusal.
- Make fun of the patient.

Providing patient-centered care means the medical assistant respects patients and their right to refuse.

> ### Professional Behaviors
> Part of being professional is protecting the healthcare facility and the providers from lawsuits that might stem from one's own actions. The medical assistant is not exempt from being named in lawsuits. Strategies to reduce the risk of lawsuits include:
> - Respecting and communicating professionally with patients
> - Working within one's scope of practice
> - Accurately and concisely documenting all patient encounters
> - Following the facility's policies and procedures

SUMMARY OF SCENARIO

Daniela enjoyed working with Bella as she studied for her midterm exam in her law class. She found that Bella had unique ways of remembering and explaining concepts. These methods helped Daniela. Daniela knew it was important for her to understand the concepts because they might appear on her national certification test.

Daniela now understands the legal importance of answering patients' calls and returning them. She knows this is important to prevent abandonment suits from patients. Daniela encourages her peers to return calls in a timely manner

and has talked with her supervisor about strategies to make the reception desk more efficient.

Thanks to Bella's help, Daniela also realizes the importance of the Patient's Bill of Rights to patients and to every healthcare professional. These rights must be upheld and respected. Medical assistants and other healthcare professionals must be sensitive when patients refuse tests, treatments, and procedures. Daniela is looking forward to studying more about the healthcare laws and learning how they affect her job.

SUMMARY OF LEARNING OBJECTIVES

1. **Discuss the balance of power in the United States and name the four types of laws.**

   The legal system of the United States is made up of both federal and state laws and is designed to allow for a balance of power. The three branches of government are the legislative, executive, and judicial branches. The four types of law are constitutional, case, regulatory and administrative, and statutory law.

2. **Compare criminal and civil law as they apply to the practicing medical assistant.**

   In criminal law, the state or federal government is the plaintiff and the defendant is the party accused. The offense is a crime, and the standard of proof is that the charge must be proved beyond a reasonable doubt. A medical assistant who gives a patient medication without a provider's order is prescribing medication, which is a criminal offense.

   In civil law, the victim is the plaintiff and the person accused is the wrongdoer. The offense can be called a tort or a breach of contract. The standard of proof requires the preponderance of evidence. A medical assistant who does a task within his or her scope of practice based on a provider's order, but does it incorrectly, may be sued.

3. **Differentiate between intentional torts and negligent (unintentional) torts.**

   In an intentional tort, the plaintiff must prove the defendant had specific intent to perform the action that caused the injury. Examples include assault, battery, and false imprisonment. Refer back to the Intentional Tort section to read more about the different types of intentional torts.

   Negligent torts are more common in healthcare because they are unintentional. The harm that is caused by negligence is the result of a person's carelessness. Negligence results when a person's conduct falls below the standard of behavior expected of a reasonable person in the same situation.

4. **Differentiate between standard of care and scope of practice for a medical assistant, define terms related to a civil lawsuit, and explain the 4 _D_s of negligence.**

   Standard of care refers to the level and type of care an ordinary, prudent healthcare professional, having the same training and experience in a similar practice, would have provided in a similar situation. The standard of care takes into account the accused person's skills and knowledge. It also considers the environment.

   The _scope of practice_ for an occupation defines the procedures, actions, and processes that individuals are permitted to perform.

   Terms related to a civil lawsuit include:
   - _Negligence:_ Failure to act as a reasonably prudent person would under similar circumstances; such conduct falls below the standards of behavior established by law for the protection of others against unreasonable risk of harm.
   - _Malpractice:_ A type of negligence in which a licensed professional fails to provide the standard of care, causing harm to a person.
   - _Statute of limitations_: Length of time legal action can be taken after an event has occurred.

- _Subpoena duces tecum:_ A legal document commanding a person to bring a piece of evidence (e.g., the plaintiff's health record) to court.
- _Subpoena:_ A court order requiring a person to appear in court at a specific time to testify in a legal case.
- _Defendant:_ An individual or business against whom a lawsuit is filed.
- _Plaintiff:_ An individual or party who brings the suit to court.
- _Deposition:_ A sworn testimony made before a court-appointed officer; it is used in the discovery process and may be used in the trial.
- _Expert witnesses:_ People who are educated and knowledgeable in the area of concern; they testify in court and provide an expert opinion on the topic of concern.
- _Fact witnesses:_ People who observed the situation and testify in court about the facts of the case.
- _Arbitration:_ The process in which conflicting parties in a dispute submit their differences to a court-appointed person (arbitrator), who submits a legally binding decision.
- _Mediation:_ The process of facilitating conflicting parties to make an agreement, settlement, or compromise.

   The 4 _D_s of negligence:
   - _Duty of care_: The healthcare professional has a legal obligation to the patient. Many times, the duty of care comes from the provider-patient relationship.
   - _Dereliction_: The healthcare professional breached (violated) the duty of care to the patient.
   - _Damages_: The patient suffers a legally recognized injury.
   - _Direct cause_: The breach of duty of care (the negligent act or lack of action) directly causes the patient's injury.

5. **Describe types of professional liability insurance.**
   - _Liability insurance_: Provides protection from claims of injuries or damage to people or property. Different types of liability insurance include:
   - _Professional liability insurance_: A type of liability coverage used by professionals to protect themselves against liability suits incurred because of errors and omissions while performing their professional services. Medical malpractice insurance protects healthcare professionals from liability related to wrongful practices resulting in injury, expense, and property damage. It also covers the cost of defending lawsuits.
   - _General liability_ or _commercial liability insurance_: A type of liability coverage purchased by companies. It protects businesses from lawsuits for property loss and bodily injury from nonemployees.
   - _Personal injury insurance_: A type of liability coverage that protects against claims related to harm other than bodily injury. Coverage can be for invasion of privacy, slander, imprisonment, and so on.

6. **Explain the five elements required for a contract to be legally binding.**

   For a contract to be legally binding, five elements must be present:
   - _Offer_: Made by one party.
   - _Acceptance_: A second party agrees to the offer.

SUMMARY OF LEARNING OBJECTIVES—*continued*

- *Consideration*: Each party exchanges something of value.
- *Legal subject matter*: The consideration must be legal.
- *Competency and capacity*: A person entering into a contract must have the legal capacity to be held liable for the contract's obligation.

7. **Describe the reasons and the steps for terminating the provider-patient relationship.**

Reasons for terminating the provider-patient relationship include:
- Retirement or moving
- Patient is not paying for the services provided
- Patient is not following or is noncompliant with the provider's treatment plan
- Patient's behavior (e.g., rude, abusive, drug seeking, not showing up for appointments)

Steps to terminate the provider-patient relationship include:
- The provider must notify the patient in writing of the withdrawal of care.
- A date must be indicated for the termination. There must be an adequate period of coverage to allow the patient to find another provider. Fifteen to 30 days is usually recommended.
- The termination letter should be sent as a certified letter with return receipt requested.
- A copy of the letter and the return receipt need to be placed or scanned into the patient health record.
- Scheduling staff should be notified of the termination date, so no appointments are made after that date.

8. **Differentiate between implied consent, expressed consent, and informed consent.**
- *Implied consent*: Consent that is inferred based on signs, actions, or conduct of the patient rather than oral communication (using words).
- *Expressed consent*: Consent that is given either by the spoken or written word.
- *Informed consent*: A legal process that ensures that the patient or guardian understands the treatment and gives consent for the treatment.

9. **List who can give consent and who cannot give consent.**

Adults of sound mind can give informed consent. Married minors, minor parents, emancipated minors, and mature minors can also give informed consent. Patients who cannot legally give informed consent include:
- Patients under the influence of alcohol or drugs
- Patients medicated with a preoperative medication that may affect their understanding (e.g., a sedative)
- A minor
- A patient who is mentally incompetent
- A patient who speaks little or no English. (An interpreter must be used for the patient to give informed consent. The interpreter will translate the information from the provider, questions from the patient, and the information on the consent form. It is important to document in the health record that an interpreter was used.)

10. **Summarize the Patient's Bill of Rights.**

The Patient's Bill of Rights provides patients with information on their rights under federal and state laws. Healthcare professionals must ensure they uphold and respect patients' rights. See Fig. 3.3 for the typical parts of the Patient's Bill of Rights.

11. **Describe licensure, certification, registration, and accreditation.**
- *Licensure* is a mandatory process established by state law that ensures a person has met the legal standards for practicing an occupation in that state.
- *Certification* is a voluntary process indicating that a person has met predetermined criteria. The certification is granted by a nongovernmental agency, such as a national association. Most certifications require educational preparation and passing the certification exam.
- Some healthcare occupations have *registration*. People working in a specific occupation have their names entered into an official registry. To become registered, a person must meet certain requirements.
- *Accreditation* is a recognition granted by a specific organization to educational, healthcare, or managed care organizations that have demonstrated compliance with standards.

PROCEDURE 3.1 | Apply the Patient's Bill of Rights

Tasks: Apply the Patient's Bill of Rights in scenarios related to choice of treatment, consent for treatment, and refusal of treatment.

Scenario 1 (Choice of Treatment): Julia Berkley (DOB 07/05/1992) saw Dr. Angela Perez during her entire pregnancy. Julia is experiencing some complications. Dr. Perez explained the choices Julia had for delivery. She stated that, with the complications, a cesarean delivery (C-section) may be the best option. Because you are working with Dr. Perez, you prepare the consent form for the C-section. You go into the exam room to have Julia sign the consent form. As you discuss the form, Julia tells you that she is fearful of a C-section and wants a vaginal delivery.

Scenario 2 (Consent for Treatment): Ken Thomas (DOB 10/25/61) sees Jean Burke, N.P., before leaving on a week-long trip out of the country. He is leaving in 3 days and wants a hepatitis A vaccine injection. The area he is traveling to has a high risk for hepatitis A. Jean Burke orders immunoglobulin for Ken, which will provide immediate protection against hepatitis A. You

Continued

prepare the injection and enter the exam room. As you are telling Ken about the side effects of the medication, he asks, "What is immunoglobulin?" You reply that it is a sterile medication made of antibodies from blood. Ken states that he is a Jehovah's Witness and cannot receive blood products.

Scenario 3 (Refusal of Treatment): Aaron Jackson (DOB 10/17/2011) is brought in by his mother for his well-child checkup. His records indicate that he is due for his first varicella vaccine injection. You bring the Varicella (Chickenpox) Vaccine VIS (vaccine information statement) and the Vaccine Authorization form to the exam room. As you start to discuss the vaccine, Aaron's mother, Patricia, interrupts you and tells you she is not interested in having Aaron get his chickenpox vaccination.

EQUIPMENT and SUPPLIES

- Patient's health records
- Patient's Bill of Rights (see Fig. 3.3)
- General Procedure Consent form (Fig. 3.4)
- Varicella (Chickenpox) VIS (available at *https://www.cdc.gov*)
- Vaccine Authorization form (Fig. 3.5)

PROCEDURAL STEPS

1. Review the Patient's Bill of Rights. Apply the Patient's Bill of Rights as you role-play each of the three scenarios.
   PURPOSE: A medical assistant needs to be knowledgeable about the facility's Patient's Bill of Rights.

FIGURE 3.4 General Procedure Consent Form.

WALDEN-MARTIN
FAMILY MEDICAL CLINIC
1234 ANYSTREET | ANYTOWN, ANYSTATE 12345
PHONE 123-123-1234 | FAX 123-123-5678

Vaccine Authorization

Last Name: _____   First Name: _____

Date of Birth: _____   Sex: ☐ Male ☐ Female

Please answer the following questions:

1. Are you sick or do you have a high fever today? (if yes, you should not receive vaccine)   ☐ Yes ☐ No ☐ Unknown

2. Are you allergic to chicken, eggs, or egg products?   ☐ Yes ☐ No ☐ Unknown

3. Have you ever has an allergic reaction to an injection?   ☐ Yes ☐ No ☐ Unknown

4. Are you pregnant, or think you may be?   ☐ Yes ☐ No ☐ Unknown

5. Do you have a blood clotting disorder or are you taking blood thinning medication?   ☐ Yes ☐ No ☐ Unknown

CONSENT AND RELEASE STATEMENT

I, THE UNDERSIGNED, WISH TO RECEIVE A ------------------- VACCINE. I CONSENT TO THE VACCINATION BEING GIVEN TO ME. I HAVE READ THE PROVIDED INFORMATION OR HAVE HAD SUCH EXPLAINED TO ME. I UNDERSTAND THE RISKS AND BENEFITS OF THIS VACCINE. I HAVE HAD AN OPPORTUNITY TO ASK QUESTIONS WHICH HAVE BEEN ANSWERED TO MY SATISFACTION. I HEREBY REQUEST THAT THE VACCINE BE GIVEN TO ME OR TO THE PERSON NAMED ABOVE FOR WHOM I AM AUTHORIZED TO MAKE THIS REQUEST.

Signature: _____   Date: _____

FIGURE 3.5 Vaccine Authorization Form.

2. Using Scenario 1, role-play the situation with a peer. You are the medical assistant. Demonstrate how a medical assistant should handle the situation. Apply the Patient's Bill of Rights to the situation by remembering the rights of the patient.
   a. Show sensitivity to the patient by being respectful and professional. Be open and accepting in your verbal and nonverbal body language.
   PURPOSE: Being open and accepting shows the patient sensitivity and respect. The medical assistant should never show any mannerisms that would pressure the patient into making a choice that is not what he or she wants.
   b. Ask the patient if she has any questions about the procedure. Let the provider know if the patient has questions.

   PURPOSE: All patient questions need to be addressed before the patient can make an informed decision on the treatment.
   c. Ask the patient what she would like to do. Based on her answer, follow up as necessary.
   PURPOSE: If the patient wants a C-section, then the consent form should be completed. If the patient wants a vaginal delivery, then no consent form will be needed unless indicated by state laws.
   d. Using the health record, document the patient's decision and the name of the provider notified.
   PURPOSE: Documenting the patient's refusal of treatment is important legally. It is also important that the medical assistant document that the provider was informed of the decision.

Continued

PROCEDURE 3.1   Apply the Patient's Bill of Rights—*continued*

3. Using Scenario 2, role-play the situation with a peer. You are the medical assistant. Demonstrate how a medical assistant should handle the situation. Apply the Patient's Bill of Rights to the situation by remembering the rights of the patient.
   a. Show sensitivity to the patient regarding his right to refuse. Be respectful and professional. Be open and accepting in your verbal and nonverbal body language. Be accepting of his beliefs and his refusal.
      PURPOSE: Being open and accepting shows the patient sensitivity and respect. The medical assistant should never show any mannerisms that would pressure the patient into making a choice that is not what he or she wants. The patient has a right to make decisions that follow his religious beliefs.
   b. When the patient refuses the medication, be respectful in your body language and words. Notify the provider.
      PURPOSE: It is important to be respectful of the patient's decision and notify the provider of the refusal.
   c. Using the health record, document the patient's decision and the name of the provider notified.
      PURPOSE: Documenting the patient's refusal of treatment is important legally. It is also important that the medical assistant document that the provider was informed of the decision.
4. Using Scenario 3, role-play the situation with a peer. You are the medical assistant. Demonstrate how a medical assistant should handle the situation.

Apply the Patient's Bill of Rights to the situation by remembering the rights of the patient.
   a. Show sensitivity to the mother of the patient by being respectful and professional. Be open and accepting in your verbal and nonverbal body language.
      PURPOSE: Being open and accepting shows the family member and the patient sensitivity and respect. The medical assistant should never show any mannerisms that would pressure the patient or guardian into making a choice that is not what he or she wants.
   b. Ask the mother if she has any questions about the vaccine. Let the provider know if the mother has questions.
      PURPOSE: All patient and parent/guardian questions need to be addressed before an informed decision can be made on the treatment.
   c. Ask the mother what she would like to do. Based on her answer, follow up as necessary.
      PURPOSE: If the parent/guardian consents to the vaccination, the Vaccine Authorization form must be completed. If the parent/guardian refuses, the provider needs to be notified.
   d. Using the health record, document the patient's decision and the name of the provider notified.
      PURPOSE: Documenting the patient's refusal of treatment is important legally. It is also important that the medical assistant document that the provider was informed of the decision.

PROCEDURE 3.2   Locate the Medical Assistant's Legal Scope of Practice

Tasks: Search online to locate the legal scope of practice for a medical assistant practicing in your state. Summarize the scope of practice.

EQUIPMENT and SUPPLIES
* Computer and printer with word processing software and internet access

PROCEDURAL STEPS

1. Using the internet, search for the medical assistant's scope of practice in your state. Read the scope of practice for your state.
   PURPOSE: Scope of practice information is available online.
2. Using the word processing software, create a short paper summarizing the medical assistant's scope of practice. Address the following points:
   a. Can medical assistants give injections? If so, what type of injections?
   b. Can medical assistants give oral, topical, and/or inhaled medications?
   c. Can medical assistants calculate drug dosages?
   d. What is the medical assistant's role with prescriptions?

   e. Describe additional duties that a medical assistant can legally perform in your state.
   f. Include the website address(es) you used for this paper.
   Note: If your instructor does not provide you with different guidelines for the paper, follow these. Create at least a one-page paper, using double line spacing and a 10 or 12 point font. Margins should be 1 inch for all sides.
   PURPOSE: Summarizing the scope of practice will help identify the duties a medical assistant can legally perform in your state.
3. After completing the paper, proofread the paper. Use correct spelling, punctuation, sentence structure, and capitalization. Make any changes required. Based on your instructor's directions, submit the paper to the instructor.
   PURPOSE: Proofreading helps to identify mistakes.

HEALTHCARE LAWS

4

SCENARIO

Daniela Garcia was recently hired as a part-time float receptionist at Walden-Martin Family Medical (WMFM) Clinic. She works with many co-workers and providers. Daniela is attending the medical assistant program at the local community college. She is currently taking a law and ethics course. She has learned about basic law concepts. She is now learning about healthcare laws. Bella, a newly certified medical assistant (CMA), has offered to help Daniela study for her law course. Bella stated that she enjoyed learning about law and its importance in healthcare.

Many of Daniela's friends find law and ethics to be less exciting than other courses. Daniela disagrees with them. She sees the value in learning about laws that impact healthcare. She realizes it will make her a better medical assistant.

The WMFM Clinic administration created policies and procedures to follow federal and state laws. Daniela has already started to see how compliance with laws impacts what she does as a receptionist. She understands the importance of following the clinic's policies and procedures. Daniela realizes that by not complying with laws, she puts her job in jeopardy. It can also raise many issues for the facility, including fines from governmental agencies. Daniela is excited to continue learning about healthcare laws.

While studying this chapter, think about the following questions:

- What is the importance of the Health Insurance Portability and Accountability Act (HIPAA)? Why should a medical assistant know about the Privacy Rule and the Security Rule?
- What is the impact of the Health Information Technology for Economic and Clinical Health (HITECH) Act to ambulatory care facilities?
- What are important healthcare laws and regulations that must be followed in the ambulatory care environment?
- What is the provider's role in compliance with public health statutes?
- What are compliance programs that address financial, employment, and environmental safety concerns?

LEARNING OBJECTIVES

1. Explain the standards of the Health Insurance Portability and Accountability Act (HIPAA) and discuss HIPAA-related terminology (including covered entities, protected health information, business associate, permission, de-identify, and limited data set).
2. Describe the Health Information Technology for Economic and Clinical Health (HITECH) Act.
3. Describe the important features of the Genetic Information Nondiscrimination Act (GINA), the Food, Drug, and Cosmetic Act, and the Controlled Substances Act.
4. Describe the Patient Protection and Affordable Care Act, the Clinical Laboratory Improvement Amendments (CLIA), the Occupational Safety and Health Act, and the Needlestick Safety and Prevention Act.
5. Discuss Good Samaritan Laws.
6. Define the Patient Self-Determination Act, Uniform Determination of Death Act (UDDA), Uniform Anatomical Gift Act (UAGA), and the National Organ Transplant Act (NOTA).
7. Describe compliance with public health statutes related to communicable diseases and to wounds of violence, abuse, neglect, and exploitation.
8. Describe compliance with reporting vaccination issues.
9. Discuss how compliance programs work, examine common compliance concerns in healthcare, follow protocol in reporting an illegal activity, and correctly complete an incident report.

VOCABULARY

abuse An action that purposely harms another person.

advance directives Written instructions about healthcare decisions in case a person is unable to make them.

breach Disclosure of protected health information without a reason or permission, which compromises the security or privacy of the information.

claims clearinghouse An organization that accepts the claim data from the provider, reformats the data to meet the specifications outlined by the insurance plan, and submits the claim.

coding system A system designed to use characters (i.e., numbers and letters) to represent something like a medical procedure or a disease.

VOCABULARY—continued

communicable diseases Diseases spread from person to person by either direct contact or indirect contact (e.g., insects).

dependent adults People between the ages of 18 and 64 who have a mental or physical impairment that prevents them from doing normal activities or from protecting themselves.

discrimination (dis krim eh NAE shuhn) Unfair treatment of another person based on the person's age, gender (sex), ethnicity, sexual orientation, disability, marital status, or other selective factors.

egress (EE gress) Leaving a place; exit route.

electronic health record (EHR) An electronic record that conforms to nationally recognized standards and contains health-related information about a specific patient. It can be created, managed, and consulted by authorized clinicians and staff from more than one healthcare organization.

electronic transaction The electronic exchange of information between two agencies to accomplish financial or administrative healthcare activities.

exploitation (eks ploi TAY shuhn) The act of using another person for one's own advantage.

harassment (hah RAS ment) Continued, unwanted, and annoying actions done to another person.

neglect Failure to provide proper attention or care to another person.

precedence (PRES i dehns) The top priority.

privileged communication Communication that cannot be disclosed without authorization of the person involved; includes provider-patient and lawyer-client communications.

retaliation (ree tal ee A shuhn) Getting back at others for something they did to you.

retribution (reh trih BYOU shuhn) Punishment inflicted on someone as vengeance for a wrong or criminal act; the act of taking revenge.

whistleblower A person (usually an employee) who reports a violation of the law within the organization. The person reports the information to the public or to a person in authority.

In this chapter, we discuss federal and state laws that impact healthcare. Typically, a few people are the "experts" on healthcare laws in an ambulatory care setting. They work with management to create policies and procedures that follow the laws:

- *Policies* are written principles that provide goals for the employees and the facility. For instance, a policy statement may indicate that patient confidentiality is protected at all times.
- *Procedures* are step-by-step directions. They provide a consistent and repetitive approach to accomplish the goal. For instance, there might be a procedure on how to update patient information while protecting the patient's privacy.

Following the laws is important. Not only does it safeguard patients, it also protects employees and the facility. Facilities that do not comply with laws can be fined and have additional penalties imposed by governmental agencies. Therefore, medical assistants need to be knowledgeable about healthcare laws.

PRIVACY AND CONFIDENTIALITY

Privacy means being free from unwanted intrusion. Privacy was one of the principles our country was built on. The word *privacy* does not appear in the Constitution, but privacy elements appear in the amendments. An *invasion of privacy* is the disclosing of private facts without the consent of the individual. An invasion of privacy is an intentional tort.

Confidentiality is a legally protected right of patients. Healthcare professionals have the duty not to disclose medical, financial, and insurance information unless authorized by the patient. Information is shared during the provider-patient relationship, so creating a trusting relationship is critical (Fig. 4.1). The patient shares sensitive, personal information with the provider, which needs to remain confidential. It cannot be discussed outside of the provider-patient relationship.

All states have laws regarding confidentiality. If the state law is stricter than the federal law, then the state law takes **precedence**. This concept is known as *state preemption*. We will examine the federal laws that relate to privacy and confidentiality in the following sections.

Health Insurance Portability and Accountability Act

With the anticipated changes in healthcare technology (e.g., the electronic health record [EHR]), Congress passed the Health Insurance Portability and Accountability Act of 1996 (HIPAA). The US Department of Health and Human Services (HHS) is the agency responsible for developing the specific requirements of the law. The HHS Office for Civil Rights (OCR) enforces HIPAA.

Before HIPAA, the billing and payment processes were slow. Nationwide, insurance companies used many different **coding**

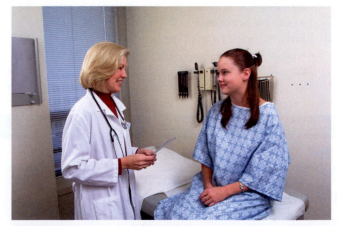

FIGURE 4.1 Patient confidentiality is the most important trust that exists between the patient and the provider.

systems. The coding systems were used to provide information on disease and treatments for payment purposes. It took months for facilities to receive insurance payments for services provided to patients. Paper transactions and paper checks were commonly used.

One of the goals of HIPAA was to simplify the electronic exchange of information. All health plans, **claims clearinghouses**, and healthcare facilities needed to be consistent with their electronic exchange of information. This meant they all needed to use the same coding systems. They also needed to follow the same requirements for the electronic exchange of information. Today, this is called *administrative simplification*. The goal is to reduce clerical burden and increase **electronic transaction** adoption.

With the increased electronic transactions, HIPAA also contained provisions for the privacy and security of the patients' information. Primary provisions of the law were stated in four standards:

- *Standard 1 related to transactions and code sets:* HHS adopted standard transactions for the electronic exchange of administrative healthcare information. This included insurance claims, payment, and insurance eligibility information. The goal was to speed up the process of identifying insurance benefits, submitting insurance claims, and receiving payment. Standard 1 also included mandating universal coding systems. Processes become more efficient with everyone using the same coding systems.
  - The *Current Procedural Terminology* (CPT) is used to code procedures and services.
  - The *International Classification of Diseases* (ICD) is used to code diseases and disorders.
- *Standard 2 related to the Privacy Rule*: Healthcare facilities, insurance companies, and others need to protect written, electronic, and oral patient health information.
- *Standard 3 related to the Security Rule*: Healthcare facilities, insurance companies, and others need to protect patient information that is electronically stored and transmitted.
- *Standard 4 related to unique identifiers:*
  - *National Provider Identifier (NPI)*: Each covered healthcare provider has a unique identification number that is used for financial and administrative transactions. The NPI is a 10-digit number.
  - *Health Plan Identifier (HPI)*: Each health plan has a unique identifier.
  - *Employer Identification Number (EIN)*: Each employer has a unique identifier issued by the Internal Revenue Service.

In addition to these provisions, HIPAA focused on insurance portability. HIPAA allows extra opportunities to enroll in health insurance plans. For instance, a person can request special enrollment if there is a loss in coverage from another policy. HIPAA prohibited enrollment discrimination based on a person's health history or genetics.

HIPAA-Related Terminology

HIPAA has many unique terms, including the following:
- *Covered entities*: Healthcare providers, health (insurance) plans, and claims clearinghouses that transmit protected health information electronically. The following box lists examples of covered entities.

Examples of Covered Entities Under HIPAA

- Providers (medical doctors, doctors of osteopathic medicine, nurse practitioners, physician assistants, etc.)
- Dentists
- Chiropractors
- Psychologists
- Nursing homes
- Pharmacies
- Ambulatory care facilities (e.g., clinics)
- Health insurance companies
- Government insurance programs (Medicare, Medicaid)
- Health maintenance organizations (HMOs)
- Claims clearinghouses
- Billing services

- *Protected health information (PHI)*: Individually identifiable health information stored or transmitted by covered entities or business associates. Includes verbal, paper, or electronic information.
- *Business associate*: A person or business that provides a service to a covered entity that involves access to PHI. Examples include legal, billing, and management services; accreditation agencies; consulting firms; and claims processing organizations.
- *Permission*: A reason for releasing or disclosing patient information under HIPAA.
- *De-identify:* To remove all direct patient identifiers from the PHI. In other words, this is the process for removing anything that can link the information back to a specific person. This process can create the limited data set (Table 4.1).
- *Limited data set*: PHI that has had all of the direct patient identifiers removed. This would include the name, contact information, Social Security number, and so on. The only information left would be health information (see Table 4.1).

CRITICAL THINKING APPLICATION 4.1
Daniela is working with Bella, a medical assistant who has been helping her with the law course. They are reviewing HIPAA. Bella asks Daniela to describe the four HIPAA standards. How might Daniela respond?

TABLE 4.1 Example of PHI Under HIPAA Grouped by Direct Patient Identifiers and Data Set Information

EXAMPLES OF DIRECT PATIENT IDENTIFIERS	EXAMPLES OF LIMITED DATA SET INFORMATION
• Personal demographic information (name, date of birth, address, phone number, Social Security number) • Payment and insurance information	• Physical or mental health conditions • Test results • Medications currently taking • Allergies

Privacy Rule

The HIPAA Privacy Rule has created national standards that protect health records and other patient information. The Privacy Rule's main purpose is to define and limit the situations in which a patient's information can be used or disclosed. The rule also describes the patients' rights over their information. Patients have the right to do the following:

- Examine their health information.
- Obtain a copy of their health records.
- Request corrections to be made if information is incorrect.

Covered entities must comply with the Privacy Rule. They must safeguard all patient information. Covered entities must ensure that business associates also keep PHI private. A written agreement detailing how the business associate will safeguard the PHI must be signed. Covered entities cannot give PHI to business associates until the agreement has been signed. Only PHI required for the job of the business associates can be given.

Legal Example: HIPAA Settlement for Lack of Business Associate Agreement

In 2015 the HHS Office for Civil Rights (OCR) investigated the Center for Children's Digestive Health (CCDH). CCDH failed to obtain a written, signed business associate agreement with Filefax. CCDH disclosed the PHI of at least 10,728 patients to Filefax. In 2017 CCDH paid the HHS $31,000 to settle the potential violations and agreed to implement a corrective action plan.

Resolution Agreement. Retrieved from *https://www.hhs.gov/sites/default/files/ra_cap _ccdh.pdf.*

The Privacy Rule lists *permissions,* or reasons that the health information can be released. The following permissions do not require written authorization from the patient to release PHI:

- *To the individual*: A covered entity can disclose PHI to the patient. If you want a copy of your health record, you can get it without completing a written authorization (record release form).

Patients and Their Health Information

It is understood that the contents of the health record belong to the patient. The physical part of the record belongs to the facility or provider. Patients own the contents and can request a copy of their own record at any time. There are state laws that regulate the release. In most cases, the patient can get a copy and can be told of his or her health information immediately. The following examples illustrate cases in which patients cannot get their information immediately:

- When a provider is treating a patient for emotional or mental conditions, the provider can exercise professional judgment to determine if the records should be released to the patient. This is known as the *doctrine of professional discretion*. The provider may feel that if the patient saw the records, more harm than good would result. For instance, you are obtaining a weight on a patient with an eating disorder. The provider's policy is that you do not share the weight with the patient. The provider makes the decision if the weight is shared. For some patients, a weight gain may harm their current success.

- Another situation in which patients cannot get health information immediately when requested relates to diagnostic tests. In the ambulatory care setting, patients have diagnostic tests done all the time. The provider must review the results before they are given to the patient. After reviewing the results, the provider instructs the medical assistant what to tell the patient. The medical assistant contacts the patient and discusses what the provider stated. After the call, the medical assistant documents the call in the patient health record.

- *Treatment, payment, and healthcare operations (TPO)*: *Treatment* relates to when the covered entity discloses PHI when coordinating or managing healthcare. For instance, you do not need to sign a written authorization for your provider to send a prescription to a pharmacy. *Payment* relates to activities related to payment or reimbursement for services. For instance, if you were not paying your bill, the healthcare facility might turn your account over to a collection agency. They would not need a written authorization from you to disclose your information. *Healthcare operations* relates to the financial, legal, quality improvement, and administrative activities that healthcare facilities need to do to run and support their business.

- *Uses and disclosures with opportunity to agree or object*: The patient can give informal permission when asked outright or can be given an opportunity to agree or object. For example, a patient comes into the exam room with a friend. You ask the patient if she wants the friend to remain. The patient can say yes or no.

- *Incidental use and disclosure*: We need to take reasonable precautions so patient information is not overheard or seen by others. The Privacy Rule does not require that we get written authorization for incidental disclosures. For instance, you take precautions, but you are overheard discussing patient PHI on the phone. There is no need for you to get a written authorization from the patient on the phone for the incidental disclosure.

- *Public interest and benefit activities*: PHI can be released when required by law, law enforcement, and for public health activities. PHI can also be released for research, organ and tissue donation, and for workers' compensation. Funeral directors, coroners, and medical examiners can also obtain PHI.

- *Limited data set*: The direct patient identifiers are removed from the PHI. The remaining information can be used for research, public health purposes, and healthcare operations.

The only permission that requires written authorization from patients is disclosing the PHI to a third party. Examples of this type of disclosure may include when the patient wants another person to be told information or when the patient wants the records transferred to another facility. This may include a life insurance company, an employer for a pre-employment health requirement, another healthcare facility, or the patient's lawyer. In both situations, the patient must sign a form allowing the information to be released. In some agencies, a *disclosure authorization form* (also called an authorization to disclose form) must be completed before information can be shared with another person. The patient must complete a *record release form* before

WALDEN-MARTIN
FAMILY MEDICAL CLINIC
1234 ANYSTREET | ANYTOWN, ANYSTATE 12345
PHONE 123-123-1234 | FAX 123-123-5678

Disclosure Authorization

Full Name: _____ Date of Birth: _____

I hereby authorize _____ to use or disclose my protected health information related to

_____

to _____

Representative's Address:

Purpose:

- I understand that I may inspect or copy the protected health information described by this authorization.
- I understand that, at any time, this authorization may be revoked, when the office that receives this authorization receives a written revocation, although that revocation will not be effective as to the disclosure of records whose release I have previously authorized, or where other action has been taken in reliance on an authorization I have signed. I understand that my health care and the payment for my health care will not be affected if I refuse to sign this form.
- I understand that information used or disclosed, pursuant to this authorization, could be subject to re-disclosure by the recipient and, if so, may not be subject to federal or state law protecting its confidentiality.

Signature of individual or Representative: _____

Date: _____

Authority or Relationship to Individual, if Representative: _____

This authorization will expire on: _____ If no date or event is stated, the expiration date will be six years from the date of this authorization.

The subject of this authorization shall receive a copy of this authorization, when signed.

FIGURE 4.2 Disclosure authorization form.

the records can be transferred. The form names can differ from facility to facility. To make things more interesting, some facilities combine the forms into one document and may call it a release of information authorization, or something similar.

The forms typically require the patient to indicate the information to be released/disclosed. The form must include the patient's name and the date of the request. The person or facility disclosing the information and receiving the information must be indicated. The form must include an expiration date. These forms also include a statement to notify patients of their right to revoke the release.

Disclosure Authorization Process. When patients request their information to be given to another person (e.g., family member, friend), the medical assistants can help. They can assist patients in completing the disclosure authorization form (Fig. 4.2). Once completed, this form must be added to the patient health record.

When a person calls requesting information on a current patient, the medical assistant should first ask the caller's name. The medical

assistant must check to see if the caller is listed on the patient's disclosure authorization form (see Procedure 4.1, p. 88). If that caller's name appears, then, per the facility's policy, the medical assistant can release information about the patient. If the caller's name is not on the form, the medical assistant

- cannot release the patient's information.
- cannot even acknowledge that that person is a patient of the facility.

Applying HIPAA rules is important when protecting a patient's privacy.

In some facilities, the patient supplies a code word or number. This is entered into the patient record. The patient gives this code to family members. When they call the staff and give the code, the staff member can provide an update on the patient. It is understood that the patient gives consent to anyone who received the code. This helps to settle the issue of who is really calling requesting information. The code system may be seen more in the ambulatory surgical departments.

Records Release Process. Patients must complete, date, and sign a (medical) records release form for their records to be transferred to another facility (Fig. 4.3; see Procedure 4.2, p. 88). No records, including images and videos, can be released without the completed form. Release forms may specifically address the release of videos and images. With these forms, patients must indicate they want these to be released. If that is not done, then the videos and images are not released.

Parts of the patient record are held at a higher level of confidentiality. Many release forms require the patient to indicate if psychotherapy notes, substance abuse information, and human immunodeficiency virus (HIV) information should be released. Such information may not be automatically released with the other records due to federal and state legislation.

Under HIPAA, psychotherapy notes are treated with higher levels of confidentiality. *Psychotherapy notes* include the patient-provider details from mental health treatment either from private, group, or family therapy. Psychotherapy notes include what the patient stated during the session and the provider's analysis of the patient's statements and the situation. Psychotherapy notes need to be stored separately from the patient paper health record. If electronic, the access to the psychotherapy notes is limited to those healthcare professionals who work in the mental health area. Additional information from the visit is not held at a higher level of confidentiality and includes prescriptions, session times, types and frequency of treatments, and results of clinical tests.

Drug and alcohol substance abuse and HIV content in patient records also are held at a higher level of confidentiality. There are many federal and state laws that relate to the privacy of these records. The federal statute called Confidentiality of Alcohol and Drug Abuse Patient Records, enforced by a division of HHS, is one example. This law restricts the release and use of patient records that include substance use diagnoses and services. State preemption applies with these privacy laws.

WALDEN-MARTIN
FAMILY MEDICAL CLINIC
1234 ANYSTREET | ANYTOWN, ANYSTATE 12345
PHONE 123-123-1234 | FAX 123-123-5678

Medical Records Release

Patient Name: _____   Date of Birth: _____
SSN: _____   Phone: _____
Address:

I, _____ authorize
to disclose/release the following information (check all applicable):

☐ All Records   ☐ Abstract/Summary
☐ Laboratory/pathology records   ☐ Pharmacy/prescription records
☐ X-ray/radiology records   ☐ Other
☐ Billing records

Note: If these records contain any information from previous providers or information about HIV/AIDS status, cancer diagnosis, drug alcohol abuse, or sexually transmitted disease, you are hereby authorizing disclosure of this information. A copy of this signed authorization must be given to the individual.

These records are for services provided on the following   _____
date(s):

Please send the records listed above to (use additional sheets if necessary):
Name: _____   Phone: _____
Address: Fax: _____

The information may be used/disclosed for each of the following purposes:

☐ At patient's request   ☐ For employment purposes
☐ For patient's health care   ☐ Other
☐ For payment/insurance

This authorization shall expire no later   _____ or upon the following event _____ , and may not
than:
be valid for greater than one year from the date of signature for medical records.

I understand that after the custodian of records discloses my health information, it may no longer be protected by federal privacy laws. I understand that this authorization is voluntary and I may refuse to sign this authorization which will not affect my ability to obtain treatment; receive payment; or eligibility for benefits unless allowed by law. By signing below I represent and warrant that I have authority to sign this document and authorize the use or disclosure of protected health information and that there are no claims or orders that would prohibit, limit, or otherwise restrict my ability to authorize the use or disclosure of this protected health information.

Patient signature _____   Date _____
(or patient's personal representative)

Printed name of patient representative _____   Representative's authority to sign for patient
                                                          (i.e. parent, guardian, power of attorney, executor)

FIGURE 4.3 Medical records release form.

CRITICAL THINKING APPLICATION   4.2
Daniela and Bella are reviewing HIPAA concepts. They start to discuss local news and a case in which a medical assistant snaps a picture of a patient record and posts it to a popular social media site. Bella asks Daniela what this act violated. How would you answer this question? Why are employee cell phones a risk in the healthcare setting?

Security Rule

HIPAA's Security Rule addresses the national standards used to protect electronic protected health information (ePHI). This rule covers the records that are created, used, received, and maintained by the covered entities. Safeguards important to ensure the security of the ePHI include the following:

- *Administrative safeguards*: The security officer is responsible for creating and carrying out security policies and procedures. Potential risks to the ePHI must be identified. Steps must be taken to prevent any issues. Cyber attackers pose a huge risk to network security.

- *Physical safeguards*: Facility, workstation, and device security must be implemented. A security officer must create procedures for the proper use of workstations and ePHI.
- *Technical safeguards*: Only authorized employees should have access to ePHI. Safeguards include audits to track activities of users with the ePHI. They also include safeguards to prevent improper alteration, destruction, or transmission of ePHI.

Legal Example: Cyber Attackers Breach Insurer's Database

In 2015 Anthem, Inc., the second largest insurer in the United States, announced that cyber attackers had breached its database. The PHI for almost 80 million people (e.g., names, birth dates, Social Security numbers, addresses, employment information, and email addresses) was compromised. Anthem agreed to pay $115 million to settle the class-action lawsuit.

Chapter 8 provides additional information on network security procedures. It is important for the medical assistant to follow the facility's electronic security procedures. Many facilities have policies to keep passwords confidential. Downloading personal documents puts the computer network at risk and thus is not allowed. Audit trails monitor who is looking at which patient's chart. If the medical assistant is not working with a specific patient, then the patient record should not be accessed. Violating this rule will cause the medical assistant to breach the patient's confidentiality and security. Many healthcare professionals, from providers to medical assistants, have breached confidentiality. They have lost their jobs and licenses or certifications. Many have also been fined.

Legal Example: HIPAA Settlement for Inappropriate PHI Access

In 2012 Memorial Healthcare System (MHS) submitted a breach report to HHS indicating that two of its employees inappropriately accessed PHI, potentially impacting 80,000 patients. Several months later MHS notified HHS of another 12 users that inappropriately accessed PHI, which potentially impacted another 105,646 individuals. As a result, some of the PHI was sold and fraudulent tax returns were filed. In 2017 MHS paid the HHS $5.5 million to settle the potential violations and agreed to implement a corrective action plan.

Resolution Agreement. Retrieved from *https://www.hhs.gov/sites/default/files/memorial-ra-cap.pdf*.

Health Information Technology for Economic and Clinical Health Act

One of the issues with HIPAA was the limited enforcement and penalties. In 2009, as part of the American Recovery and Reinvestment Act, the Health Information Technology for Economic and Clinical Health (HITECH) Act was passed. HITECH is enforced by the OCR. The HITECH Act contains provisions that increased the enforcement of the privacy and security of electronic transmission

and health information. HITECH modified HIPAA in the following ways:

- Made business associates directly liable for compliance with HIPAA.
- Prohibited the sale of PHI without the patient's authorization.
- Created a tiered violation category that included unknowing, reasonable cause, willful neglect–corrected, and willful neglect–uncorrected. Violation penalties go from $100 for each "unknowing" violation to $1.5 million per calendar year. The greater the violation, the greater the penalty amount. Individuals, healthcare agencies, and business associations could be penalized and fined.
- **Breach** notification requirements were increased. Individuals must be notified of the breach via mail or email. If the facility does not have up-to-date contact information for 10 or more patients, then a notice must be posted on the company's website for at least 90 days. If more than 500 individuals were affected, then the media and the OCR secretary must be notified. A list of breaches reported is published on the OCR website (*https://ocrportal.hhs.gov/ocr/breach/breach_report.jsf*).

It is important for the medical assistant to be aware of the importance of keeping the PHI secure. Any breaches or loss/theft of computer equipment must be reported immediately to the facility's security officer.

CRITICAL THINKING APPLICATION 4.3
Daniela and Bella are reviewing HITECH. Daniela asks Bella why it is important for large breaches to be posted on the OCR website. How would you answer this question as an employee? How would you answer as a patient of a facility that had a posting on the OCR website?

Genetic Information Nondiscrimination Act

The Genetic Information Nondiscrimination Act (GINA) became law in 2008. It modified HIPAA and increased the protection for individuals. GINA prohibits genetic discrimination in health coverage and employment.

ADDITIONAL HEALTHCARE LAWS AND REGULATIONS

This section presents additional laws that impact healthcare. Throughout the textbook, these laws and others will be discussed in more depth. This chapter introduces the more common laws that impact ambulatory healthcare.

Drug Laws
Food, Drug, and Cosmetic Act
In 1906, the Food and Drug Act became law. It prohibited the misbranding of food and drugs. It was replaced in 1938 by the Food, Drug, and Cosmetic Act, which is still enforced today. The Food and Drug Administration (FDA) enforces the act. The FDA is responsible for the safety, effectiveness, security, and quality of drugs, cosmetics, and food. Some of the areas overseen by the FDA include human and veterinary drugs, vaccines, biologic products (e.g., blood components), medical devices, food, cosmetics, dietary

TABLE 4.2   Schedules of Drugs, Substances, and Chemicals

SCHEDULE	PSYCHOLOGICAL AND PHYSICAL DEPENDENCE	EXAMPLES
I	Highest potential for abuse; drugs with no currently accepted medical use	• *Examples:* Heroin, lysergic acid diethylamide (LSD), ecstasy
II/IIN (C–II)	High level of abuse and can lead to severe psychological or physical dependence	• *Schedule II narcotics:* oxycodone (OxyContin, Percocet), fentanyl (Duragesic), codeine, morphine • *Schedule IIN stimulants:* amphetamine (Adderall), methamphetamine (Desoxyn), methylphenidate (Concerta, Ritalin LA)
III/IIIN (C–III)	Moderate to low physical dependence or high psychological dependence	• *Schedule III narcotics:* acetaminophen with codeine (Tylenol #2 or #3), buprenorphine (Suboxone) • *Schedule IIIN non-narcotics:* ketamine, anabolic steroids (e.g., Depo-Testosterone)
IV (C–IV)	Low potential for abuse relative to substances in schedule III	• *Schedule IV:* alprazolam (Xanax), clonazepam (Klonopin), diazepam (Valium), lorazepam (Ativan)
V (C–V)	Lowest potential for abuse relative to substances listed in schedule IV; contains limited quantities of certain narcotics	• *Schedule V substances:* Robitussin AC, ezogabine (Potiga)

Information obtained from the Drug Enforcement Agency (https://www.deadiversion.usdoj.gov/schedules/) on 01/08/2019.

supplies, and products that give off radiation. When you see recalls of food, cosmetics, or medications, the FDA is involved with the process.

The FDA website (*www.fda.gov*) provides useful information for the healthcare facility. The website is the resource for information and recalls on the areas overseen by the FDA. Many times, the medical assistant is responsible for maintaining the stock medications and equipment in the department. Any medications or medical devices recalled need to be removed immediately and not used. The providers should be notified of recalls.

Controlled Substances Act

The Controlled Substances Act (part of the Comprehensive Drug Abuse Prevention and Control Act of 1970) is a federal law. The US Drug Enforcement Agency (DEA) enforces the law. The DEA oversees the manufacturing, importation, possession, use, and distribution of certain drugs and chemicals. The DEA handles both illegal and legal drugs. The Controlled Substances Act has five schedules of medications. These schedules are arranged from greatest to least abuse potential (Table 4.2). State statutes also address procedures related to scheduled medications. Some scheduled medication prescriptions are handled differently, which will be discussed in Chapter 14. It is important for the medical assistant to be aware of the schedule of medications.

Each provider prescribing scheduled medications needs to have a unique DEA number. The DEA number needs to be renewed every 3 years. The medical assistant may need to assist the provider in renewing or obtaining a DEA number. This can be done at the DEA website (*www.deadiversion.usdoj.gov*).

Insurance Law
Patient Protection and Affordable Care Act

The Patient Protection and Affordable Care Act is commonly known as the Affordable Care Act. This federal statute was signed into law in 2010. The goal of the law was to provide Americans with affordable health insurance. It also attempted to reform the healthcare system and reduce healthcare spending. A few of the reforms include the following:

• Insurance coverage of preventive services and immunizations.
• People with preexisting health conditions cannot be dropped or charged more for insurance.
• Dependents can stay on their parent's insurance plan until age 26.
• Large businesses have to provide insurance to full-time workers. Small businesses are eligible for tax credits to help offer insurance coverage to their employees.
• The Physician Payments Sunshine Act (PPSA), part of the law, increases the transparency between providers, teaching hospitals, and manufacturers of medical products (e.g., drugs and medical devices). The manufacturers must report any payments and transfers of value (e.g., gifts, meals) to the Open Payments Program of the Centers for Medicare and Medicaid Services (CMS).

Medical Laboratory Regulations
Clinical Laboratory Improvement Amendments

Congress passed the Clinical Laboratory Improvement Amendments (CLIA) in 1988. CLIA establishes quality standards and regulates laboratory testing. The quality standards focus on accuracy, reliability, and timeliness of test results. The federal agencies involved with administering CLIA include:

- *The Food and Drug Administration (FDA)*: Oversees the medical laboratory tests. Categorizes the tests based on the complexity: waived, moderate, or high complexity. High complexity laboratories can perform more tests than waived complexity laboratories.
- *Centers for Medicare and Medicaid Services (CMS)*: Inspects laboratories and issues certificates. Enforces compliance with regulations.
- *Centers for Disease Control and Prevention (CDC)*: Develops standards and laboratory practice guidelines. Develops professional information and resources mostly related to health and disease topics (*www.cdc.gov*). (The CDC, a division of HHS, focuses on disease control and prevention, environmental health, and health promotion; thus, its overall mission is to improve the health of the people.)

All agencies providing clinical laboratory services, including ambulatory care laboratories, must meet the CLIA requirements. The laboratories must have a CLIA certificate to operate and must be certified by the state. Smaller ambulatory care laboratories have one of the following certificates:

- *Certificate of Waiver*: Allows the facility to perform CLIA-waived tests, which are simple and accurate with little risk for error if done correctly. A urine pregnancy test is a waived test.
- *Certificate for Provider-Performed Microscopy Procedures (PPMP)*: Allows the provider to perform only specific microscopy procedures and waived tests.

Additional certificates are obtained by larger laboratories. These laboratories perform more complex tests.

Workplace Safety Laws

Occupational Safety and Health Act

The Occupational Safety and Health Act of 1970 (OSH Act) is enforced by the Occupational Safety and Health Administration (OSHA). Based on this act, OSHA sets workplace standards and conducts inspections to ensure employee safety. Employers must comply with all of OSHA's regulations. Table 4.3 addresses the OSHA standards in healthcare.

CRITICAL THINKING APPLICATION   **4.4**

Daniela is reading about OSHA. She thinks back to what she has heard about OSHA in other businesses. What have you heard about OSHA in other businesses? Is OSHA's role in that company similar to its role in healthcare? Explain.

Needlestick Safety and Prevention Act

The Needlestick Safety and Prevention Act was signed into law in 2000. The goal of the act was to reduce the risk of healthcare workers' exposure to bloodborne diseases. The act required OSHA to update its Bloodborne Pathogens Standard. The revised standards apply to all employees with anticipated occupational exposure to blood or

---

TABLE 4.3 OSHA Standards Related to Healthcare

STANDARD	SUMMARY	EXAMPLES OF WORKPLACE APPLICATION
Bloodborne pathogens	Protects healthcare workers against the hazards caused by bloodborne pathogens.	Exposure control plans, universal precautions, safety needles, personal protective equipment, hepatitis B vaccination, and record keeping.
Hazard communication	Requires employers to provide information about the chemical hazards in the workplace. The *General Duty Clause* states that any equipment that can pose a health danger must be considered a hazard.	All chemicals are labeled. A Safety Data Sheet (SDS) must be available for each chemical in the workplace. Employees must be trained in how to handle the chemical hazards in the workplace.
Occupational exposure to hazardous chemicals in laboratories	Also called the "laboratory standard." Specifies the requirements of a Chemical Hygiene Plan (CHP).	The CHP is a written program that includes the policies, procedures, and responsibilities that protect employees from hazardous chemicals. The CHP describes the appropriate handling of chemicals in the laboratory.
Ionizing radiation	Addresses the protections needed when working with ionizing radiation (i.e., x-rays).	Signs posted where x-rays are taken. Employees wear personal radiation monitors to detect radiation amounts. X-ray rooms are built with protected areas for the employee. X-ray exposure is limited if the employee is pregnant.
Nonionizing radiation	Addresses the protections needed in place when working with nonionizing radiation (i.e., lasers).	Signs need to be posted on the door of a room where lasers are being used. Appropriate eye protection must be worn at all times by both the patient and the employees. Goal is to prevent blindness, retinal burns, and eye damage due to the radiation.
Means of egress	Addresses the exit routes in a building.	Employers are responsible for having appropriate building exit routes. Routes are posted. Exits are unlocked and clear in case of emergency.

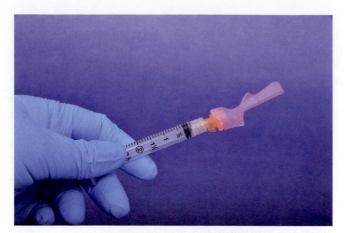

FIGURE 4.4 A safety needle device.

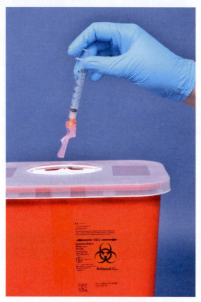

FIGURE 4.5 Used needles need to be placed in a biohazard sharps container.

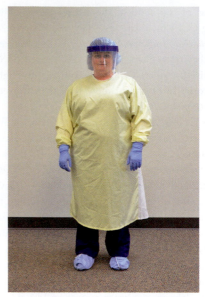

FIGURE 4.6 Personal protective equipment.

other potentially infectious materials (OPIM). The impact of this act include the following:

- Healthcare workers must use safer medical devices. For example, many needles can be capped with a special safety device after use (Fig. 4.4).
- The facility's Exposure Control Plan must include a sharps injury log documenting all instances of injuries from sharps (e.g., used needles, blades).
- Used needles, blades, and other sharps must be put in sharps disposal containers (Fig. 4.5).
- Personal protective equipment (PPE) (i.e., gloves, mask, and gown) must be worn if there is a risk of blood or body fluid exposure (Fig. 4.6).

Good Samaritan Laws

Good Samaritan laws are state laws that provide legal protection for those assisting an injured person during an emergency. If possible, the injured person needs to agree to the help. The person responding must meet the following criteria:

- Not be paid for the care given.
- Act reasonably, exercising the same standard of care (for their profession) within the limitations of the emergency.

- Not act negligently or recklessly; such action makes the responder liable for damages.

The Good Samaritan law does not mean you cannot be sued. In some states, healthcare professionals who do not assist another person in an emergency can be held liable. It is important to be aware of your state's Good Samaritan law and find out if medical assistants have an obligation to stop and provide first aid.

> **CRITICAL THINKING APPLICATION   4.5**
> Daniela is reviewing Good Samaritan laws. How might she describe these laws in terms of importance during an emergency situation?

Laws for End-of-Life Issues

A medical assistant should be aware of laws that relate to end-of-life issues. A brief summary of acts that relate to advance directives, organ donation, and determining death include:

- *Patient Self-Determination Act:* Requires most healthcare institutions to inform patients of their right to make decisions and the facility's policies respecting advance directives.
- *Uniform Determination of Death Act (UDDA):* Served as a guide for state lawmakers to create their own laws that define death.
- *Uniform Anatomical Gift Act (UAGA):* Purpose of the act was to make organ donation easier for people.
- *National Organ Transplant Act (NOTA):* Established the Organ Procurement and Transplant Network (OPTN) and also established a national registry for organ matching.

These acts will be discussed in depth in Chapter 5.

COMPLIANCE REPORTING

Healthcare agencies and employees are required to comply with all federal and state laws and regulations. There are several areas of compliance that the healthcare facility must focus on. Administrators must have policies and procedures in place for employees to report issues. Reports need to be followed up on. Documentation may need to be done for federal or state agencies regarding compliance issues. Healthcare providers also need to report specific diseases, injuries, and issues with vaccines. We will focus on compliance that occurs in ambulatory care facilities.

Compliance with Public Health Statutes

Public health statutes exist in each state to help promote the health of the residents. According to these statutes, healthcare providers have a responsibility to report specific information to various authorities, including:

- Births and deaths
- Specific diseases
- Sexually transmitted infections (STIs)
- Specific injuries related to violence
- Abuse, neglect, and exploitation

These topics will be examined closer in the following sections.

Per the HIPAA permission "public interest and benefit activities," PHI can be released when required by law, law enforcement, and for public health activities. For the mandatory reporting situations based on state statutes, the provider can release PHI without the patient's authorization.

Reportable Diseases

Reportable diseases are communicable diseases that have a significant public health impact. When a provider diagnoses a reportable disease, the state's public health department must be notified. This notification process is called disease reporting. Each state has statutes that address disease reporting. Lists of reportable diseases and reporting requirements are typically available on the state's public health department website. The following are examples of reporting levels and reporting procedures, though each state may be slightly different:

- *Urgent reporting*: For diseases such as hepatitis A, food or water disease outbreaks, pertussis (whooping cough), measles, plague, and tuberculosis. Reporting must be done immediately, usually by phone or fax.
- *Less urgent reporting*: For diseases such as sexually transmitted infections; hepatitis B, C, D, and E; legionellosis, Lyme disease, mumps, bacterial meningitis, malaria, tetanus, varicella (chickenpox), and toxic shock syndrome. Reporting may be done electronically, by mail or fax. The provider usually has up to 3 days to file the report.
- *Highly confidential reporting*: For diseases such as acquired immune deficiency syndrome (AIDS) and HIV infection. The provider may need to mail the paperwork to increase confidentiality.

Disease reporting procedures and regulations may vary by state. The medical assistant should be aware of the state's disease reporting process. The provider may ask the medical assistant to contact the public health department regarding a new reportable disease case (see Procedure 4.3, p. 89).

CRITICAL THINKING APPLICATION   4.6

Daniela is learning about public health statutes and reporting obligations of providers. Why is it important for the public health services to be notified about specific diseases?

Wounds of Violence

Most state statutes require healthcare providers to report cases of violence. Statutes vary from state to state. Typically, reportable cases include wounds caused by gunshots and stabbings; specific types of burns; and nonaccidental wounds caused by a knife, an axe, or a sharp pointed instrument. The medical assistant should be aware of the state's statutes for reporting wounds of violence. In some cases, the medical assistant may need to assist the provider in preparing documents for law enforcement for such cases.

CRITICAL THINKING APPLICATION   4.7

Daniela is learning about public health statutes and the reporting obligations of providers. Why is it important for law enforcement to be notified about cases of violence?

Child Abuse, Neglect, and Exploitation

The Federal Child Abuse Prevention and Treatment Act (CAPTA) aided the states as state statutes were drafted. The act was updated by the CAPTA Reauthorization Act of 2010. This updated act defined child abuse and neglect as follows:

1. Any recent act or failure to act on the part of a parent or caretaker that results in death, serious physical or emotional harm, sexual abuse, or **exploitation**; or
2. An act or failure to act that presents an imminent risk of serious harm.

These definitions set the minimum standard for describing child abuse and neglect. States typically address child maltreatment in both civil and criminal statutes.

All states and territories require child maltreatment to be reported. Most states mandate specific professionals to report any child maltreatment, including school personnel, social workers, healthcare providers, nurses, mental health professionals, child care providers, medical examiners or coroners, and law enforcement officers. Some states require anyone who suspects child abuse or neglect to report the situation (Table 4.4). Mandatory reporters need to provide the facts. They do not have to prove that abuse or neglect occurred. Most state statutes do not consider abuse and neglect information as **privileged communication** between the patient and the provider. This allows the provider to report the information (and thus protect the maltreated child). The medical assistant should be aware of the state statutes regarding child maltreatment. The Child Welfare Information Gateway website (*www.childwelfare.gov*) can be used as a resource for state reporting information.

CRITICAL THINKING APPLICATION   4.8

Daniela is learning about child abuse and neglect. How might she describe the difference between abuse and neglect? Why is this information important for medical assistants to know?

The Unborn Victims of Violence Act was signed into law by Congress in 2004. Prior to this act, *babies in utero* (also called fetuses) harmed or killed due to violence were not considered victims. This act considers babies in utero who are harmed or killed during certain acts of violence to be victims, and charges could be brought forth.

TABLE 4.4   Types of Child Neglect and Abuse

CHILD MALTREATMENT		DESCRIPTION
Neglect	Physical	Failure to provide adequate nutrition, clothing, shelter, and hygiene. Child has poor growth and hygiene and may hide food for later.
	Educational	Failure to enroll child in school or to home-school child. Child may have a poor school attendance record.
	Medical	Failure to provide needed care for injury, impairment, or illness. Child may have untreated injuries. May see developmental delays from lack of therapy to help with impairment.
Abuse	Physical	Bruises, fractures, or burns that are unexplained or do not match the explanation given; untreated dental or medical problems.
	Sexual	Sexual behaviors inappropriate for child's age; sexually transmitted infections, genital pain and bruising, bleeding.
	Emotional	Delayed emotional development, loss of self-confidence, social withdrawal, headaches, depression, poor school performance.

Adult Abuse, Neglect, and Exploitation

In 1965 the Older Americans Act was signed into law. The purpose of the act was to maintain the rights and dignity of the older person. It also created the Administration on Aging. Since then, several federal laws have been passed to help fund federal programs.

Abuse, neglect, and exploitation of older adults and **dependent adults** are dealt with in state statutes. All states have the following:

- Adult or elder protective services statutes that provide reporting and investigating procedures for elder abuse in the state.
- Statutes that establish a Long-Term Care Ombudsman Program that advocates for the safety and rights of long-term care facility residents.
- General criminal statutes on fraud, sexual assault, battery, and other abuses that can relate to elder abuse.

Some states require financial institutions (banks) to report suspected financial abuse or exploitation of older adults.

The state statute will dictate who are mandated reporters, when to report, and how to report the situation. Many ambulatory healthcare facilities are screening older adults to identify those who do not feel safe in their living conditions. If the medical assistant suspects abuse, neglect, or exploitation of an older person, it is important to bring it to the provider's attention. Typically, the provider is a mandated reporter under state law. If the provider suspects neglect, abuse, or exploitation, then a report needs to be filed.

State statutes on domestic violence and abuse vary. In some cases, the reporting for injuries caused by violence covers some domestic abuse situations. Some states have mandatory reporting for domestic violence. It is recommended that providers talk to the victim of the domestic violence. They should inform the person when it must be reported. In states where domestic violence is not a mandatory reporting situation, providers can encourage the victim to report the situation. Safe houses are also available in many areas for victims. Having information on local resources for domestic abuse is important in the ambulatory care setting. Providing the information in restrooms is very common. Typically, that might be the only location where the abuser does not follow the victim. It is important to remember that both men and women can be victims of domestic abuse.

Reporting Vaccination Issues

When a healthcare provider orders a vaccine to be given to a child, the medical assistant must provide the parent or guardian with a Vaccine Information Statement (VIS). This document reviews the reasons for and the risks of the vaccine. Prior to giving the vaccine, the medical assistant must have the parent or guardian sign a consent form allowing the administration of the immunization.

If a patient is having an unusual side effect from a vaccine, the provider might need to file a report with the Vaccine Adverse Event Reporting System (VAERS). Patients and families can also file a report. VAERS is a national surveillance program that monitors vaccine safety. It collects information on unusual vaccine side effects. VAERS is co-sponsored by the CDC and FDA.

In 1986 the National Childhood Vaccine Injury Act was passed. It created the National Vaccine Injury Compensation Program (VICP). This program provides compensation for children injured by childhood vaccines. The VICP lifts the burden of lawsuits from vaccine manufacturers and healthcare providers. The VIS contains information about VICP for patients' families.

Compliance Programs

A compliance program or corporate compliance is a program within a business that detects and prevents violations of state and federal laws. An effective compliance program helps protect the organization from fines and lawsuits. Most compliance programs have reporting mechanisms (i.e., a toll-free number or website) where employees can report suspected violations, suspected illegal activity, fraud, abuse, safety issues, and noncompliance issues. It is important for employees to be able to report issues without fear of retaliation and retribution. Many times, reports can be submitted anonymously.

If a medical assistant needs to report a situation, it is important to follow the healthcare facility's policies and procedures. Different reporting pathways are seen in ambulatory care settings:

- *If the facility has a compliance reporting procedure*: A report can be filed through the compliance reporting mechanisms available to the employee.
- *If the facility does not have a compliance reporting procedure*: The employee may need to report the situation using the chain

of command. This means the employee must report the issue to the supervisor. If the supervisor was involved with the situation, then the employee must report the issue to the supervisor's supervisor.

- *For employment or conflict-of-interest issues*: Some agencies require the employee to contact the human resources supervisor.

In the following sections, we will examine the more common compliance concerns in healthcare.

Financial Concerns

Financial concerns relate to financial and property theft, identity theft, conflict of interest, and fraud. Theft can be of drugs, equipment, supplies, or money. *Identity theft* occurs when someone sells or uses another person's personal information for financial gain. In healthcare, medical identity theft occurs. When a person poses as another person during a healthcare visit, this is considered medical identity theft, because the wrong person's insurance is getting billed for the services. To prevent medical identity theft, many agencies are doing the following:

- Requiring photo identification during the check-in process for visits and services
- Taking the patient's picture, which is uploaded to the electronic health record for future reference

Conflict of interest relates to any financial interest, personal or professional activity, or obligation that impacts a person's objectivity when performing the job. For instance, a provider owns stock in a pharmaceutical company. This provider then prescribes medications made by that company. The provider is benefiting from patients purchasing medications from that company.

Fraud is a deceitful action that causes another to give up something of value. Healthcare fraud is prevalent. Some experts have concluded that Medicare fraud totals more than $60 billion a year. Examples of healthcare fraud include the following:

- Providers and agencies bill for services that were not provided.
- Information is falsified for payment.
- Services are overcharged.
- Medical identification theft occurs.

The list of fraud examples is long. The Office of Inspector General of the HHS oversees fighting fraud and abuse in governmental programs. The following are federal laws that address fraud in healthcare:

- *Anti-Kickback Statute (AKS)*: Since 1972, this federal statute has prohibited intentionally receiving or giving anything of value to get referrals or generate federal healthcare program business.
- *False Claims Act (FCA)*: Originally signed into law during the American Civil War in 1863 and revised in 2010. It prohibits a person from submitting false or fraudulent Medicare or Medicaid claims for payment. Under this act, a person can bring a civil suit on behalf of the government when he or she finds others sending false claims to the government for payment. The individual can receive part of the settlement.
- *Stark Law* (also called the *Physician Self-Referral Law*): Became law in 1989 and became effective in 1992. Several revisions have occurred since then. It prohibits a healthcare provider from referring a Medicare patient for services to a facility with which the provider or the provider's immediate family has a financial relationship.
- *Healthcare Fraud Statute*: Originated in 1996 and revised in 2010. It prohibits intentionally defrauding any healthcare benefit program.

Legal Example: False Claim Act Violations

A lawsuit alleged that Berkeley Heart Lab, Inc., paid kickbacks to physicians and patients to use the company for blood testing. The kickbacks were disguised as "processing and handling" fees. Patients received kickbacks in the form of waived copayments, which they were legally required to pay for the services provided. The government also alleged that unnecessary cardiovascular tests were being charged to Medicare and TRICARE programs. Quest acquired Berkeley in 2011 and ended the practice of kickbacks. In 2017 Quest Diagnostics., Inc., agreed to pay $6 million to resolve a lawsuit by the United States.

From *United States ex rel. Mayes v. Berkeley HeartLab Inc., et al.,* Case No. 9:11-cv-01593-RMG (D.S.C.).

A medical assistant should be aware of the laws related to fraud and conflict of interest. If violations or illegal activities are noticed in the workplace, the medical assistant should follow the reporting procedures outlined in the facility's compliance program (see Procedure 4.4, p. 90). Conflicts of interest need to be reported immediately to the human resources supervisor or to your supervisor.

CRITICAL THINKING APPLICATION 4.9
Daniela and Bella are studying compliance. They start to discuss the importance of declaring a conflict of interest. Describe why being upfront and notifying administration/human resources about a conflict of interest is important in healthcare.

Employment Concerns

Employment concerns relate to discrimination, harassment, retaliation and retribution, and unfair employment practices. In many states, most medical assistant positions are considered *employment-at-will*. This means that the employer can end employment at any time for any reason. Many states recognize this concept. It also means the employee can quit at any time for any reason, though giving a 2-week notice is considered professional. Most jobs are considered employment-at-will.

Employers cannot fire an employee for an illegal reason. The employer needs to have a *just cause*, or legal reason, for firing an employee. Legal reasons could include terminations due to cutbacks in staffing or an employee's behavioral issues. A terminated employee may have an opportunity to sue if wrongful termination occurred. *Wrongful termination* means that the employer did not have just cause for firing the employee. For instance, an employee reported that fraud was occurring in the billing department at the facility. The facility then is under investigation for the fraud. The supervisor fires the **whistleblower**. Federal and state laws protect the whistleblower from retaliation and retribution.

Many federal laws regulate issues regarding employment. The following are laws that address discrimination in the workplace:

- *National Labor Relations Act*: Also called the Wagner Act of 1935. It gave the right to most workers to organize or join a union.
- *Title VII of the Civil Rights Act of 1964 (Title VII)*: Prohibits employment discrimination based on color, race, gender, religion, or national origin.

- *Age Discrimination in Employment Act of 1967 (ADEA)*: Revised several times. It protects applicants and employers 40 years and older from discrimination and includes hiring, promotion, termination, and compensation practices.
- *Rehabilitation Act of 1973*: Prohibits discrimination in employment practices based on physical or mental disabilities. This act applies to federal employers or employers that are federal contractors (provide services to the federal government).
- *Pregnancy Discrimination Act of 1978*: Amended Title VII of the Civil Rights Act of 1964. This act prohibits gender discrimination based on pregnancy.
- *Title I and Title V of the Americans with Disabilities Act of 1990 (ADA)*: Prohibits employment discrimination against qualified persons with disabilities.
- *Genetic Information Nondiscrimination Act of 2008 (GINA)*: Prohibits employment discrimination based on the person's genetic information.
- *Civil Rights Act of 1991*: Provides punitive damages in cases of intentional employment discrimination.

Legal Example: Wrongful Termination and Invasion of Privacy

The plaintiff was a security guard at Children's Hospital. He was involved in an accident while on the job. He was examined at the emergency department, given a painkiller, and released. There was no record of intoxication or impairment. The next day, while recovering at home, he was called to the hospital to submit to a drug test. The test was positive for hydrocodone, and the hospital terminated him based on its drug-free workplace policy. He had been an employee for 18 years and had a clean record with no work-related accidents or drug abuse issues. The plaintiff sued the hospital for wrongful termination, invasion of privacy, and defamation. The case went through mediation, and the hospital offered $40,000 to settle. With no resolution, the case was brought to trial. After deliberation, the 12-member jury came back with a 12–0 decision for the plaintiff. He was awarded $385,050 for past and future economic loss and $650,000 for past and future emotional distress. The total verdict for the plaintiff was $1,035,050.

From *Mckinley Nou v. Children's Hospital Central California,* (October 16, 2014) Fresno Superior Court, Case Number: 12-CECG-02169.

Legal Example: Whistleblower Retaliation

According to a complaint, psychologist Melody Jo Samuelson was hired by Napa State Hospital in California. For 2 years she received good reviews, and then she testified in a case in which she alleged that a patient had been improperly assessed as competent to stand trial. In court she indicated the hospital did not use adequate methods to analyze patients. She complained that the hospital immediately retaliated against her, and she was fired from her job. She appealed her firing and filed a whistleblower retaliation complaint. She was reinstated, but the retaliation continued, she stated. She claimed anxiety and depression as a result of the situation. She was awarded $1 million.

From *Samuelson v. California Department of Mental Health, et. al.,* No. 26-57631 (N.D.Cal. Feb. 20, 2014).

Americans with Disabilities Act and the Rehabilitation Act of 1973

People with disabilities have a right to accessible healthcare. The Americans with Disabilities Act (ADA) prohibits discrimination against individuals with disabilities in everyday activities including getting healthcare. The Rehabilitation Act of 1973 prohibits discrimination against individuals with disabilities in services that receive federal financial assistance, including healthcare services. These laws require that healthcare agencies make their services accessible to people with disabilities.

Examples of how these laws impact ambulatory care facilities:

- *Patients in wheelchairs:* These patients need to be moved to exam tables when the exam requires the patient to be lying down. Lifts and low exam tables are available to help in these situations. Patients with disabilities cannot be denied care on the grounds that accessible medical equipment is not available.
- *Patients with disabilities:* If a patient has an interpreter or a companion, it is important that the healthcare provider focus on the patient.
- *Exam table location:* Patients must have a minimum of 30 inches by 48 inches of clear space adjacent to the exam table and the accessible route out of the room. This allows individuals in wheelchairs to approach the table and be able to transfer onto it. An adjustable-height exam table should be available.
- *Accessible scales:* Special wheelchair scales and in-floor scales (built into the floor) are needed for patients with limited or no mobility.

Americans with Disabilities Act Amendments Act of 2008

The ADA Amendments Act of 2008 is also known as the ADA Amendment Act and the ADAAA. The original ADA narrowly defined disability. The ADA Amendment Act expanded the meaning and interpretation of the definition of disability. People with cancer, diabetes, attention deficit/hyperactivity disorder, learning disabilities, and epilepsy are now included. This should ensure that individuals with disabilities receive protection under the law.

The following federal laws address hours, pay, and leave in the workplace:

- *Federal Insurance Contributions Act of 1935 (FICA)*: Created a payroll tax that requires a deduction from a person's paycheck. The withheld amount and an employer contribution fund the Social Security program and a portion of Medicare.
- *Fair Labor Standards Act of 1938*: Prohibits child labor and also provides overtime pay and a minimum wage.
- *Equal Pay Act of 1963 (EPA)*: Protects against gender-based wage discrimination; equal pay for both men and women who are performing the same job at the same organization.
- *Employee Retirement Income Security Act of 1974 (ERISA)*: Sets minimum standards for pension and health plans in private industry and protects individuals in these plans.
- *Family Medical Leave Act (FMLA) of 1991*: Provides unpaid leave time for maternity, adoption, or caring for ill family members.

State laws also protect employees in different areas. For instance, state workers' compensation laws protect employees who are injured on the job. An employee may collect money to cover lost wages, medical expenses, and retraining.

A medical assistant should be aware of the employment laws. If violations are noticed in the workplace, the medical assistant should follow the reporting procedures outlined in the facility's compliance program. If no program exists, then it is important to discuss the issues with the person responsible for the human resources duties.

Interview Concerns. To prevent legal issues related to hiring practices, healthcare facilities need to stay away from specific topics during the interview process. Asking questions related to these topics can put the facility at risk for discrimination lawsuits. Examples of illegal and legal questions include:

- *Birthplace, ancestry, or national origin*: Legal to ask, "Are you eligible to work in this state?" Illegal to ask, "When did you move to the United States?"
- *Marital status, children, or pregnancy*: Legal to ask, "Are you able to work an 8 a.m. to 5 p.m. schedule?" Illegal to ask, "Who will look after your child when he is born?"
- *Health or medical history, or physical disability*: Legal to ask, "Can you perform the essential job functions of a medical assistant with or without reasonable accommodations?" Illegal to ask, "What medications are you on?"
- *Religion or religious days observed*: Legal to ask, "Can you work on the weekends?" Illegal to ask, "Where do you attend church services?"
- *Age, race, ethnicity, gender, or color*: Legal to ask, "Are you 18 or older?" Illegal to ask, "How old are you?"
- *Criminal records*: Legal to ask, "Have you ever been convicted of a crime?" Illegal to ask, "Have you ever been arrested?"

Environmental Safety Concerns

Compliance reporting also relates to environmental safety violations. Offenses can be violations of local, state, or federal regulations. The unsafe activities or practices may cause hazardous conditions that impact the health or safety of employees, patients, and others. Recall that OSHA is involved with creating a safe environment for employees. Any situation that risks the safety of employees or patients must be reported immediately.

The Occupational Safety and Health Act of 1970 gives employees the right to file a complaint with OSHA. Employees can request an OSHA inspection if they believe their workplace has safety hazards. The employee filing the report does not need to be knowledgeable about the OSHA regulations. OSHA will keep the reporting person's information confidential.

To report a safety and health issue, the employee can file an electronic form, fax or mail a report to the local OSHA office, or call the local OSHA office. Specific information and forms are available at the OSHA website *(https://www.osha.gov)*.

Incident Reports and Risk Management. When a person is injured or equipment malfunctions, most ambulatory care facilities require an incident report to be completed. An *incident report* is an internal document that needs to be completed whenever an unexpected event occurs. The purposes of the incident report are to gather information about the situation in case of a future lawsuit and to communicate

issues for risk management procedures. The medical assistant should remember these points about incident reports:

- Complete an incident report for patient complaints, medication errors, medical device malfunctions, and any injury.
- Complete the incident report clearly and accurately in pen or electronically.
- List the facts. Do not speculate or draw conclusions.
- Make sure to complete it by the end of the day the situation occurred.
- Do not mention the incident report in the patient health record. If it is mentioned, a lawyer may request a copy of the report.

Usually, the incident report is given to the supervisor to review before it is sent to the risk management team. *Risk management* involves techniques used to reduce or eliminate accidental loss to the healthcare facility. It involves identifying, assessing, and controlling risks. Risks can relate to financial issues, legal liabilities, accidents, and electronic data security threats.

Patient Safety Concerns

Patient safety concerns are of utmost importance in healthcare facilities. Even with careful practices, patients can be harmed. A patient can fall. The wrong medication may be given to the patient. The wrong procedure may be done. All issues of safety can lead to potential liability for injuries that result.

If a medical assistant is involved in a situation in which a person is harmed, it is important to do the following:

- Immediately notify the provider. This is especially important if the wrong medication was given to the patient. The provider must identify what steps need to be taken.
- Arrange to have the person seen by a provider immediately. The provider can assess the extent of the injuries and provide the required treatment. Information on the injuries and treatment will then be documented in the health record should future litigation occur.
- Complete the incident report (see Procedure 4.5, p. 91). The employee witnessing the situation should be the person completing the report if possible. The incident report communicates what occurred and provides information if future litigation occurs.
- Notify the department supervisor. The supervisor can follow up with the patient. Many agencies do not charge the injured patient for the services provided. If the wrong medication is given, many agencies do not charge for the medication and services provided.
- Notify state or federal governmental agencies regarding the injury. Some states have medical error reporting systems in place. OSHA requires agencies to record all work-related needlestick injuries and cuts from sharp objects that are contaminated with another person's blood or other potentially infectious material. The case must be reported on the OSHA 300 Log (available at *www.osha.gov*).

CLOSING COMMENTS

Patient Coaching

When you are working with older patients, questions on record release and disclosure authorization forms can be common. Years ago, such forms did not exist. Today patients may feel they have to complete forms for everything. Make sure to take time to explain why it is important to have the forms completed. Remember that some of the older patients may have difficulty reading the forms. Some may not be able to hear as well as they used to. Take time and communicate clearly and slowly with older patients. If appropriate, use simple phrases when answering their questions. If possible, help complete whatever information you can. Be patient and respectful during your interaction with patients.

Legal and Ethical Issues

During a busy day in an ambulatory care facility, the medical assistant performs many administrative and clinical tasks. It is important for the medical assistant to perform these tasks following the facility's policies and procedures. Remember that these policies and procedures are created so that the staff complies with state and federal laws. Should a medical assistant feel that a task conflicts with a law, he or she should talk with the supervisor.

Patient-Centered Care

In a patient-centered care environment, the patient is the focus. When a medical assistant does a procedure incorrectly or makes

a medication error, it is very important to immediately notify the provider and the supervisor. The provider will evaluate the situation and make a judgment on what needs to be done for the care and safety of the patient. The supervisor will help manage the situation by talking with the patient, ensuring everything is done for the patient, and eliminating charges related to the error. Being upfront and honest about the error to the provider, supervisor, and patient (per agency policy) is most important for the patient's health and safety.

Professional Behaviors

Many ambulatory care facilities do not allow medical assistants to carry personal cell phones. Limiting cell phones can decrease the chance of employees recording or taking a picture of a patient and posting something patient related on social media sites. These situations are breaches of confidentiality and can lead to HIPAA violations and settlements. Besides OCR concerns, the facility may also be sued by the patient. It is important to remember to maintain patient confidentiality. What you see and hear in the clinic, remains there!

SUMMARY OF SCENARIO

Daniela has learned a lot about healthcare-related laws. Not only did she learn about laws that healthcare professionals must follow, she also learned about employment laws. One of Daniela's assignments for her course was to identify three risks of HIPAA violations. Daniela and Bella talked about the assignment and the risks in their department.

Unattended computers that were open to the electronic health record were problems. This is especially a risk in the patient examination rooms, because each room is equipped with a personal computer for documenting. Daniela also mentioned conversations about patients in the medical assistants' station.

Sometimes she hears medical assistants discussing a patient who came in. She feels uncomfortable about those conversations and ensures she does not take part in them.

Cell phones in the workplace and frequent use of social media sites during work hours can be risks. Bella mentioned that she heard several stories of employees being terminated. The employees posted patient-related photos and information on social media sites. Bella and Daniela work hard to prevent HIPAA violations. They do not ever want to be named in a lawsuit for such violations.

SUMMARY OF LEARNING OBJECTIVES

1. **Explain the standards of the Health Insurance Portability and Accountability Act (HIPAA) and discuss HIPAA-related terminology (including covered entities, protected health information, business associate, permission, de-identify, and limited data set).**
   The four standards include:
   - *Standard 1 related to transactions and code sets:* HHS adopted standard transactions for the electronic exchange of administrative healthcare information.
   - *Standard 2 related to the Privacy Rule:* Healthcare facilities, insurance companies, and others need to protect written, electronic, and oral patient health information.
   - *Standard 3 related to the Security Rule:* Healthcare facilities, insurance companies, and others need to protect patient information that is electronically stored and transmitted.
   - *Standard 4 related to unique identifiers:* This included the National Provider Identifier (NPI), the Health Plan Identifier (HPI), and the Employer Identification Number (EIN).

   HIPAA-related terminology:
   - *Covered entities:* Healthcare providers, health (insurance) plans, and claims clearinghouses that transmit protected health information electronically.
   - *Protected health information* (PHI): Individually identifiable health information stored or transmitted by covered entities or business associates. Includes verbal, paper, or electronic information.
   - *Business associate:* A person or business that provides a service to a covered entity that involves access to PHI.
   - *Permission:* A reason for releasing or disclosing patient information under HIPAA.
   - *De-identify:* To remove all direct patient identifiers from the PHI. In other words, this is the process for removing anything that can link the information back to a specific person.
   - *Limited data set:* PHI that has had all of the direct patient identifiers removed. This would include the name, contact information, Social Security number, and so on.

2. **Describe the Health Information Technology for Economic and Clinical Health (HITECH) Act.**

   The HITECH Act contains provisions that increased the enforcement of the privacy and security of electronic transmission and health information. HITECH modified HIPAA in the following ways:

   - Made business associates directly liable for compliance with HIPAA.
   - Prohibited the sale of PHI without the patient's authorization.
   - Created a tiered violation category that included unknowing, reasonable cause, willful neglect—corrected, and willful neglect—uncorrected.
   - Breach notification requirements were increased.

3. **Describe the important features of the Genetic Information Nondiscrimination Act (GINA), the Food, Drug, and Cosmetic Act, and the Controlled Substances Act.**

   - *The Genetic Information Nondiscrimination Act (GINA)* became law in 2008. It modified HIPAA and increased the protection of individuals. GINA prohibits genetic discrimination in health coverage and employment.
   - *The Food, Drug, and Cosmetic Act* is enforced by the Food and Drug Administration (FDA). The FDA is responsible for the safety, effectiveness, security, and quality of drugs, cosmetics, and food. Some of the areas overseen by the FDA include human and veterinary drugs, vaccines, biologic products (e.g., blood components), medical devices, food, cosmetics, dietary supplies, and products that give off radiation.
   - *The Controlled Substances Act* is enforced by the U.S. Drug Enforcement Agency (DEA). The DEA oversees the manufacturing, importation, possession, use, and distribution of certain drugs and chemicals. The DEA handles both illegal and legal drugs. The Controlled Substances Act has five schedules of medications, arranged from the greatest to the least abuse potential.

4. **Describe the Patient Protection and Affordable Care Act, the Clinical Laboratory Improvement Amendments (CLIA), the Occupational Safety and Health Act, and the Needlestick Safety and Prevention Act.**

   - *Patient Protection and Affordable Care Act:* Also known as the Affordable Care Act; it was to provide Americans with affordable health insurance and attempted to reform the healthcare system and reduce healthcare spending.
   - *Clinical Laboratory Improvement Amendments (CLIA):* Establishes quality standards and regulates laboratory testing. The quality standards focus on accuracy, reliability, and timeliness of test results.
   - *Occupational Safety and Health Act of 1970 (OSH Act):* Enforced by the Occupational Safety and Health Administration (OSHA). Based on this act, OSHA sets workplace standards and conducts inspections to ensure employee safety.
   - *Needlestick Safety and Prevention Act:* The goal of the act was to reduce the risk of healthcare workers' exposure to bloodborne diseases. The act required OSHA to update its Bloodborne Pathogens Standard.

5. **Discuss Good Samaritan laws.**

   Good Samaritan laws are state laws that provide legal protection for those assisting an injured person during an emergency. The person responding must not be paid for the care given; must act reasonably, exercising the same standard of care (for their profession) within the limitations of the emergency; and cannot act negligently.

6. **Define the Patient Self-Determination Act, Uniform Determination of Death Act (UDDA), Uniform Anatomical Gift Act (UAGA), and the National Organ Transplant Act (NOTA).**

   - *Patient Self-Determination Act:* Requires most healthcare institutions to inform patients of their right to make decisions and the facility's policies respecting advance directives.
   - *Uniform Determination of Death Act (UDDA):* Served as a guide for state lawmakers to create their own laws that define death.
   - *Uniform Anatomical Gift Act (UAGA):* Purpose of the act was to make organ donation easier for people.
   - *National Organ Transplant Act (NOTA):* Established the Organ Procurement and Transplant Network (OPTN) and also established a national registry for organ matching.

7. **Describe compliance with public health statutes related to communicable diseases and to wounds of violence, abuse, neglect, and exploitation.**

   Reportable diseases are communicable diseases that have a significant public health impact. When a provider diagnoses a reportable disease, the state's public health department must be notified. This notification process is called disease reporting. Each state has statutes that address disease reporting.

   Most state statutes require healthcare providers to report cases of violence. Statutes vary from state to state. Typically, reportable cases include wounds caused by gunshots and stabbings; specific types of burns; and nonaccidental wounds caused by a knife, an axe, or a sharp-pointed instrument.

8. **Describe compliance with reporting vaccination issues.**

   When a healthcare provider orders a vaccine to be given to a child, the medical assistant must provide the parent or guardian with a Vaccine Information Statement (VIS) and have that person sign a consent form. The VIS reviews the reasons for and the risks of the vaccine.

   If a patient is having an unusual side effect from a vaccine, the provider might need to file a report with the Vaccine Adverse Event Reporting System (VAERS). VAERS is a national surveillance program that monitors vaccine safety. It collects information on unusual vaccine side effects.

9. **Discuss how compliance programs work, examine common compliance concerns in healthcare, follow protocol in reporting an illegal activity, and correctly complete an incident report.**

   A compliance program, or corporate compliance, is a program within a business that detects and prevents violations of state and federal laws. An effective compliance program helps protect the organization from fines and lawsuits. Most compliance programs have reporting mechanisms (i.e., a toll-free number or website) where employees can report suspected violations, suspected illegal activity, fraud, abuse, safety issues, and noncompliance issues.

   This chapter reviewed the following concerns in healthcare: financial, employment, environmental safety, and patient safety. The steps required to report illegal activity and complete an incident report were discussed.

PROCEDURE 4.1   Protecting a Patient's Privacy

Tasks: Apply HIPAA rules and protect a patient's privacy. Demonstrate sensitivity to a patient and his or her rights.

Scenario: Ken Thomas (date of birth [DOB] 10/25/61) saw Jean Burke, NP (nurse practitioner), this past week. He was diagnosed with acute leukemia after several tests. You work with Ms. Burke, and you were involved with arranging Ken's tests. Today, Ken's adult child, Alex Thomas, calls you. Alex wants to know what is going on with Ken. You look at Ken's health record and see that Alex is not on the disclosure authorization form or a medical records release form. Per the facility's policy, for information to be given to a patient's family, a disclosure authorization form must be completed.

 Later Ken calls and asks why you did not update Alex on his condition. He sounds upset while he is talking with you.

EQUIPMENT and SUPPLIES

- Patient record
- Disclosure authorization form (electronic or paper) (see Fig. 4.2)

PROCEDURAL STEPS

1. Using the scenario, role-play the situation with a peer. You are the medical assistant and just realized that Alex is not on the release form. Be professional and respectful as you apply HIPAA rules to the situation.
 PURPOSE: As a professional, you need to follow the law and yet be professional and respectful.
2. Inform Alex that his name is not on a disclosure authorization form. Discuss the purpose of the disclosure authorization form.
 PURPOSE: The patient must sign a disclosure authorization form and indicate who can be given information. If a person wants information but is not listed on the form, legally the medical assistant cannot give any information.
3. Explain to Alex how you would be able to give him information. Encourage Alex to talk with his father about the situation.
 PURPOSE: The medical assistant can only give information if the person's name is on the release form.

4. When Ken calls, be professional and respectful as you hear his complaints. Keep your voice even and do not raise the volume.
 PURPOSE: The release form needs to indicate where the records are being sent.
5. Inform Ken that you understand his frustration. Be sensitive to his feelings and his rights. Explain why you could not give information to Alex.
 PURPOSE: Having the patient understand that you could not legally give the information to Alex is important. Speaking in a sensitive, respectful tone may help Ken feel less frustrated with the situation.
6. Discuss with Ken how you could prepare the disclosure authorization form. Make plans for how Ken would sign the form.
 PURPOSE: Helping to come up with a solution to achieve the patient's wishes is important to solving Ken's frustration.
7. Document the phone calls with Alex and Ken. Describe the facts and the plan to complete the release form.
 PURPOSE: All phone calls with patients or related to patients should be documented. This provides an ongoing log of what occurs with the patient and can be helpful in a court of law should something come up.

PROCEDURE 4.2   Completing a Release of Records Form for a Release of Information

Tasks: Apply HIPAA rules, and complete a release of record form for a release of information.

Scenario: Aaron Jackson was seen at Walden Hospital for a high fever. You need to help Aaron's mother complete a record release form so his record from the emergency department visit can be sent to the clinic. She needs to request all records from the visit on the first of this month. The clinic information is on the form. The release will expire in 1 month.

AARON'S INFORMATION

Date of birth: 10/17/2011
Social Security number: 164-72-4618
Address: 555 McArthur Avenue
Anytown, AL 12345-1234
Phone: (123) 814-7844
Mother: Patricia Jackson

WALDEN HOSPITAL'S INFORMATION

Address: Walden Hospital
123 Healing Way
Anywhere, AL 12345-1234
Phone: (123) 814-4563
Fax: (123) 814-6544

PROCEDURE 4.2	Completing a Release of Records Form for a Release of Information—*continued*

EQUIPMENT and SUPPLIES

- Records release form (electronic or paper) (see Fig. 4.3)
- Patient record

PROCEDURAL STEPS

1. Using the medical records release form, insert the patient information (see Fig. 4.3). Add the patient's name, DOB, and Social Security number (SSN). Include the current address and phone number that is found in the patient record. If an electronic form is used, select the correct patient and the fields will auto-populate.
   PURPOSE: The patient's information is required on the form. The patient's name, DOB, and SSN are direct identifiers, which will also help the hospital identify the correct patient.
2. Complete the parts of the form that specify who authorizes the release and who is to release the information.
   PURPOSE: Depending on state law and the facility's policy, the mother's name or the child's name may be the party authorizing the release. The hospital is the party that will release the information.
3. Check the box(es) of the information that needs to be released. If required, write in what other records need to be released.
   PURPOSE: Depending on state law and the facility's policy, the "Other" location might be where substance abuse and HIV records can be specifically requested. Other forms have a specific section for the release of substance abuse and HIV records.
4. Add the date of the visit. Add the name and contact information for the facility where the records need to be sent.

PURPOSE: The release form needs to indicate where the records are being sent.
5. Indicate how the released information will be used.
   PURPOSE: This information tells the releasing facility what the information will be used for. In this situation, the provider is requesting the information for healthcare purposes.
6. Indicate when the authorization should expire. Proofread the form for accuracy. If using an electronic form, save the form to the patient record. Print the form so the mother can sign.
   PURPOSE: In some situations, this may be an ongoing release. For example, the patient may get weekly blood tests at a local clinic, and the results need to be sent to the patient's specialist.
7. During a role-play with the patient's mother, explain what the provider is requesting. Ensure she can understand and read English. Have the mother read the form.
   PURPOSE: To be legal, the mother must understand what she is signing. If she does not understand English, you will need to have a translator available to help in this situation.
8. Ask the mother if she has any questions. Answer any questions, and then explain where she needs to sign if she agrees with the documentation.
   PURPOSE: By answering questions, you can help her understand the release process. It is important to make sure she is in agreement with the form before she signs. After the mother has signed, the form will be faxed to the hospital. The signed form should be filed in the patient record or scanned and uploaded into the electronic health record.

PROCEDURE 4.3	Perform Disease Reporting

Tasks: Research the state's disease reporting public health statutes, and complete the disease reporting paperwork based on public health statutes. Document the activity in the patient's health record.

Scenario: Jean Burke, NP, received the test results for Ken Thomas. He tested positive for gonorrhea. She wants you to file the report with the public health department. Here is the information from his health record and the clinic. For any missing information, follow the instructor's directions (or, if no directions are provided for this exercise, make up the information.).

PATIENT INFORMATION

Ken Thomas
398 Larkin Avenue
Anytown, AL 12345-1234
Anycounty
k.thomas@anytown.mail
Phone: (123) 784-1118
DOB: 10/25/61
Race: Multiple races
Ethnicity: Unknown
Marital status: Single, living with Sandy Brown, who was not treated

PROVIDER AND LAB INFORMATION

Provider:
Jean Burke, NP
Walden-Martin Family Medical Clinic
1234 Anystreet
Anytown, AL 12345-1234
Phone: (123) 123-1234
Fax: (123) 123-5678
Lab:
Walden-Martin Family Medical Clinic Lab

HEALTH RECORD INFORMATION

Diagnosis: Gonorrhea
Symptoms: Started 5 days ago, greenish discharge from penis, burning with urination
Test: Urine specimen was collected yesterday; gonorrhea nucleic acid amplification test (NAAT) done yesterday, results are positive
Treatment: Patient treated today with ceftriaxone 250 mg intramuscular (IM) single dose and azithromycin 1 g orally single dose

Continued

PROCEDURE 4.3   Perform Disease Reporting—*continued*

EQUIPMENT and SUPPLIES

- Computer with internet access and printer
- Patient record (see preceding table)
- Black pen

PROCEDURAL STEPS

1. Using the internet, search for the disease reporting procedure in your state's public health department or similar facility. Read the procedure.
   PURPOSE: A medical assistant needs to be aware of the disease reporting procedure for the state.
2. Identify which form is required based on the patient's diagnosis. Print the form.
   PURPOSE: Some department of health services agencies may have several forms available on the website. It is important to use the correct form. Gonorrhea is a sexually transmitted infection.
3. Use a black pen to complete the form. Neatly complete the patient's demographic information section using the information from the health record.
   PURPOSE: All forms require the patient's name and contact information.

4. Complete the diagnosis, symptoms, testing, and treatment information.
   PURPOSE: The public health department needs information on the diagnosis, symptoms, test results, and the treatment provided.
5. Complete the rest of the form. Review the form for accuracy. Make any changes required before submitting the form to the instructor.
   PURPOSE: The form must be accurate and complete before it is sent to the public health department.
6. Document in the patient health record that the disease reporting paperwork was completed and submitted.
   PURPOSE: All activities related to the patient must be documented in the patient's health record.

07/25/20XX 11:05 a.m. The state's disease reporting paperwork for the Gonorrhea diagnosis (on 07/25/20XX) was completed and submitted as requested by Jean Burke, NP. _____ Bella Dickens, CMA (AAMA)

PROCEDURE 4.4   Report Illegal Activity

Task: Report an illegal activity in the healthcare setting following proper protocol.

Scenario: Today you witnessed a co-worker, Sally Brown, taking medical samples from the supply cabinet. You see her sticking them in her purse. She sees you and states, "This was the same medication I had to pay $200 for the last time I was sick. I don't see why we need to pay for medications when we have samples that we give free to patients. We should be able to use them also." You know the facility's professional policy prohibits taking medical samples from the sample cabinet for personal reasons.

Facility's Compliance Reporting Protocol

Walden-Martin Family Medical Clinic's Compliance Program has a phone number and email address for employees to report suspected violations, suspected illegal activity, fraud, abuse, theft, and workplace safety concerns. Concerns can be left on the voice mail or emailed without fear of retribution or retaliation. Please include as many details as possible, including dates, names, and the situation.

Any employee who seeks retribution or retaliation against another employee for reporting an offense needs to be aware of criminal penalties for such actions.

EQUIPMENT and SUPPLIES

- Computer with email and internet access or phone
- Instructor's email address or voice mail phone number
- Pen and paper
- Facility's compliance reporting protocol

PROCEDURAL STEPS

1. Read the facility's corporate compliance reporting protocol.
   PURPOSE: Prior to reporting an illegal action, the medical assistant needs to identify the facility's protocol or the reporting chain of command. (Chain of command usually begins with your supervisor, then the supervisor of your supervisor, and so on. It is recommended you start with the lowest level that you feel comfortable with.)
2. Using the paper and pen, write down the facts of what you witnessed.
   PURPOSE: Writing down the facts soon after the situation will help you to remember the details.
3. Using the paper and pen, compose the message you want to email or leave on the voice mail for the compliance office.
   PURPOSE: Composing a message will help you organize your thoughts and leave an accurate message.

PROCEDURE 4.4   Report Illegal Activity—*continued*

4. Proofread the message and make any changes required. Make sure to include the date, names of people involved, and the details of the situation.
PURPOSE: It is important to have an accurate, complete message for the compliance office. Proofreading helps to ensure the message is accurate.

5. Using your email or phone, send a message to the corporate compliance office. Use the email address or phone number provided by your instructor.
PURPOSE: To complete the reporting process, the medical assistant must contact the corporate compliance office or the required supervisor if following the chain of command.

PROCEDURE 4.5   Complete Incident Report

Task: Complete an incident report form for a medication error.

Scenario: Johnny Parker (DOB 06/15/10) saw Jean Burke, NP, for a well-child visit. Johnny is off schedule with his hepatitis B vaccine series, and today he is to get his last hepatitis B booster. You (a medical assistant) prepare the medication and give the injection in his right deltoid muscle. Later in the day you realize that hepatitis B has been out of stock for 1 week. You must have given a hepatitis A booster to Johnny. You realize that you failed to read the label three times during preparation of the medication. You report the mistake to Jean Burke, NP, and your supervisor. Your supervisor calls Lisa Parker, Johnny's mother. They will come back next week for the hepatitis B vaccine. You need to complete the incident report.

EQUIPMENT and SUPPLIES

- Incident report form (Fig. 4.7) and black pen, or computer with an internet connection and SimChart for the Medical Office (SCMO)

PROCEDURAL STEPS

1. *SCMO method:* Access SCMO and enter the Simulation Playground. If a popup window appears, select "Return to previous session with saved patient information" and click Start. On the Calendar screen, click on the Form Repository icon. Click on Office Forms on the left Info Panel and select Incident Report. *For both methods:* Accurately complete the information from the date down to the reason for the patient's visit.
PURPOSE: It is important to have accurate information regarding the date, time, location, incident type, and the reason for the visit. Giving the background information will help the reader understand what occurred.

2. *For both methods:* Specify the incident description, immediate action and outcome, and contributing factors, and fill in the prevention boxes. Provide as much detail as possible. Be honest and concise with your facts.
PURPOSE: It is important to give a clear, concise, and honest description of what occurred. It is hard to admit fault, but doing so shows your professionalism in the situation.

3. *For both methods:* Complete the reported by, position, and contact phone number sections. Your information should be in these fields. (For this exercise, make up a contact phone number.)
PURPOSE: It is important to have accurate information in these fields so that if people have questions, they can contact you.

4. *For both methods:* Complete the other persons involved, position, and contact phone number sections. Jean Burke's information should be in these fields. (Make up her contact phone number.)
PURPOSE: Having additional people listed on the form helps if questions arise about the situation. The rest of the form, from the Medical Report field to the end, needs to be completed by the provider.

5. *For both methods:* Review the form for accuracy. Make any changes required before submitting the form to the instructor. (*For the SCMO method:* Save or print the form based on your instructor's directions.)
PURPOSE: It is important to proofread the form to ensure it is accurate and complete.

Continued

PROCEDURE 4.5   Complete Incident Report—*continued*

WALDEN-MARTIN
FAMILY MEDICAL CLINIC
1234 ANYSTREET | ANYTOWN, ANYSTATE 12345
PHONE 123-123-1234 | FAX 123-123-5678

Incident Report

Date: _____	Time: _____

Incident Type: ☐ Staff   ☐ Patient   ☐ Visitor   ☐ Equipment/Property

Witness: ☐ Staff   ☐ Patient   ☐ Visitor

Department: _____	Exact Location: _____

Medical Team: _____

Patient Reason for Visit: _____	Medication Incident: ☐ Yes ☐ No

Incident Description: [box]

Immediate Actions and Outcome: [box]

Contributing Factors: [box]

Prevention: [box]

Next of kin / guardian notified / patient?   ☐ Yes   ☐ No   ☐ N/A

Medical staff notified?   ☐ Yes   ☐ No   ☐ N/A

Reported By: _____	Position: _____

Contact Phone Number: _____

Other Persons Involved: _____	Position: _____

Contact Phone Number: _____

Medical Report (Document patient's assessment and list investigations and treatments):

Provider: _____	Designation: _____
Provider Signature: _____	Date/Time: _____

FIGURE 4.7 Incident report form.

HEALTHCARE ETHICS

5

SCENARIO

Daniela Garcia was just hired as a part-time float receptionist at Walden-Martin Family Medical (WMFM) Clinic. As a float receptionist, she will be working with many co-workers and providers. Besides working, Daniela is also attending the local community college for medical assisting. She is currently taking a law and ethics course.

Daniela has completed the law part of the course. She is starting the ethics unit. Daniela grew up in a conservative family. They lived in a very small town in the Midwest. She has since relocated and finds that some of the beliefs she held as a teen are now changing as she encounters more life challenges. As she studies various topics, she has also found that what she believed to be true when she was younger is not actually true. Daniela is very interested in continuing to learn about ethics.

While studying this chapter, think about the following questions:
- What are personal and professional ethics?
- How can people separate their personal and professional ethics?
- What are the four principles of healthcare ethics?
- What are ethical issues that relate to genetics, reproductive, childhood, end-of-life, and organ donation issues?

LEARNING OBJECTIVES

1. Do the following related to ethics:
   - Define ethics and morals.
   - Differentiate between personal and professional ethics.
   - Identify the effect of personal morals on professional performance.
   - Develop a plan for separation of personal and professional ethics.
   - Recognize the impact personal ethics and morals have on the delivery of healthcare.
2. List and describe the four ethical principles in healthcare.
3. Demonstrate appropriate responses to ethical issues involving genetics.
4. Demonstrate appropriate responses to ethical issues involving reproductive issues.
5. Demonstrate appropriate responses to ethical issues involving childhood issues.
6. Demonstrate appropriate responses to ethical issues involving medical research trials.
7. Demonstrate appropriate responses to ethical issues involving end-of-life issues and discuss the theory of Elisabeth Kübler-Ross.
8. Demonstrate appropriate responses to ethical issues involving organ donation issues; discuss the Patient Self Determination Act and the Uniform Anatomical Gift Act, and define terms related to organ donation issues (advance directives, living will, medical durable power of attorney, and healthcare proxy).

VOCABULARY

bioethicists (BYE oh eth i sists) People who study the ethical effect of biomedical advances (e.g., drugs and genetic engineering).

cessation Bringing to an end.

chromosomes (KROE mah somes) Rod-shaped structures found in the cell's nucleus; they contain genetic information.

cryopreservation (KRIE oh pri zur vae shun) To preserve by freezing at low temperatures.

discipline A branch of knowledge, learning, or instruction; for instance, medicine, nursing, social work, and physical therapy.

embryo (EM bree oh) A developing organism from the moment of conception through the eighth week of development.

ethics (ETH iks) Rules of conduct that differentiate between acceptable and unacceptable behavior.

ethics committee A group composed of members from a variety of disciplines that analyze ethical issues.

evidence-based practice Healthcare practice that incorporates the most current and valid research results, thus providing the best patient care.

germline cells Sperm and egg cells.

morals (MORE ahls) Internal principles that distinguish between right and wrong.

oocyte (OO eh site) An immature ovum (egg).

personal ethics An individual's code of conduct.

resident A physician who has graduated from medical school and is finishing specialized clinical training.

somatic cells (soe MAT ik) Nonreproductive cells; they do not include sperm and egg cells.

surrogate (SUR ah git) A person who acts on behalf of another person or takes the place of another person. Examples include a surrogate mother or a healthcare agent.

As you move into healthcare, you may be faced with situations in which you do not agree with a person's decision. As a healthcare professional, you need to respect a patient's decision whether or not you agree with it.

This chapter examines **ethics**. Ethical issues are different from legal issues. What may be legal may not be ethical. Personal ethics and its impact on professional performance will be discussed. Professional ethics differs from personal ethics. This topic is explored, along with how to handle the differences. Common ethical issues in healthcare are examined. End-of-life issues, including advance directives, are also discussed.

PERSONAL AND PROFESSIONAL ETHICS

Personal Ethics

Personal ethics includes an individual's honesty, fairness, commitment, integrity, and accountability. It also includes doing what one considers to be correct.

Our **morals** tell us what is right and wrong. Our moral compass develops as we grow. Our first lessons on right and wrong come from those we live with. Our socialization and background shape our morals. For instance, if your parents instilled in you the importance of always being on time, you may grow up feeling that a person should always be on time. You may feel others are in error if they are late for an event. As we grow, our morals may change if our beliefs change. Our morals impact how we conduct ourselves or, in other words, our personal ethics.

Our personal morals impact our professional performance. If people believe in being on time, this characteristic will transfer to the work environment. Employees will be on time for work. Being timely when rooming patients will be important to employees. Having patients wait for long periods of time in the reception area will be challenging to accept. Personal ethics that align with professional characteristics will positively impact one's professional performance.

Our personal morals may also negatively impact our professional performance. Let's say a person grew up without grandparents or older adults in the family. That person may view older people as not being as knowledgeable as the younger generations. If a medical assistant had this belief, imagine how that might impact his or her professional performance. That person may not respect older adults and may view them as being useless, unimportant, or irrelevant individuals. This will impact how the medical assistant would treat an older patient. As professionals, we cannot let our personal morals negatively impact the care that we provide to patients.

> **CRITICAL THINKING** APPLICATION   5.1
>
> Daniela was working on her ethics assignment on break at the clinic. She thought about her personal ethics. She decided that some of her personal ethics would benefit her in a job. She realizes that some of her personal morals may negatively impact the care she provides to patients. She realizes that she needs to explore these morals and make some personal decisions.
>
> Think about your personal ethics and morals. What will positively influence your professional performance? What personal morals will negatively impact your professional performance?

Professional Ethics

Professional ethics are codes of conduct stated by an employer or a professional association (Table 5.1). Many employers state how employees need to conduct themselves in the workplace. This information can usually be found in the employee handbook.

Many healthcare professional associations have published professional ethics for their members. These are called codes of ethics. A *code of ethics* is a set of rules about good and bad behavior. If a member or employee violates a professional ethic, the association or agency will discipline the person. We will examine the codes for physicians and medical assistants.

Code of Ethics for Physicians

One of the most famous and oldest codes of ethics is the Hippocratic oath. The original oath has been around for longer than 2000 years.

TABLE 5.1 Differences Between Personal and Professional Ethics		
	PERSONAL ETHICS	**PROFESSIONAL ETHICS**
Definition	Individual's code of conduct	Codes of conduct stated by an employer or a professional association
Ability to change	Individuals can change their own personal ethics	Individuals cannot change these codes and must comply; codes can only be changed by employer or professional association
Accountability	On the individual	On the members and organization

I swear to fulfill, to the best of my ability and judgment, this covenant:

I will respect the hard-won scientific gains of those physicians in whose steps I walk, and gladly share such knowledge as is mine with those who are to follow.

I will apply, for the benefit of the sick, all measures [that] are required, avoiding those twin traps of overtreatment and therapeutic nihilism.

I will remember that there is art to medicine as well as science, and that warmth, sympathy, and understanding may outweigh the surgeon's knife or the chemist's drug.

I will not be ashamed to say "I know not," nor will I fail to call in my colleagues when the skills of another are needed for a patient's recovery.

I will respect the privacy of my patients, for their problems are not disclosed to me that the world may know. Most especially must I tread with care in matters of life and death. If it is given me to save a life, all thanks. But it may also be within my power to take a life; this awesome responsibility must be faced with great humbleness and awareness of my own frailty. Above all, I must not play at God.

I will remember that I do not treat a fever chart, a cancerous growth, but a sick human being, whose illness may affect the person's family and economic stability. My responsibility includes these related problems, if I am to care adequately for the sick.

I will prevent disease whenever I can, for prevention is preferable to cure.

I will remember that I remain a member of society, with special obligations to all my fellow human beings, those sound of mind and body as well as the infirm.

If I do not violate this oath, may I enjoy life and art, respected while I live and remembered with affection thereafter. May I always act so as to preserve the finest traditions of my calling and may I long experience the joy of healing those who seek my help.

Written in 1964 by Louis Lasagna, Academic Dean of the School of Medicine at Tufts University, and used in many medical schools today.

FIGURE 5.1 Modern version of the Hippocratic oath.

Some of its concepts include treating the patient, not the disease, and maintaining the patient's confidentiality. Hippocrates, often called the father of medicine, is credited for the oath. The oath is a code of ethics for physicians. Over the years, the code has been modernized (Fig. 5.1).

In 1847 the American Medical Association (AMA) adopted its Code of Medical Ethics. The code lists the values that physicians commit themselves to as they practice medicine. The AMA's current Code of Medical Ethics is available on its website (*www.ama-assn.org*). The code is a living document. This means that as medicine and technology change, the code is updated by the members. Key themes in the code include the following:

- Physicians should provide competent care and continue learning.
- Physicians should respect human dignity and human rights.
- Physicians should follow the laws, be professional, and uphold the standard of the medical profession.
- Physicians should contribute to the welfare of the community.

The Council of Ethical and Judicial Affairs (CEJA) is one of the councils within the AMA. The CEJA analyzes ethical issues in healthcare and develops ethical policies and recommendations. These recommendations, along with the Code of Medical Ethics, are used by physicians to guide their practice. The CEJA prompts AMA members to adhere to the Code of Medical Ethics.

Code of Ethics for Medical Assistants

The American Association of Medical Assistants (AAMA) developed a code of ethics that provides the principles of ethical and moral conduct for the profession.

Medical Assisting Code of Ethics

Members of AAMA dedicated to the conscientious pursuit of their profession, and thus desiring to merit the high regard of the entire medical profession and the respect of the general public which they serve, do pledge themselves to strive always to:

A. Render service with full respect for the dignity of humanity.

B. Respect confidential information obtained through employment unless legally authorized or required by responsible performance of duty to divulge such information.

C. Uphold the honor and high principles of the profession and accept its disciplines.

D. Seek to continually improve the knowledge and skills of medical assistants for the benefit of patients and professional colleagues.

E. Participate in additional service activities aimed toward improving the health and well-being of the community.

From the American Association of Medical Assistants: Medical assisting code of ethics. *http://www.aama-ntl.org/about/overview#.WSDywmjytPY.*

The AAMA has also written a Medical Assisting Creed, which can be used as a guideline for medical assistants facing complex ethical and moral issues in the course of their work. The Medical Assisting Creed supports the code of ethics by asking members to abide by ethical statements of belief. These include:

- I believe in the principles and purposes of the profession of medical assisting.
- I endeavor to be more effective.

- I aspire to render greater service.
- I protect the confidence entrusted to me.
- I am dedicated to the care and well-being of all people.
- I am loyal to my employer.
- I am true to the ethics of my profession.
- I am strengthened by compassion, courage, and faith.

The Medical Assisting Creed supports the code of ethics. The above creed can be found on the AAMA's website (*http://www.aama-ntl.org/about/overview#.WSDywmjytPY*).

It is important for the medical assistant to follow the code and the creed. The care provided to others must reflect respect for that person. The medical assistant is legally and ethically obligated to keep patient information confidential. Continual learning is critical. The medical assistant must provide the best care possible and uphold the standards of the profession.

CRITICAL THINKING APPLICATION   5.2

Daniela read the AMA Code of Medical Ethics and the AAMA Medical Assisting Code of Ethics. She notices some similarities between the codes. What similarities do you notice between the two codes?

Separation Plan

Sometimes an individual's personal ethics clashes with professional ethics. It is important to take steps to separate one's personal ethics from professional ethics.

Let's examine a few situations that might impact a medical assistant. Imagine if a medical assistant has personal beliefs that vaccines are not needed and harm individuals. This medical assistant obtains a job in a pediatric department. She is required to give vaccines numerous times a day. In this situation, her personal ethics would clash with her professional ethics. She would be professionally obligated to give the vaccines to patients. She could not share her antivaccine beliefs with patients. Due to the clash of ethics, it might be a stressful job for her.

In another situation, a medical assistant believes that everything that can be done should be done when someone is dying. Professional ethics mandate that each person has a right to make end-of-life decisions. Legally and ethically, the medical assistant must follow what the patient decides. The medical assistant cannot put pressure on the patient to change his or her decisions.

Creating a Plan

As you complete your medical assisting courses, it is important to evaluate if your personal ethics conflict with the medical assistant code of ethics.

- Are there groups of people with whom you have issues? Maybe you do not believe in their behaviors, actions, or ideas based on your morals.
- Do you have preconceived ideas about people with differing ethnicities, sexual preferences, or specific diseases?

If you identified conflicts, how might you provide respectful care to these patients? Honestly, think about your biases. How would you approach a situation if it involved your bias? Remember, the professional code of ethics supersedes your personal code. You need to follow the professional ethics of your agency and profession (see Procedure 5.1, p. 106).

Before medical assistants start applying for positions, it is important that they evaluate if personal ethics will clash with the professional ethics of an agency. If a person does not believe in vaccinations, then working in a department that gives vaccinations would not be a good job choice. If a person does not believe in abortions, then working in an agency that does abortions would not be a good choice.

CRITICAL THINKING APPLICATION   5.3

Daniela decided to create a plan to separate her personal ethics from her professional ethics. Think about your personal ethics. What steps might you take to change your personal morals so that they better align with your professional ethics? What might you do to deal with the personal ethics that conflict with the professional ethics?

PRINCIPLES OF HEALTHCARE ETHICS

Healthcare professionals have an ethical duty to their patients. Four ethical principles summarize this ethical duty. These principles include *autonomy*, *nonmaleficence*, *beneficence*, and *justice*. Technically all four of these principles should have equal weight in ethical decisions. Many times, autonomy overshadows the other three principles.

Besides healthcare professionals, **bioethicists** also use the principles of healthcare ethics. They apply these principles when they evaluate medical technology and procedures. Are the new technology advances ethical? Are these procedures ethical?

We will examine the four ethical principles. Ethical actions to meet the principles will be discussed for both the provider and the medical assistant.

Autonomy

Autonomy is the freedom to determine one's own actions and decisions. Patients have the right to make their own healthcare decisions. Providers need to tell patients of the risks and benefits of different procedures (informed consent). After being told what may be most successful, the patients can make their own decisions. The patient's decision-making process should be free from pressure or interference from others. Healthcare professionals must respect and honor the patient's decision.

The medical assistant must protect patients' privacy. It is important to respect the uniqueness, dignity, and decisions of others. This includes patients, families, and co-workers. You must also maintain your own dignity and self-respect by following these principles:

- Help to make others around you look good without minimizing yourself. Do this by being supportive and helpful to your team members.
- Refrain from being negative and whining.
- Be assertive, not aggressive, when standing up for your rights (e.g., adequate work environment, hours, and pay).
- Collaborate and cooperate with co-workers. Do not be afraid to stand up for what is right and fair.
- Avoid bringing personal issues into the workplace.

When Daniela learned about the autonomy principle and the role of the medical assistant, it reminded her of healthcare laws that she had learned about. What healthcare laws address autonomy and the healthcare professional's role?

Nonmaleficence

Nonmaleficence means to do no harm. Healthcare professionals are obligated to not inflict intentional harm on patients. By providing the appropriate standard of care, we can reduce the risk of negligence. It is important to provide competent care to patients for both legal and ethical reasons.

The medical assistant must prevent harm to others – this means to intervene when a patient is at risk (e.g., falling). It is important to make sure the environment is both physically and psychologically safe for others and that safety hazards are reported and corrected. For instance, malfunctioning equipment must never be used until fixed. Hazardous chemicals and sharps (needles) must be unavailable to patients. The medical assistant must also provide safe and competent care to all patients.

Beneficence

Beneficence means to do good. For healthcare professionals, this means promoting health in patients and assisting patients to recover from illness. Promoting health with ambulatory care patients is an important role for medical assistants. With the current focus on prevention of diseases, medical assistants help providers by identifying the immunizations and screening tests their patients need.

Justice

Justice means to treat patients fairly and give them care that is due and appropriate. This means that patients in similar situations should receive the same services and treatments.

The medical assistant must provide equal respect and courtesy to all people. Regardless of the person's skin color, sexual preference, nationality, religion, and health history, every person must be treated respectfully. It is important that medical assistants think about their biases. Do you really feel everyone is equal? Is there any group of individuals whose ideas you do not agree with? Understanding one's biases is important. If we do not identify our biases, there is a tendency to treat others differently. As healthcare professionals, we are obligated to treat everyone equally and with respect.

ETHICAL ISSUES

There are many ethical issues in healthcare. As technology and medicine evolve, additional ethical issues arise. We will examine common ethical issues, and the CEJA's recommendations will also be explained.

Genetics Issues

Each person is made up of 46 **chromosomes**, 23 from each parent. *Genes* are the basic units of heredity, or the instructions on how our bodies should develop and function. Genes provide the differences among us and the similarities in families. From genes we get our physical appearance, in addition to our susceptibility to disease. During

the process of conception and subsequent cell division, an extra chromosome (or a change in the chromosome structure) may occur, resulting in a genetic disease or disorder. Types of genetic diseases include the following:
- *Monogenic disorder:* A defective gene is inherited from one or both parents. Huntington disease, cystic fibrosis, and sickle cell anemia are examples of monogenic disorders.
- *Chromosomal disorder:* An abnormal number of chromosomes or a change in the chromosomal structure causes diseases such as Klinefelter syndrome and Turner syndrome.

With advances in technology we can now test for many genetic disorders, sometimes even on a baby in utero (e.g., fetus). There has also been a lot of research in the areas of cloning, genetic engineering, and gene therapy. Along with these advancements come ethical issues and questions. We will explore cloning and genetic engineering advancements and related ethical issues.

Cloning

Cloning is the process of creating a genetically identical biologic entity. A clone is the copy, which has the same genetic makeup as the original entity. Researchers have cloned genes, cells, tissues, and organisms. Dolly, a sheep, was the first mammal cloned. Since then at least eight different mammals have been cloned, including horses, pigs, dogs, and cats. Advocates for human cloning discuss the need for organ transplants. Opponents of human cloning address the rights of the clone.

Genetic Engineering

Genetic engineering is the manipulation of genetic material in cells to change *hereditary* traits or to produce a specific result. Genetic engineering is used in many areas, including agriculture and medicine. For instance, a lot of corn and soybeans are genetically modified to resist disease and insects. These foods may be labeled as genetically modified organisms (GMOs). In medicine, insulin, human growth hormone, and other drugs are genetically engineered. We will focus on genetic engineering in medicine.

A *genome* is the entire genetic makeup of an organism. The Human Genome Project, a 13-year international project, mapped the human genome. The entire human genome contains about 30,000 genes. The goal of the project was to gain information that will eventually lead to the prevention and treatment of many diseases. *Genomic medicine* resulted from the Human Genome Project. Genomic medicine is an emerging branch of medicine involved with using patients' genomic information as part of their clinical care. Genetic testing, pharmacogenetics, and stem cell transplants are important advances in genomic medicine. Gene therapy is currently being researched.

Genetic Testing

Genetic testing can identify issues with a person's chromosomes, genes, or proteins. More than 1000 genetic tests are available. Some of the types of genetic testing include:
- *Newborn screening:* All states have newborn screening procedures to identify genetic disorders that can be treated early in life.
- *Diagnostic testing:* Used to diagnose a specific genetic or chromosomal condition. Testing can occur prior to birth or after. Not all genetic conditions have diagnostic tests.

- *Carrier testing*: Used to determine if a person is carrying one copy of a gene mutation. Two copies of a gene mutation (one from each parent) can result in a genetic disorder in a child.
- *Prenatal testing*: Used to detect genetic or chromosomal issues with a fetus (unborn baby).
- *Preimplantation testing*: Used to detect genetic issues in **embryos** that were created using assistive reproductive technology, which will be explained later in the chapter.
- *Predictive and presymptomatic testing*: Used to detect gene mutations associated with specific disorders that occur after birth. Usually done when a patient has a family member with a genetic disorder and the patient wants to see if he or she has it also.
- *Forensic testing*: Used to identify crime or catastrophe victims, identify or rule out crime suspects, or establish biologic relationships between people (e.g., paternity)

Per the CEJA, the impact of genetics on diseases is complex. Understanding genetic counseling and helping the patient to understand the results require special skill from the provider. Genetic testing is most important when it makes a meaningful impact on the person's health. The provider ordering genetic testing should have the appropriate knowledge and expertise to counsel the patient on the findings and implications. Providers must keep genetic testing information confidential.

CRITICAL THINKING APPLICATION   5.5

When Daniela learned about genetic testing, she remembered hearing about how people could trace their relatives. She also had heard about forensic testing while watching crime drama shows. What types of genetic testing are you familiar with?

Pharmacogenetics

Pharmacogenomics is a branch of pharmacology that studies the genetic factors that influence a person's response to a medication. Based on a person's genome, pharmacogenomics can determine if a specific therapy will be effective. More than 100 medications approved by the US Food and Drug Administration (FDA) already have pharmacogenomics information available. Some of these medications include analgesics, antivirals, cardiovascular drugs, and anticancer drugs.

Stem Cell Transplants

Stem cells can *differentiate*, or develop into specialized cells (e.g., muscle, blood, or brain cells). They can *self-renew*, or make copies of themselves. The new cell can remain as a stem cell or turn into a specialized cell. Depending on where the stem cells are located, they may be constantly repairing and replacing damaged tissue (e.g., intestinal tract). In other locations, such as the heart, they only divide under special situations.

There are two main categories of stem cells: adult and embryonic. Table 5.2 describes both types of stem cells. Stem cell research has been going on since the 1960s. New technology has helped advance the research. Many researchers are excited about the potential of stem cells. Cord blood stem cell transplants have been used to treat more than 75 diseases, including cancers, anemias, metabolic disorders, and immune system disorders.

Though both types of stem cell research have ethical issues, embryonic stem cell research has greater ethical issues. Harvesting stem cells from an embryo would mean destroying the embryo. For those believing life begins at the moment of conception, this means a life is lost.

Gene Therapy

Gene therapy is currently an experimental technique that uses genes to prevent or treat diseases. With this procedure, a gene is inserted into a patient's cell. The hopes are that the new gene might do the following:
- Replace a mutated gene
- Prevent the mutated gene from functioning
- Help fight the disease

Gene or genome editing is a specific gene therapy. This technique can remove, add, or alter sections of the gene. With new technology emerging in this area, ethical issues have also arisen. Genome editing of **somatic cells** would only impact the individual. This treatment has already been used and is considered ethical. Genome editing of

TABLE 5.2	Types of Stem Cells	
	Adult Stem Cells	**Embryonic Stem Cells**
Derived from	Found in infants through adults; found in many organs and tissues including the brain, bone marrow, blood, skin, heart, teeth, testis, liver, blood vessel, and skeletal muscles. Umbilical cord blood also contains adult stem cells.	Taken from a 4- to 5-day-old human embryo
What types of cells can they become?	Variation thought to be limited; could become cell types similar to their tissue of origin. Scientists have found a way to "reprogram" some types of adult stem cells so they act like embryonic cells.	Can become all cell types
Advantages	Thought to cause fewer rejection issues with transplants if a person's own stem cells are used.	Easy to grow in a laboratory setting
Ethical issue	Risks involved with adult stem cell use are still being evaluated.	For those believing life begins at the moment of conception, removing stem cells from an embryo would mean killing a person

germline cells can cause issues that may impact future generations. Genome editing of germline cells raises ethical concerns and is illegal in the United States.

Reproductive Issues
Assistive Reproductive Technology
Infertility is the inability to get pregnant after 1 year of unprotected intercourse (sex). Infertility can affect both males and females. There are many causes of infertility. With advances in technology, assistive reproductive technology (ART) has allowed many couples to have children. Assisted reproductive technology includes all procedures that involve the handling of the eggs, sperm, or embryos. Common types of ART include:

- *In vitro fertilization:* Involves removing egg cells from a female's ovaries. The egg cells are fertilized with sperm cells outside of the body. The fertilized egg is then implanted in the uterus for pregnancy.
- *Intrauterine insemination (IUI):* Also called *artificial insemination.* Specially prepared sperm is placed into a woman's uterus using a long, narrow tube (e.g., a straw). The woman's partner's sperm or a donor's sperm can be used.
- *Surrogacy:* A woman carries and gives birth for another couple. A legal contract should be in place to protect all parties. *Traditional surrogacy* or *partial surrogacy* occurs when the egg is from a **surrogate** and the sperm is from the father. *Gestational surrogacy* or *full surrogacy* occurs when the sperm and egg come from the intended parents or are donated, and the surrogate is not related to the baby.

One of the complications of ART is multiple births. An ethical issue can arise if the success of the pregnancy may be hindered by the number of babies in utero. If this situation occurs, the provider must inform the patient of the risks with multiple births.

CEJA's opinions are that providers who offer assisted reproductive services should provide accurate advertising of their services. They need to provide all information, including success rates and costs, so patients can make an informed decision. Prospective donors need to be tested for infectious disease agents and genetic disease. Donors need to provide informed consent.

Gamete Donation. *Gamete* (egg or sperm) donation allows others who are unable to have children to do so. Many ethical issues surround gamete donation, including:

- The privacy of the donors
- The rights of the child born from the donated gamete
- The relationship of the child and the donor
- The number of donations from a single donor (the more children born from the donor's gamete, the greater the risk of the children mating and conceiving children together)
- The health of the donors and the children born from the donations
- The regulations on gamete storage
- The compensation for gamete donation (many countries do not allow payment for gamete donation; however, the US does allow it)

CEJA's opinions are that providers who participate in the gamete donation process must inform the prospective donors about the risk of the donation, the testing involved, and if the donor will receive the test results. Donors should be tested for infectious diseases and

genetic disorders. The donor should be notified that all information will be kept indefinitely. The provider should discuss the storage of the gametes, compensation, and that the state law governs the relationship between the gamete donor and the child born from the gamete.

CEJA's opinions are that providers should not allow people to donate if they have infectious diseases. The provider should also gather the donor's preferences on the use of the gametes, whether for research or reproduction. The provider should find out the donor's preferences regarding release of identifying information to any child resulting from the donor. Donors should also limit the number of pregnancies resulting from a single gamete donor.

Egg Freezing. *Egg freezing,* or *egg banking,* is the **cryopreservation** of **oocytes,** which is done to preserve the female's fertility. Egg freezing is done for a variety of reasons, including:

- Women are diagnosed with cancer and may become infertile with the cancer treatments
- Women who want to delay childbearing
- Women who object to freezing embryos

The egg retrieval process requires the patient to undergo about 9 to 10 days of hormone injections to stimulate the ovaries and assist in the ripening of multiple eggs. Once the egg retrieval is completed, the eggs are frozen until they are needed. Usually 10 to 20 eggs are retrieved.

With the freezing process, the eggs are dehydrated, and the water is replaced with a fluid that prevents ice from forming and destroying the egg. The eggs can be flash frozen or frozen using a slow process. When the patient wants to become pregnant, some of the eggs are thawed. They are fertilized and then transferred to the patient's uterus.

Ethical issues surrounding egg freezing include:
- Safety of the procedure for both the patient and any future children that result from the eggs
- Marketing practices that focus on healthy women
- Pressures from companies for women to focus on their career, freeze their eggs, and consider childbearing at a later time
- Disposition decisions, including egg-sharing options, for unused or unwanted eggs

Currently, CEJA has no published opinion on egg freezing.

Abortion
Elective abortion is the deliberate termination of a pregnancy. Abortions can be done through medications and medical procedures. Abortions raise many ethical questions and concerns. Some feel that women have the right to determine what occurs with their bodies and babies have no rights until they are born. Others feel that from the moment of conception, babies have rights.

The advancement of technology has impacted abortions. With greater technology, complex testing and treatments can occur. Surgery on babies in utero can treat health issues that in the past caused death or elected abortions. Advanced testing can diagnose issues sooner. For instance, imaging tests provide clearer pictures of babies in utero. In cases in which diagnostic tests indicate major abnormalities, providers discuss the worst-case scenarios with the parents and include termination as part of informed consent. Per the CEJA's opinion, providers are not prohibited from performing an abortion in situations in which it does not violate the law.

Childhood Issues

In most cases, parents of minor children must authorize or decline treatment. In some cases, the state may need to provide the parental authority. *Parens patriae* is Latin for "father of the country." This doctrine gives the courts the power to make decisions for people who cannot make their own decisions. Many times this doctrine is used for children or adults who are incompetent. It can be used when the parent or parents refuse healthcare for the child. The court may take over the parental rights and make decisions for the child.

There have been situations in which parents refuse procedures or treatments for their children based on religious or personal beliefs. One of the more common situations in ambulatory care is the refusal of vaccinations (see Procedure 5.2, p. 107). It is important for the medical assistant to respect the Patient's Bill of Rights. If the patient provides a reason for the refusal, the medical assistant should let the provider know. The provider should also be told of the refusal, so other procedures or treatments can be discussed if needed.

CEJA's opinion is that providers are encouraged to seek consultation with **ethics committees** in the following situations:

- The parent or guardian refuses treatment for a reversible life-threatening condition.
- There are disagreements about the minor's best interest.

The provider should only ask the courts to resolve the disagreement as the last option.

Adoption

Federal and state laws govern adoption. In healthcare, we run into adoption fairly often. Our patients may be adopted and do not know their family medical history. We need to be understanding of their situation. We may also work with pregnant women who are planning to give up their babies. Again, these are situations in which medical assistants need to be sensitive and understanding. The following are different types of adoption:

- *Adopting through an agency*: Private and public adoption agencies are regulated by the state and must be licensed to place children with adoptive parents. Public agencies usually place abandoned, orphaned, or abused children who are wards of the state.
- *Adopting independently*: The birth parents and the adoptive parents have an arrangement. Some states do not allow this type of adoption.
- *Adopting through identification*: Adoptive parents and birth parents work with an adoption agency to complete the adoption process.
- *Adopting internationally*: Adoptive parents work with an international adoption agency to adopt a child from another country. International adoption agencies must be certified by the US State Department.
- *Relative adoptions*: Relatives of a child adopt the child.
- *Closed adoptions*: There is no contact between the adoptive parents and the birth parents.
- *Open adoptions*: Adoptive parents meet and may stay in contact with the birth parents.

Safe Haven Infant Protection Laws

Safe haven infant protection laws allow a person to give up an unwanted infant anonymously. The goal is to protect unwanted babies from abuse or death. The person is not prosecuted if

- the infant is not abused.
- the infant is left at a designated location, as indicated by the state law.
- the infant is within the age limit, as indicated by the state law.

The designated locations vary by state. They may include hospitals, emergency departments, fire and police stations, and child welfare agencies. The age of the child varies. A few states allow children up to 1 year of age. Opponents of the safe haven laws voice concerns for fathers' rights and the lack of family medical history obtained. Supporters state that these laws save babies by providing a safe drop-off location and no questions asked.

Confidential Healthcare for Minors

Providers have an ethical duty to promote decision making in minor patients to the degree of the child's ability. Providers have a responsibility to protect the confidentiality of minor patients, within certain limits. We see this in the ambulatory care setting when parents wait in the reception area while minor children (usually teens) have their physical exams. Many providers feel that the minor's answers to questions on safety, sex, drugs, and alcohol may be more truthful without the presence of parents.

In some states, laws permit unemancipated minors to request and receive confidential services. These services must relate to contraception, pregnancy testing, prenatal care, and delivery services. Additional services can include prevention and treatment of sexually transmitted infections (STIs), substance use disorders, and mental illness. When the law does not grant minors decision-making authority for healthcare, CEJA's opinion is that providers should:

- Involve the parent or guardian in situations in which it is necessary to prevent harm to the patient or others.
- Involve the parent or guardian if the provider does not feel it will impact the patient's health.
- Explore reasons the minor does not want the involvement of the parent or guardian.
- Inform the minor that parents may learn of the treatment through insurance statements.
- Protect the confidentiality of the information from the minor, keeping within ethical and legal standards.

CRITICAL THINKING APPLICATION   5.6

On break one afternoon, Daniela was talking to Jan, a medical assistant. She asked Jan how she handles parents who want to find out confidential information about their children. How might you professionally and respectfully handle a phone call from a parent who is requesting confidential information on her or his child?

Research Trials

Many of the larger ambulatory healthcare facilities are involved with teaching nurse practitioner and physician assistant students and **residents** to become future healthcare providers. Typically, these facilities also are involved with research trials. These trials may relate to a treatment for a disease, such as a new surgical procedure or a new medication. Many healthcare **disciplines** use **evidence-based practice** that originated from research trials. Research on patient volunteers is critical to find new ways of treating and managing diseases and caring for patients.

Potentially, research trials place some people at risk of harm for the good of others. This could cause the exploitation of patient volunteers and is an ethical concern. Many ethical guidelines exist at local and national levels to protect patient volunteers. These guidelines were initiated based on past abuses. Some of the most influential guidelines and codes of ethics that guide clinical research include:

- *Nuremberg Code*: Originated in 1947 after the Nuremberg trials, in which Nazi doctors were convicted of crimes committed during human experiments on concentration camp prisoners. The code outlined what was legal when conducting human experiments. Several of the points included the need for voluntary consent, the results must be for the good of society, and the experiments must be based on prior knowledge and should avoid all unnecessary physical and mental suffering.
- *Belmont Report*: Written in 1976 by the National Commission for the Protection of Human Subjects of Biomedical and Behavioral Research. The report identifies basic ethical principles and guidelines regarding human subject research.
- *Declaration of Helsinki*: A landmark document regarding research ethics developed by the World Medical Association in 1964 and revised many times. This document addressed the importance of human research, the obligations of the physicians involved, the importance of informed consent and protection of the participants.

Tuskegee Study

In 1932 the Public Health Service, working with the Tuskegee Institute, researched the natural history of syphilis. They hoped to justify treatment programs for African-Americans. The study involved 399 black men with syphilis and 201 without it. The original 6-month study ended 40 years later when the Associated Press ran a story about the research study, and the public outcry led to an advisory panel investigation.

For this research study, the men had agreed freely to be examined and treated, but no informed consent was used. In compensation for the study, the men received free medical exams, free meals, and burial insurance. The men were told they were getting treated, but they did not receive proper treatment to cure syphilis even though penicillin was available in 1947.

In 1974, a $10 million settlement was reached for the study participants and their surviving family members. The settlement also included health benefits for the participants and their family members.

According to the National Institutes of Health (NIH) Clinical Center (*https://clinicalcenter.nih.gov/recruit/ethics.html*), seven main principles are involved with ethical research:

- *Social and clinical value:* It should contribute to the knowledge base of either understanding health or preventing, treating, and caring for people with a specific disease.
- *Scientific validity:* The methods used should be valid and feasible, and the study must have clear scientific objectives.
- *Fair subject selection:* The subjects recruited should be based on the goals of the study.
- *Favorable risk-benefit ratio:* Everything must be done to minimize the risk to the research subjects and to maximize the benefits. The benefits should outweigh the risks.

- *Independent review*: The study should be reviewed by an independent review panel with no vested interest to ensure that the study is ethical and to minimize potential conflicts of interest.
- *Informed consent*: To be ethical, the participants need to be informed of the purpose, methods, risks, benefits, and alternatives to the research. They need to understand the information and make a voluntary decision to participate.
- *Respect for potential and enrolled subjects*: Individuals have a right to change their minds at any time. Their information must be kept confidential, and they must be informed of information that may change their assessment of the risks and benefits of participating in the project.

Often medical assistants who are working at larger facilities may be involved with research projects. They may need to identify patients who match the project's criteria. Medical assistants may help with data collection. It is important for the medical assistant to know that all information must be kept confidential. All participants have a right to change their minds regarding their participation. Typically, the research guidelines or documents will have contact information provided if the medical assistant has questions or concerns regarding the project.

End-of-Life Issues

With the changes in healthcare and technology, more treatment options exist today to prolong a person's life. Ventilators assist the breathing process, and feeding tubes provide nutrition. Medications and defibrillators can help restart the heart. Legislation exists at the state and federal levels to help address death and dying issues. There are also many ethical questions that surround end-of-life issues.

It may sound like end-of-life issues are only addressed in the hospital. End-of-life issues also impact ambulatory care. Medical assistants may accompany providers in skilled nursing facility (nursing home) visits. Medical assistants provide ambulatory care to patients who have terminal illnesses. It is not uncommon for the medical assistant to process a referral for hospice care for a patient. The medical assistant should know the differences between palliative medicine and hospice care.

Palliative means to help relieve the symptoms of a serious illness. Palliative medicine is a subspecialty. The providers offer palliative care to patients who are seriously ill, regardless of age. The disease may be curable, chronic, or life-threatening. Palliative care focuses on the entire person. It does not provide a cure, just helps to reduce the symptoms.

Hospice is a type of palliative care for people who have about 6 months or less to live. The goal of hospice care is to allow patients who are dying to have dignity, comfort, and peace. Hospice programs not only work with the patient, but also the family. Hospice care can be provided in the hospital, skilled nursing facility, hospice center, and at home.

Working with patients who have a terminal illness can be emotionally challenging. It is important for the medical assistant to remember that patients and families go through the grieving process. The stages of grief and dying, as defined by Dr. Elisabeth Kübler-Ross, include:

- *Denial*: Person refuses to accept the diagnosis or prognosis. Defense mechanism that protects people from being overwhelmed. Disbelief and numbness may occur.

- *Anger*: Person's anger can be directed at self or others. May blame others.
- *Bargaining*: Person attempts to bargain with the higher power the person believes in (i.e., God).
- *Depression*: Person feels sadness, fear, and uncertainty. Crying and depression may occur. Person may not participate in normal activities; distances self from others.
- *Acceptance*: Person has come to terms with the situation.

Not everyone goes through all five stages, and people may not go through the stages in the order listed. Some people may switch back and forth between the stages.

Various behaviors may be seen during the grieving process including:

- Sadness, loneliness, social isolation, crying, and difficulty concentrating
- Anger, guilt, denial, and confusion
- Fatigue, numbness, and appetite changes
- Sleep changes, fatigue, and nightmares

Patient Self-Determination Act

The Patient Self-Determination Act (PSDA) became law in 1990. This act requires most healthcare institutions at the time of admission to do the following:

- Provide patients with a written document of their rights to make decisions and the facility's policies respecting advance directives.
- Ask patients if they have advance directives and document the response in the health record.

Healthcare agencies must provide advance directive training to their staff. Staff members cannot discriminate against patients who have or do not have advance directives.

Per the CEJA, providers should:

- Discuss advance care planning with all patients, regardless of health status or age.
- Explain advance directives and document in the health record information about advance care planning.
- Review advance care planning periodically with patients.

If patients present advance directive paperwork, the medical assistant needs to ensure it gets into the health record. It is not uncommon for medical assistants to provide advance directive information to patients. The medical assistant must also be familiar with the different types of advance directives.

Advance Directives. *Advance directives* are written instructions about healthcare decisions, should a person be unable to make them. Advance directives are not just for older adults to complete. It is important for everyone to consider completing advance directives. Once completed, advance directives can be modified in the future. It is important that local healthcare agencies have a copy of the person's advance directive paperwork.

Per the CEJA, providers should:

- Identify if patients have advance directives, including a healthcare proxy.
- Respect the wishes of the patient's surrogate and help the surrogate understand the patient's wishes in the advance directives.
- Seek assistance from the ethics committee if a patient lacks advance directives and is unable to communicate,

Today most states have a multiple-page document for people to complete. The document can be found online or at healthcare agencies. The document may be called *advance directives, durable power of attorney for healthcare,* or something similar. It replaces multiple documents of the past. Generally, the advance directives document contains sections for the different types of advance directives, including:

- *Living will:* Provides instructions about life-sustaining medical treatment to be administered or withheld when the patient has a terminal condition.
- *Medical durable power of attorney:* May be known by other names. Similar to a living will but includes all healthcare decisions. It lasts as long as the person is not able to make decisions. This document names a healthcare proxy and can include healthcare wishes. It can be used when the situation is not terminal.
- *Healthcare proxy:* Also called *healthcare agent* or *surrogate*. A competent adult can appoint a person (called a proxy or agent) to make healthcare decisions in the event he or she is unable to do so.
- *Organ donation:* Indicates if a person wants to donate organs.
- *Do not resuscitate* (DNR): Can be part of the living will. Indicates if the person refuses cardiopulmonary resuscitation (CPR) if he or she stops breathing or has no pulse.

The document can also include additional topics. Remember, each state has its own advance directives form for state residents to complete.

Additional Topics on Advance Directive Forms

- Life-sustaining treatments (e.g., drugs, machines, medical procedures, feeding tubes)
- Desires if permanently unconscious
- Desires with terminal condition
- Mental health treatment
- Admission to nursing home
- Unconscious and pregnant
- Pain relief
- Additional desires

Physician Orders for Life-Sustaining Treatment. Physician Orders for Life-Sustaining Treatment (POLST) can be known by similar names across the United States. It is promoted to work with advance directives. When a person is diagnosed with advanced illness or frailty, having a POLST may be recommended. The POLST is a one-page physician order sheet that indicates the care a person should receive. It should be based on the advance directives and the person's wishes.

For some people the POLST is concerning. The POLST can supersede a person's advance directives. Keep in mind that the POLST is a limited document, and some forms state that the healthcare staff should follow the orders listed before contacting the provider. Opponents to the POLST encourage patients to refuse it. They state that the provider should be contacted when the patient's condition changes, and that the advance directives in its entirety can be followed, not the summarized version listed in the POLST.

Uniform Determination of Death Act

The Uniform Determination of Death Act (UDDA) was drafted in 1981. It served as a guide for state lawmakers to create their own laws. The act provided a definition of death. A person may legally be declared dead if one of the following two events occurs:

- Irreversible **cessation** of circulatory and respiratory functions
- Irreversible cessation of all functions of the entire brain, including the brainstem

This act provided an accepted definition of death. Most states have adopted the exact wording of the UDDA. Some states have added additional regulations to their laws.

Withholding or Withdrawing Life-Sustaining Treatment

Withholding or withdrawing treatments that extend the life of a person can be emotional for the patient and family. This situation can also be ethically challenging for healthcare providers. It is important to remember that patients have the right to decline medical intervention. They can also determine when the intervention should be stopped. If the patient cannot make these decisions, it is up to the patient's surrogate.

Per the CEJA's opinion, providers should identify the patient's wishes early in the treatment. Should providers have questions regarding life-sustaining treatments, they should review the patient's advance directives, support the decisions of the patient or surrogate, and seek advice from an ethics committee.

Euthanasia

Euthanasia is the act of killing a person who is suffering from an incurable disease. It can also be called "mercy killing" because it is ending the patient's suffering. Types of euthanasia include:

- *Active euthanasia:* Killing the person using an active means (e.g., an injection).
- *Passive euthanasia:* Withholding a lifesaving treatment (e.g., feeding tube) and letting the person die.
- *Voluntary euthanasia:* The patient consents to the action.
- *Involuntary euthanasia:* The patient does not consent to the action. Patients may be unconscious or unable to communicate their wishes.
- *Self-administered euthanasia:* The patient kills himself or herself.
- *Other-administered euthanasia:* Another person kills the patient.
- *Assisted suicide/assisted euthanasia:* The patient kills himself or herself with the assistance of another person (e.g., physician-assisted suicide).

Physician-assisted suicide occurs when the provider makes available the means for a patient to end his or her life. The means can be sleeping pills in lethal doses or some other medication that impacts the breathing or heartbeat. The provider is also aware that the patient wants to commit suicide. Most states make physician-assisted euthanasia illegal. Only six states have legalized physician-assisted suicide.

Proponents state that terminally ill patients have a right to end their suffering when they want to. Opponents state that providers have a moral responsibility to keep their patients alive. Per the CEJA's opinion, physician-assisted suicide is against the fundamental nature of the healer role of the provider. Providers must respond to the patient's needs at the end of life. They should respect the patient's autonomy and provide effective communication and emotional support. Providers need to make the patient comfortable and provide adequate pain medications.

Organ Donation Issues

More than 114,000 people in the United States need a lifesaving organ transplantation. More than 74,000 people are on the active waiting list. Six people are added to the national transplant waiting list every hour. The gap between available organs and those needing organs is increasing. More people need organs than are available. On average, 20 people die each day while waiting for a transplant. There continues to be a great need for organ and tissue donations.

According to Donate Life America (*www.donatelife.net*), one organ donor can save eight lives. A cornea donation can restore the sight of two people. Donating tissue can heal the lives of 75 people. The following organs and tissue can be donated:

- *Organs:* Kidney, liver, lung, heart, pancreas, and intestines
- *Tissue:* Hands, faces, heart valves, skin, bones, tendons, bone marrow, cord blood stem cells, blood, platelets, corneas, and eyes

Cord Blood Banking

Cord blood is found in the blood vessels of the placenta and umbilical cord. It is collected after the umbilical cord has been cut at birth. Cord blood is considered a biological product regulated by the Food and Drug Administration (FDA). Currently, cord blood is only used for hematopoietic stem cell transplantation procedures. Such a procedure is used for patients with leukemias and lymphomas. The cord blood has a source of stem cells that form into blood cells. When given transplanted stem cells from cord blood, healthy blood cells regrow after chemotherapy has killed both cancer and health cells.

Collected cord blood can be frozen and stored for years. Parents may opt to store their baby's cord blood in a private bank, so it can be used in the future by the child or a close relative. Private cord banks charge fees for collection and storage. Parents could also donate the cord blood to a public bank, so it can be used for a patient who needs the hematopoietic stem cell transplant.

Living donations are becoming more common; that is, people donate organs or partial organs while living. For example, they can donate a kidney, a lobe of a lung, or a partial liver, intestine, or pancreas. Living tissue donations include skin after surgeries (e.g., abdominoplasty), bone after knee and hip replacement surgeries, bone marrow, umbilical cord blood, amnion, and blood. Both blood and bone marrow can be donated more than once. There are different types of living donations, including:

- *Directed donation:* The donor specifically names the person to receive the donation. Usually, this is a family member or someone the donor has heard about.
- *Nondirected donation:* The donor does not know the person nor is related to the person. The match is made based on the medical compatibility of the person and the donor. Both parties have the option to choose to meet the other person. If both agree and if the transplant center's policy permits it, they can meet.
- *Paired donation:* This involves at least two pairs of living kidney donors. The transplant candidates do not match the donor

they know but match the other donor, thus the organs are swapped or traded.

If a person wishes to be a potential donor at death, registering in your state is the first step. Registration is available online or through your local motor vehicle department. (For more information, go to *organdonor.gov.*) It is also important to let your family know of your wishes. Some advance directive forms also have areas where you can include your wishes.

With organ donation, justice and medical utility are factors that are balanced. Justice refers to the fair consideration of the patient's situation and medical needs. Medical utility relates to trying to increase the number of transplants performed and the survival time of patients and organs. Many factors are considered when organs are matched to patients. When an organ becomes available, patients on the waiting list are screened for blood type, height, weight, and other medical factors. The computer uses national policies to determine the order of the candidates who would be a match for the donor's organs. The right-size organ and the geographic location of the donor organ and the candidate must be considered. Children do better with pediatric donor organs. Each organ has specific factors that are also considered in the allocation. For instance, waiting time, survival benefit, and medical needs may be considered. The following sections will examine laws and ethical recommendations related to organ donation.

Uniform Anatomical Gift Act

The Uniform Anatomical Gift Act (UAGA) was enacted in 1968. All 50 states have adopted this law. The purpose of the act was to make it easier for people to donate organs. This act has been revised several times over the years. States enacted the UAGA, but differences existed between states. In 2006 the UAGA was revised to provide uniformity in organ and tissue donations across the nation. The 2006 revisions include the following:

- Clarified who can make donation decision for the patient
- Strengthened language on protecting the patient's decision on donating or not donating organs
- Established standards for donor registries, which will help match donors to recipients

The CEJA addressed organ donation. It is the opinion of the CEJA that providers should do the following:

- Avoid conflicts of interest and ensure that no members of the transplant team are involved with pronouncing the patient dead.
- Ensure the death is pronounced using accepted clinical and ethical standards.
- Ensure the transplant procedures are done by knowledgeable providers.
- Ensure the prospective recipient of the donor is fully informed about the procedure.

National Organ Transplant Act

The National Organ Transplant Act (NOTA) was passed by Congress in 1984. The act established the Organ Procurement and Transplant Network (OPTN) to be run by contract by the Secretary of Health and Human Services. The act established a national registry for organ matching. NOTA also made it a criminal action to exchange organs for transplant for something of value (e.g., money).

Xenotransplantation

With the lack of available organs and tissues, researchers are studying the use of nonhuman tissue and organs. *Xenotransplantation* is any procedure in which nonhuman cells, tissues, or organs are implanted or infused into a person.

Currently, pigs are the animals of choice for xenotransplants. Their organs are about the same size as humans, and they breed quickly. Pig heart valves are already being used to treat human heart valve issues.

CLOSING COMMENTS
Patient Coaching

When medical assistants are working with patients who are on the organ transplant waiting list, it is important for them to coach each patient on the process and encourage the patient to get emotional support. Once the patient is on the list, the transplant center will confirm the registration. If the person is removed from the list for any reason, the transplant center sends a written letter to the patient. The length of the wait is based on how sick the person is, the availability of organs that match, and the number of donors in the local area. With the organ allocation being based on many factors, a person's wait may vary. Sadly, some people's conditions deteriorate, and they are removed from the list and never get an organ.

Waiting for an organ transplant can cause a wide range of emotions. Once on the list the person is hopeful, but as the wait lengthens, the stress can increase. The same is true for the patient's family. It is important for the patient and family to get support during this time. Local or online support groups may be helpful.

Legal and Ethical Issues

It is important for the medical assistant to continue to learn about healthcare advances. New procedures, treatments, and medications are continually impacting patient care. As technology advances and healthcare changes, the medical assistant needs to remain updated on the ethical issues that surround the changes. Following the professional code of ethics, in addition to learning the CEJA's opinions on the new advances, will help guide the medical assistant's practice.

Patient-Centered Care

One of the key elements to providing patient-centered care is respecting the patient's decision and preferences. When working with ethical situations, it is important for the medical assistant to remember the Patient's Bill of Rights. Patients have the right to refuse treatment. They have the right to make their own decisions. Their decisions may not be our decisions in that situation, but we need to do what they want. It is important to respect patients and ensure their dignity during beginning-of-life issues through end-of-life issues.

Professional Behaviors

All healthcare professionals need to provide ethical, respectful care to all patients. Professional ethics guide healthcare employees on how to be ethical in their role. A medical assistant should be aware of the medical assisting code of ethics and the healthcare facility's professional ethics. The medical assistant needs to practice these professional ethics in every patient situation.

SUMMARY OF SCENARIO

Daniela has completed the ethics unit in her law and ethics course. She is excited to be done with the course. What she has learned in the ethics unit has helped her consider why she believes what she believes. She is realizing that some of her values and morals were built on information that was old or inaccurate. She needs to do some research to verify the information. Daniela feels that as she continues to learn and gain experience, her moral compass may change in the future. She hopes that this will help her to provide the best possible care to her patients.

SUMMARY OF LEARNING OBJECTIVES

1. **Do the following related to ethics:**
   - *Define ethics and morals.*
     Ethics are rules of conduct that differentiate between acceptable and unacceptable behavior. *Morals* are internal principles that distinguish between right and wrong.
   - *Differentiate between personal and professional ethics.*
     Personal ethics are individual choices and are impacted by one's morals. *Professional ethics* are created by associations for members to follow. They are also created by employers for employees to follow. A medical assistant must create a plan to separate personal and professional ethics if they conflict.
   - *Identify the effect of personal morals on professional performance.*
     Our personal morals impact our professional performance in other positive or negative ways. The chapter provided examples of both effects on our professional performance. As professionals, we cannot let our personal morals negatively impact the care that we provide to patients.
   - *Develop a plan for separation of personal and professional ethics.*
     Procedure 5.1 provides an opportunity to develop a plan for separating personal and professional ethics based on the scenario provided.
   - *Recognize the impact personal ethics and morals have on the delivery of healthcare.*
     Procedure 5.1 provides an opportunity to describe the impact of personal morals and ethics on the delivery of healthcare. It is important that medical assistants recognize the impact personal ethics and morals have on the delivery of healthcare.

2. **List and describe the four ethical principles in healthcare.**
   There are four ethical principles in healthcare:
   - *Autonomy:* The freedom to determine one's own actions and decisions
   - *Nonmaleficence:* To do no harm
   - *Beneficence:* To do good
   - *Justice:* To treat patients fairly and give them what is due to them
   These four principles need to be considered equally when evaluating ethical issues. The medical assistant has related responsibilities for each of these principles.

3. **Demonstrate appropriate responses to ethical issues involving genetics.**
   The chapter discussed the ethical issues involved with cloning, genetic engineering, genetic testing, pharmacogenetics, stem cell transplantation, and gene therapy. Many advances have occurred in genetics, and with

them many ethical issues have surfaced. Refer to each section for the ethical issues related to the topic and the CEJA's opinion for providers.

4. **Demonstrate appropriate responses to ethical issues involving reproductive issues.**
   Different types of assistive reproductive technology were discussed. Gamete donation and egg freezing were also addressed, along with abortion. Refer to the sections for the CEJA's opinion.

5. **Demonstrate appropriate responses to ethical issues involving childhood issues.**
   This chapter discussed many different types of adoption. With most adoptions, the child does not have information regarding the parents. This is important for the medical assistant to remember. Ethical issues surrounding adoption, safe haven infant protection laws, and confidential healthcare for minors were addressed. Refer to the chapter sections for the ethical issues surrounding these topics.

6. **Demonstrate appropriate responses to ethical issues involving medical research trials.**
   This chapter discussed the abuses and influential guidelines and codes of ethics for clinical research. Seven main principles are involved with ethical research, and these include social and clinical value, scientific validity, fair subject selection, favorable risk-benefit ratio, independent review, informed consent, and respect for potential and enrolled subjects.

7. **Demonstrate appropriate responses to ethical issues involving end-of-life issues and discuss the theory of Elisabeth Kübler-Ross.**
   Many ethical issues surround end-of-life issues. This chapter discussed advance directives, withholding or withdrawing life-sustaining treatment, and euthanasia. The CEJA's opinion and the ethical issues involved with each of these topics were discussed.
   The stages of grief and dying, as defined by Elisabeth Kübler-Ross, include:
   - *Denial:* Person refuses to accept the diagnosis or prognosis.
   - *Anger:* Person's anger can be directed at self or others.
   - *Bargaining:* Person attempts to bargain with the higher power the person believes in.
   - *Depression:* Person feels sadness, fear, and uncertainty.
   - *Acceptance:* Person has come to terms with the situation.
   Not everyone goes through all five stages, and people may not go through the stages in the order listed. Some people may switch back and forth between the stages.

8. **Demonstrate appropriate responses to ethical issues involving organ donation issues; discuss the Patient Self Determination Act and the**

Continued

SUMMARY OF LEARNING OBJECTIVES—*continued*

Uniform Anatomical Gift Act; and define terms related to organ donation issues (advance directives, living will, medical durable power of attorney, and healthcare proxy).

Organ donation topics, including the need for organ and tissue donors, what can be donated, and the emotional wait for an organ, were discussed. The ethical issues related to organ donation and the CEJA's opinion were explained. It is important for potential donors to talk with their family members about their wishes.

The Patient Self-Determination Act (PSDA) requires most healthcare institutions at the time of admission to do the following:

- Provide patients with a written document of their rights to make decisions and the facility's policies respecting advance directives.
- Ask patients if they have advance directives and document the response in the health record.

The Uniform Anatomical Gift Act (UAGA) was enacted in 1968, and all 50 states have adopted this law. The purpose of the act was to make it easier for people to donate organs. This act has been revised several times over the years.

Terms related to organ donation issues:

- *Living will:* Provides instructions about life-sustaining medical treatment to be administered or withheld when the patient has a terminal condition.
- *Medical durable power of attorney:* Similar to a living will but includes all healthcare decisions. Names a healthcare proxy and can include healthcare wishes.
- *Healthcare proxy:* Also called a *healthcare agent* or *surrogate*. A competent adult can appoint a person (called a *proxy* or an *agent*) to make healthcare decisions in the event he or she is unable to do so.

PROCEDURE 5.1   Develop an Ethics Separation Plan

Task: To develop a plan for separating personal and professional ethics.

Scenario: You are working at WMFM Clinic. Your provider sees many children, including teens. New state laws allow confidential healthcare for minors. The agency has now adopted policies and procedures to allow providers to see teens 16 years or older without parental consent. The teens can be seen for sexually transmitted infections (STIs) and reproductive issues (including birth control). All health records related to these visits are confidential, meaning parents cannot be told about their child's visit.

Your personal belief is that parents should always be allowed to know what is occurring with their children. They are responsible for the child until age 18, and they pay the bills. You also believe that children under 18 are too young to be in an intimate relationship with others. This type of relationship should be only for adults in a committed relationship. You do not believe in birth control.

EQUIPMENT and SUPPLIES

- Paper and pen
- Medical Assisting Code of Ethics

PROCEDURAL STEPS

1. Read the code of ethics for medical assistants. Write down key themes or phrases.
   PURPOSE: Medical assistants need to follow the code of ethics for the medical assistant professional.

2. Using the scenario, write down the professional ethics involved in the situation.
   PURPOSE: Medical assistants need to follow the laws and agency's policies and procedures. The procedures indicate how the healthcare professional needs to perform duties.

3. Using the scenario, write down the personal ethics involved in the situation.
   PURPOSE: Medical assistants need to identify their personal ethics. They need to be honest when analyzing how they think and feel about different scenarios that may occur in healthcare. Understanding one's biases is the first step in ensuring that respectful, ethical care is provided to all patients.

4. Compare the lists. Identify the personal ethics that conflict with the code of ethics and the professional ethics of the agency.
   PURPOSE: Medical assistants must identify areas where their personal ethics conflict with the code of ethics and the professional ethics of the agency. Medical assistants need to follow professional ethics. Personal ethics should not supersede professional ethics.

5. For each area of conflict, create a plan on how you will separate your personal and professional ethics. Remember, as a professional, you need to follow the professional ethics of the agency and the profession. Address how you will handle the situation and what would be your options if you were in the situation.
   PURPOSE: Medical assistants must create a plan and be aware of how they will handle situations that conflict with their personal ethics. This might mean they need to find another job. They may need to rethink their biases. Learning more about a bias can help a person identify errors in his or her thinking.

6. Describe how the personal ethics and morals in this scenario would impact the patient care.
   PURPOSE: It is important that medical assistants recognize the impact personal ethics and morals have on the delivery of healthcare.

PROCEDURE 5.2 | Demonstrate Appropriate Responses to Ethical Issues

Tasks: Identify ethical issues and demonstrate appropriate and professional responses. Recognize the impact personal ethics and morals have on the delivery of healthcare.

Scenario 1: You are working at WMFM Clinic.. You are responsible for collecting payments from patients. Mr. Smythe, who is visually impaired, paid for his visit in cash. He gives you $500 for a $402 bill. You make change and give him a receipt. At the end of the day, you notice that you have $60 more than what you should have, and some of the bills were mixed up in the cashbox. You realize you gave Mr. Smythe the incorrect amount of money.

Scenario 2: You are setting up a laceration repair tray for Dr. Martin to use. As you are preparing the sterile equipment, one of the instruments becomes contaminated. You know Dr. Martin urgently needs the tray. You do nothing about the contamination, which you realize can cause an infection. You finish setting up the tray.

EQUIPMENT and SUPPLIES

- Paper and pen

PROCEDURAL STEPS

1. Read both scenarios. Identify and write down the ethical issues involved.
   PURPOSE: It is important to identify the issues as the first step in responding to ethical situations.
2. With a peer, role-play scenario 1. Your peer should be the supervisor in this scenario. Demonstrate a professional and appropriate ethical response to this situation.
   a. Explain the situation to the supervisor.
   b. Describe how you felt the error occurred and who received the incorrect change.
   c. Explain how you would like to handle the situation and correct the error.
   PURPOSE: It is important that the medical assistant act professionally and ethically when a mistake is discovered.
3. With a peer, role-play scenario 2. Your peer should be the provider in this scenario. During the role-play, demonstrate a professional and appropriate ethical response to this situation.
   PURPOSE: It is important that the medical assistant act ethically and notify the provider when an error is made.
4. In a written response, discuss the potential implication to the patient's health related to not reporting or correcting the error.
   PURPOSE: It is important that the medical assistant realize how unethical actions impact patient care.

6

INTRODUCTION TO ANATOMY AND MEDICAL TERMINOLOGY

Daniela Garcia has just been hired as a part-time float receptionist at Walden-Martin Family Medical Clinic (WMFM). She also has just started the medical assistant program at the local community college. She is currently taking a medical terminology course and a human body and disease course. She understands that learning medical terminology is very much like learning a foreign language. She also understands that by learning the meanings of different word parts, she can easily figure out the meaning of a new medical term.

Daniela was excited to accept this position. She feels that this job would give her a foot in the door for a possible medical assistant position in the future.

It will also allow her to learn more about healthcare. Having just graduated from high school in May, she does not have a lot of previous work experience.

During her first week on the job, Daniela realizes there is a lot to learn. As a float she will be assisting in the specialty clinic, where providers from other agencies hold outreach clinics. During outreach, these providers see patients and provide specialty services not offered by WMFM providers. From patients to providers, everyone seems to use medical terminology, body-related terms, and language describing disease states. Daniela is happy to know a bit from her course, but she realizes she has a lot more terminology to learn.

While studying this chapter, think about the following questions:
- How do you decode medical terms using the CARD method?
- How do you identify combining forms, suffixes, and prefixes used in medical terminology?
- How do you apply spelling rules to medical terminology?
- How do you recognize and use terms related to the basic anatomy and pathology concepts?
- How do you describe the organization of the body?
- How do you describe body systems?
- How do you recognize and use surface anatomy, directional, and positional terms?
- How do you describe body cavities and abdominopelvic quadrants?
- What are common predisposing factors and causes of disease?

LEARNING OBJECTIVES

1. Review the origins of medical terminology and discuss the difference between decodable and nondecodable terms.
2. Describe how to decode terms using the check, assign, reverse, and define (CARD) method.
3. Use the rules given to build and spell healthcare terms.
4. Describe the structural organization of the human body.
5. Properly use surface anatomy, positional, and directional terminology.
6. Describe body cavities, abdominopelvic quadrants, and body planes.
7. Discuss the acid-base balance in the human body.
8. Discuss pathology basics, including pathology terminology, protection mechanisms, predisposing factors, and the causes of disease.

VOCABULARY

anaplastic (an uh PLAS tic) A rapidly dividing cancer cell that has little to no similarity to normal cells.

antibodies Protein substances, produced in the blood or tissues in response to a specific antigen, that destroy or weaken the antigen. Part of the immune system.

antigens Substances that stimulate the production of an antibody when introduced into the body. Antigens include toxins, bacteria, viruses, and other foreign substances.

biopsy (BIE op see) Process of viewing living tissue that has been removed for the purpose of diagnosis or treatment.

chromosomes (KROH muh sohms) Rod-shaped structures found in the cell's nucleus; they contain genetic information.

combining forms The "subjects" of most terms. They consist of the word root with its respective combining vowel.

diaphragm A broad, dome-shaped muscle used for breathing that separates the thoracic and abdominopelvic cavities.

differentiated (dif uh REN shee ayt ed) Describes the degree to which malignant tissue looks like the normal tissue it came from – poorly differentiated means it does not look like the normal tissue; well differentiated means it looks like the normal tissue.

endoscopy (en DOS kuh pee) An examination using a scope with a camera attached to the long, thin tube that can be inserted into the body.

homeostasis (hoh mee uh STAY sis) The internal environment of the body that is compatible with life. A steady state that is created by all the body systems working together to provide a consistent and unvarying internal environment.

intercellular Located between cells.

mitosis (mie TOH sis) A cell division process by which two daughter cells are formed from one parent cell; each daughter has a complete copy of the parent's chromosomes.

nondecodable terms Words used in healthcare whose definitions must be memorized without the benefit of word parts.

oncologist A specially trained doctor who diagnoses and treats cancer.

organelle Structures inside of the cell that have specific functions to maintain the cell.

pathogen A disease-causing organism.

pathologist A physician specially trained in the nature and cause of disease.

pathology The study of disease.

peristalsis (per uh STAL sis) Wavelike motion.

prefixes Word parts that appear at the beginning of terms.

suffixes Word parts that appear at the end of terms.

toxins (TOK sins) Substances created by microorganisms, plants, or animals that are poisonous to humans.

vasoconstriction Contraction of the muscles, causing narrowing of the inside tube of the vessel.

Medical terminology is a specialized vocabulary that has its roots in Greek and Latin word components. Professionals in healthcare use this terminology to communicate with each other. By applying the process of "decoding," or recognizing the word components and their meanings, you will be able to interpret literally thousands of medical terms. By using **combining forms**, **suffixes**, and **prefixes** you can break down medical terms and easily learn their meaning. This chapter presents a review of medical terminology to help you fully communicate as a healthcare professional.

This chapter also will review general anatomy, directional terms, and **pathology** terms and testing. This will help you before you start the specialty chapters of the book. Review is key to remembering and using information that has been presented in your education. Having a mastery of medical terminology, basic anatomy terms and concepts, and disease terminology and testing will give you the tools to understand the language and procedures presented in each medical specialty.

TYPES OF MEDICAL TERMS

Decodable Terms

Decodable terms are those that can be broken into their Greek and Latin word parts and given a working definition based on the meanings of those word parts. Most medical terms are decodable, so learning word parts is important. The word parts are as follows:

Combining form: Word root with its respective combining vowel.
Word root: Foundation of the medical term.
Combining vowel: A letter sometimes used to join word parts. Usually an "o" but occasionally an "a," "e," "i," or "u."
Suffix: Word part that appears at the end of a term. Suffixes are used to modify the meaning of the combining form.
Prefix: Word part that sometimes appears at the beginning of a term. Prefixes also modify the meaning of the combining form. They usually are used to further define the absence, location, number, quantity, or state of the term.

For our first examples, we will use ophthalm- (Greek) and ocul- (Latin). These combing forms both mean "eye." Both of the word

roots use an "o" as their combining vowel. Therefore ophthalmo/o and ocul/o are the combining forms related to "eye." Figs. 6.1 and 6.2 demonstrate the decoding of the terms *ophthalmology* and *extraocular*. Throughout the text, we will be using combining forms so that you will learn the appropriate combining vowel for that particular term.

Nondecodable Terms

Not all terms are composed of word parts that can be used to determine the definition. These terms are known as **nondecodable terms**. For these types of terms, the meaning must be memorized. A medical dictionary is an excellent tool to help with finding the definition of nondecodable terms. Examples of nondecodable terms include the following:

Cataract: From the Greek term meaning "waterfall." In healthcare language, this means the condition in which the lens becomes progressively opaque (loss of transparency).

Asthma: From the Greek term meaning "panting." Although this word origin is understandable, the definition is a respiratory disorder characterized by recurring episodes of paroxysmal dyspnea (difficulty breathing).

Diagnosis: The disease or condition that is determined after a healthcare provider evaluates a patient's signs, symptoms, and history. Although the term is built from word parts (dia-, meaning "through," "complete," and -gnosis, meaning "state of knowledge"), using these word parts to form the definition of diagnosis, which is "a state of complete knowledge," is not very helpful.

Prognosis: Similar to *diagnosis*, the term *prognosis* can be broken down into its word parts (pro-, meaning "before" or "in front of," and -gnosis, meaning "state of knowledge"), but this does not give the true definition of the term, which is "a prediction of the probable outcome of a disease or disorder."

Sequela: A condition that follows and is the result of an injury or disease.

Acute: A term that describes a sudden, severe onset (acu- means "sharp") of a disease.

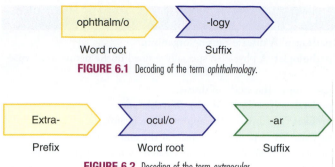

FIGURE 6.1 Decoding of the term *ophthalmology.*

FIGURE 6.2 Decoding of the term *extraocular.*

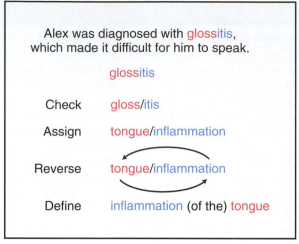

FIGURE 6.3 How to decode a medical term using the check, assign, reverse, and define (CARD) method. (From Shiland B: *Mastering healthcare terminology,* ed 5, St Louis, 2016, Elsevier.)

Chronic: Developing slowly and lasting for 6 months or longer (chron/o means "time"). Diagnoses may be additionally described as being either acute or chronic.

Sign: An objective finding of a disease state (e.g., fever, high blood pressure, rash).

Symptom: A subjective report of a disease (pain, itching).

Other types of terms that are not built from word parts include the following:

Eponyms: Terms that are named after a person or place associated with the term. Examples include the following:

Alzheimer disease, which is named after Alois Alzheimer, a German neurologist. The disease is a progressive mental deterioration.

Achilles tendon, which is a body part named after a figure in Greek mythology whose one weak spot was this area of his anatomy. Tendons are bands of tissue that attach muscles to bone. The Achilles tendon is the particular tendon that attaches the calf muscle to the heel bone. Unlike some eponyms, this one does have a medical equivalent, the calcaneal tendon.

This text presents eponyms without the possessive. This practice is in accordance with the American Medical Association (AMA) and the American Association for Medical Transcription (AAMT).

Abbreviations and Symbols

Abbreviations are terms that have been shortened to letters or numbers for the sake of convenience, such as AAMA for the American Association of Medical Assistants. Symbols are graphic representations of a term, such as @ for *at.* Abbreviations and symbols are common in written and spoken medical terminology but can pose problems for healthcare workers. The Institute of Safe Medical Practice has provided an extensive list. Each healthcare organization should have an official list, which includes the single meaning allowed for each abbreviation or symbol. Examples of acceptable abbreviations and symbols include the following:

Simple abbreviations: A combination of letters (often, but not always the first letter of significant word parts) and sometimes numbers; for example:

IM: Abbreviation for *intramuscular* (pertaining to within the muscles)

C2: Second cervical vertebra (second bone in neck)

Acronyms: Abbreviations that are also pronounceable; for example:

CABG: Coronary artery bypass graft (a detour around a blockage in an artery of the heart)

TURP: Transurethral resection of the prostate (a surgical procedure that removes the prostate through the urethra)

Symbols: Graphic representations of terms

♂ stands for male

♀ stands for female

↑ stands for increased

↓ stands for decreased

+ stands for present

− stands for absent

DECODING TERMS

Check, Assign, Reverse, and Define (CARD) Method

Using Greek and Latin word components to break down the meanings of medical terms requires a simple four-step process – the check, assign, reverse, and define (CARD) method. You need to do the following:

- *Check* for the word parts in a term.
- *Assign* meanings to the word parts.
- *Reverse* the meaning of the suffix to the front of your definition.
- *Define* the term.

Using Fig. 6.3, see how this process is applied to a medical term.

In the tables that follow, the term is in the first column and a definition is in the second column. Table 6.1 introduces six common combining forms and six common suffixes. (The use of prefixes will be introduced later.) Table 6.2 introduces six medical terms that use six different combining forms and suffixes. Success in decoding these terms depends on how well you remember the word parts presented in Table 6.1. Once you have mastered these 12 word parts, you will be able to recognize and define many other medical terms that use these same word parts.

BUILDING TERMS

Now that you've seen how terms are decoded, we will talk about how they are built. First, here are a few rules on how to spell medical terms correctly.

TABLE 6.1 Common Combining Forms and Suffixes

COMBINING FORMS	SUFFIXES
ot/o = ear	**-algia** = pain
cardi/o = heart	**-tomy** = incision
ophthalm/o = eye	**-scope** = instrument to view
nephr/o = kidney	**-logy** = study of
neur/o = nerve	**-plasty** = surgical repair
hepat/o = liver	**-itis** = inflammation

TABLE 6.2 Samples of Decodable Terms

TERM	DEFINITION
otalgia	Pain in the ear, or earache
cardiotomy	Incision of the heart
ophthalmoscope	Instrument used to view the eye
nephrology	Study of the kidney
neuroplasty	Surgical repair of a nerve
hepatitis	Inflammation of the liver

TABLE 6.3 Noun-Ending Suffixes

SUFFIX	MEANING
-icle	small, tiny
-is	structure, thing
-ole	small, tiny
-ule	small, tiny
-um	structure, thing, membrane
-y	process of, condition

Spelling Rules

With a few exceptions, decodable medical terms follow five simple rules.

1. If the suffix starts with a vowel, a combining vowel is *not* needed to join the parts. For example, it is simple to combine the combining form **hepat/o** and suffix **-itis** to build the term **hepatitis**, which means "an inflammation of the liver." The combining vowel "o" is not needed because the suffix starts with the vowel "i."
2. If the suffix starts with a consonant, a combining vowel *is* needed to join the two word parts. For example, to build a term using **neur/o** and **-plasty**, the combining vowel is used and the resulting term is spelled **neuroplasty**, which refers to a surgical repair of a nerve.
3. If a combining form ends with the same vowel that begins a suffix, one of the vowels is dropped. The term that means "inflammation of the inside of the heart" is built from the suffix **-itis** (inflammation), the prefix **endo-** (inside), and the combining form **cardi/o**. **Endo-** + **cardi/o** + **-itis** would result in *endocardiitis*. Instead, one of the "i"s is dropped, and the term is spelled **endocarditis**.
4. If two or more combining forms are used in a term, the combining vowel is retained between the two, regardless of whether the second combining form begins with a vowel or a consonant. For example, joining **gastr/o** and **enter/o** (small intestine) with the suffix **-itis**,

results in the term **gastroenteritis**. Notice that the combining vowel is *kept* between the two combining forms (even though **enter/o** begins with the vowel "e"), and the combining vowel is *dropped* before the suffix **-itis**.

5. Sometimes when two or more combining forms are used to make a medical term, special notice must be paid to the order in which the combining forms are joined. For example, joining **esophag/o** (which means esophagus), **gastr/o** (which means stomach), and **duoden/o** (which means duodenum, the first part of the small intestines) with the suffix **-scopy** (process of viewing), produces the term *esophagogastroduodenoscopy*. An esophagogastroduodenoscopy (EGD) is a visual examination of the esophagus, stomach, and duodenum. In this procedure, the examination takes place in a specific sequence (that is, esophagus first, stomach second, and then the duodenum). Thus the term reflects the direction from which the scope travels through the body (Fig. 6.4).

Suffixes

The body system chapters in this text include many combining forms that are used to build terms specific to each system. These combining forms will not be seen in other places, except as a sign or symptom of a particular disorder. Suffixes, however, are used over and over again throughout the text. Suffixes usually can be grouped according to their purposes. Tables 6.3 through 6.8 cover the major suffix categories.

Noun-Ending Suffixes

Noun endings are used most often to describe anatomic terms. Noun endings such as -icle, -ole, and -ule describe a small or tiny structure. See Table 6.3.

Adjective Suffixes

Adjective suffixes usually mean "pertaining to." For example, when the suffix **-ac** is added to the combining form **cardi/o**, the term *cardiac* is formed, which means "pertaining to the heart." Remember that when you see an adjective term, you need to see what it is describing. For example, cardiac pain is pain of the heart, and cardiac surgery is surgery done on the heart. An adjective tells only half of the story. Common adjective suffixes include the following: -ac, -al, -ar, -ary, -eal, -ic, -ous and mean pertaining to.

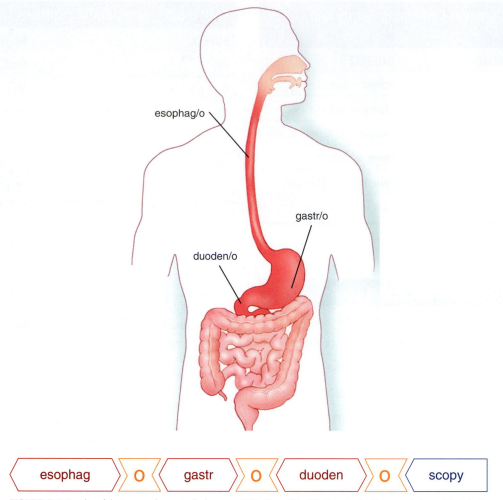

esophag/o

gastr/o

duoden/o

esophag > O < gastr > O < duoden > O < scopy

FIGURE 6.4 Decoding of the term *esophagogastroduodenoscopy* (EGD). (From Shiland B: *Mastering healthcare terminology*, ed 5, St Louis, 2016, Elsevier.)

Pathology Suffixes

Pathology suffixes describe a disease process or a sign or symptom. The meanings vary according to the conditions that they describe. See Table 6.4.

Diagnostic Procedure Suffixes

Diagnostic procedure suffixes point to a procedure that helps to determine the diagnosis. Although a few diagnostic procedures also can help to treat a disease, most are used to establish which particular disease or disorder is occurring. See Table 6.5.

Therapeutic Intervention Suffixes

Therapeutic intervention suffixes indicate types of treatment. Treatments may be medical or surgical in nature. See Table 6.6.

Instrument Suffixes

Instruments are indicated by yet another set of suffixes. Note the obvious similarities to their diagnostic and therapeutic cousins. For example, electrocardiography is a diagnostic procedure that is done to measure the electrical activity in the heart; an electrocar-

diograph is the instrument used to perform electrocardiography. See Table 6.7.

Specialty and Specialist Suffixes

Specialties and specialists require yet another category of suffixes. Someone who specializes in the study of the heart would be called a *cardiologist*. **Cardi/o** means "heart," and **-logist** means "one who specializes in the study of." See Table 6.8.

TABLE 6.4 Pathology Suffixes

SUFFIX	MEANING
-algia	pain
-cele	herniation
-dynia	pain
-emia	blood condition
-ia	condition
-itis	inflammation
-malacia	softening
-megaly	enlargement
-oma	tumor, mass
-osis	abnormal condition
-pathy	disease process
-ptosis	prolapse, drooping, sagging
-rrhage, -rrhagia	bursting forth
-rrhea	discharge, flow
-rrhexis	rupture
-sclerosis	abnormal condition of hardening
-stenosis	abnormal condition of narrowing

TABLE 6.5 Diagnostic Procedure Suffixes

SUFFIX	MEANING
-graphy	process of recording
-metry	process of measuring
-opsy	process of viewing
-scopy	process of viewing

TABLE 6.6 Therapeutic Intervention Suffixes

SUFFIX	MEANING
-ectomy	removal, resection, excision
-plasty	surgical repair
-rrhaphy	suture, repair
-stomy	new opening
-tomy	incision, cutting
-tripsy	crushing

TABLE 6.7 Instrument Suffixes

SUFFIX	MEANING
-graph	instrument to record
-meter	instrument to measure
-scope	instrument to view
-tome	instrument to cut
-tripter	machine to crush
-trite	instrument to crush

TABLE 6.8 Specialty and Specialist Suffixes

SUFFIX	MEANING
-er	one who
-iatrician	one who specializes in treatment
-iatrics	treatment
-iatrist	one who specializes in treatment
-iatry	process of treatment
-ist	one who specializes
-logist	one who specializes in the study of
-logy	study of

Prefixes

Prefixes modify a medical term by indicating a structure's or a condition's
- Absence
- Location
- Number or quantity
- State

Sometimes, as with other word parts, a prefix can have more than one meaning. For example, the prefix **hypo-** can mean "below" or "deficient." To spell a term with the use of a prefix, simply add the prefix directly to the beginning of the term. No combining vowels are needed (Table 6.9).

CRITICAL THINKING APPLICATION   **6.2**

Daniela has mastered suffixes and is ready to move on to prefixes. She concentrates most on prefixes that are similar to one another in spelling or meaning. Can you explain the difference between inter- and intra-? Para- and peri-? Ante- and anti-?

TABLE 6.9   Prefixes

PREFIX	MEANING
a-	no, not, without
an-	no, not, without
ante-	forward, in front of, before
anti-	against
dys-	abnormal, difficult, bad, painful
endo-, end-	within
epi-	above, upon
hyper-	excessive, above
hypo-	below, deficient
inter-	between
intra-	within
neo-	new
par-	near, beside
para-	near, beside, abnormal
per-	through
peri-	surrounding, around
poly-	many, much, excessive, frequent
post-	after, behind
pre-	before, in front of
sub-	under, below
trans-	through, across

SINGULAR/PLURAL RULES

Most medical terms end with Greek or Latin suffixes. Making a medical term singular or plural is not always done the same way as it is in English. Listed below are the most common singular/plural endings and the rules for using them.

- When a singular form of a word ends with -a, keep the -a and add an -e.
  - Example: singular – axilla   plural – axillae
- When a singular form of the word ends with -ax, drop the -x and add -ces.
  - Example: singular – thorax   plural – thoraces
- When a singular form of the word ends with -ex or -ix, drop the -ex or -ix and add -ices.
  - Example: singular – apex   plural – apices
  - Example: singular – cervix   plural – cervices
- When a singular form of the word ends with -is, drop the -is and add -es.
  - Example: singular – diagnosis   plural – diagnoses
- When a singular form of the word ends with -us, drop the -us and add -i.
  - Example: singular – embolus   plural – emboli
- When the singular form of the word ends with -um, drop the -um and add -a.
  - Example: singular – ovum   plural – ova
- When the singular form of the word ends with -y, drop the -y and add -ies.
  - Example: singular – biopsy   plural – biopsies
- When a singular form of the word ends with -x, drop the -x and add -ges.
  - Example: singular – larynx   plural – larynges

COMMON COMBINING FORMS

Table 6.10 lists the common combining forms in medical terminology. This is not a complete list of combining forms, but it covers the most

TABLE 6.10   Common Combining Forms

COMBINING FORM	MEANING	COMBINING FORM	MEANING
aden/o	gland	cholecyst/o	gallbladder
arteri/o	artery	chondr/o	cartilage
arthr/o	joint	col/o	large intestine, colon
aur/i	ear, hearing	coron/o	crown, heart
bacteri/o	bacteria	cut/o	skin
bi/o	living, life	cutane/o	skin
cardi/o	heart	cyst/o	bladder, sac
carp/o	wrist	dent/i	tooth
cephal/o	head	derm/o	skin
cervic/o	neck, cervix	duoden/o	duodenum

TABLE 6.10	Common Combining Forms—*continued*		
COMBINING FORM	**MEANING**	**COMBINING FORM**	**MEANING**
electr/o	electricity	path/o	disease
enter/o	small intestine	ped/o	child
esophag/o	esophagus	pharyng/o	throat
gastr/o	stomach	phleb/o	vein
gingiv/o	gums	phil/o	attraction
gloss/o	tongue	pne/o	breathing
glyc/o	glucose, sugar	pneum/o	lungs
hem/o, hemat/o	blood	psych/o	mind
hepat/o	liver	pulm/o, pulmon/o	lungs
hyster/o	uterus	rhin/o	nose
lingu/o	tongue	somn/o	sleep
lipid/o	lipid, fat	spir/o	breathing
lith/o	stone	splen/o	spleen
mamm/o	breast	therm/o	heat, temperature
muscul/o	muscle	tonsill/o	tonsil
my/o	muscle	trache/o	trachea, windpipe
nat/o	birth, born	troph/o	nourishment
nephr/o	kidney	ur/o, urin/o	urine, urinary system
neur/o	nerve	urethr/o	urethra
ophthalm/o	eye	valvul/o	valve
oste/o	bone	ven/o	vein
ot/o	ear	vertebr/o	backbone, vertebra

commonly used forms. Until you are comfortable with medical terminology, keep a list of common combining forms, prefixes, and suffixes nearby so that you can refer to it as needed.

ANATOMY REVIEW

Structural Organization of the Body

The human body is a collection of many body systems. Examples include the digestive, cardiovascular, musculoskeletal, and respiratory systems. Each system is composed of different organs. For instance, the stomach and intestines are digestive system organs. Each organ is made up of combinations of tissues, and these tissues are composed of cells. So when studying the organization of the body, it is easier to start at the level of cells and work up to the organism (human body) level.

Cells

The basic unit of life is the *cell*. Cells determine the functional and structural characteristics of the entire body. Cells are microscopic in size. They have a variety of shapes and perform a vast array of functions. A cell is covered by a plasma membrane. The cell contains cytoplasm and **organelles**. See Table 6.11 and Fig. 6.5 for the parts of the cells.

Most human cells reproduce by **mitosis**. Mitosis is a process in which one cell splits into two identical daughter cells. The two cells are genetically identical to the parent cell. Prior to the mitosis process, the cell enters the interphase stage. During this stage, the genetic information (i.e., **chromosomes**) replicate. Each sister pair of chromosomes (called *chromatids*) are joined together until they are pulled apart later in the mitosis process. The point where the two chromatids are joined is called the *centromere*. The centromere is also the attachment point for spindle fibers, which will be involved in the mitosis process. The mitosis process consists of four phases; prophase, metaphase, anaphase, and telophase.

Tissues

Tissue is a group of similar cells from the same source that together carry out a specific function. The study of body tissues is known as

TABLE 6.11   Cell Parts

CELL PARTS	DESCRIPTION
Plasma membrane	Outer covering of the cell that allows certain substances to enter the cell and blocks the entrance of other substances. Can also be called the *cell membrane*.
Cytoplasm	Gel that surrounds the nucleus and fills the cells. Organelles are suspended in the cytoplasm.
Ribosome	Organelle that makes enzymes and proteins. Contains ribonucleic acid (RNA).
Rough endoplasmic reticulum (ER)	Organelle that is a network of membranes; connects to the nucleus. The rough appearance is due to the attachment of ribosome to the ER.
Smooth endoplasmic reticulum (ER)	Tube-like organelle; function changes depending on the cell type. Functions may include calcium storage, steroid production, and lipid production.
Golgi apparatus	Processes and packages proteins and lipids produced by the cell. The cell's "processing plant."
Lysosomes	Contain enzymes which digest nutrients and other substances in the cell.
Mitochondrion	Produces energy for the cell. The cell's power plant.
Nucleus	Control center of the cell; contains chromosomes made up of deoxyribonucleic acid (DNA); carries genetic information.
Nucleolus	A small organelle inside of the nucleus; produces ribosomes.
Centrioles	Tube-like structures that help with cell division.
Cilia	Fine, hair-like extensions on the surface of the cell.
Microvilli	Small projections on the surface of the cell; increases the surface area and increases cellular absorption.
Flagellum	Single, long, whip-like extension on the surface of the cell. Used to move the cell.

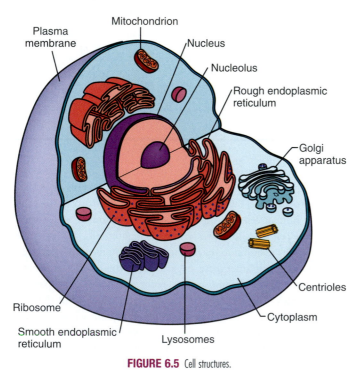

FIGURE 6.5 Cell structures.

histology. All body tissues are grouped into four types. The four types of tissue include the following:

- *Epithelial tissue*: Acts as an internal or external covering for organs. Examples of epithelial tissue include the outer layer of the skin, glands, and linings of body cavities and organs. Epithelial tissue

CRITICAL THINKING APPLICATION   **6.3**

Daniela was learning about the cell structures in school. While on break one night, she talked to Bella. Bella is a new CMA (AAMA) who just graduated. Daniela mentioned she was learning about cell parts. Bella encouraged Daniela to associate the cell parts to the things she might see in a city. For instance, she stated, "The plasma membrane could be the walls around the city." What other associations could be made between the cell structures and a city?

has the cells packed so closely together that there is little to no **intercellular** material. *Simple epithelium* is a single layer of the same-shaped cells. *Stratified epithelium* contains multiple layers of cells.

- *Connective tissue*: Supports and binds other body tissues. Examples of connective tissue include bone; blood; adipose, fibrous, and areolar tissues; and cartilage. Connective tissue is the most frequently occurring tissue in the body.
- *Muscle tissue*: Produces movement. Table 6.12 shows the classification, characteristics, and roles of the types of muscle tissue.
- *Nervous tissue*: Includes cells that provide transmission of information to control a variety of functions. Nervous tissue controls the body's functions to maintain **homeostasis**. Nervous tissue is made up of neurons (nerve cells) and supportive structures called *neuroglial cells*.

Organs

An *organ* is a structure composed of two or more types of tissue. An organ may have one or more functions. Organs are grouped within

TABLE 6.12   Classification of Muscle Tissue

CLASSIFICATION	CHARACTERISTICS	ROLE
Skeletal	Striated, voluntary	Attached to bones and produces voluntary body movements when contracted
Cardiac	Striated, involuntary	Forms the heart muscle wall
Smooth	Nonstriated, involuntary	Lines the blood vessel walls and hollow organs; allows **peristalsis** and **vasoconstriction**

body systems. An organ may be part of one or more systems. Organs can be divided into parts.

Body Systems

A *body system* is composed of several organs and their related structures. These structures work together to perform a specific function in the body. Table 6.13 summarizes the body systems, including their structures and functions.

Organism

The *organism* of the body is made up of many body systems. These work together to maintain a steady environment in the body, called *homeostasis*. If the balance is off or if the environment moves out of the normal range, diseases can occur.

To summarize the structural organization of the body, from simple to complex:

- *Cells:* The most basic unit
- *Tissues:* Groups of similar cells from the same source that carry out a specific function
- *Organ:* A structure made up of two or more types of tissues

TABLE 6.13   Summary of Body Systems

BODY SYSTEM	CELLS, STRUCTURES, AND ORGANS	FUNCTIONS
Blood	Arteries, arterioles, veins, venules, white blood cells, red blood cells, platelets, plasma	Transports materials (e.g., oxygen, nutrients) and collects wastes throughout the body; involved with fighting infection and forming clots
Cardiovascular	Heart, valves, arteries, arterioles, veins, venules	Transports materials in the blood throughout the body
Endocrine	Pituitary, pineal gland, hypothalamus, thyroid, pancreas, adrenal cortex and medulla, parathyroid, thymus, ovaries, testes	Produces hormones that circulate in the blood to target tissue that stimulates a particular action. Helps maintain homeostasis.
Gastrointestinal	Mouth, tongue, teeth, pharynx, esophagus, stomach, small intestine, large intestine, liver, gallbladder, pancreas, appendix	Breakdown, digestion, and absorption of nutrients
Integumentary	Skin, subcutaneous tissue, sweat and sebaceous glands, hair, nails, sense receptors	Protection, temperature regulation, senses organ activity
Lymphatic and immune	Lymph, lymph vessels, lymph nodes, thymus, tonsils, spleen, lymphocytes, antibodies	Maintains fluid balance; protects internal environment; provides immunity to many diseases
Musculoskeletal	Bones, joints, muscles, tendons, ligaments, cartilage	Movement, heat production, support, protection
Nervous	Brain, spinal cord, neurons, neuroglial cells, peripheral nerves, autonomic nerves	Controls body structures to maintain homeostasis; receives and processes information
Reproductive	*Female:* estrogen and progesterone, ovum, ovaries, fallopian tubes, uterus, vagina, vulva, mammary glands *Male:* testosterone, sperm, epididymis, vas deferens, prostate gland, testes, scrotum, penis, urethra	Produces hormones; reproduction
Respiratory	Nose, sinuses, pharynx, larynx, trachea, bronchi, lungs, bronchioles, alveoli	Delivers oxygen to cells and removes carbon dioxide
Sensory	Eyes, ears, taste buds, olfactory receptors, sensory receptors	Gathers information through vision, hearing, balance, taste, and smell
Urinary	Nephron unit, kidneys, ureters, bladder, urethra	Eliminates nitrogenous waste; maintains electrolyte, water, and acid-base balances

- *Body system:* Made up of several organs and their related structures
- *Organism:* Made up of many body systems that work together to maintain homeostasis in the body

CRITICAL THINKING APPLICATION   6.4

Bella's tip really helped Daniela with the cell structures. Now Daniela needs to remember the organization of the body, in order, from the simplest to the most complex. Bella encourages Daniela to create a phrase or word that would help her remember cells, tissues, organs, body system, and organism. What might be a way to remember these five items in order?

SURFACE ANATOMY TERMINOLOGY

In healthcare we use surface anatomy terminology to describe locations on the body. For instance, when you take a blood pressure reading, you need to place the stethoscope over the brachial artery in the antecubital space. The radial artery is used when you take a radial pulse. Knowing the surface anatomy terminology will help you understand what is being asked of you and will allow you to communicate professionally with others.

Anatomical position is a standard frame of reference. This means the body stands erect with the face forward, arms at the sides, palms forward, and toes pointed forward. Fig. 6.6A shows the body in anatomical position, in addition to the ventral surface anatomy. (Fig.

6.6B shows the dorsal surface anatomy.) Tables 6.14 through 6.17 provide additional information on front (ventral) and back (dorsal) surface anatomy terminology.

CRITICAL THINKING APPLICATION   6.5

As Daniela was learning about surface anatomy terminology, she tried to relate it to things she knew or had learned about in her receptionist position. For instance, *palmar* sounds like *palm* and refers to the palm of the hand. From Tables 6.14 through 6.17, which words have you heard before? How might you remember these surface anatomy terms?

POSITIONAL AND DIRECTIONAL TERMINOLOGY

Positional and directional terms are used to describe up/down, middle/side, and front/back. Many times patients will be in different positions, depending on the situation. Having a standard method to communicate directions and positions allows for clear communication between healthcare professionals. These terms are used commonly in healthcare. For example, x-rays may be taken from the front of the body to the back – an anteroposterior (AP) view, or from the back to the front – a posteroanterior (PA) view.

The *midline* of the body is an imaginary line drawn from the crown of the head down between the eyes, through the chest, and separating the legs. Several of the directional terms use the midline as a reference. See Table 6.18.

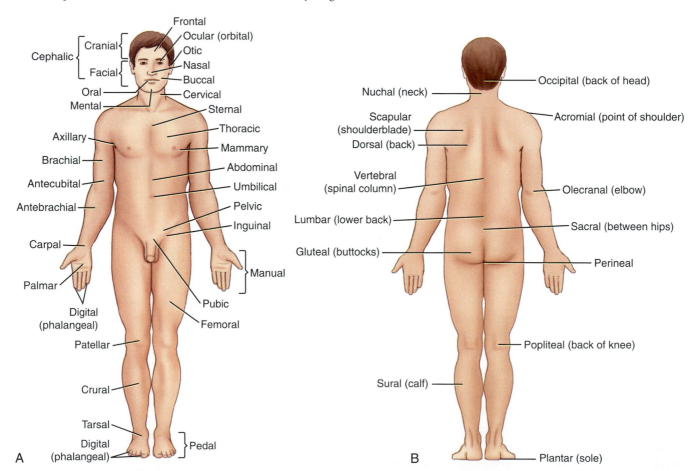

FIGURE 6.6 (A) Ventral surface anatomy. (B) Dorsal surface anatomy. (From Shiland B: *Mastering healthcare terminology,* ed 5, St Louis, 2016, Elsevier.)

TABLE 6.14 Ventral Surface Anatomy: Terms for the Head

TERM	DEFINITION
buccal	Pertaining to the cheek
cephalic	Pertaining to the head
cervical	Pertaining to the neck
cranial	Pertaining to the skull
facial	Pertaining to the face
frontal	Pertaining to the front, the forehead
mental	Pertaining to the chin, or to the mind
nasal	Pertaining to the nose
ocular	Pertaining to the eye
oral	Pertaining to the mouth
otic	Pertaining to the ear; also called *auricular*

TABLE 6.16 Ventral Surface Anatomy: Terms for Arms and Legs

TERM	DEFINITION
antecubital	Pertaining to the front of the elbow
brachial	Pertaining to the arm
carpal	Pertaining to the wrist
crural	Pertaining to the leg
digital	Pertaining to the finger/toe
femoral	Pertaining to the thigh
manual	Pertaining to the hand
palmar	Pertaining to the palm; also termed *volar*
patellar	Pertaining to the kneecap
pedal	Pertaining to the foot
tarsal	Pertaining to the ankle

TABLE 6.15 Ventral Surface Anatomy: Terms for the Trunk

TERM	DEFINITION
abdominal	Pertaining to the abdomen
axillary	Pertaining to the armpit
coxal	Pertaining to the hip
deltoid	The triangular muscle covering the shoulder joint
inguinal	Pertaining to the groin
mammary	Pertaining to the breast
pelvic	Pertaining to the pelvis
pubic	Pertaining to the pubis
sternal	Pertaining to the breastbone
thoracic	Pertaining to the chest; also called *pectoral*
umbilical	Pertaining to the umbilicus

TABLE 6.17 Dorsal Surface Anatomy Terms

TERM	DEFINITION
acromial	Pertaining to the acromion (highest point of shoulder)
dorsal	Pertaining to the back
gluteal	Pertaining to the buttocks
lumbar	Pertaining to the lower back
nuchal	Pertaining to the neck, especially the back of the neck
olecranal	Pertaining to the elbow
perineal	Pertaining to the perineum; the perineum is the space between the external genitalia and the anus
plantar	Pertaining to the sole of the foot
popliteal	Pertaining to the back of the knee
sacral	Pertaining to the sacrum
scapular	Pertaining to the scapula
sural	Pertaining to the calf
ventral	Pertaining to the belly side
vertebral	Pertaining to the spine

CRITICAL THINKING APPLICATION 6.6

Bella continues to help Daniela on breaks during work. Today, Daniela is learning directional terms. Bella encourages Daniela to repeat the term and definition as she points to that part of her body. How else might Daniela learn the directional terms and the opposite pairs?

TABLE 6.18   Positional and Directional Terms

TERM	DEFINITION
anterior	Pertaining to the front
ventral	Pertaining to the belly side
posterior	Pertaining to the back
dorsal	Pertaining to the back of the body
superior	Toward the head
cephalad	Toward the head
inferior	Toward the tail
caudad	Toward the tail
medial	Pertaining to the middle (midline)
lateral	Pertaining to the side
ipsilateral	Pertaining to the same side
contralateral	Pertaining to the opposite side
unilateral	Pertaining to one side
bilateral	Pertaining to two sides
superficial (external)	On the surface of the body
deep (internal)	Away from the surface of the body
proximal	Pertaining to near the origin
distal	Pertaining to far from the origin
dextrad	Toward the right
sinistrad	Toward the left
afferent	Pertaining to carrying toward a structure
efferent	Pertaining to carrying away from a structure
supine	Lying on one's back
prone	Lying on one's belly

BODY CAVITIES

The body contains cavities, or hollowed areas, that are filled with organs. The body is separated into the dorsal (posterior) and ventral (anterior) body cavities. The *dorsal body cavity* protects nervous system organs. It contains the cranial cavity and the spinal cavity. The *ventral body cavity* is divided into the thoracic and abdominopelvic cavities. The **diaphragm** creates a physical separation between the thoracic and the abdominopelvic cavities. Table 6.19 summarizes the structures found in each body cavity.

Abdominopelvic Quadrants and Regions

The abdominopelvic cavity is extensive. To help describe a location in the abdominopelvic area, either the four quadrants or the nine regions can be used. Descriptions that focus on the quadrants are

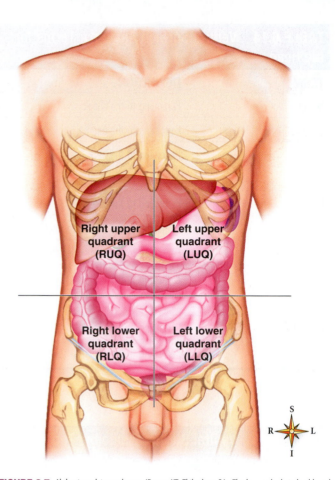

FIGURE 6.7 Abdominopelvic quadrants. (Patton KT, Thibodeau GA: *The human body in health and disease*, ed 7, St Louis, 2018, Elsevier.)

simpler to understand and may be used with patients. The regions are more specific and are typically used by healthcare providers.

With the abdominopelvic quadrants, an imaginary line is drawn down the midline of the body. A horizontal line is drawn across the abdominopelvic cavity, intersecting at the naval (Fig. 6.7). These quadrants are referred to as either right or left and upper or lower. Typically, the abbreviations are used when documenting information about the patient. The four quadrants, and their contents, are as follows:

- *Right upper quadrant* (RUQ): Right lobe of the liver, gallbladder, right kidney, small intestine (duodenum), large intestine (ascending and transverse colon), and head of the pancreas
- *Left upper quadrant* (LUQ): Stomach, spleen, left lobe of the liver, pancreas, left kidney, and large intestine (transverse and descending colon)
- *Right lower quadrant* (RLQ): Appendix, cecum, right ovary, right ureter, right spermatic cord, large intestine (ascending colon), and right kidney
- *Left lower quadrant* (LLQ): Small intestine, large intestine (descending and sigmoid colon), left ovary, left ureter, left spermatic cord, and left kidney

The nine abdominopelvic regions lie over the abdominopelvic cavity. They provide a more specific location than the quadrants. Refer to Fig. 6.8 and Table 6.20 for the nine regions and the related organs.

TABLE 6.19   Body Cavities

MAIN BODY CAVITIES	SUBCATEGORIES	DESCRIPTION
Dorsal body cavity	Cranial cavity	Contains the brain; surrounded and protected by the cranium (skull)
	Spinal cavity	Contains the spinal cord; surrounded and protected by the vertebrae (bones of the spine)
Ventral body cavity	Thoracic cavity	Contains the heart, lungs, esophagus and trachea (windpipe); protected by the ribs, the sternum (breastbone), and the vertebrae (backbones)

	Abdominopelvic cavity	Can be divided as follows:
		    Abdominal cavity — contains the abdominal organs (e.g., stomach, liver, gallbladder, intestines).
		    Pelvic cavity — contains the urinary bladder and the reproductive organs
		Nothing separates the abdominal and pelvic cavities.

TABLE 6.20   Abdominopelvic Regions With the Underlying Organs

Right Hypochondriac Region Liver, gallbladder, right kidney	**Epigastric Region** Kidneys, pancreas, liver, stomach	**Left Hypochondriac Region** Stomach, liver, left kidney, spleen
Right Lumbar Region Small intestine, large intestine (ascending colon), liver, right kidney	**Umbilical Region** Small intestine, large intestine (transverse colon), pancreas, stomach	**Left Lumbar Region** Small intestine, large intestine (descending colon), left kidney
Right Iliac Region Appendix, small intestine, large intestine (cecum and ascending colon)	**Hypogastric Region** Small intestine, large intestine (sigmoid colon), bladder	**Left Iliac Region** Small intestine, large intestine (descending and sigmoid colon)

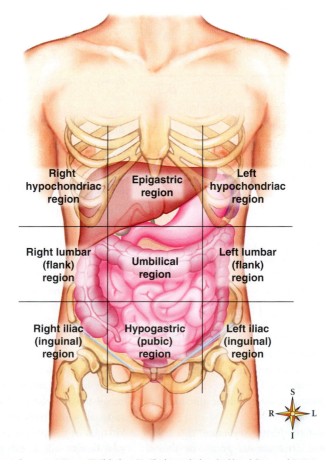

FIGURE 6.8 Abdominopelvic regions. (Patton KT, Thibodeau GA: *The human body in health and disease*, ed 7, St Louis, 2018, Elsevier.)

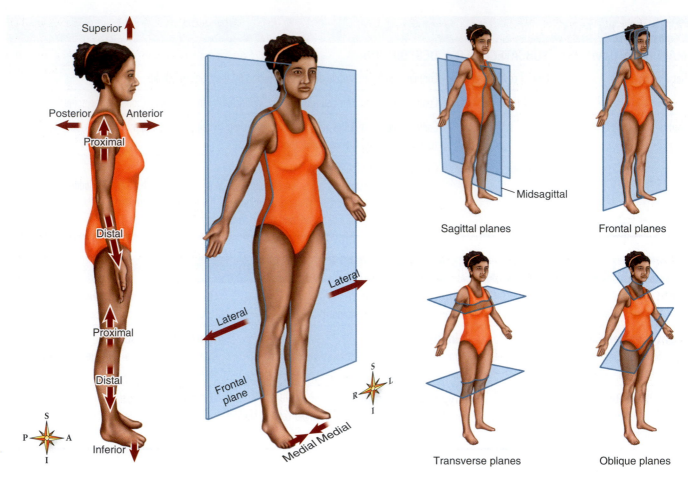

FIGURE 6.9 Body planes. (Patton KT, Thibodeau GA: *The human body in health and disease*, ed 7, St. Louis, 2018, Elsevier.)

CRITICAL THINKING APPLICATION   **6.7**

Tonight Bella is helping Daniela practice positional and directional terms with the regions. Bella asks Daniela the following questions:
- What regions are lateral to the umbilical region?
- What regions are superior to the lumbar regions?
- What region is medial to the hypochondriac regions and superior to the umbilical region?
- What region is inferior to the umbilical region?
- What regions are lateral to the sides of the hypogastric region?

What should Daniela's answers be to these questions?

BODY PLANES

Another way of describing the body is by dividing it into planes. *Planes* are imaginary cuts or sections through the body. The use of plane terminology is common when diagnostic imaging of the body is discussed (e.g., computed tomography [CT] or computerized axial tomography [CAT] scan). Diagnostic imaging will be discussed in more detail later in the chapter.

A *midsagittal plane,* or *median plane,* separates the body into equal right and left halves. The *coronal plane,* or *frontal*

plane, divides the body into front and back portions. The *transverse plane,* or *horizontal plane,* divides the body horizontally into an upper part and a lower part. An *oblique plane* uses a diagonal cut through the body. See Fig. 6.9 for illustrations of the body planes.

ACID-BASE BALANCE

The *pH* is important to review because it affects body homeostasis. pH refers to the acid-base level of a solution on a scale of 1 to 14. A neutral pH is 7. An acidic solution has a pH less than 7 and contains more hydrogen ions. A base, or alkaline solution, has a pH greater than 7 and contains fewer hydrogen ions. To maintain homeostasis, the body attempts to keep the pH between 7.35 and 7.45. To maintain the acid-base range in the body, the concentration of hydrogen ions must remain constant. If the pH moves outside of this range, serious illness or even death can occur.

The pH of our bodies can change based on the food we eat, the air we breathe, and the urine we excrete. To help maintain the pH range, the urinary system, the respiratory system, and chemical buffers must all work together. *Buffers* (e.g., bicarbonate) work to prevent changes in the pH. If there are more hydrogen ions, lowering the pH, buffers will absorb some of the hydrogen ions. This will raise the pH. If the pH is too high, the buffers will "donate" hydrogen ions, bringing the pH down to the normal range.

The respiratory system regulates the carbon dioxide (CO_2) in our blood. CO_2 in the blood can combine with water to form the buffer bicarbonate. If a person *hyperventilates* (breathes rapidly), the CO_2 levels in the blood decrease, which also causes a decrease in the bicarbonate levels in the blood. This causes the pH of the body to rise.

The urinary system also has a role in acid-base levels. The kidneys can absorb more base or more acid, depending on what the body needs for homeostasis. The kidneys can also produce bicarbonate if needed.

PATHOLOGY BASICS

Pathology is the study of diseases. In the ambulatory care setting, many patients' visits relate to the diagnosis or treatment of one or more disease processes. As a person ages, it is common to have more than one chronic illness. Having an understanding of common diseases is important for medical assistants. The body system chapters that follow will cover the most common diseases impacting the system discussed. This chapter provides you with the basics to help you understand the concepts discussed in future chapters. Common pathology terminology, protective mechanisms in the body, predisposing factors for disease, and causes of disease will be discussed.

Pathology Terminology

As you learn more about diseases, you will notice different terms used. Here is a list of terms commonly used when discussing pathology:

- *Disease*: A specific illness with a recognizable group of signs and symptoms and a clear cause (e.g., infection, environment).
- *Syndrome*: A group of signs and symptoms that occur together and are associated with a condition.
- *Disorder*: A disruption of the function or structure of the body. Many times the words *disorder* and *disease* are used interchangeably in healthcare.
- *Prevalence*: How often the disease occurs.
- *Incidence*: Reflects the number of newly diagnosed people with the disease.
- *Morbidity*: Illness.
- *Mortality*: Death.
- *Acute*: A severe, sudden onset of a disease.
- *Chronic*: A disease, disorder, or syndrome that lasts longer than 6 months.

The upcoming chapters will discuss common diseases in each body system. For most of the diseases, the following sections will be discussed. It is important for the medical assistant to be familiar with the terminology used:

- *Etiology*: The cause of the disorder or disease.
- *Sign*: An indicator that is measured or observed by others; also called *objective data*. Examples of signs include redness, swelling (edema), blood pressure, and pulse.
- *Symptom*: An indicator that is only perceived by the patient; also called *subjective data*. Examples include pain, headache, dizziness, and nausea. Many times *signs* and *symptoms*

are used interchangeably, but there is a difference in their definitions.

- *Diagnostic procedures*: Tests and procedures that are used to help diagnose or monitor a condition. See Table 6.21 and Figs. 6.10 and 6.11 for common diagnostic procedures.
- *Treatments*: Management of a disease or disorder; they can include follow-up care and home treatments (e.g., medications, special diets, testing).

CRITICAL THINKING APPLICATION   6.8

Daniela is struggling to remember the difference between signs and symptoms. What might be ways to remember these two terms? What are some examples of signs and symptoms?

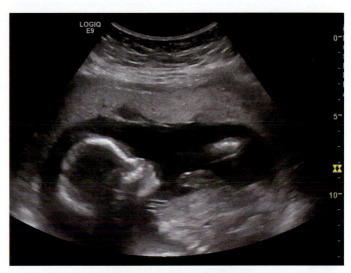

FIGURE 6.10 Two-dimensional fetal ultrasound.

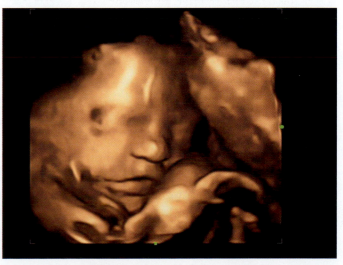

FIGURE 6.11 Three-dimensional fetal ultrasound.

TABLE 6.21   Common Diagnostic Procedures and Tests in Ambulatory Healthcare

PERFORMED BY/TYPE OF TEST	PROCEDURE	DESCRIPTION
Medical Laboratory Blood Tests	Blood glucose	Used to detect high or low blood sugar (glucose)
	C-reactive protein (CRP)	Detects inflammation
	Complete blood count (CBC)	Measures red blood cells (RBCs) and white blood cells (WBCs), hemoglobin (Hgb), hematocrit (HCT), and platelets; CBC with differential test provides a breakdown of the number of each type of white blood cell
	Comprehensive metabolic panel (CMP)	Includes different tests that evaluate, for instance, liver function, kidney function, glucose, and electrolytes
	Electrolyte panel (Lytes)	Used to check for electrolyte (e.g., sodium, potassium, chloride) imbalances
	Erythrocyte sedimentation rate (ESR)	Used to measure the degree of inflammation in the body
	Follicle-stimulating hormone (FSH)	Measures the follicle-stimulating hormone, a reproductive hormone
	Glycated hemoglobin test or hemoglobin glycosylated test (HbA1C or A1C)	Measures the average blood glucose (sugar) over 2 to 3 months
	Lipid profile	Used to check cholesterol and triglycerides
	Liver function panel	Measures specific proteins and enzymes to provide information on the liver's functioning; also called the *hepatic function test*
	Partial thromboplastin time (PTT), prothrombin time (PT), and international normalized ratio (INR)	Measures blood clotting time
	Thyroid-stimulating hormone (TSH) test	Measures the amount of thyroid-stimulating hormone in the blood; also part of the thyroid panel, which includes additional tests
Medical Laboratory Tests	Culture and sensitivity (C&S)	Culture detects organism in body fluid (e.g., blood, sputum, urine) and sensitivity testing to determine antibiotics that would inhibit organism growth
	Fecal immunochemical test (FIT)	Uses antibodies to detect human hemoglobin protein
	Guaiac fecal occult blood test (gFOBT)	Used to detect blood in stool
	Stool parasitic examination (O&P)	Used to detect ova and parasites in the stool
	Urinalysis (UA)	Detects abnormalities in the urine that can be used to diagnose many conditions
Endoscopy	Arthroscopy	An arthroscope is inserted through a small incision to view a joint
	Bronchoscopy	A bronchoscope is inserted through the mouth to visualize the trachea and bronchi
	Capsule endoscopy	A camera in a capsule is swallowed and provides pictures of the gastrointestinal tract
	Colonoscopy and sigmoidoscopy	An endoscope is inserted through the anus and used to visualize the large intestine and colon
	Colposcopy	A colposcope is inserted into the vagina to visualize the cervix and vagina
	Cystoscopy and ureteroscopy	An endoscope is inserted into the urethra to look at the urinary system
	Endoscopic retrograde cholangiopancreatography (ERCP)	An endoscope is inserted into the mouth and passed to the duodenum; a thin tube, called a *catheter*, is passed through the endoscope and is used to inject dye into the ducts that lead to the pancreas and gallbladder, then x-rays are used to detect narrowing of structures
	Esophagogastroduodenoscopy (EGD)	An endoscope is inserted through the mouth to visualize the lining of the esophagus, stomach, and duodenum (small intestine)

TABLE 6.21	Common Diagnostic Procedures and Tests in Ambulatory Healthcare—*continued*	
PERFORMED BY/TYPE OF TEST	**PROCEDURE**	**DESCRIPTION**
Imaging Procedures	Computed tomography (CT, CAT) scan	A computerized x-ray imaging modality that provides axial and three-dimensional scans; the patient lies on a table that slides into the circular device that takes the x-rays
	Fluoroscopy	Direct observation of an x-ray image in motion
	Magnetic resonance imaging (MRI)	An imaging modality that uses a magnetic field and radiofrequency pulses to create computer images of both bones and soft tissues in multiple planes
	Nuclear scans	A radioactive substance is injected or ingested and then is detected by a special camera as it moves through a body structure
	Positron emission tomography (PET) scan	Imaging test that uses a radioactive drug (tracer) to show the activity of tissues and organs

	Ultrasound (US) (also called *sonography*)	A transducer is moved over the body and sends out high-frequency sound waves; waves bounce off tissues and the transducer captures the waves:
		    2D US: creates a flat, two-dimensional picture
		    3D US: creates a three-dimensional (3D) picture
		    4D US: creates a 3D picture with sound and motion
		    Doppler US: assesses blood flow through blood vessels

	X-ray (also called *radiograph*)	Uses electromagnetic waves to take pictures of the inside structures of the body; creates black-and-white images based on the amount of radiation that is absorbed:
		    White areas: absorb more radiation (e.g., bones)
		    Gray areas: absorb less (e.g., soft tissue and fat)
		    Black: absorbs none (e.g., air)
		Different views can be ordered:
		    PA (posteroanterior) films: x-ray passes from the back to the front of the person
		    AP (anteroposterior) films: x-ray passes from the front to the back of the person

	Contrast media	Can be used with x-rays, CT, MRI, and US to improve the clarity of the soft tissue picture; ingested, administered by enema, or by injection (via blood vessels) and eliminated via the urine or stool; common contrast media include:
		    X-rays and CT scans: barium and iodine
		    MRIs: gadolinium
		    US: saline (salt water) and air

Predisposing Factors

Predisposing factors are risk factors for disease. These factors make it more likely or increase the risk that the person may develop the disease or condition. Some predisposing factors can be changed to reduce the risk of developing a disease, whereas others cannot be changed. Predisposing factors include the following:

* *Hereditary or genetic factors*: Certain diseases can be inherited, or members of a family can have a higher-than-normal risk for getting a specific disease.

* *Age*: Certain diseases occur in childhood, whereas others occur more often in older adults. Some diseases occur due to changes in the body structures with age. For instance, the ear structures are different in an infant compared with an older person. Degenerative diseases occur in older generations due to the wear and tear on the structures.

* *Gender*: Certain diseases occur specifically, or more often, in one gender than the other. For instance, testicular cancer impacts males. whereas uterine cancer affects females. Sometimes both genders may get a disease, but one gender has a higher risk factor. Women are at higher risk for breast cancer than men.

- *Environmental factors*: Certain diseases are more common when a person has been exposed to pollutants in the air, land, or water. Though pesticides can reduce the risk of disease (e.g., West Nile viral infection and rabies), exposure to certain pesticides has been found to increase the risk of cancer.
- *Lifestyle*: Stress, poor diet, infrequent exercise, or abusing nicotine, alcohol, or drugs can increase the risk for disease.

CRITICAL THINKING APPLICATION   **6.9**

While on break at work, Daniela works on an assignment. She needs to determine which predisposing factors could be changed and how they could be changed. What could be her answers?

Causes of Disease

Disease can result from a change in homeostasis or can be the result of the body's response to a perceived threat. There are several common causes of disease, including genetics, infectious **pathogens**, inflammatory processes, immunity, nutritional imbalance, trauma and environmental agents, and neoplasms. The following sections describe these causes.

Genetics

Each person is made up of 46 chromosomes, which carry genetic information (genes). We get 23 chromosomes from each of our parents. *Genes* are the basic units of heredity, or the instructions on how our bodies should develop and function. Genes provide the differences among us and the similarities in families. From genes we get our physical appearance and our susceptibility to disease.

Recall that chromosomes are found in the cell's nucleus. During the process of conception and the cell division that follows, an extra chromosome or a change in the chromosome structure may occur. A genetic disease may result from a chromosomal error or from the patient inheriting a defective gene from either parent. Types of genetic disease include the following:

- *Monogenic disorders*: A defective gene is inherited from one or both parents. See Table 6.22 for information on genetic diseases and how a child could develop a disease.
- *Chromosomal disorders*: An abnormal number of chromosomes or a change in the chromosomal structure causes a disease such as Klinefelter syndrome or Turner syndrome.

Infectious Pathogens

Many microorganisms are *nonpathogenic*, which means they do not cause disease. They can be found in our body, maintaining the homeostasis. Other microorganisms are *pathogenic*, which means disease causing (Table 6.23). These pathogens enter our bodies through direct contact, indirect contact, or by vectors (Table 6.24).

When a pathogen enters our body and starts to multiply, we have an infection. Changes occur in our body, yet we do not feel any different. This is the *incubation period*. It starts at the time of exposure

---

TABLE 6.22   Genetic Diseases

NEEDED FOR DEVELOPMENT OF DISEASE OR TRAIT	EXAMPLES OF GENETIC DISEASES
One copy of the defective dominant gene	Huntington disease
Two copies (one from each parent) of the defective recessive gene	Cystic fibrosis Tay-Sachs disease Sickle cell anemia Phenylketonuria (PKU)

---

and ends when the signs and symptoms appear. The incubation period is different for each disease. For instance, strep throat has an incubation period of 2 to 5 days, whereas varicella (chickenpox) has an incubation period of 14 to 16 days. As our body tissues become damaged from the infection, we start to see the signs and symptoms. This is when disease occurs.

Some diseases are *noncommunicable*. They cannot be transmitted from one person to another. For instance, a person with tetanus cannot spread the disease to another person. Other diseases are *communicable*. These diseases are transmitted from one person to another. If a communicable disease is known to be easily transmitted, it is called a *contagious disease*. Strep throat and influenza are examples of contagious diseases. For instance, people with strep throat are contagious from the start of the fever until they have been on the appropriate antibiotics for 24 hours. The period during which a disease can spread to another is called the *contagious period*. It is important for people in healthcare to understand the ways diseases are spread. Taking required precautions will minimize your risk of "catching something" from your patients.

CRITICAL THINKING APPLICATION   **6.10**

At school, Daniela learned about the transmission of pathogens. As a receptionist, she sees a lot of sick people stopping at her desk. She encourages those who cough to wear a mask. Hand sanitizer and tissue are also available. Thinking about disease transmission, why are these three items important in the prevention of disease?

Inflammatory Response

The inflammatory response is the body's efficient way of protecting itself. Inflammation occurs when the tissues are injured. The five key signs of inflammation are redness (erythema), swelling (edema), pain, warmth, and loss of function. The injury could be the result of bacteria, trauma, heat, toxins, or other causes. The cells damaged release chemicals called *histamine*, *prostaglandins*, and *bradykinin*. These chemicals cause the following responses:

- Blood vessels at the site dilate. This causes more local blood flow. With the increase in blood flow, redness and warmth occur in that area.

TABLE 6.23 Common Pathogens

PATHOGEN	DESCRIPTION	RELATED DISEASES
Fungi	Yeast and molds; only a few cause fungal disease or mycoses	Tinea corporis (ringworm) Tinea pedis (athlete's foot) Thrush
Protozoa	One-celled organisms	Trichomoniasis Malaria Amebic dysentery
Viruses	Smallest microorganism; requires a host cell to multiply	Common cold Measles, mumps Chickenpox, influenza
Bacteria	Single-celled organisms; classified by shape: bacilli (rod shaped), spirilla (spiral shaped), cocci (dot shaped) Many disease-causing bacteria produce **toxins** that create the illness	Bacilli: tuberculosis, whooping cough, *Escherichia coli*, salmonella Spirilla: cholera, syphilis, Lyme disease Cocci: gonorrhea, meningitis, strep throat
Helminths	A group of larger parasites that enter the body and live off the food you eat	Pinworms, tapeworms, flukes
Ectoparasites	A parasite that lives on the outside of the body	Lice, scabies

TABLE 6.24 Modes of Transmission for Pathogens

MODES OF TRANSMISSION	DEFINITION	EXAMPLES OF DISEASES
Direct contact	Susceptible person comes in contact with an infected person; spread occurs via contact with blood, body fluids, and excretions (e.g., stool, urine, and saliva). Methods of direct contact include: • Person to person (sneezing, touching, coughs) • Animal to person (being bitten or scratched or handling animal waste) • Mother to unborn child	Influenza Pertussis Chickenpox Rabies Gonorrhea Tuberculosis
Indirect contact	Spread occurs through contact with a contaminated object (e.g., water, food, drinking glass, airborne transmission).	*Escherichia coli* Botulism
Vectors (insects)	Most blood-sucking insects consume the disease-causing microorganism from one host and transmit it during a "meal" to another host.	Mosquitoes: yellow fever, malaria, West Nile fever, Zika Ticks: Lyme disease, tick-borne encephalitis, rickettsial diseases Fleas: plague, rickettsiosis

• Blood vessel walls allow more white blood cells and plasma to move out of the vessel into the surrounding tissues. The white blood cells work to protect the cells and clean up the dead tissue. The extra fluid from the blood causes swelling, pain, and loss of movement. For instance, if an injury occurs in your finger joint area, the swelling may be so great that it prevents you from moving your finger.

Even though the inflammatory process can be efficient, it can also be the cause of disease. *Autoinflammatory diseases* (e.g., familial Mediterranean fever) differ from autoimmune diseases, which will be described later in the chapter. Autoinflammatory diseases result from a genetic mutation that causes the inflammatory process to activate without a reason. The person may experience recurring brief attacks of pain and fever, and blood work indicates systemic inflammation.

Immunity Disorders

Our immune system protects our bodies against potentially harmful substances. Our immune system "remembers" the **antigens** from diseases and responds with specific **antibodies**. The antibodies destroy or attempt to destroy the harmful substances. Similar to autoinflammatory conditions, at times the immune response can work against us. These malfunctions are classified as follows:

- *Allergies*: Reactions occur if a person is exposed to a food (e.g., milk, tree nuts, peanuts, eggs, soy, and wheat), pollen, dust mites, mold, pet dander, inhalants, or other substances.
- *Autoimmunity*: The immune system does not recognize the body's own antigens and starts attacking itself. Rheumatoid arthritis, lupus, and psoriasis are examples of autoimmune disorders.
- *Immunodeficiency*: This is caused by a deficiency in one or more of the immune system's key players, such as white blood cells (e.g., B cells and T cells). A person with immunodeficiency has impaired resistance to infections.

Nutritional Imbalances

Nutritional imbalances include too little or too much of a nutrient. Nutritional imbalances can impact growth and disease and can result in death. The following are causes of nutritional imbalances:

- *Vitamin and mineral deficiencies:* Some of these deficiencies can be caused by alcoholism, disease, dietary deficiencies (and poverty), weight loss surgery, and metabolic disorders.
- *Vitamin and mineral excesses:* Vitamin excesses can occur when a person takes too much of a vitamin. The water-soluble vitamins (vitamins B and C) pass through the body fairly quickly. The fat-soluble vitamins (vitamins A, D, E, and K) can accumulate in the body. This can lead to toxic conditions. Mineral excess can be caused by diet, medication, or a metabolic error.
- *Obesity:* Causes include the following:
  - Eating too many calories
  - Getting too little exercise
  - Having an endocrine or a metabolic condition
    Obesity can increase a person's risk for other diseases, including heart disease, diabetes, hypertension (high blood pressure), and stroke.
- *Starvation:* Eating too little food can result from disease or poverty.
- *Trauma and environmental agents:* Trauma from auto accidents, violence, falls, and other events can cause disease. Common traumatic injuries include fractures, lacerated and ruptured organs, bleeding, neck and spinal injuries, and head injuries. Psychological trauma can also cause disorders.

Environmental changes, such as severe heat or cold and extremes of atmospheric pressures, can impact health. Poisonings, insect and animal bites, burns, electric shocks, and near drownings can also cause diseases.

NEOPLASMS

When cells grow quicker than normal or do not die as fast as they should, an abnormal mass is created. This mass is called a *neoplasm,* or *tumor*. Tumors can be *benign* (noncancerous) or *malignant* (cancerous). Table 6.25 shows the difference between benign and malignant tumors.

There are more than 100 different types of cancer. Cancers are classified based on the type of tissue from which they originate. See Table 6.26 for the classifications of cancer. (See also Figs. 6.12 and 6.13.)

As the malignant cells grow, they can break through the *basement membrane*. This delicate membrane separates the epithelial cells from connective tissues. Once this occurs, the cancerous cells can invade blood and lymph vessels. The circulating fluid (blood, lymph fluid) can then carry the cancerous cells to another location in the body. Thus cancerous cells from the primary (or original) tumor can

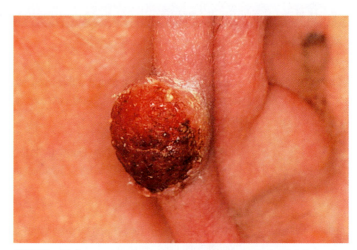

FIGURE 6.12 Squamous cell carcinoma on the ear. (From McCance KL, Huether SE: *Pathophysiology: the biologic basis for disease in adults and children,* ed 6, St. Louis, 2010, Mosby.)

TABLE 6.25	Differences Between Benign and Malignant Tumors	
CHARACTERISTIC	**BENIGN TUMOR**	**MALIGNANT TUMOR**
Cellular structure	Same as surrounding tissue	**Anaplastic** changes and poorly differentiated
Type of growth	Grows within a "shell" (encapsulated)	Infiltrates and *metastasizes*; spreads to distant site(s) in the body via the bloodstream or lymph system
Rate of growth	Usually slow; rarely fatal	May be slow, rapid, or very rapid; almost always fatal if left untreated
Destruction of localized tissue	None	Common; invades and takes over the surrounding tissue

TABLE 6.26   Classification of Cancer

CLASSIFICATION	DESCRIPTION	DISEASE EXAMPLES
Carcinoma Types:	Impact skin, lungs, breast, colon, prostate	
Squamous cell carcinoma	Derived from squamous epithelium	Squamous cell carcinoma of the lung
Adenocarcinoma	Derived from an organ or a gland	Gastric adenocarcinoma
Sarcomas	Impact connective tissue (bones, muscle, cartilage, blood vessels, and fat)	Osteosarcoma, chondrosarcoma, hemangiosarcoma, mesothelioma, and glioma
Lymphomas Types:	Impact lymphatic tissue (vessels, nodes, and organs, including the spleen, tonsils, and thymus gland)	
Hodgkin lymphoma	Diagnosed by the detection of Reed-Sternberg cell, a cell specific only to this disease	
Non-Hodgkin lymphoma	All other lymphomas with the exception of Hodgkin lymphoma	
Leukemia	Impacts the bone marrow, causing lots of abnormal blood cells to be created	Acute myelocytic leukemia
Myeloma	Impacts the plasma cells (a type of white blood cell) in the bone marrow	Multiple myeloma
Mixed tumors	Combination of cells from within one classification or between two cancer classifications	Teratocarcinoma, carcinosarcoma

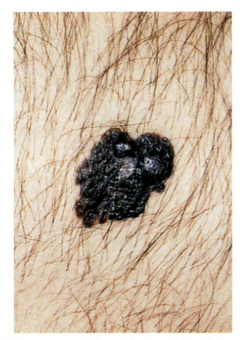

FIGURE 6.13 Malignant melanoma on the arm. (From Damjanov I: *Anderson's pathology,* ed 10, St. Louis, 2000, Mosby.)

metastasize to another location in the body, creating a secondary tumor.

If a provider suspects a patient may have cancer, a number of blood tests and imaging tests will be ordered. A **biopsy** may be performed. The surgeon may also take a biopsy of nearby lymph nodes so the tissue can be checked for malignant cells. Based on the diagnostic results, the **oncologist** or **pathologist** will grade and stage the cancer.

Grade refers to how abnormal the malignant cells look. If the malignant cells and tissues closely resemble normal cells and tissue, the tumor is called "well **differentiated**." These are more slow-growing tumors. If the malignant cells and tissues do not look like normal cells and tissue, they are called "undifferentiated" or "poorly differentiated." The microscopic look of the cell is graded using 1, 2, 3, or 4 to indicate the appearance. Grade 1 means well-differentiated, or the cells and organization of the malignant tissue look close to those of normal tissue. Grade 2 means moderately differentiated, or the tissue does not look like normal tissue; the cells are growing at a faster rate than normal. Grades 3 and 4 do not look like normal tissue and tend to spread quicker.

Stage refers to the extent of the cancer, including the size and if it has spread. A cancer is staged in this manner. Several staging systems are used, and various factors must be taken into consideration with staging systems:

- Location of the tumor
- Type of cell
- Size of the tumor
- If it has spread to nearby lymph nodes

TABLE 6.27	Stages of Cancer: 0 to IV System
STAGE	DESCRIPTION
Stage 0	Abnormal cells are present; no spreading has occurred.
Stages I, II, and III	Malignancy is present. The number is greater for larger tumors and tumors that have spread to nearby tissues.
Stage IV	Cancer has metastasized.

TABLE 6.28	Stages of Cancer: Defined by Terms
STAGE	DEFINITION
In situ	Abnormal cells are present; no spreading has occurred.
Localized	Cancer cells are present; no spreading has occurred.
Regional	Cancer has spread to nearby lymph nodes, organs, or tissues.
Distant	Cancer has metastasized.
Unknown	Not enough information is available.

- If it has spread to other locations in the body
- Tumor grade, or how abnormal the cells look compared with normal cells and how quickly the tumor grows and spreads

The TNM staging system is widely used. The letters T, N, and M will be followed by a number or letter. For instance, a patient may have T1N0M0. It is important to have an understanding of what this means:

T: Refers to the size and extent of the primary tumor
- TX: Primary tumor cannot be measured
- T0: Primary tumor cannot be found
- T1, T2, T3, and T4: Refer to the size and extent of the primary tumor; the higher the number, the larger or more extensive the tumor

N: Refers to the number of nearby lymph nodes impacted by the malignant cells
- NX: Nearby lymph node cancer cannot be measured
- N0: No cancer in the nearby lymph nodes
- N1, N2, and N4: Refers to the location and quantity of nearby lymph nodes that have cancer; the higher the number, the more nodes are impacted

M: Refers to whether the tumor has metastasized
- MX: Metastasis cannot be measured
- M0: No metastasis has occurred
- M1: Metastasis has occurred

Other systems can be used in healthcare to stage cancer. Tables 6.27 and 6.28 provide two additional methods. This information will help you understand references to cancer.

CLOSING COMMENTS

Patient Coaching

Putting medical terminology into understandable language is important for every patient. Many patients will benefit from having medical terms put into simpler, everyday language. Choose your words carefully. Describe body parts, systems, and procedures in language that is clear and understandable to your patient. Ask your patients to repeat instructions back to you so that you know that they are clear on all instructions. Listen to your patient and be open and willing to answer any questions that are within a medical assistant's scope of practice. Have written instructions available whenever possible.

Legal and Ethical Issues

Communication is key to providing the best possible patient care and serving the patient in an ethical manner. Using proper terminology, spelling, and pronunciation will help you inform your patients in a useful way. Being certain that your patients are clear on all instructions is vital. If patients don't receive clear instructions, they may make mistakes in preparing for diagnostic procedures, taking medication, or following treatment or therapy regimens. Clear communication is essential.

Patient-Centered Care

Understanding medical terminology, basic anatomy, and basic pathology allows the medical assistant to help his or her patients in very real ways. The medical assistant can "translate" medical terms into day-to-day language. Medical assistants who can describe procedures in everyday terms help their patients understand what will happen during a procedure and may put a patient's mind at ease. Knowing what to expect helps relieve fear of the unknown.

Professional Behaviors

Having a good understanding of the structural organization of the body will help as you learn about each body system. Knowing how medical terminology relates to body organization, cavities, quadrants, regions, and planes is important for accurate communication. As a medical assistant, you will be communicating with providers and peers. Using correct medical terminology and having a strong understanding of the body systems will help you communicate effectively in the ambulatory care setting.

SUMMARY OF SCENARIO

Daniela continues in her position as a float receptionist. She is gaining a lot of experience in the Walden-Martin Family Medical Clinic. She is excited to be able to understand so many medical terms. When she comes across a new term, she is now able to decode it by breaking it down into word parts. With her knowledge of the most common prefixes and suffixes, she can get a general idea of what the term means even if she does not know the meaning of all the word parts. She can already see how she will be able to use her knowledge of medical terminology in other classes in her medical assistant program.

Bella continues to help Daniela study for her medical terminology and human body courses. Daniela really appreciates the study tips and reviewing assistance that Bella gives her. Some of her favorite ways to study these courses include the following:

- Making flashcards with the term or word part on one side and the definition on the other. Bella warned her to keep the definition short and simple.

For nonmedical terminology, she learned more when she wrote her own definition. She realized the tests did not always use the exact words used in the textbook.

- Daniela realized that she learned better when she listened to the content. So she recorded herself going through her flashcards and review sheets. She found that if she stated the term or question and then paused, when she listened she could fill in the blank before hearing the answer.
- Lastly, Daniela learned that she sometimes felt she knew the content but was not always sure until it came to the test. So she decided to test herself on the content during her study times to see what she really knew.

Daniela is very excited that she will soon complete her human body and disease course and medical terminology course. She is also excited to apply the study practices she is learning to her future medical assistant courses.

SUMMARY OF LEARNING OBJECTIVES

1. **Review the origins of medical terminology and discuss the difference between decodable and nondecodable terms.**

   Medical terminology is a specialized vocabulary that has its root in Greek and Latin word components. Decodable terms are those that can be broken into their Greek and Latin word parts and given a working definition based on the meanings of those word parts. Most medical terms are decodable, so learning word parts is important. The word parts are as follows: **Combining form:** Word root with its respective combining vowel. **Word root:** Foundation of the medical term. **Combining vowel:** A letter sometimes used to join word parts. Usually an "o" but occasionally an "a," "e," "i," or "u." **Suffix:** Word part that appears at the end of a term. Suffixes are used to modify the meaning of the combining form. **Prefix:** Word part that sometimes appears at the beginning of a term. Not all terms are composed of word parts that can be used to determine the definition. These terms are known as **nondecodable terms**. For these types of terms, the meaning must be memorized.

2. **Describe how to decode terms using the check, assign, reverse, and define (CARD) method.**

   Using Greek and Latin word components to break down the meanings of medical terms requires a simple four-step process — the check, assign, reverse, and define (CARD) method. You need to do the following:
   - *Check* for the word parts in a term.
   - *Assign* meanings to the word parts.
   - *Reverse* the meaning of the suffix to the front of your definition.
   - *Define* the term.

   Fig. 6.3 shows how this process is applied to a medical term.

3. **Use the rules given to build and spell healthcare terms.**

   With a few exceptions, decodable medical terms follow five simple rules:
   1. If the suffix starts with a vowel, a combining vowel is not needed to join the parts.

   2. If the suffix starts with a consonant, a combining vowel is needed to join the two word parts.
   3. If a combining form ends with the same vowel that begins a suffix, one of the vowels is dropped.
   4. If two or more combining forms are used in a term, the combining vowel is retained between the two, regardless of whether the second combining form begins with a vowel or a consonant.
   5. Sometimes when two or more combining forms are used to make a medical term, special notice must be paid to the order in which the combining forms are joined.

   Prefixes and suffixes are also used to build medical terms. See Tables 6.1 through 6.10 for an overview of prefixes, suffixes, and root words used in medical terminology.

4. **Describe the structural organization of the human body.**

   The human body is a collection of many body systems. In studying the organization of the body, you will see that it follows this order, from most simple to most complicated: cells make up tissues, tissues make up organs, organs make up systems, systems work together to make up the human body.

5. **Properly use surface anatomy, positional, and directional terminology.**

   In healthcare we use surface anatomy terminology to describe locations on the body. Anatomical position is a standard frame of reference. This means the body stands erect with the face forward, arms at the sides, palms forward, and toes pointed forward. Fig. 6.6A shows the body in anatomical position. Tables 6.14 through 6.17 provide additional information on front (ventral) and back (dorsal) surface anatomy terminology.

   Positional and directional terms are used to describe up/down, middle/side, and front/back. The *midline* of the body is an imaginary line drawn from the crown of the head down between the eyes, through the chest, and separating the legs. Several of the directional terms

Continued

use the midline as a reference. See Table 6.18 for more information on positional and directional terms.

6. **Describe body cavities, abdominopelvic quadrants, and body planes.**
   The body is separated into the dorsal (posterior) and ventral (anterior) body cavities. The *dorsal body cavity* protects nervous system organs. It contains the cranial cavity and the spinal cavity. The *ventral body cavity* is divided into the thoracic and abdominopelvic cavities. The diaphragm creates a physical separation between the thoracic and the abdominopelvic cavities. Table 6.19 summarizes the structures found in each body cavity.

   With the abdominopelvic quadrants, an imaginary line is drawn down the midline of the body. A horizontal line is drawn across the abdominopelvic cavity, intersecting at the naval (Fig. 6.7). These quadrants are referred to as either right or left and upper or lower. The four quadrants are as follows: *Right upper quadrant* (RUQ), *Left upper quadrant* (LUQ), *Right lower quadrant* (RLQ), *Left lower quadrant* (LLQ).

   The nine abdominopelvic regions lie over the abdominopelvic cavity. They provide a more specific location than the quadrants. Refer to Fig. 6.8 and Table 6.20 for the nine regions and the related organs.

   Another way of describing the body is by dividing it into planes. *Planes* are imaginary cuts or sections through the body. The use of plane terminology is common when discussing diagnostic imaging. A *midsagittal plane,* or *median plane,* separates the body into equal right and left halves. The *coronal plane,* or *frontal plane,* divides the body into front and back portions. The *transverse plane,* or *horizontal plane,* divides the body horizontally into an upper part and a lower part. An *oblique plane* uses a diagonal cut through the body. See Fig. 6.9 for illustrations of the body planes.

7. **Discuss the acid-base balance in the human body.**
   pH refers to the acid-base level of a solution on a scale of 1 to 14. A neutral pH is 7. An acidic solution has a pH less than 7 and contains more hydrogen ions. A base or alkaline solution has a pH greater than 7 and contains fewer hydrogen ions. To maintain homeostasis, the body attempts to keep the pH between 7.35 and 7.45. To maintain the acid-base range in the body, the concentration of hydrogen ions must remain constant. If the pH moves outside of this range, serious illness or even death can occur. To help maintain the pH range, the urinary system, the respiratory system, and chemical buffers must all work together. *Buffers* (like bicarbonate) work to prevent changes in the pH.

8. **Discuss pathology basics, including pathology terminology, protection mechanisms, predisposing factors, and the causes of disease.**
   Pathology is the study of diseases. Pathology terminology includes the following terms:
   - Disease, syndrome, disorder, prevalence, incidence, morbidity, mortality, acute, chronic, etiology, sign, symptom, diagnostic procedures, and treatments.

   Protection mechanisms are ways that the body guards itself from disease and death.
   - Mechanisms include the inflammatory response and immunity.

   Predisposing factors are risk factors for disease. Some predisposing factors include:
   - Hereditary or genetic factors, age, gender, environmental factors, and lifestyle

   Disease can result from a change in homeostasis or can be the result of the body's response to a perceived threat. There are several common causes of diseases, including genetics, infectious pathogens, inflammatory processes, compromised immunity, nutritional imbalance, trauma and environmental agents, and neoplasms. See Tables 6.22 through 6.28 for additional information.

PATIENT COACHING

7

SCENARIO

Suzanne Peterson, CMA (AAMA), has worked for Walden-Martin Family Medicine (WMFM) Clinic for 5 years. Her favorite part of her job is coaching patients on health topics, diagnostic tests, and treatment plans. Her patients know they can contact Suzanne if they have questions between appointments. Suzanne answers the questions she can and also talks with the providers for other questions. She feels that it is very important for patients to understand how to self-manage their conditions and to know when to contact their providers.

Over the years, Suzanne has seen the role of the medical assistant expand. She has learned the importance of screening patients during the initial interview. The information that she enters into the electronic health record is then used to collect data on how well the clinic provides patient care. She has also learned the importance of patient care coordinators. She hopes WMFM Clinic implements a care coordinator program soon.

While studying this chapter, think about the following questions:

- What are basic concepts of teaching and learning? What are the domains of learning? How can a medical assistant adapt coaching to patients?
- What are types of disease prevention coaching?
- What are types of health maintenance coaching?
- What coaching should a medical assistant do for common diagnostic tests?
- What coaching can be done for treatment plans?
- What is the medical assistant's role with coordination of care, navigation, and community resource referrals?

LEARNING OBJECTIVES

1. Describe the medical assistant's role as a coach.
2. List and describe the stages of grief; also, discuss how the health belief model helps to explain what factors influence a person's health beliefs and practices.
3. Describe the three domains of learning.
4. Explain how a medical assistant can adapt coaching to the patient.
5. Describe the teaching-learning process.
6. Discuss how a medical assistant can coach on disease prevention.
7. Describe how a medical assistant can coach on health maintenance and wellness, including different types of self-exams and screenings.
8. Describe how a medical assistant can coach on diagnostic procedures and treatment plans.
9. Describe care coordination and patient navigation, develop a list of community resources, and facilitate referrals.

VOCABULARY

adherence (ad HEER ehns) The act of sticking to something.
anhedonia (an hee DOE nee ah) The inability to feel or experience pleasure during a pleasurable activity.
cessation (se SAY shuhn) Bringing to an end.
compliance (kuhm PLIE ahns) The act of following through on a request or demand. Patient compliance sounds negative, thus patient adherence is now being used.

patient navigator A person who identifies patients' barriers, works closely with the healthcare team and patients, and guides the patients through the healthcare system; may also be called *care coordinator*.

Healthcare is changing, and the role of the medical assistant is changing too. Some of the current challenges in healthcare include the following:

- Pressure to reduce cost
- Shorter primary care provider visits, yet an increased need for data collection to incorporate patient interviews and outcome measurements (e.g., test results)
- Patients leaving the facility not understanding what they were told
- An unwillingness on the part of patients to adhere to treatment plans (e.g., not taking medication or not taking it correctly, not making lifestyle changes that would improve their health)

Many experts have researched ways to reduce these challenges. Several studies have examined patient medication **adherence** or **compliance.** *Medication adherence* means patients are taking the right dose at the right times as prescribed by the provider. Research has shown that medication adherence with chronic diseases is low. This leads to the progression of the disease and more medical visits for the patient. Ultimately, nonadherence to medication is increasing the cost of healthcare.

Why is it that patients do not take their medication correctly? This question has been a focus of many studies. Common reasons include the following:

- Forgetfulness and confusion on how to take it
- Side effects and cost of the medication
- Feeling it is not helping

Research has shown that many patients are confused after seeing their providers. Patients do not always understand the treatment plan designed to manage their conditions. Confusion about medication and home care is prevalent. Many patients are not able to manage their disease adequately between provider visits; thus, their condition worsens. To solve this problem, ambulatory care facilities are moving toward coaching and care coordination. This chapter focuses on the medical assistant's role in coaching and care coordination.

COACHING

Coaching provides patients with skills, knowledge, support, and confidence to manage their disease between provider visits. One study found that coaching by medical assistants increased the patients' compliance with medication regimens and lifestyle changes. Coaching is extremely valuable for patients. The medical assistant can coach patients in many areas, including the following:

- *Disease prevention:* Provide patients with information on preventing the disease or the spread of disease. Medical assistants can provide information on hygiene practices, recommended vaccines, and nicotine **cessation.**
- *Health maintenance:* Provide patients with information on routine screenings and show patients how to do self-exams (e.g., foot, breast, and oral self-exams).
- *Diagnostic tests:* Instruct patients prior to diagnostic tests. This can include special preparation (e.g., fasting and bowel cleansing preparations).
- *Treatment plans:* Instruct patients on home care and follow-up as ordered by the provider. Research has shown that coaching

can help patients understand information from the visit. It can ensure patients understand how they need to proceed and addresses any concerns before patients leave the facility. Coaching educates patients on self-management of diseases, thus increasing compliance with the treatment plans.

- *Specific needs:* Patients have unique concerns. These can include personal, family, social, financial, and culture-related issues. By listening and asking questions, the medical assistant can help address their specific needs. By closely working with the patient, the medical assistant can provide emotional support and create a bond with the patient. This bond helps the patient feel comfortable. With encouragement, the patient may be more willing to call the medical assistant with questions and concerns between visits.
- *Community resources:* By listening to patients and by asking questions, the medical assistant can identify patients' unique needs. Patients have many needs that affect their health. For instance, if a patient has a limited income, does the patient purchase the prescribed medication, or food? Community resources exist to address many needs, including low-cost medications, food banks, transportation, medical supplies, assisted living, and so on.

This chapter provides information on specific aspects of patient education required for these coaching areas. But first, let's examine health beliefs and practices and how to adapt education to patients' needs.

MAKING CHANGES FOR HEALTH

Often, healthcare professionals see patients who do not comply with the treatment plan. They may not take the prescribed medication, or maybe they do not make the recommended lifestyle changes. If the diagnosis is life-threatening or life-changing, grief and loss can occur. Other times, patients may not perceive the change as necessary. The following sections examine theories that may explain why patients do not comply with the treatment plan.

Stages of Grief

Elisabeth Kübler-Ross studied people's reactions to death and dying. She found that people experienced similar stages. Over the years, these stages have been applied to grief and loss. When a patient and the family get a life-threatening or life-changing diagnosis, they can feel grief and loss. People go through the stages of grief in their own way and at their own pace (Table 7.1). This process can take weeks to months. Patients may not be open to making the recommended changes. Healthcare professionals may view this as the patient not wanting to comply with the treatment plan. Sometimes a patient has to accept a diagnosis before compliance occurs. It is important for the medical assistant to adapt interactions to help with the stages of grief.

CRITICAL THINKING APPLICATION   **7.1**

Suzanne has seen many patients dealing with grief. Why might a patient who is grieving not adhere to a treatment plan?

TABLE 7.1 Stages of Grief and Dying

STAGE	DESCRIPTION	ADAPTIVE INTERACTIONS
Denial	Refuses to accept the fact (i.e., diagnosis or prognosis). May refuse to discuss the diagnosis. May not remember the health coaching. Denial is a defense mechanism that allows the person to ignore what is happening.	Provide handouts that explain the disease and treatment. Encourage family member(s)' support with the treatment. Provide online and community resources (i.e., support groups).
Anger	Anger can be directed at self or others. Anger can surface at unrelated times and be directed toward unrelated issues.	Use therapeutic communication techniques (e.g., reflection) to acknowledge the patient's feelings about the issue. Recognize the real cause of the anger.
Bargaining	Attempts to bargain with the higher power the person believes in (i.e., God). Sometimes the patient will bargain with the provider to make lifestyle changes at a later time.	Work with the healthcare team regarding the bargaining requests. Help provide opportunities where the patient can make decisions.
Depression	People feel sadness, fear, and uncertainty. They may grieve the loss of their health or independence. They may dread the change that is occurring.	Encourage the use of community and healthcare resources to help ease the change process for the patient and family members.
Acceptance	Has come to terms with situation.	Provide coaching on aspects of the disease and self-care management.

Health Belief Model

The health belief model helps explain what factors influence a person's health belief and practices. The first part of this model deals with a person's perception of his or her chance of developing a disease. Some examples include the following:

- Jess is in her 20s and has lost her mother, sister, and grandmother to breast cancer. She feels her chance of developing breast cancer is significant.
- Sam has an older brother with heart disease that is being managed by medication, diet, and exercise. Sam blames the disease on his brother's stressful job. Sam does not have a stressful job, so he feels he will not get heart disease. Even

though Sam receives education on a heart-healthy lifestyle, he ignores the information.

The second part of this model deals with a person's perception of the severity of the disease. A person's perception is influenced by the following:

- Personal factors (e.g., age, gender, race, employment)
- Social factors (e.g., peers, personality, family)
- Perceived threats of the disease
- Cues to action (e.g., mass media campaigns, social media, advice from family, friends, and healthcare providers and professionals)

In the prior examples, Jess has lost three family members to breast cancer. She perceives breast cancer as being a severe disease. Sam, on the other hand, may not perceive the severity of heart disease, because his brother's heart disease is being managed.

The third part of the model focuses on whether the person will take preventive action. A person weighs the benefits of and barriers to taking the preventive actions. For example, Jess may decide to have a double mastectomy as a preventive strategy. For many it may seem severe, but for Jess, she is willing to take such a preventive action. Sam, on the other hand, may not see the benefit of following a heart-healthy lifestyle. He may feel that he has to "give up" his current lifestyle and make changes.

Because a medical assistant coaches patients on preventive actions, it is important to remember the model. Start with identifying if the person perceives he or she is at risk for a disease. Exploring the patient's beliefs and educating the patient on the facts, in addition to getting rid of the myths, can be helpful. Discussing the severity of the disease or what the disease can lead to is the next important step. Finally, offering the patient help in eliminating or diminishing the barriers and helping the person see the benefits of the preventive action are important.

CRITICAL THINKING APPLICATION 7.2

Suzanne has had patients state they do not want to give up their lifestyle and follow the provider's recommendations for better health. How might a medical assistant address this issue with a patient?

BASICS OF TEACHING AND LEARNING

Domains of Learning

Learning is the process of gaining new knowledge or skills through instruction, experience, or study. We learn new information in three different ways or *domains*: cognitive, psychomotor, and affective. These domains are discussed in the coming sections.

Cognitive Domain

The *cognitive domain* of learning involves the mental processes of recall, application, and evaluation. We learn new information by listening to what is said and by reading written words. Many experts believe we have three ways to store memories:

- *Sensory stage:* For a memory to be created, we must pick up something from our senses (e.g., touch, hearing, sight). Our senses are constantly picking up perceptions. Many will be forgotten in a split second. We will pay attention to just a few, and they will move to the short-term memory. The deciding factor between what is forgotten and what moves into the short-term memory is based on its importance to us.

- *Short-term memory:* This is our temporary working memory. If nothing is done with the memory, it will fade within 30 seconds. The short-term memory can only handle about seven units of information at once. By chunking information into meaningful units or attaching it to something we already know, we can increase the amount in our short-term memory.
- *Long-term memory:* The more we use short-term memories, the quicker they enter our long-term memory. We can add endless memories to our long-term memory, but without use (recall), those memories can fade.

Our goal for patient education is to put the information into patients' long-term memory. Not everything we tell the patient will be picked up and remembered. We hope the important information will be. The following tips can be used to help patients remember critical information:

- *Present the information at an appropriate level for the patient.* Most studies show that patient education literature should be at a sixth-grade reading level. According to the US National Library of Medicine's website MedlinePlus, patient educational materials should be between a seventh- and eighth-grade reading level. If the patient's primary language is not English, then a lower reading level is needed.
- *Build on the patient's prior knowledge about the topic.* Start by finding out what the patient knows about the topic. Clarify any inaccurate information and then provide new information that builds on the existing knowledge.
- *Present information in small chunks, in a clear well-organized manner.* Do not overwhelm the patient; keep to the facts and keep it simple. For complex topics, meeting with the patient over several days may help the patient to retain the information.
- *Provide the information in two different ways* (e.g., verbally discuss it and provide a written handout) (Fig. 7.1).
- Tell the patient "this is important to remember" and repeat important information several times during the session. Be aware

that if everything is "important to remember," nothing will be remembered. Do not overuse this strategy.
- *Have the patient teach back the information you provided.* This allows you to check what the patient recalls and if it is accurate. Teaching back also helps the patient remember the information even more.

Table 7.2 provides strategies to use for the cognitive domain. The *barriers* or reasons learning does not occur effectively are also listed. These barriers are important for the medical assistant to limit if possible.

Psychomotor Domain

The *psychomotor domain* is the "doing" domain. We learn new skills and procedures by watching demonstrations and assisting with something. Many people would prefer to attempt a skill versus reading about it or discussing it. They learn best through the psychomotor domain. Table 7.2 provides some barriers to the psychomotor domain.

Some tips to help patients remember critical information include the following:

- Provide written step-by-step directions for the patient to follow and then take home.

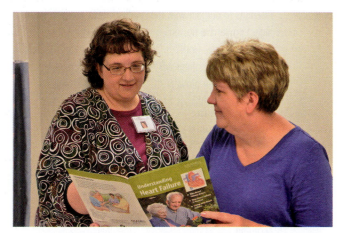

FIGURE 7.1 Provide patients with handouts to take home.

TABLE 7.2	Strategies to Use and Barriers for the Three Domains of Learning			
DOMAIN	INVOLVES	TEACHING STRATEGIES TO USE	BARRIERS TO LEARNING	STRATEGIES TO ADAPT TO BARRIERS
Cognitive	Learning new concepts and information	Discussion, written information, online videos, computer instruction	Memory or cognition issues; language barriers	Keep it simple. Provide easy-to-read handouts. Use an interpreter and provide handouts in the patient's primary language if possible.
Psychomotor	Learning new skill or procedure	Demonstration and return demonstration	Tremors and paralysis; sensory limitations (e.g., visual impairment, hearing impairment)	Use adaptive equipment, such as a magnifying glass and a magnifier for syringes.
Affective	A change in attitude or emotions that will influence the person's behavior	Discussion, role-play, and simulations	Anxiety, denial, pain, fatigue, or stress, cultural customs, previous experience, and poor coping skills	Provide analgesics as ordered by the provider, help to minimize barriers, provide home instructions, and include additional family member(s) if possible.

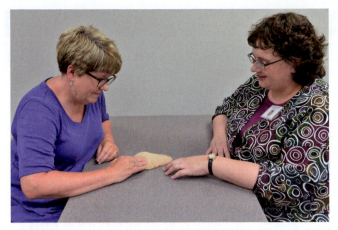

FIGURE 7.2 Having a patient do a return demonstration or "teach back" the skill allows the medical assistant to check the patient's knowledge and skills for accuracy.

- Give timely feedback on the person's performance.
- Have the patient "teach back" the skill to check for accuracy (Fig. 7.2).
- Repeated practice doing the skill helps with recall and retention of the steps.
- Make sure to use the equipment and supplies the patient will be using at home.

Affective Domain

The *affective domain* is the "feeling" domain. It includes our feelings, emotions, values, and attitudes. Our emotions and values are very important. They affect our motivation, confidence, and priorities. When our personal values conflict with the new information presented, a barrier to learning can occur. Pain is another example of an affective barrier. If you are instructing a patient on wound care and he is in pain, he may not remember what you said. Additional barriers to the affective domain are listed in Table 7.2.

Make sure that you address (as much as you can) any affective domain barriers prior to educating a patient. If another family member accompanied the patient, it can be helpful to instruct both the patient and the family member (Fig. 7.3). Written home instructions should also be given.

Adapting Coaching to the Patient

When coaching patients, it is important to recognize that they are individuals. One way of presenting new information to a patient may not work for another patient. It is important for the medical assistant to consider the barriers to learning and possible ways to help the patient overcome those barriers. It is also important for the medical assistant to remember the patient's developmental level and possible cultural diversity issues that may impact learning.

Developmental Level

As we grow and develop, our thought processes and behaviors change. We learn differently. We can understand more complex concepts than when we were younger. It is important for the medical assistant to consider the person's developmental level when coaching. For instance, young children are concrete thinkers. What you say is what they believe you will do. For example, if you say, "I am going to take

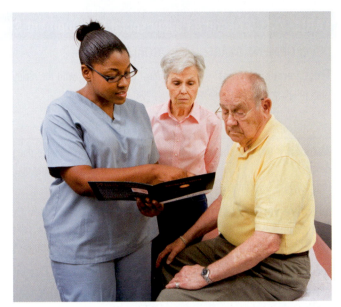

FIGURE 7.3 Teaching the family member along with the patient can provide the patient with more support.

your blood pressure," a 2-year-old child would have no idea what you are going to do. If you say, "I am going to give your arm a hug," then the child may have a better understanding of what you are going to do. Coaching techniques you use for teens will be different from those you use with older adults. Also, referencing materials as you talk can be helpful to the patient.

Erikson's psychosocial developmental stages can be useful when considering the developmental level of patients. Understanding the goal of each stage can help a medical assistant to coach patients in that age group. Table 7.3 provides coaching tips based on the developmental stages.

CRITICAL THINKING APPLICATION   **7.3**

In the family practice environment, Suzanne sees patients of all ages. Explain why the methods she uses with 2-year-old children should differ from those she uses when working with teens. What strategies could she use when coaching both of these populations?

Cultural Diversity

Culture is the set of behaviors, ideas, and customs shared by a specific group of people, which distinguishes the members from other people. Some characteristics of a culture group may include its language, religious beliefs, geographic origin, ethnicity, history, sexual orientation, and socioeconomic class. Culture can be learned from prior generations and passed on to future generations. It is dynamic and evolving. Our culture frames and shapes how we feel about our health and the world around us. Factors affected by a person's culture that healthcare professionals should consider include the following:

- Role of the family and community: Who makes the healthcare decisions? Who pays for the healthcare? Who needs to be present during healthcare discussions?

TABLE 7.3   Erikson's Psychosocial Development Stages With Coaching Tips

DEVELOPMENT STAGE	GOALS OF STAGE	COACHING TIPS
Trust versus mistrust (age range 0–1.5 years [*infancy*])	Must develop trust, with the ability to mistrust should the need arise.	Use a calm, soothing voice, hold child securely. Involve the parent(s) as much as possible. Keep routines consistent as much as possible (if it is time for the infant to eat, allow the child to eat unless eating/drinking is restricted for a medical reason).
Autonomy versus shame and doubt (age range 1.5–3 years [*toddler*])	Must explore and manipulate things in their "world" to develop autonomy and self-esteem.	Use simple, familiar words. Allow child to handle equipment and make choices. Use play to teach the child.
Initiative versus guilt (age range 3–6 years [*preschool*])	Encourage to try new activities. Must assume responsibilities and learn new skills. Will make child feel purposeful and increase self-esteem.	Use familiar words and simple explanations and demonstrations. Allow the child to handle equipment and make choices. Explain a procedure as the child would sense it (e.g., how it feels, looks).
Industry versus inferiority (age range 6–12 years [*school age*])	Must seek to finish tasks. Recognition for accomplishments is important.	Use engaging simple tools to communicate information (videos, gaming software, and pamphlets). Encourage discussion, questions, and making choices. Use concrete terms (with pictures and diagrams) when explaining procedures.
Identity versus role confusion (age range 12–18 years [*adolescence*])	To know whom you are as a person and how you fit into the world around you. Creates a meaningful self-image.	Provide privacy and independence. Encourage responsible decision making. Encourage discussion and questions. Address how a procedure might affect the adolescent's appearance. Promote honest discussion about lifestyle issues.
Intimacy versus isolation (age range 18–25 years [*young adult*])	Can vary. Develops friendships; takes on commitments.	Identify motivating factors. Find out what they know about the topic; correct any inaccuracies. Build on prior information. Listen to their concerns and provide resources as needed.
Generativity versus stagnation (age range about 25–60 years [*middle adulthood*])	Achieve a balance between the concern for the next generation (having a family) and being self-absorbed.	
Ego integrity versus despair (age range 60 or older [*late adulthood*])	Reflect on one's life and come to terms with it instead of regretting the past.	Communicate with dignity and respect. Use simpler language. Speak clearly. Allow time to respond. Find out what they know about the topic; correct any inaccuracies. Build on prior information. Listen to their concerns and provide resources as needed.

- Religion: What are the beliefs about illness? Will the person's religious beliefs affect adherence to the treatment?
- Views on health, wellness, death, and dying
- Views on complementary therapies (e.g., chiropractic care, massage) and *alternative therapies* (other practices used in place of conventional medicine)
- Views on gender roles and relationships
- Beliefs related to food, diet, illness and health
- Beliefs regarding sexuality, fertility, and childbirth

In the United States, disease conditions are seen as more of a scientific situation. Science plays a major role in medicine. Many other cultures take more of a *holistic* approach. A holistic view focuses on the interrelationship among the physical, mental, social, and spiritual aspects of the person's life. A holistic approach is broader than a scientific approach to health and illness.

Many cultures have similar practices, such as:
- *Coining* and *spooning*: Rubbing a silver coin or spoon vigorously on the skin. These practices leave red marks on the skin. Do not confuse the marks with signs of abuse.
- *Cupping*: Applying suction to the skin, which can leave marks. Do not confuse these marks with signs of abuse.
- *Acupressure*: Applying firm pressure on specific points on the body.
- *Acupuncture*: Inserting fine needles into *acupuncture points* (specific sites on the body).

It is important to remember that not every member of the same culture has the same health beliefs. Differences are typically seen between the generations. The healthcare professional should not assume patients have specific health beliefs. Being aware of possible cultural beliefs and practices of a group is important. It can help the medical assistant ask related questions to identify a patient's beliefs and practices.

Cultural Differences

African Americans
- Extended family and church play important roles.
- May have a key family member who must be consulted on healthcare decisions.
- Older members may look at their health as being up to God's will, although younger members seek health screening and treatments as needed.

Cambodians
- Good health means the person is balanced; believe in the balance of hot and cold.
- Illness may be seen as punishment for sins in a past life.
- Typically use traditional healing practices before seeking conventional medicine. May use herbs, cupping and coining, acupuncture and acupressure.
- They may not be interested in preventive care and screenings.

Chinese
- May use acupuncture, massage, and herbs, seeking care from traditional practitioners for less severe illnesses.
- Respectful of elders, teachers, and healthcare professionals. May affect how a person interacts and discusses health topics with the healthcare professional. The person may not ask questions or discuss concerns.

Hispanics/Latinos
- May have strong family and religious beliefs. Family is respected and plays an important role. May view an illness as God's will.
- May use home remedies or folk healer's advice over conventional medicine.
- Sickness is caused by a person having too much heat or cold. Foods and herbs are used to bring back the balance. (Heat and cold are not temperature related.) Cold diseases have more unseen symptoms, such as a chest cold and an earache. Hot diseases have more visible symptoms, such as vomiting, fever, and sore throat.
- Males often answer questions and give consent. Make sure to address the patient also. Friendliness and respectfulness are very important.

Hmong
- Lack words in native language for medical terms and some body organs.
- May seek care from folk medicine doctors and shaman.
- Herbs, massage, coining or spooning, and cupping can be used.
- Accessories may be worn around wrists, necks, or ankles for health or religious reasons.

- Respecting older family members is very important. Often oldest male in the family is the decision maker. Extended family is very important.
- Eye contact is considered rude.
- Touching the head of a child is not accepted. The head is considered sacred.

Native Americans
- May place a lot of value in family and spiritual beliefs.
- State of health occurs when living in total harmony with nature. Illness is the imbalance between the person and nature.
- May use a traditional tribal medicine person.
- Often avoid direct eye contact out of respect and concern for the loss of one's soul.

Russians
- May view healthcare with some mistrust, based on past experience.
- May not be used to asking questions and participating in a discussion with a provider.
- Some practice home remedies and bonki. *Bonki* is practiced by pressing glass cups against the person's shoulders to ease the symptoms. Bruising can occur, which should not be confused with abuse.
- Family likes to receive news about patient's condition and prognosis and may not give bad news to the patient. This lessens the person's anxieties and promotes calmness.

Somali
- Believe that individuals do not prevent illness, which is only done through prayer and living a life according to their religion.
- Use traditional spiritual healers.
- May not take medication if they feel healthy.
- Healthcare decisions are made by the family, and the father gives consent for procedures.
- Male and female circumcisions are performed; being uncircumcised means the person is unclean.

Vietnamese
- Illness is often explained by mystical beliefs.
- Health is the balance between the hot and cold poles that govern the bodily functions.
- Use alternative therapies, such as acupuncture, coining, spooning, and cupping.

CRITICAL THINKING APPLICATION 7.4

In the family practice environment, Suzanne sees patients from a variety of cultures. If you worked in a similar place, what would you do if you noticed red circles on a child's back? You are unsure as to what caused the circles.

Communication Barriers

Coaching patients with communication barriers can be a challenging process. Hearing, vision, and language barriers are common in healthcare. It is estimated that 2% of people in the United States have a visual impairment, 3% have a hearing impairment, and 9% have limited English proficiency. It is important to overcome these barriers when coaching patients.

For healthcare agencies accepting federal funds, the Civil Rights Act requires that all patients have equal access to services. People with vision, hearing, or speech impairments use different ways to communicate. The Americans with Disability Act requires effective communication with patients who have impairments. This may mean offering a qualified medical interpreter or other interpretation services free of charge. Large-print materials and written instructions are also required. Translated written materials are needed for non-English-speaking patients.

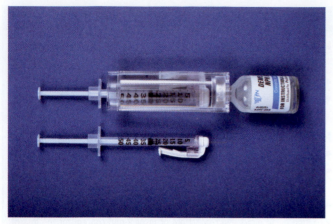

FIGURE 7.4 Syringe magnifiers are used by people with visual impairments. The magnifiers increase the size of the calibration markings on the syringes.

The following sections provide tips for communicating with patients. It is important to listen to patients concerning what works best for them.

Patients Who Have Impaired Vision. When working with patients who have impaired vision, it is important to ensure the room has adequate light. Position the patient so he or she does not have to look directly toward the light source. Make sure the patient is wearing glasses or contacts if needed. When teaching a patient with impaired vision, the following are important:

- Consider the impact of color contrast and glare on the materials used. Use a large black and white font (>14 point font) or electronic copy that can be enlarged. Use bold markers for handwritten information.
- Ask the patient how he or she prefers the information. Provide the patient with large-print directions or brochures.
- Have adaptive equipment available or information on resources for such equipment. For instance, you need to show a patient how to draw up insulin using a syringe. Having a syringe magnifier can help the patient see the calibration markings on the syringe (Fig. 7.4).
- Face the patient directly. Make eye contact. Use a normal tone of voice.
- Gestures and other nonverbal cues are not as helpful with visual impairments.
- Encourage the patient to use his or her own magnification aids.

Patients Who Have Impaired Hearing. When teaching a patient with impaired hearing, the following are important:

- Face the person when speaking.
- Determine if the person has better hearing in one ear over the other. Position yourself so your voice is close to that side.
- If the patient has a hearing aid, encourage the patient to use it.
- Use a low-pitched voice, and speak clearly, slowly, and distinctly. Pause between sentences or phrases. Speak naturally; do not shout. Limit medical terms.
- Say the person's name before you begin a conversation.
- Keep your hands away from your face when talking.
- If an interpreter is present, look at the patient, not the interpreter.
- Limit extra noises in the environment.

- Attempt to rephrase or find a different way to say something if the patient has difficulty understanding a phrase.
- Provide important information in writing.
- Have the person repeat back important information.

Patients Who Have Language Barriers. When teaching a patient who has a language barrier, the following are important:

- Address the patient by his or her last name (e.g., Mrs. Martinez, Mr. Nguyen).
- Be respectful and courteous.
- Use simple phrases. If medical terminology must be used, make sure to define it for patients.
- Use an interpreter or an interpretation service. Focus on the patient and not on the interpreter.
- Use translated materials.
- Pictures and models can be helpful during the coaching session.

Teaching-Learning Process

Teaching opportunities vary greatly in ambulatory care. Sometimes a patient wants to know what a certain medication is for. Other times, the medical assistant needs to coach a patient on a diagnostic test.

Always take a moment to look over any information you provide to patients. Make sure you know the content before you review it with the patient. Providing information that conflicts with the handout will confuse the patient.

The medical assistant should start the coaching process by finding out what the patient knows about the topic. A simple way to do this is by asking a few questions, such as, "Have you had an ultrasound before? If so, what do you remember about it?" This helps the medical assistant identify what the patient knows. From there the medical assistant can begin teaching.

Other coaching sessions will be lengthy because more complex topics are being taught. These coaching sessions should be well planned so the time is used efficiently. Using the teaching-learning process requires the following steps:

- *Assessing the learning needs*: What does the patient need to learn? How ready is the patient for learning? What are the patient's motivations and concerns? What is the patient's learning style? It is important to identify the patient's *learning goals* or the main reason for learning the content.
- *Determining teaching priorities*: It is important to prioritize what the patient needs to learn first. When there is a lot of content to learn, the medical assistant must prioritize the most important topics and address those. Other topics will be addressed on another day. To determine the priorities, ask what information does the patient need to maintain his or her health until the next meeting?
- *Planning the teaching process:* When planning, determine what teaching aids and strategies will be used. The teaching strategies and aids used must be appropriate for the content being taught. For instance, demonstrating how to give an injection and having the patient give a return demonstration will be more useful than just discussing the steps of giving an injection.
  - *Teaching aids* are materials that will be used. These can include brochures, online resources, health-related apps, videos, posters, models, and drawings. Be sure to consider the patient's individual needs (e.g., primary language, developmental level, barriers to learning). For patients with lower reading levels or English as a second language, using more pictures can be helpful.

- *Teaching strategies* are ways the information will be given. For skills, demonstration and role-play with demonstration are effective strategies. Discussion, videos, and internet sites can be helpful for teaching about a disease, diagnostic tests, or treatment.
- *Implementing the teaching process*: It is important to start with the basics and build from there. Keep the information simple, focused, and appropriate for the individual patient. Reinforce important information. If teaching a skill, make sure to have the equipment available that the patient will use at home. This will promote the patient's comfort with the task.
- *Evaluating the patient's learning*: After teaching important points, have the patient summarize what you stated. Keeping the patient involved will help him or her to retain more information. Throughout the teaching session, make sure to ask the patient for feedback on if he or she understands what you are discussing. Instead of just saying, "Do you understand?" Ask specific questions to evaluate the patient's learning; for example, "What are four symptoms of low blood sugar?" Summarize the important points at the end of the teaching session. Answer any questions the patient may have. Identify areas in which the patient needs more information. If there will be more than one session, summarize what will occur during the next meeting
- *Documenting the teaching-learning process*: It is important to document the content taught to the patient, how the patient responded, evidence that the patient learned the content, handouts given, and any plans for follow-up. Make sure to include the provider's name and any adaptations you made to individualize the teaching/learning experience. Evidence may include statements such as, "Pt safely and accurately walked 20 feet using the walker." "Pt stated six signs and symptoms of hypoglycemia."

Tips on Patient Education Materials

Guidelines to follow if you are responsible for developing or ordering educational supplies include:

- The material should be written in lay language at a sixth- to eighth-grade level to promote understanding.
- Good pictures can help patients understand the information.
- Information should be well organized and clearly described.
- All material should be checked for accuracy. (Providers will request to approve the information ahead of time.)
- Handouts should be attractive and professional.
- Copies should be available in languages other than English when possible and in large print for visually impaired clients.
- Do not use disease information literature from medical and pharmaceutical companies that includes advertising of their products. (This type of information can create confusion, if the patient is not using the product advertised.)

COACHING ON DISEASE PREVENTION

Medical assistants coach patients of all ages on disease prevention. It is important to help patients understand ways to prevent diseases in their lives (see Procedure 7.1, p. 152). Common disease prevention coaching by age group includes the following:

- School-age children: Teaching about handwashing and cough etiquette.
- Teens and adults: Teaching about ways to prevent sexually transmitted infections (STIs) and the risks of using cigarettes, smokeless tobacco, and e-cigarettes.
- All age groups: Coaching patients and parents on the vaccines recommended for that specific age (see Procedure 7.1, p. 152). Childhood immunization schedules can be found on the website for the Centers for Disease Control and Prevention (CDC), https://www.cdc.gov/vaccines/schedules/downloads/child/0-18yrs-child-combined-schedule.pdf. Common adult vaccines usually include the following:
- Influenza yearly
- Tetanus and diphtheria (Td) every 10 years and substitute tetanus, diphtheria, and acellular pertussis vaccine (Tdap) once.
- Recombinant zoster vaccine (RZV), Shingrix, two doses for adults age 50 or older; or Zoster vaccine live (ZVL), Zostavax, one dose for adults age 60 or older.
- 13-Valent pneumococcal conjugate vaccine (PCV13), one dose usually after age 65 unless given before based on the patient's health.
- 23-Valent pneumococcal polysaccharide vaccine (PPSV23 or PPSV), one to two doses, depending on patient's health
- Additional vaccines can be given based on the situation (e.g., traveling or job related); adulthood immunization schedules can be found on the CDC's website, *https://www.cdc.gov/vaccines/schedules/downloads/adult/adult-combined-schedule.pdf*

Cough Etiquette

- When coughing or sneezing, turn away from others and cover your mouth and nose with a tissue. If a tissue is not available, cough or sneeze into your elbow or upper sleeve.
- Discard the tissue in the nearest waste container.
- Sanitize hands with an alcohol-based hand sanitizer or wash hands.

How to Prevent Sexually Transmitted Infections

- Abstinence (not having any type of sex) is the most reliable way to prevent STIs.
- Long-term mutual monogamy (an agreement to be sexually active with just one person) with an uninfected partner is also a reliable way to prevent STIs.
- Reducing the number of partners reduces the risk. All partners need to be tested.
- Use latex condoms, although they are not 100% effective.
- Avoid sharing underwear and towels.
- Wash after intercourse.
- Avoid anyone with a genital rash, sore, discharge, or other symptoms.
- Get vaccinated for hepatitis B and human papillomavirus (HPV).

Health Risks Associated With Cigarettes, Smokeless Tobacco, and E-Cigarettes

Tobacco smoke contains more than 7000 chemicals, of which 250 are harmful and at least 69 can cause cancer. One in five deaths are related to smoking. According to the Centers for Disease Control and Prevention (CDC), smokers are more likely to develop heart disease, lung cancer, and strokes. Smoking can cause problems in all parts of the body.

Secondhand smoke causes lung cancer, strokes, low-birth-weight babies, and heart disease. Children exposed to secondhand smoke have increased risks of sudden infant death syndrome (SIDS), ear infections, bronchitis, pneumonia, colds, and asthma.

Quitting has numerous health advantages for the smoker:

- Blood pressure and heart rate begin to return to normal.
- Within a few hours, carbon monoxide levels in the blood decline.
- Within a few weeks, circulation improves and abnormal respiratory systems (e.g., cough, wheezing) decrease.
- One year after quitting smoking, the cardiovascular risks decrease sharply.
- Two to 5 years after quitting, the risk for stroke returns to nonsmoker level.
- Five years after quitting, the risk of cancer of the esophagus, bladder, throat, and mouth is cut in half.
- Ten years after quitting, the lung cancer risk decreases by 50%.

The CDC reports that at least 28 cancer-causing chemicals have been found in smokeless tobacco (e.g., chew and dip). Smokeless tobacco can cause cancer of the mouth, pancreas, and esophagus.

According to the US surgeon general, e-cigarettes heat liquids to form an aerosol that is then inhaled. Many people call this *vaping*. The liquids typically contain nicotine, flavorings, and other additives. E-cigarettes are considered tobacco products because they contain nicotine that comes from tobacco. The nicotine makes e-cigarettes addictive. The additives can pose health risks.

There are many resources available to help smokers quit, including online resources (*https://smokefree.gov*) and the National Cancer Institute's Smoking Quitline at 1–877–44U–Quit. Local resources are usually available. Healthcare providers can discuss medications that can be helpful.

From the Centers for Disease Control and Prevention (CDC). *https://www.cdc.gov/tobacco/infographics/health-effects/index.htm#smoking-risks*; Office of the US Surgeon General: Know the risks. *https://e-cigarettes.surgeongeneral.gov/*. Accessed October 21, 2018.

CRITICAL THINKING APPLICATION   7.5
Suzanne has seen many patients who smoke. Describe how a medical assistant should discuss cessation with a patient who uses nicotine.

COACHING ON HEALTH MAINTENANCE AND WELLNESS

Often with health maintenance and wellness, the provider establishes standing orders for specific education to be given based on the patient's history or age. When the medical assistant rooms a patient, a health history is obtained, and screening questions are asked. Based on the patient's answers, the medical assistant may need to provide coaching on specific topics per the provider's standing orders. For instance, a patient states she smokes 1 pack of cigarettes daily. The provider's standing order for smokers requires the medical assistant to provide information on the hazards of tobacco use and resources for quitting. Another example would be a patient who is turning 45. Because colon cancer screenings typically start at age 45, the provider's standing order would be to provide this information to the patient.

The following sections discuss self-exams that can be taught to patients and the screenings that are commonly done. The medical assistant completes some screenings, whereas others require the medical assistant to educate the patient on the tests to be performed.

Self-Exams

The purpose of self-exams is to identify changes in one's body. Sometimes these changes can be the first sign of a disease. Self-exams are typically done monthly. To help maintain a person's health, the early diagnosis of a disease such as cancer is important.

Breast Self-Exam

Breast cancer can affect both females and males, though males are at a lower risk. Breast cancer is the second most common cancer in females after skin cancer. The risk of breast cancer increases with age. About one in eight women will have invasive breast cancer. Typically, the survival rate is higher the earlier the cancer is diagnosed.

According to the American Cancer Society, research has not shown a benefit for patient or provider breast exams when women are also getting mammograms. It is recommended for women with an average risk of breast cancer to start having yearly mammograms between ages 45 and 50. It is important for all women to know what is normal with their breasts. Any abnormality should be reported to their provider. Some providers still recommend a monthly breast self-exam (BSE) to be done after the menses.

Testicular Self-Exam

According to the American Cancer Society, males at any age can develop testicular cancer. About 50% of those diagnosed are between 20 and 34 years of age. It is estimated that 1 in 263 males will get testicular cancer. If the cancer is found early (before it has spread), there is a good chance of a cure. The American Cancer Society recommends that providers perform a testicular exam as part of a routine physical exam. Some providers recommend that after puberty (around age 15) males should do a monthly testicular self-exam (TSE) after a shower.

Skin Self-Exam

Skin cancer is the most common type of cancer in the United States. The three most common types of skin cancer are basal cell, squamous cell, and melanoma. Basal cell and squamous cell carcinomas are curable. Melanoma is more dangerous and can cause death. These three types of skin cancers are caused by overexposure to ultraviolet (UV) light. UV exposure comes from the sun, tanning beds, and sun lamps. UV rays are an invisible kind of radiation that penetrates and changes skin cells.

Certain people have more risk than others for skin cancer. Experts recommend monthly skin self-exams. It is important to watch for changes in moles. To remember how moles may change, use the ABCDE rule (Table 7.4). Any change in moles, including in the size, shape, color, elevation, or symptom (e.g., bleeding, itching, or crusting), should be reported immediately (Fig. 7.5).

When doing the monthly skin check, start at the scalp and work toward the soles of the feet. Use mirrors to exam the back of the ears and the back. Many people miss mole changes on the back of their ears. When examining hands and feet, make sure to check between the fingers and toes and to check the nail beds. Check all skin surfaces. Document the location of the moles and their appearances. Any changes seen, or any suspicious-looking mole, should be reported to the provider immediately.

TABLE 7.4	Early Warning Signs of Malignant Melanoma: ABCDE Rule
Asymmetry	One half of the mole does not match the other half.
Border	The edges of the mole are blurred or irregular.
Color	The mole is not the same color throughout and has shades of tan, brown, black, red, white, or blue
Diameter	The mole is larger than 6 mm, about the size of a pencil eraser or pea; but it could be smaller.
Evolving	The mole changes over time.

Risk Factors for Skin Cancer

- Skin that is lighter than normal skin color; burns, freckles, or reddens easily; becomes painful in the sun
- Family or personal history of skin cancer
- History of sunburns (especially early in life) or indoor tanning
- Exposure to sun through work or play
- Green or blue eyes
- Red or blond hair
- Certain types and a large number of moles

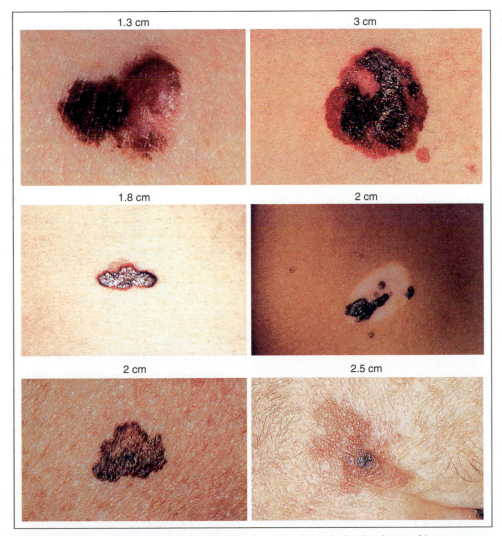

FIGURE 7.5 Malignant melanomas. Note the presence of the ABCDE characteristics. (From Rothrock J: *Alexander's care of the patient in surgery*, ed 14, St Louis, 2011, Mosby.)

Oral Cancer Self-Exam

Oral cancer includes cancer of the lips, tongue, throat, salivary glands, pharynx, larynx, and sinuses. Most oral cancers occur after age 40. It is estimated that more than 40,000 new cases of oral cancer are diagnosed yearly with almost 9,000 related deaths. Early detection is important for oral cancer. Here are some facts about oral cancer:

- Men get oral cancer twice as often as women.
- Using tobacco, drinking alcohol, or having oral human papillomavirus (HPV) are risk factors for oral cancer.
- About 25% of those with oral cancer had no risks.

Oral cancer screening is routinely done by the dentist and should occur every 6 months. It is important for people to do a monthly oral cancer self-exam. Any changes in appearance or sores that do not heal should be reported to the dentist immediately. According to the American Dental Hygienists Association, an oral cancer self-exam consists of looking for lumps and color changes and then feeling for lumps and swelling. To do an oral cancer self-exam, follow these steps:

- Check the head and neck for lumps, bumps, or swelling. Is one side of the face larger than the other?
- Check the skin on the face for changes. Is there a color change? Are there sores, moles, or growths?
- Check for any lumps or tenderness in the neck.
- Check the upper and lower lip for sores and color changes. After the visual inspection, feel for any changes in texture or lumps.
- Check the inner cheek for any color changes (red, white, or dark patches). Then palpate the cheeks with a thumb on the outside and a finger inside. Are any lumps found?
- Check the roof of the mouth for lumps and color changes. Feel for any lumps.
- Check the floor of the mouth using your tongue for any lumps or color changes. Examine all angles. Feel the tongue with a finger for any lumps or tenderness.

Symptoms of Oral Cancer

- White or red patches in the mouth or on the gums, tongue, or lips
- Numbness or pain in the mouth; pain with chewing or talking
- Long-term hoarseness or sore throat
- Swelling in the jaw area or constant earache
- Bleeding in the mouth or a long-term sore
- Feeling of a lump or something stuck in the throat

Regular Screenings

Medical assistants in primary care typically need to talk with patients about the recommended regular screenings for different diseases. Suggested times for screenings are based on an adult with an average risk. If a patient has family members with the disease, that person may have a higher than normal risk. This means the patient may need to be screened earlier and more often than other adults. Regular preventive screenings are summarized by age in Table 7.5 and include the following:

- *Blood pressure*: Patients at higher risk include African Americans, those who are overweight, and those with previously higher than normal blood pressure readings.

- *Bone density*: This screening provides information on the strength of the patient's bones and if the patient has osteoporosis. Women have a higher risk than men, and it increases with age.
- *Cholesterol*: Adults with a family history of high cholesterol levels or who have high cholesterol need more frequent testing.
- *Colorectal cancer screening*: The American Cancer Society recommends that regular screening start at age 45. Screening can either be stool based or visual exams (Table 7.6).
- *Dental exam*: The American Dental Association recommends a dental exam and cleaning yearly. Dental health can affect the overall health of the body.
- *Dilated eye exam*: It is important to have a dilated eye exam if a person has a risk of eye disease (e.g., glaucoma). The CDC recommends dilated eye exams for the following individuals:
  - Patients with diabetes (recommended annually)
  - African American patients age 40 years or older (recommended every 2 years)
  - Patients older than 60 years of age (recommended every 2 years)
  - Patients with a family history of glaucoma (recommended every 2 years)
- *Lung cancer screening*: Patients who are 55 to 80 years old, have a history of heavy smoking, and are currently smoking or quit in the previous 15 years should be screened for lung cancer. (Heavy smoking means smoking one pack of cigarettes a day for 30 years or two packs for 15 years.)
- *Mammogram*: This x-ray of the breasts helps to identify breast cancer. The American Cancer Society recommends women ages 40 to 44 have the option to have annual mammograms. Women ages 45 to 54 should have annual mammograms, and those age 55 years or older should have mammograms every 2 years.
- *Pap test*: This test is used to identify cervical cancer.
- *Prostate cancer*: Risk factors include being 50 years old or older, being African American, exposure to Agent Orange, and having a father, brother, or son who had prostate cancer. No specific test exists for prostate cancer. The digital rectal exam (DRE) and the prostate-specific antigen (PSA) test are used. The provider may offer either test after age 50. Frequency is based on the patient's history.
- *Blood glucose test*: Adults should be screened for Type 2 diabetes mellitus every 3 years or sooner, depending on their medical history.

CRITICAL THINKING APPLICATION   **7.6**

Suzanne has seen more providers ordering the fecal immunochemical test (FIT) over the guaiac fecal occult blood test. What are the advantages of the FIT test?

One-Time Screenings

The medical assistant may also need to coach patients on one-time screening as indicated by the provider. People are recommended to have the following screenings at least once, unless a person's risk is greater than average:

- *Abdominal aortic aneurysm*: Males between 65 and 75 years of age who have smoked at one time in their lives should receive

TABLE 7.5   Preventive Recommendations

	AGE 18–39	AGE 40+
Blood Pressure	Every 3–5 years	Age 40+: every year
Bone Density		Age 65+: Females: every 2 years
Cholesterol	Every 5 years	
Stool-based Tests (gFOBT, FIT, iFOBT)		Age 45–75: annually Age 75+: individual decision
Stool-based Test (MT-sDNA [Cologuard])		Age 45–75: every 3 years Age 75+: individual decision
Colonoscopy		Age 45–75: every 10 years Age 75+: individual decision
Dental exam	Yearly	
Dilated eye exam		Age 60+: every 2 years
Lung Cancer Screening		Age 55–80: those who meet the criteria: annual low-dose computed tomography (LDCT)
Mammogram		Age 45–54: every year Age 55 or older: every 2 years
Pap Test	Females age 21–29: every 3 years Age 30–65: every 3 years or every 5 years if having an HPV test Over 65: individual decision	
Prostate Cancer (DRE or PSA test)		Males age 50+: individual decision
Blood Glucose Test	Every 3 years or more frequent if patient has hypertension or obesity	

From Healthfinder.gov. *https://healthfinder.gov/HealthTopics/Category/doctor-visits*; the American Cancer Society. *https://www.cancer.org*.

this screening. This population has the highest risk of having an abdominal aortic aneurysm (AAA).

- *Human immunodeficiency virus (HIV) screen (blood test):* People 15 to 65 years old need to get an HIV test at least once in their lifetime. All pregnant women need to be tested. People with a high risk for HIV should have testing annually, if not more often. High-risk factors include multiple sexual partners, sexual partners who have or may have HIV, and those who use injectable illegal drugs.
- *Hepatitis C:* This condition is passed through blood from an infected person. A person with risk factors should be tested. Risk factors for hepatitis C include the following:
  - Born between 1945 and 1965
  - History of a blood transfusion or organ transplant before 1992
  - Use of injected illegal drugs
  - Has chronic liver disease, HIV, or AIDS

Additional Screenings

When rooming patients, medical assistants have to perform different screenings. Either the patient's age or the patient's responses will trigger the need for the screening. Screenings have increased throughout the years. This is due to increased data collection requirements and focusing on prevention and quality patient care. Common screenings include the following:

- *Alcohol misuse screening:* Drinking in moderation means that females have no more than one drink a day and males have no more than two drinks per day. (An alcoholic drink is classified as a 12-oz bottle of beer, a 5-oz glass of wine, or a 1.5-oz shot of liquor.) Drinking more than the recommended daily amount may lead to health issues.
- *Nicotine or tobacco screening:* Various tools are used. Tools typically focus on whether or not tobacco products are used, how much is used per day, the history of use, and quitting behaviors (e.g., strategies used in the past or thoughts of quitting).
- *Drug abuse screening:* Various tools are used. Tools focus on prescription drug use for nonmedical reasons and illegal drug use. Tools are designed differently, but it is important to identify any history of or recent drug abuse. Common signs of drug abuse include the following:
  - Poor hygiene; changes in eating and sleeping patterns
  - Loss of interest in favorite things
  - Very energetic, talking fast, very sociable
  - Tired, sad, nervous, agitated, and bad moods
  - Missing school, work, or appointments

TABLE 7.6   Common Colorectal Cancer Screenings

TEST	TESTING FREQUENCY	DESCRIPTION	PATIENT PREPARATION
Guaiac fecal occult blood test (gFOBT)	Age 45–75: every year Age 75–85: individual decision based on health of the person and prior screening history	A fecal specimen is examined for occult or hidden blood, which may indicate gastrointestinal (GI) bleeding. Intestinal bleeding may be an indicator of colon cancer. Stool samples are collected by the patient and returned to the medical laboratory for testing.	For 7 days prior to the test must not take vitamin C supplements, aspirin, or nonsteroidal anti-inflammatory medications (e.g., ibuprofen, naproxen, and indomethacin). Many foods can create false positives. For 3 days before the test, do not eat red meat and raw fruits or vegetables (e.g., horseradish, turnips, broccoli, melons, and radishes).
Fecal immunochemical test (FIT) (also called immunochemical fecal occult blood test [iFOBT])	Age 45–75: every year Age 75–85: individual decision based on health of the person and prior screening history	A fecal specimen is examined for human hemoglobin protein, which may indicate GI bleeding and cancer. Stool samples are collected by the patient and returned to the medical laboratory for testing.	No dietary restrictions are required.
Multi-targeted stool DNA test (MT-sDNA [Cologuard])	Age 45–75: every 3 years Age 75+: individual decision Used in place of the gFOBT and FIT	A fecal specimen is examined for blood. Computer analysis looks at the DNA in the stool, checking for cancer and precancerous cells. Positive results should lead to a colonoscopy. Stool samples are collected by the patient and returned to the medical laboratory for testing.	No patient preparation is required.
Colonoscopy	Age 45–75: every 10 years Age 75+: individual decision	An endoscopy is inserted through the anus and used to visualize the colon.	Usually clear liquids the day before the test. No red liquids allowed. Laxatives and/or enema(s) are used to clean the bowel. May have food and fluid restrictions prior to the test.
Computed tomography (CT) colonography or virtual colonoscopy	Age 45–75: every 5 years	A small tube is inserted into the rectum. The lower colon is inflated with gas. CT images are taken of the colon and rectum.	
Flexible sigmoidoscopy	Age 45–75: every 5 years or every 10 years with yearly FIT	A sigmoidoscope is inserted into the rectum and most of the sigmoid colon. Requires patient dietary and colon preparation.	

- Spending money excessively
- Slowed reaction time, paranoid thinking
- *Intimate partner violence screening*: This screening covers domestic abuse. It is important to remember that both males and females can be victims of domestic abuse. Many psychological and health problems come from violence, including substance abuse, obesity, depression, brain trauma, pregnancy complications, and chronic pain. Intimate partner violence includes controlling behaviors, physical abuse, sexual abuse, and emotional or verbal abuse.
- *Elderly safety screening*: These screening tools focus on how safe the older person feels at home. The tools screen for abuse and neglect.
- *Functional status screening*: Several tools are available for primary care providers to use for older patients. By using a functional status screening tool, the provider obtains information on the patient, such as the following:

- Physical functions with daily activities (e.g., grooming, bathing, walking, and eating)
- Psychological health (e.g., mood and anxiety)
- Role function (e.g., employed or volunteer)
- Social function (e.g., interacting with others or isolating self)
- *Depression screening*: Several tools are used to screen for depression. The screening tools ask questions related to moods, thoughts, and feelings. The number of questions will vary depending on the tools. For instance, the Patient Health Questionnaire–2 (PHQ-2) asks two questions that focus on the frequency of depressed mood and **anhedonia** over the previous 2 weeks. If the patient screens positive, then the Patient Health Questionnaire–9 (PHQ-9) is given to see if the patient meets the criteria for a depressive disorder (Fig. 7.6). (The first two questions of the PHQ-9 are the two questions on the PHQ-2 tool.)

PATIENT HEALTH QUESTIONNAIRE-9 (PHQ-9)

Over the last 2 weeks, how often have you been bothered by any of the following problems? (Use "✓" to indicate your answer)	Not at all	Several days	More than half the days	Nearly every day
1. Little interest or pleasure in doing things	0	1	2	3
2. Feeling down, depressed, or hopeless	0	1	2	3
3. Trouble falling or staying asleep, or sleeping too much	0	1	2	3
4. Feeling tired or having little energy	0	1	2	3
5. Poor appetite or overeating	0	1	2	3
6. Feeling bad about yourself — or that you are a failure or have let yourself or your family down	0	1	2	3
7. Trouble concentrating on things, such as reading the newspaper or watching television	0	1	2	3
8. Moving or speaking so slowly that other people could have noticed? Or the opposite — being so fidgety or restless that you have been moving around a lot more than usual	0	1	2	3
9. Thoughts that you would be better off dead or of hurting yourself in some way	0	1	2	3

FOR OFFICE CODING ___0___ + _____ + _____ + _____

=Total Score: _____

If you checked off any problems, how difficult have these problems made it for you to do your work, take care of things at home, or get along with other people?

Not difficult at all	Somewhat difficult	Very difficult	Extremely difficult
☐	☐	☐	☐

FIGURE 7.6 Example of a depression screening tool: Patient Health Questionnaire–9 (PHQ-9).

• *Peripheral neuropathy screening*: Screening questions focus on loss of feeling or a "pins and needles" sensation in the feet and hands. Besides asking the patient screening questions, the medical assistant may also need to do a monofilament foot test and coach the patient on foot care.

Types and Signs of Elder Abuse and Neglect

• *Physical abuse*: Fractures, rope marks, cuts, bruising, dislocations, broken glasses, giving too little or too much medication, bleeding, and sudden changes in the person's personality or behavior
• *Sexual abuse*: Unexplained sexually transmitted infections, bruising in the genital region, and reports from the older person
• *Emotional abuse*: Not communicating, withdrawn, agitated, and symptoms that mimic dementia
• *Neglect*: Malnutrition, dehydration, lack of proper living conditions, and failing to treat health problems
• *Abandonment*: Leaving the person in a public place
• *Financial abuse*: Stealing from the older person, forging signatures on financial transactions, and any other illegal action that represents a financial loss for the older person

COACHING ON DIAGNOSTIC TESTS

It is important for the medical assistant to provide the necessary teaching for diagnostic and laboratory tests ordered for patients. For tests to be completed, the patient needs to be prepared. Some tests require fasting, whereas others do not. The medical assistant needs to provide answers to these questions:

• What is the test?
• Where does the patient need to go for the test? When is the test scheduled?
• Does the test require fasting? If so, for how long? If no foods or beverages can be consumed, does this include water?
• Should patients continue or stop taking their medications? This may require a discussion with the provider.

It is important to give patients the correct answers. Tables 7.7 and 7.8 provide information on common imaging procedures and medical laboratory tests. Remember, patient preparation may vary based on the facility.

CRITICAL THINKING APPLICATION   7.7

Sometimes Suzanne has a patient who refuses to follow the preparation steps for a diagnostic test. How might you handle this situation?

TABLE 7.7   Common Patient Instructions for Imaging Procedures

PROCEDURE	DESCRIPTION	COMMON PATIENT INSTRUCTIONS
X-ray	X-ray particles pass through the body, and an image is recorded. Many different types of x-rays.	Provide overview of test and why it is being done. Screen for pregnancy. X-rays are painless, although some body positions may be uncomfortable. Patients may be asked to hold the breath during the procedure to get a clear x-ray.
Computed tomography scan (CT scan, CAT scan)	Uses x-rays to create pictures of cross sections of the body. Several types of CT scans exist; each may have different preparations. Patient will lie on a narrow table that slides into the center of the CT scanner. The x-ray beam will rotate around the patient, creating separate images (slices) of the body.	Provide overview of test and why it is being done. May require an intravenous (IV) or oral contrast medium. If so, • Check allergies (contrast medium and iodine). • Check if patient has kidney disease or is on dialysis. • Nothing by mouth (NPO) for 4–6 hours before test. • Address if medications need to be stopped. • IV contrast medium may cause a slight burning feeling and a metallic taste in the mouth; flushing can occur.
Magnetic resonance imaging (MRI)	Uses powerful magnets and radio waves to create images of the body. Does not use radiation. Several types of MRIs exist; may have different preparations. Patient will lie on a table. The machine makes loud noises. No metal is allowed in the room.	Provide overview of test and why it is being done. May require contrast (see CT scan contrast medium information). May require being NPO for 4–6 hours Must identify if patient is claustrophobic (afraid or anxious of close spaces). Due to strong magnets, must screen for artificial heart valves, brain aneurysm clips, heart pacemaker or defibrillator, cochlear (inner ear) implants, recent artificial joint, vascular stents, or history of working with metal. Must remove all metal from patient including removable dental work (e.g., plates).
Mammography	An x-ray picture of the breasts used to find tumors. The breast will be compressed on a flat surface for the x-ray.	The patient should not use any perfume, deodorant, powders, or ointments on the arms or breast on the day of the test. These products may interfere with the results of the x-ray. The patient will need to undress from the waist up. All jewelry from the neck and chest area needs to be removed. Screen for pregnancy, breastfeeding, or if the patient has had a breast biopsy.
Positron emission tomography (PET) scan	Imagining test that uses an IV radioactive substance (tracer) to identify disease in the organs and tissues. Patient will lie on a table that slides into the tunnel shaped PET scanner.	May require patient to be NPO for 4–6 hours (with exception of water) before the scan. Medications may be held (check with the provider). IV tracer will be given, which may cause a sharp sting. Afterward the patient needs to rest for 1 hour. During the test, the patient must lie still to prevent blurry images. Screen for claustrophobia, pregnancy, and allergies to contrast medium and iodine.
Ultrasound (US)	Uses high-frequency sound waves to create the image of the organs and structures.	May require special preparation based on the type of US done. Patient will need to expose the area. A clear, water-based gel is applied to the skin, and a transducer (handheld probe) moves over the area.

COACHING ON TREATMENT PLANS

Many facilities have the medical assistants meet with the patients after the providers finish. The medical assistants review the treatment plan with the patients. They answer any questions, explore any issues the patients may have, and provide additional instructions. As mentioned, this type of coaching has been shown to increase patients' compliance with the treatment plans. Additionally, it provides patients with a lifeline should they have questions or concerns at home.

Medical assistants coach patients on treatments to do at home. These could include taking medications, caring for casts and splints, applying hot or cold therapy, and using assistive devices. Besides these treatments, the medical assistant may also need to help coordinate the patient's care for additional treatments such as physical, occupational, or massage therapies. This section focuses on common treatments and important information for patients to know.

Medication Administration at Home

It is important for patients to know how to take medications at home. This includes the following questions:

• When should the patient take the medications and how should he or she take them?

TABLE 7.8	Patient Instructions for Common Medical Laboratory Tests	
TEST	**USE**	**COMMON PATIENT PREPARATION**
Creatinine	Used to monitor kidney health and disease.	May need to fast overnight. May need to refrain for eating meat for a period of time, as it could increase the creatinine level.
Glucose tests	Used to determine the blood glucose level.	For a fasting glucose test, the patient needs to be NPO (with exception of water) for at least 8 hours. Other glucose tests may require fasting and eating at specific times.
Lipid profile	Used to monitor cholesterol levels and treatment.	May require NPO (with exception of water) prior to the test.
Pap test	Used to screen for cervical cancers and some uterine or vaginal infections.	Do not schedule the test during the menstrual period. For 48 hours prior to the test: • Refrain from sexual intercourse. • Do not use vaginal creams or foams. For 24 hours prior to the test: • Do not douche or tub-bathe.

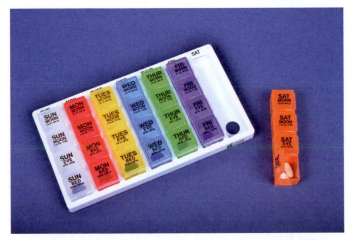

FIGURE 7.7 Daily medication boxes can help patients remember to take their medications.

in each box based on the administration time. Some have boxes for morning, noon, and night medications.

If patients are receiving injections at home, they will need to know how to safely dispose of the needles. Patients can dispose of needles in biohazard sharps containers. These containers are available at local pharmacies and medical supply stores. An internet search can identify local sites that take biohazard sharps containers from patients. Some drug companies have mail-back programs for specific medications. (For more information, visit *https://safeneedledisposal.org.*)

• Do the medications need to be taken on an empty stomach?
• Can they be taken with the other medications?
• Do they need to be taken at bedtime?

Some patients are on a lot of medications. It is important that the medications are taken correctly. When updating the patient's current medications list, it is common to find discrepancies. The patient can be taking the medication differently than how it was ordered. Any discrepancy found needs to be communicated to the provider.

The medical assistant may coach the patient on the proper ways to take medication. Sometimes the medical assistant may need to help patients find ways to remember to take medications. Many patients use medication boxes that they, a family member, or a pharmacy set up. The boxes typically are arranged for 7 days a week with one or more boxes per day (Fig. 7.7). The medications are placed

Discarding Medications at Home

It is important to encourage patients to discard expired, unwanted, or unused medications. This will help prevent misuse and theft. To get rid of controlled substances, take the medications in their original prescription bottles to a medicine take-back facility. Usually, Drug Enforcement Administration (DEA) representatives are available to take control of the controlled substances. Another option is to contact a DEA-authorized collector. The DEA's website has more information on both programs (*https://www.deadiversion.usdoj.gov*).

If these programs are not available, some medications are labeled with specific disposal instructions. Many times, the label recommends flushing controlled substances down the sink or toilet. The website for the Food and Drug Administration (FDA) contains a complete list of medications that can be discarded by flushing (*www.fda.gov*).

If the label does not indicate flushing, then mix the medications in an unpalatable substance (dirt, used coffee grounds, or kitty litter). Place the mixture in a plastic bag. Seal and discard it in the household trash. Make sure all personal information and the prescription number have been scratched out on empty pill bottles.

CARE COORDINATION

Care coordination provides personalized patient- and family-centered care in a team-based environment. Advantages of care coordination include the following:

- Greater efficiency with providing patient care
- Reduced costs
- Greater patient care
- Individualized patient guidance and services
- Encourages patients to focus on goals and self-management
- Reduces hospital emergency department visits and readmissions
- Ensures the patient's needs and preferences for healthcare services are met

The care coordinator communicates between the patient and the healthcare team. Care coordinators ensure patients get timely care and do not fall through the cracks. In the ambulatory care setting, care coordination can be set up in different ways. It has been shown to be successful in primary and specialty care areas. The overall goals include:

- Help patients understand why and what services are needed
- Schedule and sequence appointments
- Provide instructions and directions to patients
- Ensure that test results are available to the providers during patient appointments
- Communicate the patient's needs and concerns to providers

A **patient navigator** (also called a *patient advocate*) has been described as a type of care coordinator. The navigator program was established at the Harlem Hospital Center in 1990. The goal was to assist cancer patients in accessing quality healthcare. Based on the success of patient navigators, the Patient Navigator, Outreach and Chronic Disease Prevention Act of 2005 funded additional positions. Today, patient navigators typically guide chronically ill patients through the healthcare system. They identify patients' financial, cultural, physical, and emotional barriers. Then, they work closely with the healthcare team and the patients to ensure barriers are eliminated and patients get timely care.

In the ambulatory care setting, medical assistants can be care coordinators. A person must have strong interpersonal skills to be successful as a care coordinator. The medical assistant must listen to the patient and family to identify their needs and concerns. The care coordinator must be compassionate yet provide firm guidance with patients who are difficult.

Possible areas involved with care coordination can include the following:

- Interview patients to identify their needs and barriers to wellness and healthcare.
- Provide patients with resources based on their needs and barriers.
- Schedule and sequence appointments.
- Make sure the required information is communicated to and from specialty departments.
- Assist with reducing language barriers by identifying bilingual providers and translators.
- Discuss special needs patients have with their healthcare team.
- Identify community resources, which may include the following:
  - Transportation and medical equipment
  - Adult daycare, assistive living, and long-term care

- Educational programs and support groups
- Low-cost medication programs
- Low-cost preventive screening and immunizations

Procedure 7.2 on p. 153 describes the process of creating a current list of community resources and referring patients or family members.

CLOSING COMMENTS

It is an exciting time to become a medical assistant. The medical assistant's role is changing to meet healthcare needs. Studies have shown that medical assistants play an important role in coaching and helping patients comply with treatment and lifestyle changes. It is important for the medical assistant to coach the patient in a manner that helps the patient understand and retain the information. Adapting the coaching to the patient's communication barriers, developmental stage, and cultural practices will help the patient complete the treatment plan.

Patient Coaching

With the advances in technology, patient education materials are no longer available just on paper. Apps can help providers explain procedures and diseases to patients. YouTube links and other websites provide videos and information on diseases, procedures, and treatments.

When you use patient education materials from apps and online sites, it is important to use only provider-approved sites. The information must be current and from a reputable source. Possible online websites for patient education materials include the following:

- National Institutes of Health (NIH) from the US Department of Health and Human Services (*https://www.nih.gov/health-information*)
- Centers for Disease Control and Prevention (CDC) (*https://www.cdc.gov/*)
- MedlinePlus from the US National Library of Medicine (*https://medlineplus.gov/*)
- American Diabetes Association (ADA) (*http://www.diabetes.org/*)
- American Heart Association (AHA) (*https://www.heart.org/en/health-topics*)
- Drugs.com (*https://www.drugs.com/*)
- Mayo Clinic (*https://www.mayoclinic.org/*)
- Cleveland Clinic (*http://my.clevelandclinic.org/health/*)
- Stanford Health Care (*http://healthlibrary.stanford.edu/resources/bodysystems/*)
- Familydoctor.org from the American Academy of Family Physicians (*https://familydoctor.org/*)

Legal and Ethical Issues

After coaching a patient on a topic, it is important for the medical assistant to document the teaching. The medical assistant should indicate what the provider ordered for coaching, materials used, and general topics taught. The medical assistant should also document an evaluation statement regarding the learning.

Evaluating a patient's learning can be done through several methods, including asking the patient questions regarding the content or having the patient teach back the skill or content. The purpose of the evaluation is to determine if the patient accurately understood the information or skill. The evaluation method and the patient's response should be documented in the medical record for legal purposes.

Patient-Centered Care

Just by the design, care coordination helps provide patients with individual assistance. Patients who feel well cared for and who feel comfortable talking with their healthcare team stay with their provider. It is estimated that care coordination will increase in popularity in the coming years. This model of care will also promote exceptional customer service in healthcare.

Professional Behaviors

When coaching patients, the medical assistant must observe the patient's nonverbal and verbal communication. It is important for the medical assistant to listen to the patient and be open to questions from the patient. If the medical assistant does not know the answers to questions or if the questions are outside the medical assistant's scope of practice, the provider should be notified.

SUMMARY OF SCENARIO

During Suzanne's yearly review with her supervisor, she mentions that she is interested in becoming a care coordinator. She and the supervisor discuss how the program might assist the providers and patients. Suzanne agrees to research the role and bring a proposal to her supervisor in the coming weeks. The supervisor would then take it to the provider meeting and discuss the care model with all of the WMFM providers. Both Suzanne and her supervisor are excited to pursue changes in the practice and to continue to provide patients with the best possible care.

SUMMARY OF LEARNING OBJECTIVES

1. **Describe the medical assistant's role as a coach.**
   Coaching provides patients with skills, knowledge, support, and confidence to manage their disease between provider visits. The medical assistant can coach patients in many areas, including disease prevention, health maintenance, diagnostic tests, treatment plans, specific needs, and community resources.

2. **List and describe the stages of grief; also, discuss how the health belief model helps to explain what factors influence a person's health beliefs and practices.**
   The stages of grief include denial (refuses to accept the fact), anger at one's self or others, attempts to bargain, depression, and acceptance. Table 7.1 described adaptive interactions for each stage.
   The first part of the health belief model deals with a person's perception of his or her chance of developing a disease. The second part of this model deals with a person's perception of the severity of the disease. The third part of the model focuses on whether the person will take preventive action. A person weighs the benefits and barriers of taking the preventive actions.

3. **Describe the three domains of learning.**
   We learn new information in three different ways, or *domains*: cognitive, psychomotor, and affective. The *cognitive domain* of learning involves mental processes of recall, application, and evaluation. The *psychomotor domain* is the "doing" domain. We learn new skills and procedures by watching demonstrations and assisting with something. The *affective domain* is the "feeling" domain. It includes our feelings, emotions, values, and attitudes. Our emotions and values are very important.

4. **Explain how a medical assistant can adapt coaching to the patient.**
   It is important for the medical assistant to consider the barriers to learning and possible ways to help the patient overcome those barriers. It is also important for the medical assistant to remember the patient's developmental level. Erikson's psychosocial developmental stages are described in Table 7.3. Understanding the goal of each stage can help a medical assistant to coach patients in that age group. Learning about cultural differences can help the medical assistant ask related questions to identify a patient's beliefs and practices. Besides developmental levels and cultural differences, the medical assistant may also need to adapt to communication barriers, including impaired vision, impaired hearing, and language barriers. Review the related sections in the chapter for more information on each of these areas.

5. **Describe the teaching-learning process.**
   The medical assistant should start the coaching process by finding out what the patient knows about the topic. From there the medical assistant can begin teaching. For lengthy coaching situations, the medical assistant should plan so the time is used efficiently. Using the teaching-learning process requires the following steps:
   - Assessing the patient's learning needs
   - Determining teaching priorities
   - Planning the teaching process
   - Implementing the teaching process
   - Evaluating the patient's learning
   - Documenting the teaching-learning process

6. **Discuss how a medical assistant can coach on disease prevention.**
   Medical assistants coach patients of all ages on disease prevention. These topics can include hand washing and cough etiquette; STI prevention; the risks of cigarettes, smokeless tobacco, and e-cigarettes; and vaccines recommended for specific age groups.

7. **Describe how a medical assistant can coach on health maintenance and wellness, including different types of self-exams and screenings.**
   Often with health maintenance and wellness, the provider establishes standing orders for specific education to be given based on the

Continued

SUMMARY OF LEARNING OBJECTIVES—*continued*

patient's history or age. Based on the patient's answers to the health history and screening questions, the medical assistant may need to provide coaching on specific topics per the provider's standing orders. The medical assistant can provide coaching on self-exams, including breast, testicular, skin, and oral cancer. Besides self-exams, the medical assistant can provide coaching on regular screenings, on-time screenings, and additional screenings, such as tobacco screening and alcohol misuse screening.

8. **Describe how a medical assistant can coach on diagnostic procedures and treatment plans.**

    It is important for the medical assistant to provide the necessary teaching for diagnostic and laboratory tests ordered for patients. For tests to be completed, the patient needs to be prepared.

    Many facilities have the medical assistants meet with the patients after the providers finish. The medical assistants review the treatment plan

with the patients. They answer any questions, explore any issues the patients may have, and provide additional instructions.

9. **Describe care coordination and patient navigation, develop a list of community resources, and facilitate referrals.**

    Care coordination provides personalized patient- and family-centered care in a team-based environment. The care coordinator communicates between the patient and healthcare team. A patient navigator (also called a *patient advocate*) has been described as a type of care coordinator. Patient navigators typically guide chronically ill patients through the healthcare system. They identify patients' financial, cultural, physical, and emotional barriers. Then, they work closely with the healthcare team and the patients to ensure barriers are eliminated and patients get timely care. Procedure 7.2 on p. 153 describes the process of creating a current list of community resources and referring patients or family members.

PROCEDURE 7.1   Coach a Patient on Disease Prevention

Tasks: Coach a patient on the recommended vaccinations for his or her age. Adapt coaching for the patient's communication barrier and developmental life stage. Document the coaching in the patient's health record.

Scenario: You are working with Dr. David Kahn. You need to room Charles Johnson (date of birth [DOB] 03/03/1958), and his record indicates he has not been seen in several years. Charles has significant hearing loss, and he communicates by signing. His wife interprets for him. You look in his health record and see that he is due for influenza, Td, and recombinant zoster (shingles) vaccines. Per the provider's request (order), you need to coach adult patients on potential vaccines they are due for during the initial rooming process.

Directions: Role-play this scenario with two peers.

EQUIPMENT and SUPPLIES

- Vaccine Information Statements (VIS) (available at *http://www.immunize.org/vis/*)
- Patient's health record

PROCEDURAL STEPS

1. Wash hands or use hand sanitizer.
   PURPOSE: Hand sanitization is an important step for infection control.
2. Greet the patient. Identify yourself. Verify the patient's identity with full name and date of birth. Explain what you will be doing.
   PURPOSE: It is important to identify the patient in two different ways to ensure that you have the correct patient. Explaining the procedure can make the patient feel more comfortable and helps to reduce anxiety.
3. Arrange the chairs so the patient can see both you and the person signing. Speak slowly. Pause as needed to allow person signing to finish with the last statement. Look at the patient when communicating.
   PURPOSE: The medical assistant must focus on the patient and not the person signing or the interpreter. Speaking slowly and pausing allows the person to sign what you are saying.

4. Use simpler language when talking. Speak clearly. Communicate with dignity and respect. Allow time for the patient to respond. Listen to the patient's concerns.
   PURPOSE: When working with older patients, it is important to treat them with respect and dignity. Listening is important.
5. Ask the patient if he has received vaccines somewhere else over the past few years.
   PURPOSE: It is important to verify that the health record is accurate.
   Scenario Update: *The patient has not seen any healthcare providers over the past few years. The only vaccines received were given at this facility.*
6. Describe the vaccines that are due. Use the VIS for each vaccine as you coach the patient on the purpose of the vaccine.
   PURPOSE: The VIS is written for patients and describes the vaccine, disease(s) it prevents, and adverse reactions (side effects).
   Scenario Update: *The patient knows the shingles vaccine is not covered and costs more than $200. He refuses the shingles vaccine, and he does not believe in getting the influenza vaccine. He is interested in getting the Td vaccine.*

PROCEDURE 7.1 Coach a Patient on Disease Prevention—*continued*

7. Ask the patient which vaccines he is interested in getting. If he refuses, be respectful of his choice. Any reason he gives for the refusal should be communicated to the provider.
PURPOSE: Patients have the right to refuse. Any treatment refused must be communicated to the provider.

8. Document the coaching in the patient's health record. Include the provider's name, what was taught, how the patient responded, and any vaccines refused.
PURPOSE: It is important to document the procedure in the health record to show it was done.

07/16/20XX 1305 Per Dr. Kahn's order, instructed pt on the RZV, influenza, and Td vaccines. Pt stated he was not interested in the influenza vaccine or the RZV. He also stated his insurance wouldn't cover the RZV, and he didn't have the money to pay for it. He is interested in receiving the Td vaccine. Reviewed the Td VIS (07/15/20XX) with the patient. Pt stated he understood and would call if he had any issues. Due to pt's hearing impairment, pt's wife interpreted for pt during the visit._____ Suzanne Peterson CMA (AAMA)

PROCEDURE 7.2 Develop a List of Community Resources and Facilitate Referrals

Tasks: As a patient navigator, develop a current list of community resources that meet the patient's healthcare needs. Discuss the resources with the patient and facilitate referrals to the chosen resources.

Scenario 1: Robert Caudill (DOB 10/31/1940) was just diagnosed with dementia. He currently lives with his daughter, Ruby, who works full time. Ruby is feeling overwhelmed with being his only caregiver and realizes that she needs to find someone to care for her father while she is working.

Scenario 2: Leslie Green (DOB 08/03/03) just tested positive for pregnancy. She does not feel that she has a support system to help her make decisions.

Scenario 3: Ella Rainwater's husband of 30 years died suddenly 1 month ago. Ella (DOB 07/11/1959) stated that she feels alone and has no one to talk to. Her daughter feels that Ella needs the support of others who have gone through the same thing.

Directions: Role-play these scenarios with two peers.

EQUIPMENT and SUPPLIES

- Computer (with internet) or a telephone book
- Paper and pen
- Community Resource Referral Form or other referral form
- Patient's health record

PROCEDURAL STEPS

1. Using the scenarios, identify the possible types of community resources that would assist each patient or family. Identify three different types of resources (e.g., medical equipment, support group) that would meet each patient's needs.
PURPOSE: A variety of community resources are available for patients and families who are dealing with chronic illnesses and death. Such resources range from daycare, meals, transportation, medical equipment, assistive living, support groups, to reduced costs for medications.

2. Using the internet or the phone book, identify two local resources for each of the three kinds of resources (i.e., find two assistive living resources, two medical equipment suppliers, etc.). Make a list of six resources for the patient and family. Include the following:

a. Organization's name
b. Address and contact information
c. Summary of the services provided
d. Cost and other relevant information
PURPOSE: As the patient navigator or care coordinator, it is important for you to provide patients and families with the contact information for various community resources. This information can help the family find the best solution for the situation.

3. *Role-play the scenario indicated by the instructor.* Provide the patient or family member with the list of six resources. Describe the services offered and any costs.

4. Allow the patient or family member time to review the services. Answer any questions.
PURPOSE: It is important that the patient and family members understand the services available.

5. Use professional, tactful verbal and nonverbal communication as you work with the patient or family member.
PURPOSE: Patients and family members are more apt to respond positively to assistance if the medical assistant's communication is professional, empathetic,

Continued

PROCEDURE 7.2   Develop a List of Community Resources and Facilitate Referrals—*continued*

and tactful. Talking down to patients or acting superior are unprofessional behaviors that negatively impact the working relationship with patients.

6. *Role-play making the community referrals.* Have the patient or family member decide on two or more services they are interested in. Complete the referral document. Have the patient provide any additional information required on the form. Call the community resource agency and provide the referral information to the representative (a peer).

Note: Some community referrals (e.g., support groups) will require the patient to make contact and not the healthcare professional.

PURPOSE: The referral document is used by many organizations to capture the patient's preferences and to help process the referral.

7. Document the patient education and the referrals in the health record.

PURPOSE: It is important to document all patient interactions and referrals in the health record.

8

TECHNOLOGY

SCENARIO

Christiana was a clinical medical assistant at Walden-Martin Family Medical (WMFM) Clinic. She had been working as a clinical medical assistant for 5 years. She helped with diagnostic tests and treatment procedures. Christiana enjoyed providing patient care, but she wanted to use more of the administrative skills she had learned. She is organized and enjoys challenges and technology.

When a front office position opened up, Christiana moved into the administrative role. She is now the lead administrative medical assistant. Besides performing her administrative duties, Christiana is now responsible for the clinic's computer system. She is excited to continue to learn the administrative role and the computer system.

While studying this chapter, think about the following questions:

- What are the common types of hardware and software used in an ambulatory care facility?
- What is the medical assistant's role regarding maintaining computer hardware?
- How can a medical assistant apply infection control principles to a workstation?
- What are the principles of ergonomics that apply to a computer workstation?
- What are computer network security procedures?

LEARNING OBJECTIVES

1. Describe types of personal computers used in ambulatory care facilities.
2. Discuss the difference between input and output hardware, list examples of each type of hardware, describe computer storage devices, and list examples for each category of computer storage device. Also, discuss cloud storage.
3. Describe how to maintain computer hardware and explain infection control procedures with computer hardware.
4. Identify principles of ergonomics that apply to a computer workstation.
5. Identify questions to ask when purchasing hardware.
6. Differentiate between system software and application software and provide examples of each.
7. Differentiate between practice management software, electronic health records, and electronic medical records. Also, discuss hybrid health records.
8. Discuss HIPAA's Security Rule safeguards and list examples of each type of safeguard.
9. Discuss technologic advances in healthcare.
10. Describe how to identify reliable health websites.

VOCABULARY

boot The process of starting or restarting a computer when the operating system is loaded.

business associate A person or business that provides a service to a covered entity that involves access to PHI. Examples include legal, billing, and management services; accreditation agencies; consulting firms; and claims processing organizations.

claim An itemized statement of services and costs from a healthcare facility submitted to the health (insurance) plan for payment.

computer network A system that links personal computers and peripheral devices to share information and resources.

computer on wheels (COW) A wireless mobile workstation; also called a *workstation on wheels* (WOW).

covered entity (KUV er ed EN ti tee) A healthcare facility, healthcare provider, pharmacy, health (insurance) plan, or claims clearinghouse that transmits protected health information electronically.

data server Computer hardware and software that perform data analysis, storage, and archiving; also called a *database server*.

decryption (dee KRIP shun) The computer process of changing encrypted text to readable or plain text after a user enters a secret key or password.

VOCABULARY—continued

docking station Also known as a universal port replicator; this hardware device allows laptops to connect with other devices, making it into a desktop computer.

downtime The interval of time during which something, such as hardware or software, is not functioning.

drive A computer device that reads data from and may write data to a storage medium.

dumb terminal A personal computer that does not contain a hard drive and allows the user only limited functions, including access to software, the network, or the internet.

electronic health record (EHR) An electronic record that conforms to nationally recognized standards and contains health-related information about a specific patient. It can be created, managed, and consulted by authorized clinicians and staff from more than one healthcare organization.

electronic medical record (EMR) An electronic record of health-related information about an individual that can be created, gathered, managed, and accessed by authorized clinicians and staff members within a single healthcare organization. An EMR is an electronic version of a paper record.

electronic transaction The electronic exchange of information between two agencies to accomplish financial or administrative healthcare activities.

e-prescribing The use of electronic software to communicate with pharmacies and send prescribing information. It takes the place of writing a prescription by hand and giving it to a patient; most new or refill prescriptions can be submitted electronically, cutting down on fraud and errors.

ethernet (EE thuhr net) A communication system for connecting several computers so information can be shared.

file A collection of data or program records stored as a unit with a specific name.

hackers Unauthorized users who attempt to break into computer networks.

hardware Physical equipment of the computer system required for communication and data processing functions.

interface An interconnection between systems.

interoperability The ability to work with other systems.

intranet (IN trah net) A private computer network that can only be accessed by authorized people (e.g., employees of the facility that owns the network).

malware (MAL wair) Malicious software designed to damage or disrupt a system (e.g., a virus).

media (ME de ah) Types of communication (e.g., social media sites); with computers, the term refers to data storage devices.

modem (MOE duhm) Peripheral computer hardware that connects to the router to provide internet access to the network or computer.

no-show To fail to keep an appointment without giving advance notice.

operating system System software; it acts as the computer's software administrator by managing, integrating, and controlling application software and hardware. Windows is an example.

output device Computer hardware that displays the processed data from the computer (e.g., monitors and printers).

patient portal A secure online website that gives patients 24-hour access to personal health information using a username and password.

point-of-care Something designed to be used at or near where the patient is seen; point-of-care tools and apps are resources for the provider to use when working directly with the patient.

practice management software A type of software that allows the user to enter demographic information, schedule appointments, maintain lists of insurance payers, perform billing tasks, and generate reports.

privacy filters Devices attached to the monitor that allow visualization of the screen contents only if the user is directly in front of the screen; also called *monitor filters* or *privacy screens*.

protected health information (PHI) Individually identifiable health information stored or transmitted by covered entities or business associates. Includes verbal, paper, or electronic information.

revenue (REV eh noo) Money collected for providing a product or service.

secondary storage devices Media (e.g., jump drive, flash drive, hard drive) capable of permanently storing data until they are replaced or deleted by the user.

security risk analysis Identification of potential threats of computer network breaches, for which action plans for corrective actions are instituted.

software A set of electronic instructions to operate and perform different computer tasks.

stylus (STI luhs) A pen-shaped device with a variety of tips that is used on touchscreens to write, draw, or input commands.

telehealth Refers to remote clinical services and nonclinical services, such as provider training, meetings, and continuing education.

When technology was first used in healthcare, it was used in the business departments. Computer **software** was used for billing and accounting procedures, registration processes, and scheduling.

With the advent of computer technology, what used to take hours to do, now takes minutes. Data is collected once, entered, and used for many purposes. Computer software increases accuracy and efficiency and saves money.

When **electronic health records (EHRs)** were introduced, agencies implemented software to increase the accuracy and efficiency of patient care. The federal government provided financial incentives to use EHRs instead of paper medical records. Currently healthcare workers use "smart" devices for quicker access to information to provide better patient care.

Communication has also changed over the years. Patients use emails and text messages to contact their providers. To help ensure confidentiality, administrators have created tighter network security procedures. Today, medical assistants must be more computer savvy than ever before to meet technologic demands. They must follow procedures to safeguard the privacy and security of patients' records.

COMPUTERS IN AMBULATORY CARE

Many clinics are using electronic technology in both administrative and patient care areas. Paper medical charts are being replaced with EHRs or used with the EHR. Technology has increased the efficiency of the office environment. It has made patient information and resources quickly accessible to healthcare staff. Medical assistants need to learn and use computers and technology.

Personal Computer

A personal computer (PC) is a single-user electronic data processing device. Types of personal computers include:

- *Desktop computer*: A larger unit designed for use on a desk. It is used by employees who primarily perform word processing, data entry, and business tasks (e.g., scheduling, bookkeeping, and billing).
- *Laptop computer*: A thin, lightweight, wireless, portable PC with a keyboard; it may include a touchscreen. With the recent trend toward reducing the size and weight of laptops, they are often called *notebooks*, because they are a smaller, lighter computer compared to a laptop. Laptops are used by providers and medical assistants in patient exam rooms and at workstations.
- *Tablet PC*: A thin, lightweight, wireless, portable PC that functions with a touchscreen (Fig. 8.1). The most popular **operating systems** include Android and iOS. Tablets are used by providers and medical assistants in patient exam rooms and at workstations. There are several types of tablet PCs, including:
  - *Slate-style tablet*: A thin, portable computer with no keyboard. External keyboards are available for many slate-style tablets.

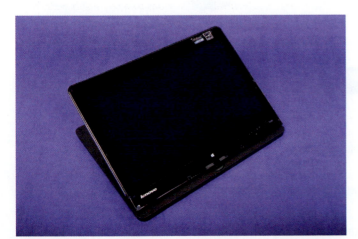

FIGURE 8.1 Tablet computers and other new computers have touchscreen panels that allow users to easily enter data.

- *Convertible tablet*: Usually allows the user to use the touchscreen or the physical keyboard. The display can rotate and cover the keyboard, making it appear like a tablet; or, the keyboard makes it look like a small laptop (e.g., notebook).
- *Hybrid tablet*: May also be called a *hybrid* or *convertible notebook*; has a removable display, making it look more like a slate tablet.

The PC accepts, stores, and processes data. After processing the information, it generates the data output in a specific form.

The personal computer is a system unit. All other forms of physical equipment used with the PC are called *peripheral devices*. The PC and peripheral devices are **hardware**. Computer hardware can be divided into the following categories: input devices, **output devices**, internal components, **secondary storage devices**, and network and internet access devices. The following sections describe these categories.

CRITICAL THINKING APPLICATION 8.1

When Christiana transitioned into the administrative role, Dr. Kahn hired Michaela as the new clinical medical assistant. Recently the healthcare facility switched from using desktop computers to tablet computers when working with patients in the exam rooms. How might Christiana's experience using the desktop computer in the exam rooms be different from Michaela's use of the tablet computer? Thinking of the patient's perception, which technology might a patient prefer the medical assistant to use? Why?

Input Devices

An *input device* is any peripheral hardware that allows the user to provide data to the computer. Many types of input devices are available on the market. This discussion focuses on those typically used in the ambulatory care setting. Common input devices include keyboards, mice and other pointing devices, touchscreens, webcams, cameras, microphones, scanners, and signature pads.

Keyboard. Keyboards are the most common input devices. The QWERTY keyboard is the standard keyboard for computers. (Q-W-E-R-T-Y are the first six letters, from left to right, just below the number keys on the keyboard.) A wide variety of keyboards are available, including standard, internet, wireless, and ergonomic. Keyboards may have special keys that perform the same functionality as the buttons on Web pages. Numeric keypads are also a feature on many keyboards. Ergonomic keyboards reduce repetitive strain injuries by minimizing muscle strain. These keyboards allow the user's hands to be in a natural position when typing. The two most common ergonomic keyboards are the split-key models and the waved or curved key layout (Fig. 8.2).

Keyboards typically have the following categories of keys:
- *Typing*: Include the numeric and alphabetic keys used for typing.
- *Numeric*: Numeric keypads in the same position as calculators.
- *Function*: The 12 keys at the top of the keyboard. Each key has a specific purpose. Some software programs allow the function keys to be programmed to complete a specific function.
- *Control*: Allow movement of the cursor and the screen; include Home, End, Insert, Delete, Page Up, Page Down, Control, Escape, Alternate, and four arrow keys.
- *Special purpose*: Include Enter, Shift, Caps Lock, Num Lock, Space Bar, Print Screen, and Tab keys.

Mouse and Touchpad. The mouse is one of the most common input devices. It makes screen navigation much simpler than using the keyboard. A mouse is a palm-sized box with a laser sensor that tracks the movement of the user's hand. It sends those messages back to the computer. The mouse is used to move the pointer (cursor) on the screen. The mouse may have left and right buttons with a wheel in between to help with cursor/pointer navigation and functionality. With a trackball mouse, the user moves the enlarged ball on the top of the mouse to control the pointer (Fig. 8.3). Other types of mice work like touchpads.

Touchpads are becoming more popular on laptops. They are touch sensitive. Touchpads move the pointer based on the user's finger movements. The functionality of touchpads can vary. Some have left- and right-click buttons like those on a mouse. Other touchpads have a finger tap or click sequence for the left- and right-click action.

CRITICAL THINKING APPLICATION   **8.2**

Christiana's keyboard looks different from Dr. Kahn's keyboard in his office. Why might Christiana have a different keyboard?

Touchscreen. A touchscreen is different from a touchpad. A touchscreen allows a person to interact with the computer by touching the display screen with a finger or **stylus.** Touchscreens can vary, which means the compatible stylus can vary (Table 8.1).

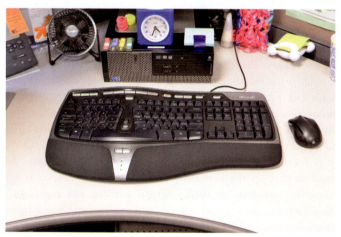

FIGURE 8.2 Ergonomic keyboards have different appearances, yet they all reduce repetitive strain injuries.

Camera, Webcam, and Microphone. Cameras, wireless webcams, and microphones are commonly seen in ambulatory care settings. Cameras are used to capture images of patients before and after surgery. Cameras may also be used to take a picture of a wound. These images are uploaded into the patient's health record. Regardless if a picture is taken in the medical facility or sent by the patient to the provider using the **patient portal**, the images must remain confidential. Patients must sign a release form before the image can be given to others.

Providers can use webcams, microphones, and internet video chat software to see patients who are at a distance from the healthcare facility. The remote diagnosis and treatment of patients using technology is called *telemedicine*.

Webcams and microphones are also used for meetings and continuing education opportunities. Microphones can be used for dictating notes into a patient's health record. Voice recognition software provides instant transcription into the patient's record.

CRITICAL THINKING APPLICATION   **8.3**

Dr. Kahn works with a home health agency. Patients and nurses can communicate with him using the internet, microphones, and webcams. How does this technology benefit the patient?

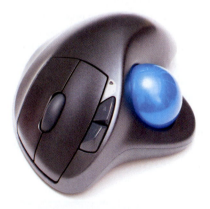

FIGURE 8.3 A trackball mouse uses a large ball to control the movement of the cursor/pointer.

TABLE 8.1	Types of Touchscreens	
TYPE OF TOUCHSCREEN	**DESCRIPTION**	**FOUND IN**
Resistive	Responds to the touch of almost anything that can generate pressure (e.g., finger, plastic stylus, rubber-tip stylus).	Many handheld electronic devices
Capacitive	Responds to the electrical characteristics of a finger. Requires a specialized stylus that has more surface area at the point.	Smart phones and other electrical devices
Surface acoustic wave	Responds to an inaudible wave of sound that is created on the screen from a finger. A stylus with a rubber or soft tip the size of a pencil eraser is required.	Kiosks and ordering screens

Scanner. Scanners in the healthcare setting have become more popular since the use of EHRs has increased. Old medical records are scanned, and the images are uploaded into the patient's EHR. Scanners convert images to digital text through a process called *optical character recognition* (OCR). Scanners available include the following:

- *Handheld scanner:* Used in healthcare to scan identification (ID) bands prior to medication administration and procedures; may also be used for managing the inventory of supplies with the use of bar codes.
- *ID card scanner:* May have other names, including insurance card scanner. Used at the reception desk to scan insurance cards, driver's licenses, etc. Usually information is then saved in the **practice management software** for billing purposes.
- *Sheet-fed scanner:* Also called an *automatic document feeder* (ADF) scanner. Used to scan loose sheets of paper. May be used to scan test result documents to import into the patient's EHR.
- *Flatbed scanner:* Has a glass panel on which the documents are placed for scanning. May also be used to scan test result documents for importing into the EHR.

Signature Pad. In many ambulatory care settings, signature pads are used in the reception area and in the exam rooms (Fig. 8.4). Patients need to sign several documents, including an Authorization for Release of Medical Information, consent forms, and the Notice of Privacy Practices (NPP). Patients sign the signature pad. The signature is then imported into the EHR as part of the patient's permanent health record.

Output Devices

The data entered into the computer are processed by the computer. The processed data are displayed using *output devices*. Common output devices in the healthcare setting include monitors, printers, and speakers.

Monitor. Monitors display the output as images. Images are created by tiny dots called *pixels*. The higher the number of pixels, the sharper the image. The most common monitor is the liquid crystal display (LCD) monitor. These monitors are easier on the eyes. They also use less electricity. LCD monitors are smaller and lighter than older monitors. Some clinics use LCD monitors in the reception area. Patients can read documents on the monitor before signing the signature pad.

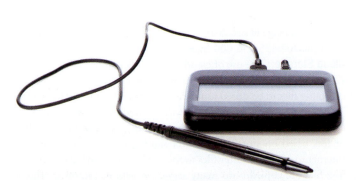

FIGURE 8.4 Signature pads allow patients' signatures to be imported into the electronic health record or practice management software.

Printer. Printers produce the output on paper. Inkjet and laser printers are the two most common types. Inkjet printers create the images by spraying small drops of ink on the paper. Advantages of inkjet printers include their high-quality printing, and they are inexpensive to purchase. Disadvantages when compared to laser printers include the increased frequency of changing the ink cartridges, which gets expensive, and the slower rate of printing.

A laser printer uses a laser, electrical charges, and toner to produce images on paper. Advantages of laser printers over inkjet printers include their high-speed printing, high-quality output, and quality graphics. Laser printers can also support many fonts and font sizes. Toner cartridges are changed less often than inkjet printers. The initial cost of laser printers is more expensive than inkjet printers, which is a disadvantage.

CRITICAL THINKING APPLICATION   8.4

Christiana frequently prints documents, including billing statements, appointment reminders, and receipts for payment. What type of printer might be the most economical to use in the reception area? Why?

Speaker. Speakers for electronic devices come in all shapes and sizes. Typically, speakers are built into the devices used (e.g., monitor, laptop, and tablet). Speakers and sound cards (which will be discussed in a later section) are needed to get sound from the computer.

Internal Components

For desktop personal computers, the internal components are found in the tower or case. Medical assistants would not need to open up the tower or case to problem-solve a computer issue. This may void warranties on the computer equipment. The need to learn about internal components relates more to purchasing hardware and software. Table 8.2 includes some of the internal components that may be of interest when purchasing new hardware or software.

Secondary Storage Devices

Secondary storage devices, or **media**, are capable of permanently storing data. With many types, the user can write over the existing data or delete the data. These devices can be considered removable, internal (such as the hard drive previously discussed), or external. The computer needs a secondary storage device to allow the user to save data. Without a storage device, the computer would be considered a **dumb terminal**. Dumb terminals provide the user access to software, the network, or the internet. They do not allow the user to save data to the hard drive of the computer.

CRITICAL THINKING APPLICATION   8.5

Christiana would like to have a small patient education space in the reception area. She would like to have a computer with internet access for patients so they can access health information. Christiana knows that cost is a factor in a small healthcare facility. The computer would have to be reasonable and reliable. What technology options might she propose to Dr. Kahn?

TABLE 8.2   Internal Components of a Personal Computer

INTERNAL COMPONENT		DESCRIPTION	ROLE
Central processing unit (CPU)		Processor or "brains" of the computer; sits on the motherboard	Interprets and executes commands from the software (program)
Primary memory	Read-only memory (ROM)	Contains read-only memory that has hardwire instructions. Not lost if power is cut, since a small long-life battery supports it.	Used to **boot** a computer
	Cache memory	Provides temporary use of information; contains data and instructions for opened programs	Allows programs to operate more quickly and efficiently
	Random access memory (RAM)	Main working memory; lost if power is turned off	Used for loading and running programs. Without enough RAM, the computer must go to the hard **drive** to read the data, which is a slower process.
Hard drive		"Hard drive," or C drive, of computer; includes the hard disc drive (HDD) and the hard drive as one unit	Reads and writes on the hard disc; provides the largest amount of permanent storage for the computer
Optical drive		Saves data on removable storage devices	Reads or reads and writes (save) data on optical discs (e.g., Blu-ray discs [BDs])
Sound card		Also called *audio card* or *audio adapter*	Allows audio information to be sent to speakers or headphones
Video card		Also called *graphic card* or *video adapter*	Allows the computer to send graphic information to output devices (monitor or projectors)
Universal Serial Bus (USB) port		Most common type of connector device that allows hardware to be plugged into the computer	Allows hardware to connect to the computer

Types of Storage Devices. The computer storage devices are categorized as:

- *Magnetic storage device*: One of the oldest types of storage; uses magnetic technology to read and write data to the device. Examples of magnetic storage devices include the internal hard drive and portable hard drive.
- *Optical storage device (optical disc)*: Uses lasers and lights to read and write data onto optical storage devices. *Recordable only* means that data can only be saved once to the disc (e.g., CD-R disc). *Read/write* (RW) allows data to be saved, rewritten (resaved), and deleted many times (e.g., CD-RW). Examples of optical storage devices include the Blu-ray disc (BD), compact disc (CD), and digital versatile/video disc (DVD).
- *Flash memory device*: Portable device that has become cheaper and has gained larger storage capacity over the years; connects to the USB port in the computer. Examples of flash memory devices include the jump drive (also called the *USB flash, data stick, pen drive, keychain drive, travel drive,* or *thumb drive*), memory card, memory stick, and solid-state disc or drive (SSD).

The capacity of storage devices is also a consideration. The storage capacity is measured in bytes. A *byte* is usually considered a character, such as a number, letter, or symbol. To simplify communication, the storage size is often estimated (Table 8.3). Over the years the capacity of storage devices has increased, and the cost of storage has decreased.

TABLE 8.3   Terms for Data Storage Capacity

SIZE	BYTE EQUIVALENT
1 kilobyte (KB)	1024 bytes
1 megabyte (MB)	1024 KB (about 1 million bytes)
1 gigabyte (GB)	1024 MB (about 1 billion bytes)
1 terabyte (TB)	1024 GB (about 1 trillion bytes)

Flash drives range in size. Some now can hold more than 250 gigabytes (GB), or 268,435,456,000 bytes.

Cloud Storage. The use of cloud storage is becoming more popular. *Cloud storage* is also called *file sharing* or *online storage*. It allows computer files to be stored using the internet and a third-party service. To get started, a person signs up with a cloud storage service. Many companies allow free minimal storage. Others charge monthly fees or fees based on storage size. After signing up, individuals use the internet to send computer files to the service company's **data servers**. The files are copied onto many servers in various locations. This is called *redundancy*. It allows the information to be accessible even if one server goes down and needs repairs.

Cloud systems are gaining in popularity, because they allow any authorized user (e.g., an employee with a password) the ability to access the healthcare facility's computer environment from any location with Web access and through a wired or wireless connection. The access can occur at any time. For instance, a patient calls the healthcare facility's after-hours number and leaves a message with the answering service. No matter the location, the provider on call can use the cloud to access the EHR when talking with the patient.

Network and Internet Access Devices

Most healthcare facilities have their own private network, or **intranet**. The intranet allows the employees to communicate with each other and access shared files. Local intranets are generally secure because only authorized personnel can access the network.

The computers and output devices are usually all connected to the facility's private network. An intranet may only be limited to the *local area network* (LAN). The local area network can span one building or multiple buildings. Some healthcare agencies have multiple locations over a large area. They may use *wide area network* (WAN) technology, which consists of two or more LANs. LAN and WAN technology can use telephone lines or fiberoptic cables that increase the speed of transmission.

A *router* must be used to allow multiple devices to be on the same network. Most routers used today have wireless connectivity. A router is peripheral hardware that looks like a small box. Many routers have antennas and use the **ethernet.** The router allows multiple computers and other devices (e.g., smart devices) to use the same network to send and receive information.

For the **computer network** to have internet access, the ambulatory care facility must do the following:

- Subscribe to an internet service provider (ISP)
- Have its router connected to a **modem**

Most routers have a specific port that is designed to connect to the ethernet port of a cable or digital subscriber line (DSL) modem. DSL is a high-speed internet service. It uses a modem to translate the computer's digital signals into voltage that is then sent over telephone lines.

Usually, healthcare facilities have a separate network for guests that provides free internet. This protects the facility's main network, which stores confidential patient information. Nonemployees should never have access to the facility's main network.

MAINTAINING COMPUTER HARDWARE

Larger facilities usually have their own information technology (IT) department. The IT staff provides technology assistance and helps maintain the equipment. Other facilities will use external IT support companies or train an employee to handle IT issues.

The medical assistant's role involves preventing computer problems and keeping the hardware clean. To prevent computer problems, the hardware should be located on a stable, even surface, away from heat sources. The ventilation slots should be clear, allowing air to flow into the device to cool the components. The medical assistant should ensure the cables and electric cords are securely plugged in. To prevent accidental spills, liquids and food should be kept away from the hardware. The following box discusses routine cleaning for computer hardware.

Routine Cleaning for Computer Hardware

Before cleaning the computer or peripheral components, turn off and unplug the device. Refer to the operator's manual for cleaning instructions:

- If liquids spill on the keyboard, unplug the keyboard. Tip the keyboard upside down to drain out the liquid. Let the keyboard dry overnight. Sticky liquids are more apt to damage the keyboard.
- Use a damp, lint-free cloth to wipe the hardware's casing to remove the grime and dirt.
- Wipe clean all vents and air holes.
- Spray a household glass cleaner on a lint-free cloth, and then wipe the glass monitor screen. Do not spray liquid directly on a component, as the liquid may drip into the device.
- Use a lint-free cloth dampened with water to clean nonglare or antiglare screens.
- Spray a disinfectant on a lint-free cloth or use a disinfectant cloth to disinfect the keyboard.
- Use compressed air dusters (i.e., pressurized air in a can) to blow the dirt out of the keyboard (Fig. 8.5).

When you are working with a disc, handle it with care and hold it by the outer edge or center hole. Keep discs clean and dust free. Use a clean, lint-free cloth to clean a disc. Wipe in a straight line from the center of the disc toward the outer edge. Store them in cases. Keep discs and flash drives out of sunlight and extreme heat or high-humidity environments. To prevent flash drive data loss, unplug the flash drive after it is finished writing or reading data.

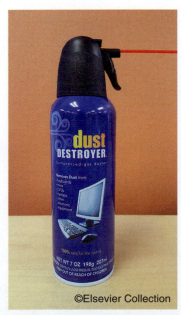
©Elsevier Collection

FIGURE 8.5 Compressed air dusters provide an efficient means of removing the dust and dirt from keyboards.

Infection Control Procedures for Computer Hardware

Many electronic devices are routinely touched by healthcare professionals and patients during the day. One study reported finding several types of harmful bacteria on keyboards. Some types could live for days or months on the keyboard surface. Another study found that keyboards in patient exam rooms were only disinfected 2% of the time, whereas the recommendation was on a daily basis.

Kiosks are being used more often in the reception area for checking in (Fig. 8.6). To help with infection control, some manufacturers are using antimicrobial coatings on kiosks and touchscreens. Some of these coatings kill 99% of all microbes. Clean Touch technology streams a UV-C light across the kiosk's touch surface for 30 seconds after the user steps away. This kills 99.9% of the bacteria and viruses on the kiosk's touch surface. Not all kiosks have infection control features.

It is important for ambulatory care facilities to have procedures for disinfecting technologic devices, including kiosks, keyboards, mice, signature pads, and styluses. Procedures should follow the recommendations from the manufacturers. Usually nonabrasive disinfectant (hospital grade) wipes or specially made wipes (e.g., antibacterial kiosk wipes) are recommended. Some of the infection control practices for technologic devices include:

- Disinfect keyboards daily. Keyboards should also be disinfected when they are contaminated with blood or visibly soiled. Using a disinfectant wipe, clean the surface using friction for 5 seconds.
- Healthcare professionals should wash hands or use hand sanitizer before and after using the keyboard.

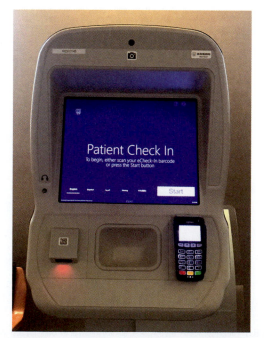

FIGURE 8.6 Many healthcare facilities use kiosks in the reception area.

- Gloves should not be worn during computer use.
- Touchscreen computer monitors and signature pads should be cleaned and disinfected daily per the manufacturer's guidelines. Avoid applying excessive force to screens.
- Plastic covers can be used to enclose keyboards and other devices. These covers should be disinfected daily.

COMPUTER WORKSTATION ERGONOMICS

It is important to arrange the computer workstation correctly to avoid the risk of repetitive stress injuries. Poor posture and straining can cause physical stress and injury to the body. This results in workers' compensation claims for treatment and services. Ergonomics is the field of study that involves reducing strain and injuries by improving the workstation design.

For an ergonomically friendly workstation, the following are important:

- The torso and neck should be vertical and in line.
- The feet need to be flat on the floor or on a footrest (Fig. 8.7A).
- The backrest should help support the upper body; the backrest lumbar support area should be fitted to the small of the back (Fig. 8.7B; see Procedure 8.1, p. 172).
- The seat should be the appropriate size and height to accommodate the person's body build so that there is no added pressure on the back of the knees or thighs.
- The armrest should support the forearms with the shoulders in a relaxed position (Fig. 8.7C).
- For standing workstations, the legs, torso, head, and neck should be vertical and in line. One foot can be elevated on a step.
- The monitor should be directly in front of the person with the top of the monitor at or just below eye level.
- Use a document holder so that documents are placed at the same distance and height as the monitor (Fig. 8.7D).
- Use an ergonomic split-key or waved keyboard. Place the keyboard at a height and an angle that allow the wrists to be in a neutral position.
- The work surface and mouse should be at elbow level for typing. Your wrist should be supported by a foam wrist rest (Fig. 8.7E).
- Headsets should be used by those answering frequent phone calls to prevent muscle strain.

Whether you are standing or sitting at a workstation, it is important to change positions every 30 minutes. If you are sitting, adjustments can be made to chairs or backrests. Stretching your fingers, arms, and torso is important. Frequently look away from the computer to a distant object to prevent eyestrain. Stand up and walk around for a few minutes. Preventing repetitive stress injuries is important for all computer users.

PURCHASING COMPUTER HARDWARE

In small ambulatory care facilities, the medical assistant may help the provider with computer hardware purchases. In larger facilities, the IT department purchases and installs computer hardware. If the medical assistant is helping with the purchase, identifying the

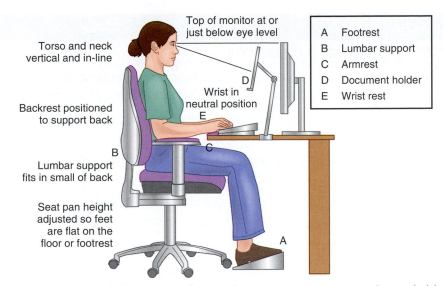

Top of monitor at or just below eye level

Torso and neck vertical and in-line

Backrest positioned to support back

Lumbar support fits in small of back

Seat pan height adjusted so feet are flat on the floor or footrest

Wrist in neutral position

A	Footrest
B	Lumbar support
C	Armrest
D	Document holder
E	Wrist rest

FIGURE 8.7 Medical assistants should use an ergonomically correct workstation to prevent repetitive stress injuries. Equipment that helps create this type of workstation includes a footrest (A), a lumbar support (B), an armrest (C), a document holder (D), and a wrist rest (E).

equipment needed is important. The following box lists possible questions to ask regarding hardware purchases.

Possible Questions to Ask for Hardware Purchases

- For computers:
  - Who will use it? What will be done on the computer? What operating system and other types of application software will be required? Usually, a software indicates the amount of memory required to run it. This needs to be taken into consideration when purchasing a new computer.
  - Does the computer need to be portable or will a desktop work? If a laptop is selected, will a docking station be needed?
  - What size processor is needed? The larger the processer, the quicker the processor will run. What type and size of a hard drive is needed? HDD (hard disc drives) are cheaper and larger, but slower compared to an SSD (solid-state drive).
  - What amount of RAM is needed? RAM keeps the computer working at fast speeds.
- For printers: What will it be used for? How often will it be used?
- For keyboards: Will an ergonomic version be needed? Will the numeric keyboard be needed? Does it need to be wireless?

Installing Hardware

If the medical assistant is installing the computer hardware, it is important to read the directions. If you are connecting cables, make sure they are properly placed and securely plugged in. Many computers will automatically detect the connected hardware and start the installation process. Other times you may be required to load the hardware software using the installation directions.

SOFTWARE USED IN AMBULATORY CARE

For hardware to work, the computer must have software. The terms *software* and *program* are mostly synonymous. Programs existed before software. A program is a sequence of instructions. It is written in a language understood by the computer. It directs the computer to perform a specific task. Software contains several programs that together perform a function. Web browsers, email, games, spreadsheets, and word processors are all types of software.

The two main categories of software are system software and application software. *System software* is a collection of programs that operate and control the computer. The system software loads on the computer. It operates in the background while application software is used. Operating systems and utility software are two types of system software (Table 8.4).

Application software (also called an *application, app,* or *application program*) allows the user or other applications to perform specific tasks. Application software may consist of a single program or a collection of programs. A collection can be called a *software package* or *system*. In the ambulatory care facility, several types of application software are used, including practice management software and electronic health records (see Table 8.4).

Practice Management Software

Practice management software (PMS), sometimes called *medical practice management* (MPM) software, is used to run the day-to-day business side of the ambulatory care facility. This software **interfaces** with the EHR software, and each must work with the other (**interoperability**). Information is passed between the practice management software and the EHR software. For instance, a new patient calls for an appointment. During the scheduling process, the person's information is entered into the practice management software. Certain elements of the person's information then move into the EHR software, creating a new health record, without requiring any additional time or action on the part of a medical assistant.

Practice management software is used for scheduling appointments, new patient registration, billing, coding, and managing finances.

TABLE 8.4 Types of Software

MAIN CATEGORY	TYPES OF SOFTWARE	DESCRIPTION
System software	Operating system	Acts as the computer's software administrator by managing, integrating, and controlling application software and hardware. Windows is an example.
	Utility software	Helps the computer function. Examples include file managers, screensavers, backup software, and clipboard managers.
Application software	Anti-malware software	Used to protect computers against viruses (malware), which damage the computer. An example is AVG AntiVirus Free.
	Database software	Allows the user to work with large amounts of data stored in the program. Examples include Microsoft Access, practice management software systems, and EHR software.
	Desktop publishing software	Used to create flyers and newsletters. An example is Microsoft Publisher.
	Presentation software	Used to create slides and handouts for presentations. Microsoft PowerPoint and Google Slides are examples.
	Spreadsheet software	Used to manage numbers, data, and expenses. Microsoft Excel and Google Sheets are examples.
	Telecommunication software	Used to email patients and vendors. An example is Microsoft Outlook, which is also a personal information manager software. Besides email, it includes a calendar, contact manager, task manager, and so on.
	Word processing software	Used to compose letters and documents. Examples include Microsoft Word, Google Docs, and Corel WordPerfect.

Some of the more useful features of many practice management software programs include:

- *Claim denial management and electronic claim submission*: Insurance **claims** from patient visits and procedures are submitted electronically using the claim submission feature. The claim denial management feature detects if there are errors on the claim before the submission, thus preventing rejections and a loss of **revenue**.
- *Financial and management reporting*: This feature allows for customized reports to be made based on the business activities of the facility. Some of these reports may include the number of patients who **no-show** for appointments or the amount of revenue each provider brought into the business.
- *Scheduler*: This allows for customization of schedules, adding in providers' out of office times and other events. This feature is used to schedule patient appointments and procedures.
- *Medical coding or encoder*: All visits, procedures, and diagnoses need to be coded. Many practice management software programs include coding features that allow the user to easily select diagnostic and procedural codes when processing billing charges.
- *Insurance eligibility verification*: This allows the staff to verify patients' insurance benefits quickly.

Electronic Health Record and Electronic Medical Records

Many people use the terms **electronic medical record (EMR)** and electronic health record (EHR) interchangeably. However, there is a significant difference between these two types of software. When patients' records became electronic (or computerized), they were called *electronic medical records*. The EMR software contains limited

information, usually related to medical treatment for one healthcare facility. The EMR was a digital version of the paper medical record.

The electronic health record has advantages over the EMR. The EHR allows sharing of information with other providers outside the facility, including medical laboratories, nursing homes, hospitals, and specialists. The information from all types of healthcare providers can be stored in the EHR, enhancing functionality and patient care.

Hybrid Health Record

Prior to the introduction of EHRs and EMRs, healthcare facilities had paper medical records. Once a facility moved toward electronic records, the choice had to be made on how to handle the paper records. Some facilities undertook the time and expense to scan all of the patients' paper records and upload the documents into the electronic record. Other facilities decided to keep the paper medical records, scan and upload only certain documents, and add all future patient information to the electronic health record. When facilities use both systems – paper and electronic – they have a *hybrid health record* (HHR).

Working with a hybrid health record requires well-thought-out policies and procedures. Ultimately, it needs to be clear where all records are stored. When records are scanned (*document imaging*) and uploaded, they need to be placed in the correct location in the EHR, and they also must have relevant headings and subheadings. These are critical for providers and other healthcare professionals to find the images of the scanned records.

COMPUTER NETWORK PRIVACY AND SECURITY

Vast quantities of confidential information are stored in computer **files**. Electronic security is becoming more important today. Many healthcare facilities have had their network computer systems compromised by **hackers** and **malware**. Unsecured patient and employee confidential information can lead to identity theft and other criminal actions.

The Health Insurance Portability and Accountability Act (HIPAA) and the Health Information Technology for Economic and Clinical Health Act (HITECH) require privacy, security, and confidentiality of patient records. These acts mandate training and procedures to be used in healthcare facilities to keep electronic records safe. Administrators and employees must work together to keep the computer network safe.

Security Rule

With the anticipated changes in healthcare technology (e.g., the EHR), Congress passed the Health Insurance Portability and Accountability Act of 1996 (HIPAA). (HIPAA is discussed at length in Chapter 4.) Given the increase in **electronic transactions**, HIPAA included provisions for the privacy and security of the patients' information. Primary provisions for privacy and security were stated in two standards:

- *Standard 2 related to the Privacy Rule*: Healthcare facilities, insurance companies, and others need to protect written, electronic, and oral **protected health information (PHI)**.
- *Standard 3 related to the Security Rule*: Healthcare facilities, insurance companies, and others need to protect the patient information that is electronically stored and transmitted.

Of these two standards, the Security Rule will be discussed in more depth in the following sections.

HIPAA's Security Rule addresses the national standards used to protect electronic protected health information (ePHI). This rule covers the records that are created, used, received, and maintained by the covered entities. Administrative, technical, and physical safeguards are important to ensure the security of the ePHI.

Administrative Safeguards

The administrative safeguards include administrative policies, procedures, and actions to manage the security measures to protect ePHI. The facility must identify a *security officer*, an employee who takes on the role to develop and implement policies and procedures that address the Security Rule requirements. The security officer has the responsibility of ensuring the facility's compliance with the HIPAA Security Rule. Besides having a security officer, the facility must have additional administrative safeguards, including:

- *Policies and procedures for assessing and managing risk to ePHI*: The facility must develop, document, and implement policies and procedures and also have a process for periodically reviewing them. Policies and procedures must address all electronic devices and programs that contain ePHI and all users who have access to ePHI. They must also address the review of information system activity (e.g., who is looking at what information).
- **Security risk analysis**: Potential threats to the computer system security are identified, the likelihood of such occurrence is determined, and additional safeguards are implemented. The facility should have a plan of action in place in case a threat occurs.
- *Risk management program to prevent against the impermissible use and disclosure of ePHI*: The facility must protect against unauthorized or inappropriate access to ePHI. Unauthorized

access may include employees and nonemployees. Policies and procedures must include disciplinary measures for unauthorized employee access. These policies and procedures are usually given to employees during orientation, and they may be required to sign a document indicating that they were notified of them.
- *Implementation of employee training*: Employers must provide privacy and security training to new employees. Periodic refresher courses are important for current staff.
- *Execution of business associate agreements*: The healthcare facility (or **covered entity**) must have a signed agreement from a **business associate** regarding security of confidential information before any ePHI can be given.

Physical Safeguards

The physical safeguards include the physical measures, policies, and procedures used to protect the computer network and related buildings and equipment from hazards and unauthorized access. These safeguards include:

- *Security policies and procedures*: The healthcare facility must implement policies and procedures that protect the agency and the equipment from unauthorized physical access, tampering, or theft. The facility should use surveillance cameras and alarms. Computers should have identification numbers and security cables for added protection.
- *Inventory of equipment*: The facility needs to have an inventory of all workstation equipment, portable devices, and medical devices that use, collect, or store ePHI.
- *Workstation security*: These safeguards protect the workstation computer from unauthorized access (Table 8.5). Software such as the EHR allows each user to have an electronic signature, thus indicating what the person entered. When an unauthorized user gets access to a logged-in workstation, information can be looked at or added to the software (e.g., patient health record). Such activity will appear to be done by the logged-in employee, not the unauthorized user.
- *Access restrictions*: The facility must limit what staff members can see on the computer based on job description. Not all staff members have the same access in software programs, such as EHRs and practice management software.

> **CRITICAL THINKING** APPLICATION   8.7
>
> As is the case in many small healthcare facilities without an IT department, Christiana must assume a leadership role with the EHRs. She has administrator rights, which means she can assign different levels of access for the various staff members. In such a small healthcare facility, what other security measures should she consider using to ensure the privacy of EHRs? What resources might she use to implement the security measures identified?

Technical Safeguards

Only authorized employees should have access to ePHI. Technical safeguards include technology and policies and procedures that protect the ePHI and the access to it. These safeguards include:

- *Encryption*: Software used to encode or change the information into nonreadable or *encrypted data* (also called *cipher text*), thus preventing unauthorized users from reading the information.

An authorized user must enter a password for **decryption** to occur and make the text readable again.

- *Data backup*: Depending on the size of the facility, the network may be backed up once to several times a day. *Backing up* is a process in which the network files are copied either using an external hard drive, a server, or an online backup system. To protect the data from a disaster in the medical facility, it is important to store the backup files offsite. When computer data are compromised, either by errors, natural causes (e.g., floods, storm damage), or human causes (e.g., fires, hackers, and malware), the data can be restored using the offsite backup copy.

- *Cloud backup services:* Many healthcare facilities contract with cloud backup services, which copy the network data on a routine basis to protect against data loss. Cloud backup services are like cloud storage services in regard to the access of the data anytime and anywhere. Backup companies do not typically provide file sharing services. When computer data are compromised, either by errors, natural causes (e.g., floods, storm damage), or human causes (e.g., fires, hackers, and malware), the data can be restored using the backup copy.

Additional technical safeguards are listed in Table 8.6.

All facilities that are using EHRs and/or practice management software need to have **downtime** policies and procedures with related supplies available. When the network or a specific software is not available for use, the facility still needs to function. When the network or software is usable, then all the patient information collected during the downtime period must be entered into the system.

TABLE 8.5   Workstation Security

PHYSICAL SAFEGUARD	DESCRIPTION
Passwords	Each user should have a strong password, which has more than eight characters and uses a random combination of uppercase and lowercase letters, numbers, and symbols. Frequently change the password and use different passwords for different software. Do not share passwords.
Privacy filters	Use over monitors to prevent others from seeing the information.
Log-out procedures	Users need to log out of the network when leaving a workstation. A logged-in unsupervised workstation allows others to view confidential information. It can also allow individuals to document in an EHR using your electronic signature.

CRITICAL THINKING APPLICATION   **8.8**

Some healthcare facilities store network backup copies in fireproof safes onsite. Why is it important to store the backup copy offsite? What would be the advantage of using a data backup internet service that has several data storage locations around the country?

CONTINUAL TECHNOLOGIC ADVANCES IN HEALTHCARE

Patients are seeing more technology in healthcare settings today. Receptionists are wearing Bluetooth headsets. These headsets allow them to be more mobile when answering phone calls (Fig. 8.8). Bluetooth is a short-range wireless communication technology. It uses short-wave radio frequencies to interconnect wireless electronic devices such as phones and headsets.

TABLE 8.6   Additional Technical Safeguards

TECHNICAL SAFEGUARDS	DESCRIPTION
Audit trail	Record of computer activity used to monitor users' actions within software, including additions, deletions, and viewing of electronic records.
Authentication	Each employee with network access must log in using a unique password. The security officer should be able to see the employee's activity in the network and individual software.
Automatic log-off	After a period of inactivity, the workstation logs off.
Firewall	A program or hardware device that acts as a barrier or filter between the network and the internet. Data coming from the internet must pass through the firewall. Data that do not meet the firewall criteria are not allowed into the network.
Monitoring of log-in activity	Multiple incorrect log-in attempts are flagged, and many times the account is locked. Prevents hackers from cracking passwords.
Unique user identification	Each employee is assigned a unique name or number for identifying and tracking user identity. This allows the security officer to see the individual's activity on the system.
Virus protection software	Also called *antivirus* or *anti-malware software;* used to detect and remove malware. Examples include Norton and AVG Anti-Virus.

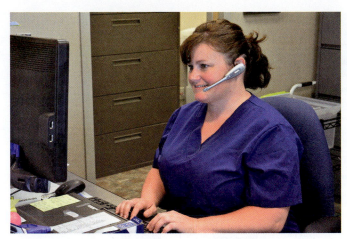

FIGURE 8.8 Bluetooth headsets are helpful for receptionists and other healthcare employees who frequently answer or make phone calls.

For HIPAA compliance, sign-in sheets are being replaced by sign-in kiosks. Some facilities have patients enter health information using the kiosk or a tablet computer. Some clinics use a camera to take the patient's picture for identification. The health information and the photo are then added to the EHR. Receptionists have card readers to use for collecting payment from patients using credit or debit cards. The card reader machines can be mounted on the computer monitor or are stand-alone units. Many have a printer feature that allows the receptionist to present the patient with a paper receipt.

Many healthcare facilities provide patients with wristbands that have bar code technology. This practice started in the hospital and is now moving into the ambulatory care setting. The wristband is scanned before diagnostic tests are done or medications are administered. This scanning process creates an automatic entry in the patient's EHR. This process is another step in ensuring the patient's safety and accuracy in billing.

Ambulatory surgery centers and walk-in clinics use patient tracking systems in both the reception area and the patient care area. Patients sign in or are signed into the system. Their names go into the queue. For confidentiality purposes, patients may be given a unique number. As patients move from one area of the facility to another, their progress shows on monitors in the reception area. This keeps family members informed of their progress. Patients awaiting appointments or laboratory services can see their number move up in the queue or can observe current wait times. These tracking systems provide cost-effective ways to promote patient satisfaction while improving flow and efficiency.

Many healthcare facilities are using biometrics to log into the network. There are many types of biometrics used, including facial or voice recognition, a palm vein, or a fingerprint. Biometric data is unique and is used to provide additional security to the network.

In the exam room, healthcare workers are using more technology to provide better patient care. Some clinics use wireless mobile workstations, called **computers on wheels (COWs)** or workstations on wheels (WOWs). Providers and medical assistants use tablets, smart devices, and wearable computing devices to access EHRs and online resources. **Point-of-care** tools and apps are available for providers to use in the exam room with the patients. This technology gives providers the latest clinical information. Apps are available to provide

patients with visuals of surgical procedures, disease processes, and anatomic structures.

Wearable computing devices allow healthcare employees to access medical records and information while moving around and providing patient care. Mobile devices and apps help providers to make quicker decisions with a lower rate of error and improved patient care outcomes. With advances in Bluetooth smart technology, more medical equipment can work with apps on smart devices.

Because it uses diagnostic imaging to provide detailed information on internal structures, three-dimensional (3D) printing has become popular in healthcare. Implants, medical devices, and prosthetics can be customized for a patient instead of using a generic model. Surgeons use 3D printing to help with virtual surgical planning. Magnetic resonance imaging (MRI) and computed tomography (CT) create detailed pictures of internal structures. An exact replica of the person's internal structures is created using 3D printing. The replica is used as the surgeons rehearse complicated surgical procedures prior to surgery.

With advancements in EHR software and practice management software, new features and programs are being used. **E-prescribing** allows providers to send prescriptions to the pharmacy electronically (Fig. 8.9). With voice-recognition software, providers can dictate notes directly into the patient's EHR. Computerized provider/physician order entry (CPOE) software allows orders for medical laboratory tests, diagnostic tests, and medications to be entered into the computer. In many healthcare facilities, licensed healthcare providers and credentialed medical assistants use CPOE. This improves the efficiency of ordering tests and medications. Some healthcare agencies hire medical scribes. A *medical scribe* enters patient data into the EHR while the provider examines and treats the patient.

Over the years, mobile testing devices (e.g., blood glucose monitor, blood pressure monitor) have been developed to save patient results. At an appointment, the test results are then transferred into the patient's electronic health record. New technology is allowing for *remote patient monitoring* (RPM), a type of **telehealth**. With RPM, a patient performs a routine test at home and sends the test results to the healthcare provider in real-time, instead of waiting for an appointment. Other examples of telehealth include:

- *Live (synchronous) videoconference:* An audiovisual conference between the patient and the healthcare provider
- *Store-and-forward (asynchronous) videoconference:* The patient transmits a recorded health history to the healthcare provider
- *Mobile health (mHealth):* The patient receives general education information, targeted texts, and information on disease outbreaks from the healthcare provider.

With all the advances in technology, medical assistants need to remain flexible and willing to adapt to technologic changes in the workplace. Medical assistants must also ensure the privacy and confidentiality of patients' records and information.

CRITICAL THINKING APPLICATION 8.9

Christiana had considered applying for a medical scribe position at a local healthcare facility before she was promoted to lead administrative medical assistant. Why would a strong background in EHR be important for a medical scribe position?

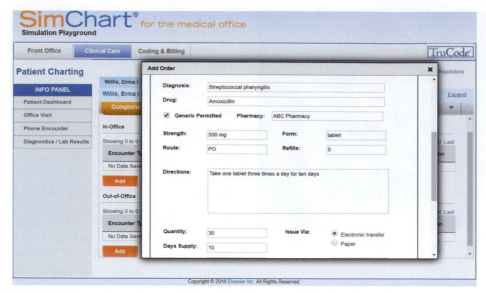

FIGURE 8.9 With e-prescribing, providers can enter the prescription information into the EHR and send it to the pharmacy. The pharmacist can easily read the information, which reduces the chance of errors.

CLOSING COMMENTS

Patient Coaching

Often, medical assistants need to research health-related topics for patients. The internet has many sites that offer information. The medical assistant must only use websites that are reliable and respected (Table 8.7). The following points should be considered when identifying reliable health websites:

- Government websites (.gov) and educational institution websites (.edu) can be trusted.
- Large, respected healthcare and educational agencies (e.g., Mayo Clinic, Cleveland Clinic, Johns Hopkins) usually have many reliable health-related resources.
- Wikipedia is not reliable.

If you are reviewing .com or .org websites, evaluate for bias and accuracy (see Procedure 8.2, p. 172). Research the site by identifying these factors:

- What is the mission or purpose of the website? Who supports or runs the website? Is advertising present on the website pages?
- Is the information current or less than 3 years old?
- What is the source of the information? Who is the author of the content? Does a panel of healthcare experts (doctors, nurses, etc.) review the content?
- Do you need to provide your personal information to view the pages? If so, what will the site do with your personal information?

When the medical assistant finds information, it is important to verify the content with the provider before using the materials to coach patients. The medical assistant may also be asked by patients for reputable sites for health education literature. Having a list of reputable websites for commonly seen conditions may be a timesaver for the medical assistant.

Legal and Ethical Issues

With the electronic health record, it is easy to view one's own health record and that of family and friends. Most healthcare facilities do not allow employees to view their own health records. Viewing family and friends' health records without a job-related reason is a breach of confidentiality. Audit trails can be done to identify what records a person views and who views a specific patient's record. Many examples can be found in which high-profile individuals were victims of confidentiality breaches. Regardless of their position, employees have been suspended for viewing records without job-related reasons. It is important for medical assistants to remember that others can view their activities in the EHR, and the consequences of breaches can include jail time, fines, and loss of a job.

Patient-Centered Care

One of the features of patient-centered care is coordination and integration of care. It is essential for healthcare facilities to have downtime procedures and policies when the EHR is not functioning. Most of the time, EHR system upgrades and maintenance occur when outside of the normal ambulatory care hours. Unexpected downtimes during times patients are seen can create chaos if policy, procedures, and supplies are unavailable. With the EHR and PMS being used for accessing lab results, prior patient information, scheduling appointments, billing, and prescriptions, everyday tasks cannot be done.

With EHR unavailability, errors can occur, including duplicate or missed testing, duplicated or missed medications, and so on. With patient safety being most critical, the Safety Assurance Factors for

TABLE 8.7   Patient Education Websites

ORGANIZATION	WEBSITE	DESCRIPTION
National Institutes of Health (NIH)	www.nih.gov/health-information	Provides information on diseases, including causes, symptoms, and treatments. Also contains Spanish-language materials.
American Diabetes Association	www.diabetes.org/ www.diabetesfoodhub.org/	Provides information on diabetes, living with diabetes, food, and fitness. Provides recipes, a meal planner, and other resources.
Mayo Clinic	www.mayoclinic.org/	Provides easy-to-read information on diseases, symptoms, diagnostic tests, and treatments.
Centers for Disease Control and Prevention (CDC)	www.cdc.gov	Provides information on diseases and conditions. It is a great resource for people who are traveling to other countries.
Johns Hopkins Medicine	www.hopkinsmedicine.org/ patient-education/index.html	Provides information on diseases, treatments, and prevention. Also includes additional tools for patients to learn about managing chronic conditions.
Cleveland Clinic	my.clevelandclinic.org/health	Provides information on diseases, treatments, procedures, drugs, supplements, diagnostic tests, videos, and tools for patients.
Drugs.com (information comes from many healthcare sources)	www.drugs.com	Provides information about medications and tools (e.g., pill identifier, symptom checker, and medication record).
MedlinePlus (hosted by NIH and U.S. National Library of Medicine)	medlineplus.gov	Provides information on health topics, medications, and supplements. Also includes health and surgery videos, health check tools, and interactive games. Offers information in more than 40 languages.
Familydoctor.org (hosted by American Academy of Family Physicians)	Familydoctor.org	Contains information on diseases and conditions, drugs, procedures, and devices, along with prevention and wellness.
American Heart Association	www.heart.org	Includes heart disease information, management, and prevention. Also includes a tracking tool for blood pressure, weight, and exercise.
American Cancer Society	www.cancer.org	Provides information on different cancers, treatment, and support.

EHR Resilience (SAFER) guides (*www.healthit.gov*) recommend the following practices for facilities:

- Hardware that runs the EHR should be duplicated, and an electric generator with sufficient fuel should be available to back up the EHR during power outages.
- Paper forms need to be available during downtime to replace key EHR functions.
- Backup must be done.
- Downtime policies and procedures need to include accurate patient identification and continuity of operations with regard to patient safety and critical business operations.
- Training and testing of scenarios of downtime and recovery procedures should be done.

Once the EHR system is available, all the downtime documentation and activities need to be added to the EHR. Policies and procedures must address how this is done in a timely and accurate fashion to prevent any future issues.

Professional Behaviors

When a medical assistant is using computers while interacting with others, it is important to focus on the customer. Often, the customer feels forgotten. The employee's attention seems to be on the computer. Being attentive to our customers is important. Remember that your customers in healthcare can be co-workers, providers, patients and their family members, and vendors. It is critical that you use eye contact and body language that show your customers you are really listening. Body language that indicates listening includes the following:

- Turning your head and upper body toward the speaker
- Leaning forward
- Tilting your head and nodding
- Smiling (if appropriate in the situation)

SUMMARY OF SCENARIO

Christiana has learned a great deal about the healthcare facility's computer network. She is implementing more security measures. She is training staff members to log out of their workstations before leaving the computer. She is also working with a local IT company to increase the network's protection against unauthorized users. She has contracted with an online backup service to protect the network files.

Christiana enjoys her new position and knows that she will need to stay up to date on technologic advances and privacy mandates. She plans to do this by reading online articles and attending continuing education events. She understands that learning is an ongoing process that will help her to become the professional she strives to be.

SUMMARY OF LEARNING OBJECTIVES

1. **Describe types of personal computers used in ambulatory care facilities.**

   Types of personal computers include:
   - Desktop computer: A larger unit designed for use on a desk.
   - Laptop computer: A thin, lightweight, wireless, portable PC with a keyboard; may include a touchscreen panel.
   - Tablet PC: A thin, lightweight, wireless, portable PC that functions with a touchscreen. There are several types of tablet PCs, including slate style, convertible, and hybrid tablets.

2. **Discuss the difference between input and output hardware, list examples of each type of hardware, describe computer storage devices, and list examples for each category of computer storage device. Also, discuss cloud storage.**

   An input device is any peripheral hardware that allows the user to provide data to the computer. Common input devices include keyboards, mice and other pointing devices, touchscreens, webcams, cameras, microphones, scanners, and signature pads.

   The data entered into the computer are processed by the computer. The processed data are displayed using output devices. Common output devices in the healthcare setting include monitors, printers, and speakers.

   The computer storage devices are categorized as:
   - *Magnetic storage device:* One of the oldest types of storage; uses magnetic technology to read and write data to the device. Examples of magnetic storage devices include internal hard drive and portable hard drive.
   - *Optical storage device (optical disc):* Uses lasers and lights to read and write data onto optical storage devices. Examples of optical storage devices include Blu-ray disc (BD), compact disc (CD), and digital versatile/video disc (DVD).
   - *Flash memory device:* Portable device that has become cheaper and has larger storage capacity over the years; connects to the USB port in the computer. Examples of flash memory devices include jump drive, memory card, memory stick, and solid-state disc or drive (SSD).

   Cloud storage is also called *file sharing* or *online storage*. It allows computer files to be stored using the internet and a third-party service.

3. **Describe how to maintain computer hardware and explain infection control procedures with computer hardware.**

   The IT staff, whether internal or external, will provide technology assistance and help maintain the equipment. The medical assistant should help to prevent computer problems and keep the hardware clean, including routinely cleaning computer hardware.

   It is important for ambulatory care facilities to have procedures for disinfecting technology, including kiosks, keyboards, mice, and signature pad stylus. Procedures should follow the recommendations from the manufacturers. Usually nonabrasive disinfectant (hospital grade) wipes or specially made wipes (e.g., antibacterial kiosk wipes) are recommended. Some of the infection control practices for technology include:
   - Disinfect keyboards daily. Keyboards should also be disinfected when they are contaminated with blood or visibly soiled. Using a disinfectant wipe, clean the surface using friction for 5 seconds.
   - Healthcare professionals should wash hands or use hand sanitizer before and after using the keyboard.
   - Gloves should not be worn during computer use.
   - Touchscreen computer monitors and signature pads should be cleaned and disinfected daily per the manufacturer's guidelines. Avoid applying excessive force to screens.
   - Plastic covers can be used to enclose keyboards and other devices. These covers should be disinfected daily.

4. **Identify principles of ergonomics that apply to a computer workstation.**

   To have an ergonomically friendly workstation, the following are important:
   - Torso and neck should be vertical and in line.
   - Feet need to be flat on the floor or on a footrest.
   - The backrest should help support the upper body in the upright position, and the backrest lumbar support area should be fitted to the small of the back.
   - The seat should be the appropriate size and height to accommodate the person, and the armrest should support the forearms with the shoulders in a relaxed position.
   - For standing workstations, legs, torso, head, and neck should be vertical and in line. One foot can be elevated on a step.

- The monitor should be directly in front of the person with the top of the monitor at or just below eye level.
- The work surface and mouse should be at elbow level for typing. Your wrist should be supported by a foam wrist rest.
- Use a headset, document holder, and an ergonomic split-key or waved keyboard.

5. **Identify questions to ask when purchasing hardware.**

There are a variety of questions to ask when purchasing hardware. For example, for computers, it's necessary to know who will be using the computer, what will be done on the computer, and what operating system will be used. For printers, it's important to know what it will be used for and how often it will be used. For keyboards, you need to know if a numeric keyboard is needed, if it needs to be ergonomic, and if it needs to be wireless.

6. **Differentiate between system software and application software and provide examples of each.**

The two main categories of software are system software and application software. System software is a collection of programs that operate and control the computer. The system software loads on the computer. It operates in the background while application software is used. Operating systems and utility software are two types of system software.

Application software allows the user or other applications to perform specific tasks. Application software may consist of a single program or a collection of programs. Examples of application software include anti-malware, database, desktop publishing, presentation, spreadsheet, telecommunication, and word processing.

7. **Differentiate between practice management software, electronic health records, and electronic medical records. Also, discuss hybrid health records.**

Practice management software (PMS), sometimes called *medical practice management* (MPM) software, is used to run the day-to-day business side of the ambulatory care facility. Practice management software is used for scheduling appointments, new patient registration, billing, coding, and managing finances. Some of the more useful features of many types of practice management software include claim denial management and electronic claim submission, financial and management reporting, a scheduler, medical coding or an encoder, and insurance eligibility verification.

When patients' records became electronic (or computerized), they were called *electronic medical records* (EMR). The EMR software contains limited information, usually related to medical treatment for one healthcare facility. The EMR was a digital version of the paper medical record.

The electronic health record (EHR) has advantages over the EMR. The EHR allows sharing of information with other providers outside the facility, including medical laboratories, nursing homes, hospitals, and specialists. The information from all types of healthcare providers can be stored in the EHR, enhancing functionality and patient care.

Hybrid health records result when facilities use both paper and electronic health records. When a practice works with hybrid health records, it is important to have well-thought-out policies and procedures.

8. **Discuss HIPAA's Security Rule safeguards and list examples of each type of safeguard.**

HIPAA's Security Rule addresses the national standards used to protect electronic protected health information (ePHI). This rule covers the records that are created, used, received, and maintained by the covered entities. Administrative, technical, and physical safeguards are important to ensure the security of the ePHI.

The administrative safeguards include administrative policies, procedures, and actions to manage the security measures to protect ePHI. The facility must identify a security officer, who oversees compliance with the Security Rule. Additional administrative safeguards include:

- Policies and procedures for assessing and managing risk to ePHI
- Security risk analysis
- Risk management program to prevent impermissible use and disclosure of ePHI
- Implementation of employee training
- Execution of business associate agreements

The physical safeguards include the physical measures, policies, and procedures used to protect the computer network and related buildings and equipment from hazards and unauthorized access. These safeguards include:

- Security policies and procedures
- Inventory of equipment
- Workstation security, including passwords, privacy filters, and log-out procedures
- Access restrictions

Technical safeguards include technology and policies and procedures that protect the ePHI and access to it. These safeguards include:

- Encryption and data backup
- Audit trails
- Authentication and unique user identification
- Firewalls and virus protection software
- Monitoring of log-in and automatic log-off

9. **Discuss technologic advances in healthcare.**

This chapter addressed the use of technology in the ambulatory care facility, including in the reception and patient care areas. Technologic advances impact administrative and clinical medical assistants, along with providers.

10. **Describe how to identify reliable health websites.**

The following points should be considered when identifying reliable health websites:

- Government websites (.gov) and educational institution websites (.edu) can be trusted.
- Large respected healthcare and educational agencies (e.g., Mayo Clinic, Cleveland Clinic, Johns Hopkins) usually have many reliable, health-related resources.
- Wikipedia is not reliable.

A list of reliable health websites was provided in the chapter. If reviewing .com or .org websites, evaluate for bias and accuracy. Research the site by identifying these factors: the mission or purpose; age of material, source of information, and the need to provide personal information.

PROCEDURE 8.1   Prepare a Workstation

Tasks: Perform infection control procedures and create an ergonomically friendly workstation.

EQUIPMENT and SUPPLIES

- Nonabrasive disinfectant (hospital grade) wipes or specially made wipes for computer hardware or wipes as indicated by the keyboard manufacturer
- Gloves (if required for using wipes)
- User guide for keyboard or facility's infection control procedure for computer hardware
- Desktop computer with adjustable monitor
- Office chair with an adjustable seat, armrest, and backrest
- Footrest (if needed)
- Foam wrist rest
- Document holder (optional)
- Hand sanitizer (optional)

PROCEDURAL STEPS

1. While sitting in the chair, adjust the backrest so it supports the upper body and the lumbar support area fits to the small of the back. Adjust the seat pan height so the feet are flat on the floor or footrest. Adjust the armrest to support the forearms with the shoulders in a relaxed position.
   PURPOSE: The backrest should support the back. The chair height should not add pressure on the back of the knees or thighs, while allowing the feet to be flat on the floor or footrest.

2. Adjust the monitor so it is directly in front of the person and the top of the monitor is at or just below the eye level. If using a document holder, position it so it is at the same distance and height as the monitor.
   PURPOSE: The correct position of the monitor helps to reduce neck muscle discomfort.

3. Place the keyboard at a height and an angle to allow the wrists to be in a neutral position. Position the mouse so it is at elbow level for typing. Support the wrists with a foam wrist rest.
   PURPOSE: Supporting the wrists prevents repetitive stress injuries.

4. While sitting with your torso and neck vertical and in line, identify if everything is positioned correctly and comfortably. Make any adjustments as needed.
   PURPOSE: For ergonomics, the torso and neck need to be vertical and in line. Slouching is not considered ergonomically friendly and can lead to discomfort and potential injuries.

5. Using the keyboard user guide or the facilities infection control procedure for computer hardware, determine the product to use to disinfect the keyboard. Apply gloves if needed. Using a disinfectant wipe, clean the surface using friction for 5 seconds in each area. Discard gloves if worn.
   PURPOSE: Use only the cleaning products recommended by the manufacturer or the facility when cleaning computer hardware.

6. Wash hands or use hand sanitizer before using the keyboard.
   PURPOSE: Hand sanitization is an important step for infection control.

PROCEDURE 8.2   Identify a Reliable Patient Education Website

Tasks: Research a disease or condition and evaluate a patient education website.

EQUIPMENT and SUPPLIES

- Computer with internet access, word processing software, and printer

PROCEDURAL STEPS

1. Select a disease or condition. Using the internet, find a website with information about the disease or condition. Do not use a website listed in this chapter.

2. Identify the mission or purpose of the website, who supports or runs the website, and whether there is advertising present on the page. If advertising is present, is the advertising mixed in with the content or text?
   PURPOSE: Understanding the mission or purpose of the website, along with who runs or supports it, will help identify if the website is reliable.

3. Identify if the information is current or less than 3 years old.
   PURPOSE: Healthcare content changes quickly, and it is important to have current information.

4. Identify the author(s) and the person's background. Does a panel of healthcare experts review the content?
   PURPOSE: The content is more reliable if an expert is the author or if it is reviewed by experts in the field.

5. Identify if a person needs to enter personal information to view pages of the website. If so, what does the website's host do with the personal information?
   PURPOSE: It is important to identify if the host will keep the personal information private or if the information will be sold to other companies.

6. Compose a one-page paper on your findings. Use double line spacing and a 12-point font size. Include the website you used. Discuss if the website is reliable and if the content is updated. Proofread and spell-check your document prior to printing it.
   PURPOSE: Professional documents need to be spell-checked and proofread.

WRITTEN COMMUNICATION

9

SCENARIO

Christiana Zwellen is a certified medical assistant (CMA) at Walden-Martin Family Medical (WMFM) Clinic. She had been working as a clinical medical assistant for 5 years. She helped with diagnostic tests and treatment procedures. Christiana enjoyed providing patient care, but she wanted to use more of the administrative skills she had learned. She is organized and enjoys challenges and technology. When a front office position opened up, Christiana moved into the administrative role. She is now the lead administrative medical assistant. Her role involves answering phones, scheduling appointments, greeting patients, and processing correspondence to patients. She is also responsible for reviewing the clinic's emails. Patients are encouraged to use email to communicate with providers using the patient portal. Christiana has seen an increase in the number of daily emails. She answers those that pertain to appointments. Other emails are forwarded to the providers or their clinical medical assistants. Christiana is excited to continue to learn the administrative role.

While studying this chapter, think about the following questions:
- What are the guidelines for using capitalization and punctuation in business communication?
- How are numbers written in business communication?
- What are the components of a business letter?
- What are the formats for business letters and memorandums?
- Why are templates used for business communication?
- What is the etiquette for professional emails?
- What postal services are used in the ambulatory care facility?

LEARNING OBJECTIVES

1. Recognize elements of fundamental writing skills. Also, explain the guidelines for using capitalization, numbers, and punctuation in business communication.
2. List and describe each component of a professional business letter.
3. Summarize the formats for business letters.
4. Describe the purpose of templates in professional communication.
5. Discuss memorandums and describe the etiquette for professional emails.
6. Describe how to complete a HIPAA compliant fax cover sheet.
7. Describe how to address envelopes and fold business documents for mailing.
8. Describe commonly used postal services in the ambulatory care facility.
9. Explain the medical assistant's role with incoming mail.

VOCABULARY

authorized agent A person who has written documentation that he or she can accept a shipment for another individual.

bonded A term describing employees for whom an employer has obtained a fidelity bond from an insurance company, which will cover losses from any dishonest acts (e.g., embezzlement, theft) committed by those employees.

electronic health record (EHR) An electronic record that conforms to nationally recognized standards and contains health-related information about a specific patient. It can be created, managed, and consulted by authorized clinicians and staff from more than one healthcare organization.

girth The measurement around something; when referring to mail, it is the measurement around the middle of the package that is being shipped.

media (ME de ah) Types of communication (e.g., social media sites); with computers, the term refers to data storage devices.

portrait orientation The most common layout for a printed page; the height of the paper is greater than its width.

practice management software A type of software that allows the user to enter demographic information, schedule appointments, maintain lists of insurance payers, perform billing tasks, and generate reports.

template (TEM plit) A document or file that has a preset format; this is used as a starting point when composing something and saves from recreating it each time it is used.

termination letters Documents sent to patients explaining that the provider is ending the physician-patient relationship and the patient needs to see other providers.

zone A region or geographic area used for shipping.

Communication has changed over the years. Many people have moved from writing letters to sending emails and text messages. Social **media** sites have gained popularity. Many of these changes have affected the ambulatory care environment. Patients use emails and text messages to contact their providers. To help ensure confidentiality, administrators have created tighter network security procedures. Restrictions on employee social media postings have also been added.

Today, medical assistants must be more computer savvy than ever before to meet technologic demands. As discussed in Chapter 8, they must follow procedures to safeguard the privacy and security of patients' records. The need for proper grammar, punctuation, and word use is greater than ever as medical assistants communicate using letters and electronic technology.

FUNDAMENTALS OF WRITTEN COMMUNICATION

Written communication from an ambulatory care facility is a reflection on the provider and the facility. Medical assistants commonly compose emails and letters to patients and vendors. A poorly worded message or incorrect punctuation in a letter or an email gives the reader a negative impression of the sender and thus the clinic. A medical assistant needs to know how to properly write a letter or message to others. It is important that the sentence structure, grammar, spelling, and tone of the message are professional.

Parts of Speech

A *noun* is a word or phrase for a person, place, thing, or idea. A *common noun* names a general group of people, places, things, and ideas (e.g., *desk, office*). A *proper noun* names a specific person, place, or thing (e.g., *Zachary, Boston*). A proper noun should start with a capital letter. A *pronoun* is a word that takes the place of a noun (e.g., *I, he, she, it,* and *they*) and is not capitalized unless it is at the beginning of a sentence.

A *verb* is a word or a phrase that shows action or a state of being (e.g., *talks, walks, is,* and *are*). The *subject* in a sentence is a noun, pronoun, or set of words that performs the verb action. A sentence requires at least one main clause, which contains an independent subject and verb and expresses a complete thought. A *fragment* is a phrase without a main clause and is a major error in writing (Table 9.1). It is important to make sure the subject and verb agree. A singular subject (e.g., *provider, patient*) must be matched with a singular verb (e.g., *is, reads, goes*). A plural subject (e.g., *providers, patients*) must be paired with a plural verb (e.g., *are, read, go*) (see Table 9.1).

TABLE 9.1	Common Grammatical Errors	
ERROR	**INCORRECT**	**CORRECT**
Fragment or incomplete sentence	*Greeted patients before she updated their information.*	*The receptionist always greeted patients before she updated their information.*
Nonagreement of subject and verb	*The medical assistant talk to the patient.* *The patients is waiting for the doctor.*	*The medical assistant talks to the patient.* *The patients are waiting for the doctor.*

Many sentences also contain the following:

- *Dependent clauses*: Often begin with words such as *although, since, when, because,* and *if.* A dependent clause needs an independent clause (e.g., subject and verb) to be a complete sentence. (Example: The receptionist immediately notified the clinical medical assistant *because the patient felt sick.*)
- *Phrase*: A group of words without a subject or verb. (Example: *A warm exam room* helps keep the patient comfortable during a physical exam.)
- *Adjective*: A word or group of words that describes a noun or pronoun; may come before or after the noun or pronoun it describes. (Example: The *warm* room was full of patients.)
- *Adverb*: A word or group of words that answers how, where, when, or to what extent, thus further describing a verb, adjective, or other adverbs. (Example: The patient spoke *softly*.)
- *Preposition*: A word that indicates a relationship or a location between a noun or pronoun and the rest of the sentence. Commonly used prepositions include *near, beside, about, to, with, by, after,* and *in.* (Example: The student sat *beside* the receptionist.)

CRITICAL THINKING APPLICATION   9.1

Christiana needs to compose a letter. How can she be sure she does not have any incomplete sentences in her letter? What parts of speech are required for a complete sentence?

Appropriate Use of Words

When medical assistants compose professional communications, it is important to use language the reader will understand. Refrain from slang, generational terms, and abbreviations used with electronic communication. These can cause miscommunication with the reader. The medical assistant should know the proper use of commonly confused words and misused phrases (Table 9.2). *Homonyms* (i.e., words that sound alike) and may not be identified by the software's spell-checker, which can lead to mistakes (Table 9.3). Commonly misused words and phrases include:

- Anyway (not *anyways*)
- Supposed to (not *suppose to*)
- Toward (not *towards*)
- Used to (not *use to*)

A common mistake in communication is a mismatch between the noun and pronoun number. When referring to plural nouns, use plural pronouns. Plural pronouns include *we, us, you, they,* and *them*. When referring to singular nouns, use singular pronouns. Singular pronouns include *I, me, you, she, her, he, him,* and *it*. For example, "When the receptionist answers the phone, they need to be polite." The *receptionist* is a singular noun, but *they* is a plural pronoun. The noun and pronoun should agree in number, as in this example: "When receptionists answer the phone, they need to be polite."

To ensure that the message is clear to the reader, make the following adjustments if necessary:

- Refrain from using two negatives in the same sentence.
- Refrain from using vague expressions or overusing the same words within a paragraph.
- Avoid using run-on sentences, which contain several independent clauses together without the required punctuation.

TABLE 9.2 Commonly Confused Words

WORDS	EXAMPLES
As: used in comparisons	She is *as* fast as he is on the keyboard.
Has: to possess, own, or experience	The medical assistant *has* increased his keyboarding speed by using the computer every day.
Lie: to recline or rest on a surface	I *lie* down to sleep.
Lay: to put or place	I *lay* down the book.
Set: to put or place	She *set* the gown on the table for the patient.
Sit: to be seated	*Sit* on the table when you have changed into a gown.
Who: refers to people; he or she did an action	*Who* placed the order for supplies?
Whom: refers to him or her	Mike saw *whom* yesterday?
That: refers to people, things, and groups of people	The letters *that* are on the printer need to be signed.
Which: refers to things or groups	The letters, *which* are on the printer, need to be signed.
Like: means "similar to"	The child is *like* her mother.
As: means "in the same manner" and requires a verb	He works *as* a phlebotomist.
Farther: refers to a measurable distance	The healthcare facility is *farther* away than I thought.
Further: refers to an abstract length	*Further* research is needed before we purchase a new computer.

TABLE 9.3 Meanings of Common Homonyms

HOMONYMS	EXAMPLES
Affect (verb): to influence or transform	The outbreak of influenza will *affect* our patients.
Effect (noun): a result, outcome, consequence, or appearance	The *effect* of influenza was devastating to the city.
Accept (verb): to receive	Will you *accept* this certified letter?
Except (preposition): excluding	She mailed all the envelopes, *except* the certified letter.
Than (conjunction): used to compare	The receptionist was busier *than* the clinical medical assistant.
Then (adverb): tells when	The receptionist finished registering the patient and *then* she scheduled the appointment.
There (adverb): indicates place	*There* were 25 chairs in the reception area.
Their (pronoun): indicates possession	*Their* children remained in the reception area.
They're (contraction): they are	*They're* the only patients in the reception area.
Your (pronoun): indicates possession	*Your* new job is in pediatrics.
You're (contraction): you are	*You're* working in pediatrics today.
To (preposition): indicates direction, action, or condition	She went *to* answer the phone.
Too (adverb): means "also"	The medical assistant's phone was ringing, *too*.
Two (noun): number	Her phone has *two* lines.
Where: to, at, or in what place	*Where* did the patient go?
Were (verb): past tense plural of "be"	*Were* you finished?
Wear (verb): to have something on your body	*Wear* the gown, please.

Proper spelling, use of words, and sentence structure are important because they reflect on the writer and the healthcare facility.

Capitalization

Part of composing written communication is using correct capitalization and punctuation. As mentioned earlier, errors can reflect poorly on the writer and the facility. Professional documents should contain correct capitalization, appropriate punctuation, and the right number format.

The first letter of the first word in a sentence or question should be capitalized. The pronoun "I" is always capitalized. The first letter of proper nouns, including names of people, months, institutions, organizations, countries, and national nouns and adjectives (e.g., *French, British*), should be capitalized. Common nouns (e.g., girls, women, boys, men) should not be capitalized unless the word is the first word of a sentence.

Punctuation

A sentence can end with one of three types of punctuation: a period (.), a question mark (?), or an exclamation point (!). Use a period for a sentence that makes a statement. Use a question mark after a direct question. Use an exclamation point for sentences that express strong emotion. An exclamation point is rarely used in professional written communication. All punctuation goes inside a closing quotation mark (e.g., "Thank you for coming in today.").

Commas are frequently used in written communication. The following are rules regarding comma use:

- Use before a coordinator (*and, but, yet, nor, for, or, so*) that links two main clauses. Do not use a comma before a coordinator that links two names, words, or phrases. (Example: The last patient left, and the receptionist locked the door.)
- Use to separate items in a list of three or more things. (Example: The medical assistant escorted the mother, the father, and the child to the exam room.)
- Use to separate two interchangeable adjectives. (Example: The patient was a strong, healthy child.)
- Use after certain words at the start of a sentence (i.e., *yes, no, hello*). (Example: Yes, the bill was correct.)
- Use to set off the name or title or an expression that interrupts the flow of the sentence. (Examples: Will you, Michaela, want an appointment in two weeks? I am, by the way, very excited about the job opportunity.)
- Use after a dependent clause that starts a sentence. (Example: If you have any questions, let me know.)
- Use to separate the day from the year. (Example: May 24, 20XX)
- Use to separate the city from its state. *(This rule does not apply when addressing envelopes.)* (Example: Madison, Wisconsin)
- Can be used to separate Sr. or Jr. from the person's name, but this is not mandatory. (Example: Bob Smith, Sr., has arrived for his appointment.)
- Use after a degree or title and to enclose the degree or title if it appears in a sentence. (Example: John Williams, MD, will be the speaker for the event.)
- Use to set off nonessential words or phrases. (Examples: Christiana, the newest secretary, has arrived. My brother, Keith, has an appointment to see Dr. Smith.)
- Use with direct quotations. (Example: She stated, "I have waited too long.")

A semicolon (;) is a common punctuation mark used in professional letters and documentation. The semicolon is used before certain words (*however, therefore, for example*). It is also used when separating phrases in a series (e.g., "The provider is running late; however, our first two patients canceled this morning."). A colon (:) is used to introduce a series of items either in the sentence or bulleted list. A colon is also used after the greeting or salutation in a professional letter.

Quotation marks (" ") are used to set off direct quotes. They are used frequently when documenting a patient's chief complaint, the main reason for the patient's visit. An apostrophe (') is used to show

ownership. To show plural possession, the apostrophe is placed after the "s" (e.g., patients').

These are the most common punctuation marks used in professional correspondence and in charting in a patient's health record. Using the correct words and punctuation marks is important when you are composing written correspondence. To reduce the risk of errors, the medical assistant should do the following:

- Perform a spelling and grammar check.
- Proofread the document.
- Double-check the recipient's address.

Many times, the reader develops an impression of the writer, the employer, and the healthcare facility based solely on written correspondence.

Writing Numbers

A few rules apply to writing numbers. Spell out all numbers at the beginning of a sentence. Hyphenate all compound numbers from 21 to 99 (e.g., twenty-three) and all written-out fractions (e.g., two-thirds). For numbers with four or more digits, use commas (e.g., 1,234). It is not advised to include a decimal point or a dollar sign when writing out sums less than a dollar (e.g., 23 cents). Use *noon* and *midnight* instead of 12 p.m. and 12 a.m. The format for a.m. and p.m. can vary.

WRITTEN CORRESPONDENCE

Medical assistants are responsible for communicating with vendors or supply companies. They are also required to send written communication to patients and other providers, as directed by their provider-employers. Knowing how to compose a professional letter is an important skill for medical assistants. To compose a letter, you must know the correct content and location for the parts of the letter. Creating an email requires that the writer follow business etiquette guidelines.

Parts of a Professional Letter

A professional letter uses 8.5 × 11-inch paper or letterhead paper. Letterhead paper is 20- to 24-lb. bond paper (e.g., the thicker the paper, the larger the lb. bond number). The letter typically has 1-inch margins on all four sides, though shorter letters may use larger margins. The entire letter should be written using single line spacing. Consistency in line spacing is important for a professional appearance. The font should be simple and easy to read, such as Times New Roman or Calibri, in a 10- or 12-point size. Limit the use of boldface and italics in the letter.

Sender's Address

The sender's address is usually located in the letterhead (Fig. 9.1). Most facilities use preprinted letterhead paper. Letterhead can also be created at the top of the document using the word processing software's header tool. The letterhead may or may not include the provider's name. It should have the clinic's name, street address or post office box, city, state, and ZIP code. Some letterheads have additional contact information, such as phone numbers, website address, and an email address.

If letterhead is not used for a professional letter, the sender's address is placed at the left margin, 1 inch from the top of the

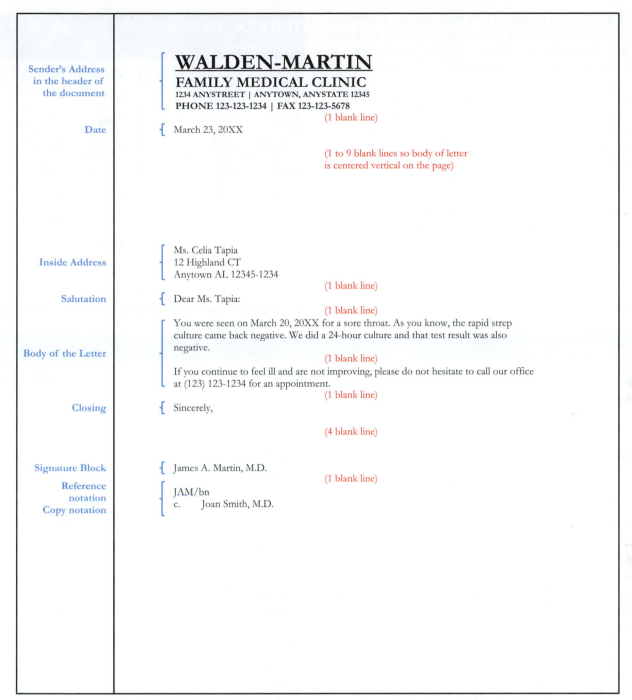

FIGURE 9.1 **Business Letter Format.** When a medical assistant types a letter for a provider, that provider must sign the letter after it has been printed.

document. Use single spacing and include the facility's address. Do not include the sender's name because that is in the closing section of the letter.

Date

All professional letters must include a date. The date is located either at the left or right margin or starts at the center point of the document (see Fig. 9.1). The location depends on the type of letter format used. When using letterhead, the date line starts on the second line after the letterhead. If letterhead is not used, the date line starts on the second line below the sender's address. In either situation, there should

be one blank line between the date and the last line of the letterhead or sender's address.

When keying (typing) the date, write out the name of the month, then the number of the day, followed by a comma and the four-digit year. Make sure to have a blank space between the month and the day and after the comma (e.g., May 14, 20XX). Do not use "th" or "st" after the day (e.g., May 14th, 20XX).

Inside Address

The inside address starts between the second to the tenth line, below the date line. The placement depends on the length of the letter (see

Fig. 9.1). If the body of the letter is long, leave one blank line between the date and the inside address. If the body is short, add up to nine blank lines between the date line and the first line of the inside address. The goal is to have the body of the letter centered vertically on the page.

The inside address is always left justified. It includes the recipient's name and title on the first line. The next lines include the department and healthcare facility name. The last lines include the street address, followed by the city, state, and ZIP code. Always address the letter to a specific person. If the letter relates to a minor, address the letter to the patient's guardian. When writing out the person's name, include the person's personal title (e.g., Miss, Ms., Mrs., Mr., or Dr.). If you are unsure of a woman's title preference, use Ms.

Use the US Postal Service format and abbreviations for the address (Table 9.4). No comma is needed between the city and state. Use the two-letter abbreviations for the states. For all other abbreviations in the address, use only approved abbreviations. For international addresses, key (type) the name of the country in capital letters on the last line.

TABLE 9.4 US Postal Service Standard Street Abbreviations

WORD	ABBREVIATION	WORD	ABBREVIATION
Alley	ALY	Drive	DR
Avenue	AVE	Estate	EST
Boulevard	BLVD	Highway	HWY
Bridge	BRG	Parkway	PKWY
Bypass	BYP	Road	RD
Center	CTR	Route	RTE
Circle	CIR	Street	ST
Court	CT	Terrace	TER
Crossing	XING	Way	WAY

State Abbreviations

STATE	ABBREVIATION	STATE	ABBREVIATION
Alabama	AL	New Jersey	NJ
Alaska	AK	New Mexico	NM
Arizona	AZ	New York	NY
Arkansas	AR	North Carolina	NC
California	CA	North Dakota	ND
Colorado	CO	Ohio	OH
Connecticut	CT	Oklahoma	OK
Delaware	DE	Oregon	OR
Florida	FL	Pennsylvania	PA
Georgia	GA	Rhode Island	RI
Hawaii	HI	South Carolina	SC
Idaho	ID	South Dakota	SD
Illinois	IL	Tennessee	TN
Indiana	IN	Texas	TX
Iowa	IA	Utah	UT
Kansas	KS	Vermont	VT
Kentucky	KY	Virginia	VA
Louisiana	LA	Washington	WA
Maine	ME	West Virginia	WV
Maryland	MD	Wisconsin	WI
Massachusetts	MA	Wyoming	WY
Michigan	MI	**FEDERAL DISTRICT AND**	
Minnesota	MN	**MAJOR TERRITORIES**	**ABBREVIATION**
Mississippi	MS	American Samoa	AS
Missouri	MO	District of Columbia	DC
Montana	MT	Guam	GU
Nebraska	NE	Northern Mariana Islands	MP
Nevada	NV	Puerto Rico	PR
New Hampshire	NH	U.S. Virgin Islands	VI

From: *Two-Letter State and Possession Abbreviations* from USPS.com at https://pe.usps.com/text/pub28/28apb.htm. Accessed January 10, 2019.

Reference Line

The reference line may be used occasionally. It starts on the second line below the inside address at the left margin. The salutation then is placed on the second line below the reference line. The purpose of the reference line is to refer to a specific item, such as a file, case number, or product number. It provides easy reference for the reader and sender (e.g., Reference: Invoice #44549).

Salutation

The salutation is the greeting. It starts on the second line below the inside address. It is always left justified (see Fig. 9.1). For business letters, the salutation should be formal. "Dear" is followed by the person's title and name and then ends with a colon (e.g., Dear Mr. Smith:). Sometime the person's first name may be added (e.g., Dear Mr. Ted Smith:). If the person's gender is not known, use the first and last name without the title (e.g., Dear Chris Smith:). The phrase "To Whom It May Concern" can be used if a person's name is not known.

Subject Line

The subject line is not used very often. The purpose of the subject line is to state the main subject of the letter. It is left justified and placed on the second line below the salutation. The body of the letter starts on the second line below the subject line. The subject line should be composed using boldface, underlining, or all capital letters to draw the reader's attention (SUBJECT: ORDER NO. 45677-93).

Body of the Letter

The body of the letter starts on the second line below the salutation (see Fig. 9.1). The body is single spaced and either left justified or left justified with the first word of each paragraph indented based on the letter format used. There should be one blank line between paragraphs.

The body of the letter contains the content of the letter. The first paragraph is a friendly opening and states the purpose of the letter. The remaining paragraphs support the purpose of the letter and should be concise. The final paragraph may request a specific action.

Closing

The closing is positioned vertically in the same position as the date (see Fig. 9.1). There should be one blank line between the last line of the body of the letter and the closing. The first word should include a capital letter. Remaining words in the closing should be in lowercase. Typically, "Sincerely" is used; more formal closings include "Yours truly" or "Very truly yours." The word or phrase is followed by a comma.

Signature Block

The signature block includes the signature, typed name, and title of the sender. There should be four blank lines between the closing and the typed name and credentials of the sender. This space allows the person to sign the letter. The person's title is capitalized and is located on the line directly below the typed name (e.g., Director of Walden-Martin Family Medical Clinic). If the medical assistant types the letter for a provider, the provider must sign the letter after it has been printed (see Fig. 9.1).

CRITICAL THINKING APPLICATION 9.2

Christiana is composing several letters. Who would sign each of the following letters?
- A letter to a patient indicating her test results
- A letter to a vendor asking for specific pricing for a new computer
- A letter to a referring physician, thanking him for the patient referral

End Notations

Several items may be noted on the letter after the signature block. This may vary among healthcare facilities.

- *Reference notation*: Notes the initials of the person who composed the letter in uppercase followed by the initials of the person who keyed (typed) the letter in lowercase (see Fig. 9.1). A colon (:) or a forward slash (/) divides the two sets of initials (e.g., MR:bn, MR/bn). This notation should be left justified on the second line below the last line of the signature block.
- *Enclosure/attachment notation*: Indicates the number of documents or attachments that accompany the letter. The enclosure notation is left justified. It starts on the second line below the reference notation. If the reference notation is not present, the enclosure notation is placed on the second line below the last line of the signature block. The enclosure notation can be typed in several ways. It can be indicated with either "Enclosure" or "Enc." If more than one enclosure is sent, the number of enclosures or the names of the enclosures should be indicated.
- *Copy notation* (c.): Used to notify the letter's recipient who else received a copy of the letter. The "c" is left justified and goes on the line immediately following the last notation. It is then followed by a period. Use the tab tool to move a half-inch before typing the person's name (e.g., c. John Smith). Additional names should be aligned vertically on the document.
- *Blind copy* (bc.): Used if the sender does not want the recipient to know a copy was sent to another person. The format is the same as it is for "c.," but the "bc." is added only to the office copy of the letter. It is not listed on the letter going to the recipient.

Suggested Styles for an Enclosure Notation

Any of the following three formats can be used to indicate that an enclosure is included with the letter:
Enclosures: 2
Enclosures (2)
Enclosures:
1. Draft of the policy statement
2. Invoice #45433

CRITICAL THINKING APPLICATION 9.3

For the letters that Christiana will sign, should she include a reference notation at the bottom of the letter? Why or why not? For the letters prepared by Christiana and signed by Dr. Walden, should she add the reference notation? Why or why not?

TABLE 9.5	Business Letter Formats
LETTER TYPE	**FORMAT WITH VARIATIONS**
Full block format	• Left justify all elements
Modified block format	• Center point or right justify date, closing, and signature block • Left justify all other elements
Semi-block format (or modified block with indented paragraphs)	• Center point or right justify date, closing, and signature block • Left justify all other elements • Indent all paragraphs 5 spaces
Simplified letter format	• No salutation or closing • Signature comes right after the body, followed by the sender's name in all capital letters • Left justify all elements

Continuation Pages

Letterhead is not used for subsequent pages of a letter. The subsequent pages should be on paper that matches in weight and color. Each sheet after the letterhead must have a heading that includes these elements on separate lines: the recipient's name, the page number, and the date. The name should be on the first line below the top margin, and all three elements should be left justified.

> Ms. Celia Tapia
> Page 2
> March 23, 20XX

Business Letter Formats

Four main formats are used to compose a business letter. The formats vary slightly in the position of certain elements of the letter (Table 9.5). The line spacing between the elements remains the same. It is important for a medical assistant to be able to compose a professional letter.

Full Block Letter Format

The full block format is the most common type of business letter (Fig. 9.2A; see Procedure 9.1, p. 191). All elements are left justified. This means the elements start at the left margin of the document. Typically, for business letters, "closed" punctuation is used. *Closed punctuation* means the document is typed using the punctuation marks described earlier in this chapter. Closed punctuation gives the letter a professional appearance.

Informal full block–formatted letters can use open punctuation. *Open punctuation* means that minimal punctuation is used in the letter. The body is the only part of the letter that contains the normal grammatical punctuation. No punctuation appears in the sender's or inside addresses, date, salutation, and closing. This is a current trend with electronic technology and letters produced by word processing. Open punctuation should not be used with professional letters.

Modified Block Letter Format

The body and the inside address are left justified with the modified block format. If letterhead is not used, the sender's address is also left justified. The date, closing, and the signature block start either at the center point of the document or are right justified (see Procedure 9.2, p. 192). If the center point is used, all three elements must start at that point (see Fig. 9.2B). The text flows toward the right margin. The three elements vertically line up in the document. When you use the right justified technique, the text for these three elements finishes in a vertical line at the right margin.

Semi-Block Letter Format

The semi-block letter format can also be called the modified block with indented paragraphs (see Fig. 9.2C). The semi-block format resembles the modified block format with the three elements (i.e., date, closing, and signature block) right justified or starting at the center point of the document. The difference with the semi-block format is the indented paragraph, or paragraphs, in the body of the letter. The paragraphs should be indented five spaces (see Procedure 9.3, p. 193).

Simplified Letter Format

The simplified letter format is not used as often in healthcare. This format does not use a salutation and closing (see Fig. 9.2D). The signature comes immediately after the body of the letter. The sender's name is keyed in capital letters. With this letter format, the elements are left justified except for the sender's information in the header. The line spacing is the same as in the other formats.

Templates

A **template** is a sample letter or email that can be personalized for each patient. Many word processing and **practice management software** programs have prebuilt letter templates. These templates can be used, or a medical assistant can design a template. For routine communication with patients (e.g., normal laboratory results or appointment reminders), a template can be used to save time composing the entire letter or email each and every time.

Some templates allow the user to merge patient data to customize such things as the address, date of the visit, provider's name, and so on. Practice management software, the **electronic health record (EHR)**, or word processing software can be used to merge the patient's data into the letter template. This creates an individualized letter and is an efficient method of providing a customer-friendly document for a patient.

Memorandums

Memorandums, or memos, are communication documents shared within a healthcare facility. They address one topic and provide a message to the reader. Use the **portrait orientation** for the document, single line spacing, and 1-inch margins. Memorandums typically have four headings:

- **TO**: Include the name of the recipient or recipients and omit the titles (e.g., Mr., Mrs.). With many recipients, each name can be followed by a comma, or each name can be on its own line.
- **FROM**: Include the name of the sender of the memo. It is optional if the sender initials the memo before it is sent.

A

WALDEN-MARTIN
FAMILY MEDICAL CLINIC
1234 ANYSTREET | ANYTOWN, ANYSTATE 12345
PHONE 123-123-1234 | FAX 123-123-5678

August 23, 20XX

Ms. Celia Tapia
12 Highland CT
Anytown AL 12345-1234

Dear Ms. Tapia:

You were seen on August 22, 20XX and had a hepatitis B titer done. Your titer showed that you are immune to hepatitis B.

If you have any questions, please do not hesitate to call our office at (123) 123-1234.

Sincerely,

James A. Martin, M.D.

JAM/cz
c. Joan Smith, M.D.

B

WALDEN-MARTIN
FAMILY MEDICAL CLINIC
1234 ANYSTREET | ANYTOWN, ANYSTATE 12345
PHONE 123-123-1234 | FAX 123-123-5678

August 23, 20XX

Ms. Celia Tapia
12 Highland CT
Anytown AL 12345-1234

Dear Ms. Tapia:

You were seen on August 22, 20XX and had a hepatitis B titer done. Your titer showed that you are immune to hepatitis B.

If you have any questions, please do not hesitate to call our office at (123) 123-1234.

Sincerely,

James A. Martin, M.D.

JAM/cz
c. Joan Smith, M.D.

C

WALDEN-MARTIN
FAMILY MEDICAL CLINIC
1234 ANYSTREET | ANYTOWN, ANYSTATE 12345
PHONE 123-123-1234 | FAX 123-123-5678

August 23, 20XX

Ms. Celia Tapia
12 Highland CT
Anytown AL 12345-1234

Dear Ms. Tapia:

You were seen on August 22, 20XX and had a hepatitis B titer done. Your titer showed that you are immune to hepatitis B.

If you have any questions, please do not hesitate to call our office at (123) 123-1234.

Sincerely,

James A. Martin, M.D.

JAM/cz
c. Joan Smith, M.D.

D

WALDEN-MARTIN
FAMILY MEDICAL CLINIC
1234 ANYSTREET | ANYTOWN, ANYSTATE 12345

August 23, 20XX

ABC Medical Suppliers
545 Supply Ave
Anytown AL 12345-1234

Reference: PO #45938

The packing slip for this order indicated that 2 cases of non-sterile gauze sponges 4"x4", 10 packs (item #1583) were included in the box but were not. The box did contain 2 cases of sterile gauze sponges, though they were not ordered.

Please let me know how you would like to handle this situation. I can be reached at (123) 123-1234.

Thank you.

CHRISTIANA ZWELLEN CMA

FIGURE 9.2 **(A)** Full block letter format. **(B)** Modified block letter format with the three elements starting at the center point of the document. **(C)** Semi-block letter format with the three elements right justified. **(D)** Simplified letter with a reference line.

TO:	Staff
FROM:	James Martin, M.D.
DATE:	December 15, 20XX
SUBJECT:	Holiday Office Hours

The office will be closed at noon on December 24, 20XX through December 26th. We will reopen at our normal time on December 27, 20XX. We will then close at 3 p.m. on December 31st for the holiday and will reopen at our normal time on January 2, 20XX.

FIGURE 9.3 Format for a memorandum.

- **DATE**: Spell out the month and follow it with the day and year (e.g., May 23, 20XX).
- **SUBJECT**: Include the topic of the memo.

The headings are left justified with a blank line between each header (Fig. 9.3). Boldface and capital letters are used for the headings, and a colon (:) follows the heading. The information should be in regular font, with a mix of capital and lowercase letters (see Procedure 9.4, p. 194). The information should be aligned vertically down the page, using the tab tool in the word processing software. The date should be written out as indicated for professional letters.

The headings may be separated from the body of the memo by a centered black line. The line should extend from 2 inches to the entire width of the page. Whether or not the line is used, there should be two or three blank lines separating the headers from the body of the memo. The body of the memo should be single line spaced and left justified. If it consists of multiple paragraphs, skip a single line between paragraphs. The content in the body of the letter should be clear, concise, and informative. The writer does not need to add a closing or signature. Special notations, including reference, copy, and enclosures, can be added to the bottom of the memo. They should be formatted as indicated in the End Notations section.

Professional Emails

The use of electronic communication among ambulatory care center staff and with patients is increasing. Medical assistants need to know how to compose a professional email (see Procedure 9.5, p. 194). Following email etiquette is important for maintaining a customer-friendly environment. Tips on writing customer-friendly emails include the following:

- When sending the email to several people, separate each email address by a semicolon (;).
- Add an email address to the cc line if another person needs to receive a courtesy copy of the email.

- If a copy of the email needs to be sent to another person, without the recipient knowing, add the address to the bc line. Blind copying is used on a selected and limited basis.
- Make sure to include a subject on the subject line. Delete any messy FWD: or RE: RE: strings.
- Start with a greeting (salutation). It should include a formal greeting followed by the person's title and name (e.g., "Good morning, Mr. Jones," "Dear Mr. Jones,").
- Be courteous, polite, and respectful in your words and tone. Maintain the appropriate level of formality in the email. Be gracious, using expressions such as "please" and "thank you."
- Refrain from using all capital letters. Many people consider all capital letters to be "shouting" in emails.
- Write out the entire word, and refrain from using abbreviations and emoticons.
- Use proper capitalization, grammar, sentence structure, and punctuation. Check the spelling in the email before sending it. Most email software has a spell-checker.
- Be concise, accurate, and clear in your message.
- Always end your email with "Thank you" or "Sincerely" and your complete name. For business emails, include contact information after your name. The contact information should include the healthcare facility's address, phone number, and fax number.
- Leave white space (i.e., one blank line) between the salutation, paragraphs, and your complete name.
- Zip large attachments before sending the files. *Zip* is a computer program that compresses a file or folder, making it smaller and easier to send. The receiver uses an unzip program to extract the contents.
- Many email programs have features such as (!) urgent or a response box that sends an email back to the sender when the email is opened by the recipient. Use the urgent feature only for crucial emails.

- Forward messages with caution. When forwarding messages, always read the content and ensure no confidentiality will be breached.

Some healthcare facilities may also include language in emails related to confidentiality and whom to contact if the email was sent to the wrong address. Medical assistants must adhere to the facility's confidentiality rules when communicating with or about patients. Copies of email communications should be uploaded to the patient's EHR for a permanent record of the electronic communication.

EHR software frequently contains clinical messaging or clinical email features. This feature is an email within the EHR. The clinical messaging feature provides secure communication for healthcare employees to converse about the patient. For instance, the message may be sent from the receptionist to the medical assistant regarding a patient who called requesting a refill. The medical assistant can then follow up with the provider regarding the refill.

CRITICAL THINKING APPLICATION   **9.4**

Christiana answers emails from patients. How might her responses differ from her personal emails to her family and friends?

CRITICAL THINKING APPLICATION   **9.5**

Christiana receives an email from a patient that is in all capital letters. How might she perceive the situation with the patient? How could she verify her perceptions? How should she handle this situation?

Faxed Communication

Fax (short for facsimile) machines send and receive documents using the phone lines. In the healthcare facility, the fax machine may be part of a copy machine, or the computers may have software that allows faxes to be sent and received. As communications technology has advanced, the use of fax machines has decreased, but they are still an important piece of equipment in the ambulatory care center.

When sending a fax, the medical assistant must adhere to rules established by the Health Insurance Portability and Accountability Act (HIPAA) and the Health Information Technology for Economic and Clinical Health Act (HITECH). Healthcare facilities usually have a required face sheet (the first sheet) that includes confidentiality language, which instructs the recipient, if he or she is not the intended party, to contact the sender (Fig. 9.4). The sender usually discusses how to destroy the records to maintain confidentiality. Besides the confidentiality statement, the face sheet should include the contact information for the sender and recipient, the date, and the total number of pages (see Procedure 9.6, p. 195).

WALDEN-MARTIN
FAMILY MEDICAL CLINIC
1234 ANYSTREET | ANYTOWN, ANYSTATE 12345
PHONE 123-123-1234 | FAX 123-123-5678

Fax

To: _____   From: _____

Company: _____   Phone: _____

Fax: _____   Date: _____

Phone: _____

Pages: _____

Re: _____

CONFIDENTIAL NOTICE

The material enclosed with this facsimile transmission is confidential and private. The material is the property of the sender and some or all of the information may be protected by the Health Insurance Portability & Accountability Act (HIPAA). This information is intended exclusively for the addressed person or agency indicated above. If you are not the intended individual or entity of this information, you are hereby notified that any use, duplication, circulation, or transmission of the information is strictly prohibited under state and federal law. Please notify the sender immediate using the telephone number indicated above.

FIGURE 9.4 A HIPAA compliant fax cover sheet.

MAIL
Envelopes

Business letters should be enclosed in standard #10 business-sized envelopes. Standard #10 envelopes measure 4.125 × 9.5 inches. Business envelopes are available with a few variations, including the type of flap, preprinted return address, and presence or absence of a window. The window envelope and the #6¾ envelope, which measures 3⅝×6½ inches, may be used for billing statements to patients. The envelopes can be white, manila, or made of recycled paper.

Addressing Envelopes

When the automated mail processing machine at the post office reads the envelope, it reads the bottom line of the recipient's address (i.e., city, state, and ZIP code) before moving up and reading the next line. To ensure timely delivery, use the following tips when addressing mail:

- Key (type) the envelope using a simple black font of at least 10 points in size. Use all capital letters and no punctuation marks (Fig. 9.5).
- Put one space between the city and state and two spaces between the state and ZIP code.
- If you cannot fit the suite or apartment number on the same line as the delivery address, put it on the line above the delivery address, not below it.

- Use ZIP code + 4 code (e.g., 55555-1111) as often as possible. This allows the piece of mail to be directed to a more precise location than when just using the ZIP code.
- Do not put anything (e.g., logo, slogan, attention line) below the last line of the delivery address. The machine will read it, and your letter may be misrouted or delayed.
- Use only approved US Postal Service abbreviations.

Folding Documents

Depending on the envelope size, the folding process may be different. It is important to fold the document neatly, as this is seen by the reader.

When using a #10 envelope, fold the letter by pulling up the bottom end until it reaches just below the inside address or two-thirds of the way up the letter (Fig. 9.6). Crease at the fold. Then, fold the top of the letter down so that it is flush with the bottom fold and crease the paper. For window business envelopes, fold the letter in a Z pattern. With the letter's print side facing up, place the envelope over or under the top third of the letter (Fig. 9.7). Fold the bottom edge of the paper up to the bottom edge of the envelope and crease at the fold. Then, remove the envelope and flip the letter over so the backside of the document is facing up. Fold the top of the letter down to the prior crease line and crease at the fold. The letterhead and recipient's addresses should then be visible. Place the letter in the envelope so that the recipient's address shows through the window.

Return Address
Use same format as the delivery address

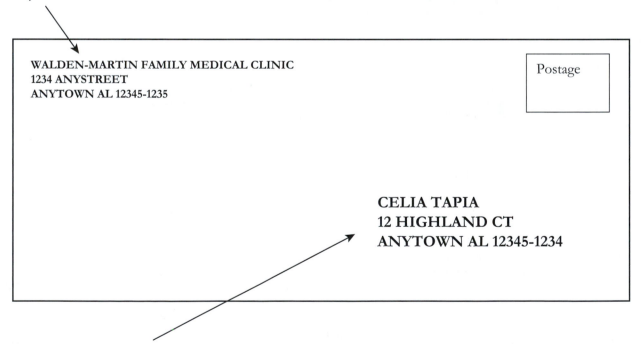

WALDEN-MARTIN FAMILY MEDICAL CLINIC
1234 ANYSTREET
ANYTOWN AL 12345-1235

Postage

CELIA TAPIA
12 HIGHLAND CT
ANYTOWN AL 12345-1234

Delivery Address
1st line: Recipient's name
2nd line: Company name
3rd line: Post Office box or street address, including Apartment or Suite number
4th line: City, State (2 letter abbreviation), ZIP code

FIGURE 9.5 Address format for an envelope.

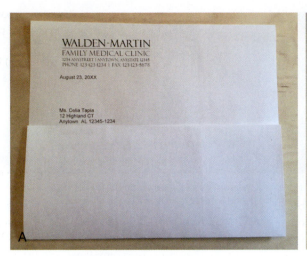

FIGURE 9.6 (A) For a #10 envelope, fold the bottom to just below the inside address and crease at the fold. **(B)** Fold the top edge down to meet the bottom edge and crease at the fold.

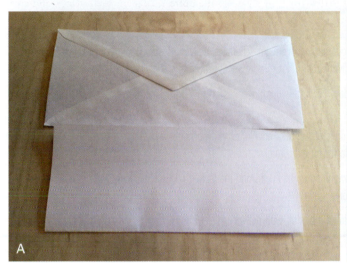

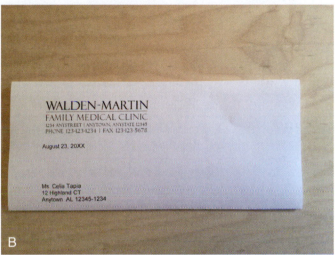

FIGURE 9.7 (A) For a window envelope, with the print side facing up, place the envelope over or under the top third of the letter. Fold the bottom edge up to meet the bottom edge of the envelope. Crease at the fold. **(B)** With the letter print facing down, fold the top down to the first crease line. Crease at the fold. When the letter is folded, the inside address is visible.

When using a #6½ envelope, fold the letter by pulling up the bottom end until it is ½ inch from the top edge of the document (Fig. 9.8). Crease at the fold. Then, fold the document vertically starting at the right edge. Bring the right edge two-thirds of the way across the width of the document and crease the paper. Then bring the left edge to the right edge and crease at the fold. Flip the document so the left edge is on the bottom and insert into the envelope.

Postage

After addressing the envelope, you must add postage prior to mailing the letter. The postage depends on the weight, size, urgency for arrival, delivery **zone**, and services required (Table 9.6). For the ambulatory care facility, there are several postage options for mailings, including:

- *Print postage labels on USPS.com*: Can print Priority Mail Express and Priority Mail shipping labels on the facility's printer.
- *Permit imprints*: For bulk mailing (200 or more envelopes); requires a fee and permit. Print postage information on the envelope and pay for postage when mailing is sent.

TABLE 9.6   US Postal Service Domestic Shipping Sizes

DOMESTIC SHIPPING	HEIGHT (inches)	LENGTH (inches)	MAXIMUM THICKNESS (inches)
Postcard	3.5–4.25	5–6	0.016
Letter	3.5–6.125 (61/8)	5–11.5	0.25
Large envelopes	6.125–12	11.5–15	0.75
Packages	Maximum length plus **girth**: 108 in (130 in for standard post)		

FIGURE 9.8 (A) For a #6¾ envelope, bring the bottom edge of the document to ½ inch from the top edge. Crease at the fold. **(B)** Fold the document vertically. Bring the right edge two-thirds of the way across the width of the document and crease the paper. **(C)** Bring the left edge to the right edge and crease at the fold.

TABLE 9.7	Summary of the US Postal Service's Domestic Services
TYPE	**DESCRIPTION**
Priority mail express	Very expensive; 7-days-a-week delivery service with guaranteed overnight scheduled delivery. Insurance is included. For letters and packages up to 70 lb. Cost based on weight and delivery zone. Flat rate boxes available.
Priority mail	Expensive; delivery within 3 days. Insurance is included. For letters and packages up to 70 lb. Cost based on weight and delivery zone. Flat rate boxes available.
First-class mail	Most commonly used service. Provides delivery in 3 days or less. For envelopes and packages weighing up to 13 oz. Cost based on size, shape, and weight. Add-on services are available for an extra fee.
USPS retail ground	Delivery in 2–8 days. Used for oversized packages weighing up to 70 lb. and measuring up to 130 inches in combined girth and length. Cost based on weight, shape, and delivery zone.
Media mail	Use for sending books, electronic media, and educational material, with delivery in 2–8 days. Cost based on weight.

- *Precanceled stamps*: Complete permit, place precanceled stamps on envelopes and mail. Cannot return unused stamps.
- *Postage meter printing*: Lease a postage meter, pay the fee, and print postage directly on the mail or on a meter tape.

The US Postal Service (USPS) website (*www.usps.com*) provides valuable resources for addressing and shipping mail. It allows you to buy stamps, schedule a pickup, calculate the shipping costs, look up ZIP codes, and track sent mail.

The medical assistant will use different types of mail services for the healthcare facility's business. It is crucial to understand the different services. For routine mail, the healthcare facility will use First-Class Mail. Table 9.7 summarizes the USPS domestic services available.

The USPS also has a host of optional services that can be added to the standard services for an additional fee. Table 9.8 summarizes additional services available. It is important to note that healthcare facilities use certified mail and return receipt. When using certified mail combined with return receipt, the facility gets a mailing receipt showing the date when the item was mailed. It also gets additional information on when the delivery occurred and the

recipient's signature. Many state laws mandate that **termination letters** be sent by certified mail with return receipt (Fig. 9.9A). The mailing receipt, the return receipt, and a copy of the letter are uploaded into the EHR or filed in the paper medical record (Fig. 9.9B). These items provide proof the law was followed if there is ever a question. For a complete list of services, refer to the USPS website.

Private Delivery Services

The USPS only handles a portion of the mail delivered in the United States. Private companies have grown by offering competitive rates and additional services compared with USPS. Some companies provide national and international services, but others are more locally based. FedEx, UPS, and DHL are very popular national options for shipping letters and packages. Some offer onsite pickup.

Larger cities have courier services that have become popular options for local deliveries. Some companies have drivers who are **bonded** and trained to handle all aspects of delivery from medical to hazardous deliveries. Some of the services provided include the following:

TABLE 9.8   Optional Services Provided by the US Postal Service

OPTIONAL SERVICE	DESCRIPTION
Standard insurance	Protects against loss or damage. Cost is based on the item's declared value.
Registered mail	Used to protect expensive items. Mailed item can be insured up to the maximum amount. A mailing receipt is given; upon request, an electronic verification of delivery or delivery attempt can be sent.
Certified mail	Mailing receipt provides evidence the letter was mailed and combined with the return receipt shows delivery information and the recipient's signature.
Signature confirmation	Provides date and time of delivery or when delivery attempt was made, along with the recipient's signature. Copy of delivery record is available upon request.
Return receipt	Provides an automatic electronic or mailed delivery record showing the recipient's signature.
Adult signature restricted delivery	Addressee or **authorized agent** must verify identity and age (i.e., must be over 21); must sign for delivery.
Restricted delivery	Addressee or authorized agent must verify identity and must sign for delivery.
Certificate of mailing	Provides evidence (i.e., date and time) when an item was mailed. (Limited service because it does not provide evidence of the delivery.)
US Postal Service tracking	Provides updates as an item is being shipped. Will include date and time of delivery or attempted delivery.
Special handling	Used to get preferential handling when shipping very unusual items or items that need extra care.
Collect on delivery (COD)	Recipient pays for merchandise and shipping when the package is received.
Hold for pickup	Option to pick up item from a specified post office within 15 days, depending on service selected.

- Pickup and delivery of medical specimens (e.g., they take patient laboratory samples to a medical laboratory for testing).
- Transportation of health records and documents from one location to another, complying with HIPAA requirements.
- Pickup and delivery of deposits to the bank, with return of cash if requested.

The goal for the healthcare facility is to use a mail/courier company that provides the most efficient service at the best price. The medical assistant may have to research the delivery services available in the area to identify the best fit for the facility.

CRITICAL THINKING APPLICATION   9.6

The providers would like to use an offsite laboratory to process specimens. Christiana would like to have a local courier service pick up specimens and deliver them to the offsite laboratory. When researching potential delivery couriers for this activity, what factors should Christiana consider?

Incoming Mail

The medical assistant's responsibility with incoming mail will vary. In large facilities, designated mailroom employees handle incoming mail and the mail is delivered to each department. The administrative medical assistant sorts the department mail. In smaller facilities, the medical assistant handles all aspects of the incoming mail.

Mail can be collected at the post office or be delivered to the healthcare facility. The medical assistant must sort the mail following the facility's procedure for incoming mail. Providers may request the incoming mail be placed on their desks. In larger departments, mailboxes are used for each person in the department (Fig. 9.10). The medical assistant can easily sort the mail and place it in the individual mailboxes. The mailboxes need to be safe and secure. They should not be in a patient care area.

If there is a question as to who should get a piece of mail, it is important to ask. If there is a question about opening something, it is better to not open it and ask the provider or office manager. If mail is accidentally opened that should not have been, the medical assistant should tape the envelope shut. A note should be included with the envelope to indicate that it was accidentally opened. The note should include the person's name who opened it and the date. The facility will have a procedure for handling the mail while the provider is on vacation.

CRITICAL THINKING APPLICATION   9.7

Christiana sorts the mail for the healthcare facility. Because the facility is small, the staff does not use the mailbox system. Mail has gotten lost after she placed it on the providers' desks. What other options can Christiana implement to prevent mail from getting lost or misplaced on the providers' desks?

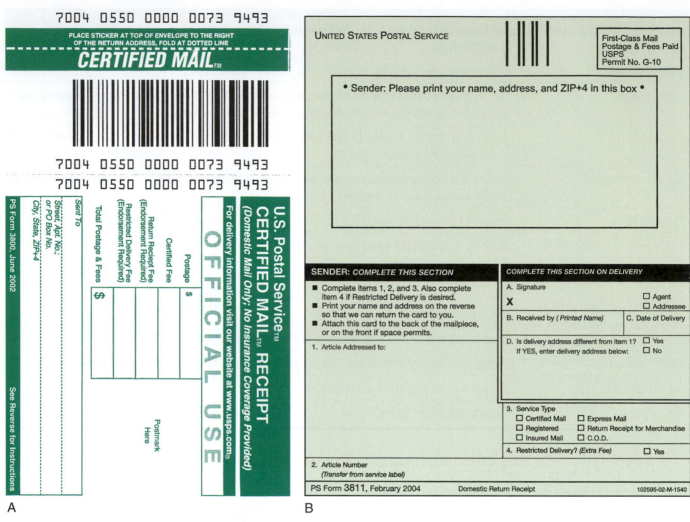

7004 0550 0000 0073 9493

**PLACE STICKER AT TOP OF ENVELOPE TO THE RIGHT
OF THE RETURN ADDRESS, FOLD AT DOTTED LINE**

CERTIFIED MAIL™

7004 0550 0000 0073 9493

7004 0550 0000 0073 9493

OFFICIAL USE

U.S. Postal Service™
CERTIFIED MAIL™ RECEIPT
(Domestic Mail Only; No Insurance Coverage Provided)

For delivery information visit our website at www.usps.com®

Postage $

Certified Fee

Return Reciept Fee
(Endorsement Required)

Restricted Delivery Fee
(Endorsement Required)

Total Postage & Fees $

Postmark
Here

Sent To

Street, Apt. No.;
or PO Box No.

City, State, ZIP+4

PS Form 3800, June 2002   See Reverse for Instructions

UNITED STATES POSTAL SERVICE

First-Class Mail
Postage & Fees Paid
USPS
Permit No. G-10

• Sender: Please print your name, address, and ZIP+4 in this box •

SENDER: *COMPLETE THIS SECTION*

■ Complete items 1, 2, and 3. Also complete item 4 if Restricted Delivery is desired.
■ Print your name and address on the reverse so that we can return the card to you.
■ Attach this card to the back of the mailpiece, or on the front if space permits.

1. Article Addressed to:

COMPLETE THIS SECTION ON DELIVERY

A. Signature
X
☐ Agent
☐ Addressee

B. Received by (*Printed Name*)   C. Date of Delivery

D. Is delivery address different from item 1?   ☐ Yes
If YES, enter delivery address below: ☐ No

3. Service Type
☐ Certified Mail   ☐ Express Mail
☐ Registered   ☐ Return Receipt for Merchandise
☐ Insured Mail   ☐ C.O.D.

4. Restricted Delivery? *(Extra Fee)*   ☐ Yes

2. Article Number
(Transfer from service label)

PS Form 3811, February 2004   Domestic Return Receipt   102595-02-M-1540

A   B

FIGURE 9.9 (A) Receipt for certified mail. Attach the bottom portion of the receipt to the top of the package or envelope, just to the right of the return address. **(B)** Return receipt used to provide an automatic electronic or hardcopy record showing the recipient's signature.

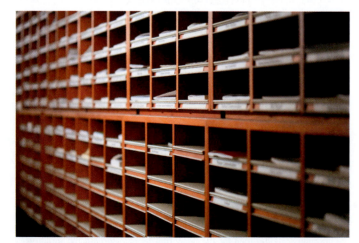

FIGURE 9.10 Mailboxes offer an efficient way to sort and store mail for individuals in the department. (Photo copyright calion/iStock/Thinkstock.)

CLOSING COMMENTS

Legal and Ethical Issues

When sending letters and emails to patients, the medical assistant must ensure that a copy is added to the patient's health record. If a copy is not added to the record, then it appears that the patient was never sent a letter or an email. Legally this can be a major issue for the healthcare facility. Having a "paper trail" of communication to the patient helps to provide evidence that the staff notified the patient about test results and updates in the patient care plan.

Patient-Centered Care

When patients are having a diagnostic test, it is important to let the patient know prior to the test when he or she will be given the results. It is also helpful to patients to let them know if the communication will be via a phone call, an email, or a letter. When a patient is waiting for a potentially life-changing diagnosis, waiting for the news is stressful. The medical assistant should help to ensure that test results are given to the patient as soon as possible and in the manner the patient was told they would be (e.g., via an email or a call).

Professional Behaviors

When communicating by email, it is important to watch one's tone. Sharp phrases or capitalizing complete words can give the reader a sense that the sender was yelling. The medical assistant should:

- Always maintain a professional tone throughout the letter or email even if the patient was not.
- Have another staff member read an email if the medical assistant is concerned that the message may be perceived in a manner other than what is intended.
- Never send an email response when not in the office or angry. Wait until the emotions have calmed down before sending an email. Often it is hard to be professional when one is so emotional.

SUMMARY OF SCENARIO

Since her promotion, Christiana has learned many helpful administrative procedures. She has also been implementing changes in the administrative area. Her first change was to email, rather than mail, appointment reminders. She uses the appointment reminder feature of the practice management software when emailing the notifications to patients. Not only does this save time, but it also saves postage costs. Christiana has also learned how to create letter and memo templates. She uses templates to notify patients about laboratory and diagnostic test results. She continues to create custom letters for patients, yet she saves time by using predesigned templates. Christiana enjoys her new position, and she understands that learning is an ongoing process that will help her to become the professional she strives to be.

SUMMARY OF LEARNING OBJECTIVES

1. **Recognize elements of fundamental writing skills. Also, explain the guidelines for using capitalization, numbers, and punctuation in business communication.**

   This chapter reviewed the parts of speech, including a noun, verb, subject, adjective, adverb, and so on. It is important to write using complete sentences and not fragments. The medical assistant should know the proper use of commonly confused words and misused phrases.

   Part of composing written communication is using correct capitalization and punctuation. Proper nouns, "I," and the first letter of the first word of a sentence or question need to be capitalized. The chapter content also discussed the correct uses for punctuation. Lastly, the medical assistant should remember the rules of writing numbers, including hyphenating all compound numbers from 21 to 99 and spelling out all numbers at the beginning of a sentence.

2. **List and describe each component of a professional business letter.**

   The following are components of the professional business letter:
   - *Sender's address*: Is usually in the letterhead of the document.
   - *Date*: Needs to be written out using the month, day, and year format.
   - *Inside address*: Includes the recipient's name, title, and address.
   - *Reference line*: Used occasionally to refer to a specific item (e.g., case number).
   - *Salutation*: The greeting needs to be formal for business letters.
   - *Subject line*: Used occasionally to state the main subject of the letter.
   - *Body of the letter*: Contains the message.

   - *Closing*: Usually, "sincerely" is used.
   - *Signature block*: Provides information on the sender, including the signature, typed name, and title.
   - *End notations* include:
     - *Reference notation*: The initials of the sender are followed by the initials of the person who keyed the letter. A colon or forward slash separates the initials.
     - *Enclosure/attachment notation*: Indicates the number of the documents or attachments that accompany the letter.
     - *Copy notation*: Indicates who received a copy of the letter.
     - *Blind copy*: Indicates who received a blind copy of the letter; only shows on the office copy of the letter.

3. **Summarize the formats for business letters.**
   - *Full block format*: Left justify all elements
   - *Modified block format*: Center point or right justify date closing, and signature block; left justify all other elements
   - *Semi-block format*: Center point or right justify date closing, and signature block; left justify all other elements; and indent all paragraphs 5 spaces.
   - *Simplified format*: Does not use the salutation and closing. The sender's name is in all capital letters.
   - *Memorandum* (memo): Includes "TO," "FROM," "DATE," and "SUBJECT" in the header, and the body is below the header.

Continued

SUMMARY OF LEARNING OBJECTIVES—*continued*

4. **Describe the purpose of templates in professional communication.**

   A template is a sample letter or email that can be personalized for each patient. For routine communication with patients (e.g., normal laboratory results or appointment reminders), a template can be used to save time composing the entire letter or email each and every time.

5. **Discuss memorandums and describe the etiquette for professional emails.**

   Memorandums, or memos, are communication documents shared within a healthcare facility. They address one topic and provide a message to the reader. They typically have four headings: to, from, date, and subject.

   Tips on writing customer-friendly emails include the following:
   - Make sure to include a subject on the subject line. Delete any messy FWD: or RE: RE: strings.
   - Start with a greeting (salutation). It should include a formal greeting followed by the person's title and name (e.g., "Good morning, Mr. Jones," "Dear Mr. Jones,").
   - Be courteous, polite, and respectful in your words and tone. Maintain the appropriate level of formality in the email. Be gracious, using expressions such as "please" and "thank you."
   - Refrain from using all capital letters. Many people consider all capital letters to be "shouting" in emails.
   - Write out the entire word, and refrain from using abbreviations and emoticons.
   - Use proper capitalization, grammar, sentence structure, and punctuation. Check the spelling in the email before sending it. Most email software has a spell-checker.
   - Be concise, accurate, and clear in your message.
   - Always end your email with "Thank you" or "Sincerely" and your complete name. For business emails, include contact information after your name. The contact information should include the healthcare facility's address, phone number, and fax number.
   - Leave white space (i.e., one blank line) between the salutation, paragraphs, and your complete name.
   - Zip large attachments before sending the files. *Zip* is a computer program that compresses a file or folder, making it smaller and easier to send. The receiver uses an unzip program to extract the contents.
   - Many email programs have features such as (!) urgent or a response box that sends an email back to the sender when the email is opened by the recipient. Use the urgent feature only for crucial emails.
   - Forward messages with caution. When forwarding a message, always read the content and ensure no confidentiality will be breached.

6. **Describe how to complete a HIPAA compliant fax cover sheet.**

   When sending a fax, the medical assistant must adhere to HIPAA and HITECH rules. Healthcare facilities usually have a required face sheet (the first sheet) that includes confidentiality language, which instructs the recipient, if he or she is not the intended party, to contact the sender. See Procedure 9.6 for details on completing a HIPAA compliant fax cover sheet.

7. **Describe how to address envelopes and fold business documents for mailing.**

   When addressing an envelope, type the address using a simple black font of at least 10 points in size. Always put one space between the city and state and two spaces between the space and ZIP code. Use only US Postal Service abbreviations.

   Procedures 9.1 through 9.3 discuss how to fold a document when using a #10 envelope. Procedure 9.2 discusses how to fold a letter when using a window envelope. Procedure 9.3 discusses how to fold a letter when using a #$6\frac{3}{4}$ envelope.

8. **Describe commonly used postal services in the ambulatory care facility.**

   The medical assistant will use different types of mail services for the healthcare facility's business. For routine mail, the healthcare facility will use First-Class Mail. Table 9.7 summarizes USPS domestic services available. It is important to note that healthcare facilities use certified mail and return receipt. When using certified mail combined with return receipt, the facility gets a mailing receipt showing the date when the item was mailed. Many state laws mandate that termination letters be sent by certified mail with return receipt.

9. **Explain the medical assistant's role with incoming mail.**

   The medical assistant's responsibility with incoming mail will vary. In large facilities, designated mailroom employees handle incoming mail and the mail is delivered to each department. The administrative medical assistant sorts the department mail. In smaller facilities, the medical assistant handles all aspects of the incoming mail.

PROCEDURE 9.1   Compose a Professional Business Letter Using the Full Block Letter Format

Tasks: Compose a professional letter using technology. Use the full block letter format and closed punctuation. Address the envelope and fold the letter.

Scenario: Jean Burke, NP (nurse practitioner), has requested that you compose a letter to the parent (Lisa Parker) of Johnny Parker (date of birth [DOB]: 06/15/2010) to let her know that Johnny's throat culture from last Wednesday was negative. If he is not improving or if she has any questions, she should call the office. Lisa Parker's address is 91 Poplar Street, Anytown, AL 12345-1234. You are working at Walden-Martin Family Medical Clinic. The healthcare facility's address is 1234 Anystreet, Anytown, AL 12345. The phone number is 123-123-1234 and the fax number is 123-123-5678.

EQUIPMENT and SUPPLIES

- Patient's health record
- Computer with word processing software and printer
- Paper
- #10 envelope

PROCEDURAL STEPS

1. Obtain the intended recipient's contact information and determine the message you want to convey. Using the computer and word processing software, compose the letter using the full block letter format. Use 1-inch margins on all four sides, portrait orientation, and use single line spacing throughout the letter. Use an easy-to-read font (e.g., Times New Roman or Calibri), in a 10- or 12-point size.
   PURPOSE: Determining the message gives you a focus when composing the letter. You will need the recipient's information to create the letter.

2. Create a letterhead in the header of the document. Include the clinic's name, street address or post office box, city, state, and ZIP code.
   PURPOSE: The information in the letterhead provides the reader contact information for the clinic.

3. Key (type) the date starting at the left margin. Have one blank line between the date line and the last line of the letterhead.
   PURPOSE: All letters require a date for legal purposes.

4. Key the inside address starting at the left margin and use the correct spelling and punctuation. Leave one to nine blank lines between the date and the inside address, to center the body of the letter on the page.
   PURPOSE: The body of the letter must be centered vertically from the top to the bottom of the document. More blank lines can be added to move the body to the correct location.

5. Key the salutation starting at the left margin and use the correct spelling and punctuation. Leave one blank line between the inside address and the salutation.
   PURPOSE: A proper greeting sets the tone of the letter.

6. Use your critical thinking skills to compose a concise, accurate message. Type the message in the body of the letter starting at the left margin. Leave one blank line between the salutation and the first line of the body and then between each paragraph of the body. The message should be clear, concise, and professional. Use proper grammar, punctuation, capitalization, and sentence structure.
   PURPOSE: Proper grammar helps to convey the message accurately and professionally.

7. Key a proper closing starting at the left margin and use the correct spelling and punctuation. Leave one blank line between the last line of the body and the closing.
   PURPOSE: The closing helps end the message with a professional tone.

8. Key the signature block starting at the left margin and use the correct spelling and punctuation. Leave four blank lines between the closing and the signature block. If you are preparing the letter for a provider, you must include a reference notation.
   PURPOSE: The signature block provides the reader with the name of the sender of the letter. The reference notation identifies who typed the letter.

9. Spell-check and proofread the document. Check for the proper tone, grammar, punctuation, capitalization, and sentence structure. Check for proper spacing between the parts of the letter. Make any final corrections. Print the document.
   PURPOSE: The spell-checker identifies only certain errors; proofreading helps you find incorrect word use, improper tone, and errors in formatting.

10. Address the envelope, using either the computer and word processing software or a pen and following the correct format.
    PURPOSE: Following the post office guidelines on format helps prevent a delay in delivery of the letter.

11. When using a #10 envelope, fold the letter by pulling up the bottom end until it reaches just below the inside address or two-thirds of the way up the letter. Crease at the fold. Then, fold the top of the letter down so that it is flush with the bottom fold and crease the paper.
    Note: If the provider needs to sign the letter, the letter is folded afterwards.
    PURPOSE: The letter must be neatly folded.

12. File a copy of the letter in the paper medical record or upload an electronic copy of the letter to the electronic health record (EHR).
    PURPOSE: A copy of all correspondence should be kept in the patient's health record.

PROCEDURE 9.2   Compose a Professional Business Letter Using the Modified Block Letter Format

Task: Compose a professional letter using technology. Use the modified block letter format (with the center point option). Address the envelope (if needed) and fold the letter.

Scenario: Julie Walden, MD, has requested that you compose a letter to Carl C. Bowden (DOB: 04/05/1954) to let him know that his hepatitis C laboratory test was negative. If he has any questions, he should call the office. His address is 19 Beale Street, Anytown, AL 12345-1234. You are working at Walden-Martin Family Medical Clinic. The healthcare facility's address is 1234 Anystreet, Anytown, AL 12345. The phone number is 123-123-1234 and the fax number is 123-123-5678.

EQUIPMENT and SUPPLIES

- Patient's health record
- Computer with word processing software and printer
- Paper
- #10 envelope or window business envelope

PROCEDURAL STEPS

1. Obtain the intended recipient's contact information and determine the message you want to convey. Using the computer and word processing software, compose the letter using the modified block letter format. Use 1-inch margins on all four sides, portrait orientation, and use single line spacing throughout the letter. Use an easy-to-read font (e.g., Times New Roman or Calibri), in a 10- or 12-point size.
   PURPOSE: Determining the message gives you a focus when composing the letter. You will need the recipient's information to create the letter.

2. Create a letterhead in the header of the document. Include the clinic's name, street address or post office box, city, state, and ZIP code.
   PURPOSE: The information in the letterhead provides the reader contact information for the clinic.

3. Key (type) the date starting at the center point of the document. Have one blank line between the date line and the last line of the letterhead.
   PURPOSE: All letters require a date for legal purposes.

4. Key the inside address starting at the left margin and use the correct spelling and punctuation. Leave one to nine blank lines between the date and the inside address, to center the body of the letter on the page. If using a window business envelope, adjust the address position to fit the window.
   PURPOSE: The body of the letter must be centered vertically from the top to the bottom of the document. More blank lines can be added to move the body to the correct location.

5. Key the salutation starting at the left margin and use the correct spelling and punctuation. Leave one blank line between the inside address and the salutation.
   PURPOSE: A proper greeting sets the tone of the letter.

6. Use your critical thinking skills to compose a concise, accurate message. Type the message in the body of the letter starting at the left margin. Leave one blank line between the salutation and the first line of the body and then between each paragraph of the body. The message should be clear, concise, and professional. Use proper grammar, punctuation, capitalization, and sentence structure.
   PURPOSE: Proper grammar helps to convey the message accurately and professionally.

7. Key a proper closing starting at the center point of the document. Use the correct spelling and punctuation. Leave one blank line between the last line of the body and the closing.
   PURPOSE: The closing helps end the message with a professional tone.

8. Key the signature block starting at the center point of the document. Use the correct spelling and punctuation. Leave four blank lines between the closing and the signature block. If you are preparing the letter for a provider, you must include a reference notation.
   PURPOSE: The signature block provides the reader with the name of the sender of the letter. The reference notation identifies who typed the letter.

9. Spell-check and proofread the document. Check for the proper tone, grammar, punctuation, capitalization, and sentence structure. Check for proper spacing between the parts of the letter. Make any final corrections. Print the document. If needed, address the envelope, using either the computer and word processing software or a pen and following the correct format.
   PURPOSE: The spell-checker identifies only certain errors; proofreading helps you find incorrect word use, improper tone, and errors in formatting.

10. When using a #10 envelope, fold the letter by pulling up the bottom end until it reaches just below the inside address or two-thirds of the way up the letter. Crease at the fold. Then, fold the top of the letter down so that it is flush with the bottom fold and crease the paper. For window business envelopes, have the letter's print side facing up and place the envelope over the top third of the letter. Fold the bottom edge of the paper up to the bottom edge of the envelope and crease at the fold. Then, remove the envelope and flip the letter over and fold the top of the letter down to the prior crease line and crease at the fold. Place the letter in the envelope so that the recipient's address shows through the window.
    Note: If the provider needs to sign the letter, the letter is folded afterwards.
    PURPOSE: The letter must be neatly folded.

11. File a copy of the letter in the paper medical record or upload an electronic copy of the letter to the electronic health record (EHR).
    PURPOSE: A copy of all correspondence should be kept in the patient's health record.

PROCEDURE 9.3   Compose a Professional Business Letter Using the Semi-Block Letter Format

Task: Compose a professional letter using technology. Use the semi-block letter format (with the right justified option). Address the envelope and fold the letter.

Scenario: Julie Walden, MD, has requested that you compose a letter to Amma Patel to let her know that her thyroid test was normal, but her vitamin D level was low. Dr. Walden would like Amma to take 15 mcg of vitamin D each morning. She can purchase this over the counter. She needs to have her vitamin D rechecked in 6 months. She can call to schedule the blood test closer to that time. If she has any questions, she should call the office. Her address is 1346 Charity Lane, Anytown, AL 12345-1234. You are working at Walden-Martin Family Medical Clinic. The healthcare facility's address is 1234 Anystreet, Anytown, AL 12345. The phone number is 123-123-1234 and the fax number is 123-123-5678.

EQUIPMENT and SUPPLIES

- Patient's health record
- Computer with word processing software and printer
- Paper
- #10 envelope or #6 3/4 envelope

PROCEDURAL STEPS

1. Obtain the intended recipient's contact information and determine the message you want to convey. Using the computer and word processing software, compose the letter using the semi-block letter format. Use 1-inch margins on all four sides, portrait orientation, and use single line spacing throughout the letter. Use an easy-to-read font (e.g., Times New Roman or Calibri), in a 10- or 12-point size.
   PURPOSE: Determining the message gives you a focus when composing the letter. You will need the recipient's information to create the letter.

2. Create a letterhead in the header of the document. Include the clinic's name, street address or post office box, city, state, and ZIP code.
   PURPOSE: The information in the letterhead provides the reader contact information for the clinic.

3. Right justify and key (type) the date. Have one blank line between the date line and the last line of the letterhead.
   PURPOSE: All letters require a date for legal purposes.

4. Key the inside address starting at the left margin and use the correct spelling and punctuation. Leave one to nine blank lines between the date and the inside address, to center the body of the letter on the page.
   PURPOSE: The body of the letter must be centered vertically from the top to the bottom of the document. More blank lines can be added to move the body to the correct location.

5. Key the salutation starting at the left margin and use the correct spelling and punctuation. Leave one blank line between the inside address and the salutation.
   PURPOSE: A proper greeting sets the tone of the letter.

6. Use your critical thinking skills to compose a concise, accurate message. Type the message in the body of the letter starting at the left margin. Leave one blank line between the salutation and the first line of the body and then between each paragraph of the body. Each paragraph should be indented five spaces. The message should be clear, concise, and professional. Use proper grammar, punctuation, capitalization, and sentence structure.

   PURPOSE: Proper grammar helps to convey the message accurately and professionally.

7. Right justify and key a proper closing. Use the correct spelling and punctuation. Leave one blank line between the last line of the body and the closing.
   PURPOSE: The closing helps end the message with a professional tone.

8. Right justify and key the signature block. Use the correct spelling and punctuation. Leave four blank lines between the closing and the signature block. If you are preparing the letter for a provider, you must include a reference notation.
   PURPOSE: The signature block provides the reader with the name of the sender of the letter. The reference notation identifies who typed the letter.

9. Spell-check and proofread the document. Check for the proper tone, grammar, punctuation, capitalization, and sentence structure. Check for proper spacing between the parts of the letter. Make any final corrections. Print the document.
   PURPOSE: The spell-checker identifies only certain errors; proofreading helps you find incorrect word use, improper tone, and errors in formatting.

10. Address the envelope, using either the computer and word processing software or a pen and following the correct format.
    PURPOSE: Following the post office guidelines on format helps prevent a delay in delivery of the letter.

11. When using a #10 envelope, fold the letter by pulling up the bottom end until it reaches just below the inside address or two-thirds of the way up the letter. Crease at the fold. Then, fold the top of the letter down so that it is flush with the bottom fold and crease the paper. When using a #6 3/4 envelope, pull the bottom edge of the letter up until it is 1/2 inch from the top edge of the document and crease at the fold. Bring the right edge two-thirds of the way across the width of the document and crease the paper. Then bring the left edge to the right edge and crease at the fold. Flip the document so the left edge is on the bottom and insert the letter into the envelope.
    Note: If the provider needs to sign the letter, the letter is folded afterwards.
    PURPOSE: The letter must be neatly folded.

12. File a copy of the letter in the paper medical record or upload an electronic copy of the letter to the electronic health record (EHR).
    PURPOSE: A copy of all correspondence should be kept in the patient's health record.

PROCEDURE 9.4   Compose a Memorandum

Task: Compose a professional memorandum.

Scenario: You are asked by the supervisor to compose a memo that can be posted in the department. You are to remind the staff about the department meeting next Tuesday, at noon in the conference room. Staff can bring their lunches, and beverages will be provided.

EQUIPMENT and SUPPLIES

- Computer with word processing software and printer
- Paper

PROCEDURAL STEPS

1. Determine the message you want to convey. Using the computer and word processing software, compose the memo. Use 1-inch margins on all four sides, portrait orientation, and use single line spacing throughout the memo. Use an easy to read font (e.g., Times New Roman or Calibri), in a 10- or 12-point size.
   PURPOSE: Determining the message gives you a focus when composing the memo.
2. Left justify the headers and use boldface and capital letters, followed by a colon. Headers include TO, FROM, DATE, and SUBJECT. Leave one blank line between each header.
   PURPOSE: Boldface and capital letters allow the headers to stand out to the reader, making it easier to read the information.
3. Key (type) the information following the headers in regular font, using a mix of capital and lowercase letters. Using the tab tool, align the information vertically down the page. Key (type) the date as indicated for professional letters.
   PURPOSE: Aligning the information helps the memo look professional.
4. Add a centered black line between the headers and the body (optional). Leave two to three blank lines between the headers and the body of the memo.
   PURPOSE: The line and extra blank lines helps to separate the message in the body from the headers.
5. Key the message in the body of the memo. Left justify the content in the body and use single line spacing. Use proper grammar and correct spelling and punctuation. With multiple paragraphs, skip a single line between paragraphs.
   PURPOSE: For professional communication, it is important to use proper grammar and correct spelling and punctuation.
6. The content of the message in the body of the memo is written clearly, concisely, and accurately. Add special notations as needed.
   PURPOSE: Special notations may be used if the memo contains enclosures and so on.
7. Spell-check and proofread the document. Check for the proper tone, grammar, punctuation, capitalization, and sentence structure. Check for proper spacing between the parts of the memo. Make any final corrections. Print the document.
   PURPOSE: The spell-checker identifies only certain errors; proofreading helps you find incorrect word use, improper tone, and errors in formatting.

PROCEDURE 9.5   Compose a Professional Email

Task: Compose a professional email that conveys the message to the reader clearly, concisely, and accurately.

Scenario: Aaron Jackson (DOB: 10/17/2011) has an appointment at 11 a.m. next Thursday. Send his guardian an appointment reminder via email. Aaron will be seeing David Kahn, MD. The guardian should bring in any medications Aaron is currently taking. You are working at Walden-Martin Family Medical Clinic. The healthcare facility's address is: 1234 Anystreet, Anytown, AL 12345. The phone number is 123-123-1234 and the fax number is 123-123-5678. Your instructor will supply you with the guardian's name and email address.

EQUIPMENT and SUPPLIES

- Patient's health record
- Computer with email software

PROCEDURAL STEPS

1. Obtain the intended recipient's contact information and determine the message you want to convey.
   PURPOSE: This gives you a focus when composing the email. You will need the recipient's information to create the email.
2. Using the computer and email software, key (type) in the recipient's email address. If the email has two recipients, use a semicolon (;) after the name of the first recipient. Double-check the email addresses for accuracy.
   PURPOSE: If the email address is incorrect, the email will not get to the recipient.
3. Key in a subject, keeping it simple but focused on the contents of the email.
   PURPOSE: In many email software packages, the user can search for emails using the subject field. Keeping the subject simple and focused makes it easier for the user to find the message.

PROCEDURE 9.5 Compose a Professional Email—*continued*

4. Key a formal greeting, using correct punctuation.
PURPOSE: A proper greeting sets the tone of the letter.
5. Key the message in the body of the email using proper grammar, punctuation, capitalization, and sentence structure. Avoid abbreviations. The message should be clear, concise, and professional.
PURPOSE: Using proper grammar and avoiding abbreviations will convey the message accurately and professionally.
6. Finish the email with closing remarks.
PURPOSE: In the closing, you can thank the recipient or encourage him or her to follow up with concerns or questions. This gives the email a professional tone.
7. Key a closing, followed by your name and title on the next line. Include the clinic's name and contact information below your name.
PURPOSE: The email clearly states who is sending it.
8. Spell-check and proofread the email. Check for proper tone, grammar, punctuation, capitalization, and sentence structure. Check for proper spacing between the parts of the email.

PURPOSE: White space or spacing between the elements of an email helps separate the parts of the email, making it easier to read.
9. Make any final revisions, select any features to apply to the email, and then send it.
PURPOSE: If the email is urgent (!), that feature should be selected before you send the email. If you require a confirmation email when the email is opened, this feature can also be selected.
10. Print a copy of the email to be filed in the paper medical record or upload an electronic copy of the email to the patient's electronic health record (EHR).
PURPOSE: A copy of all correspondence should be kept in the patient's health record.

PROCEDURE 9.6 Complete a Fax Cover Sheet

Task: Complete a fax cover sheet clearly and accurately.

Scenario: Lisa Parker, mother of Johnny Parker (DOB: 06/15/2010), requested his immunization history be sent to Anytown School, attention: Susie Payne. The school's phone number is 123-123-5784, and the fax number will be supplied by your instructor. The release of medical records has been completed and signed by Lisa, Johnny's guardian/mother. Your phone number is the main clinic number listed on the header of the fax cover sheet.

EQUIPMENT and SUPPLIES
- Document to be faxed (optional)
- Fax machine and fax number (optional)
- Pen
- Fax cover sheet (see Fig. 9.4)

PROCEDURAL STEPS
1. Using a pen and the fax cover sheet, clearly and accurately write your name, phone number, and the date.
PURPOSE: The information must be clearly written so the reader can identify who sent the fax.
2. Clearly and accurately write the name of the person receiving the fax. Also include the company, fax number, and the phone number.
PURPOSE: Being accurate with the information is important so it gets to the correct person.

3. Write the number of pages. The cover sheet must be counted in the total.
PURPOSE: It is important to have an accurate count of the total number of sheets faxed.
4. Complete Re: by indicating the subject of the fax. Be general with the subject and refrain from including anything confidential.
PURPOSE: It is important to be general when writing the subject. No confidential information should appear in the Re: line.
5. Proofread the fax cover sheet. Verify the name, agency, and contact information of the recipient. Verify the document(s) being sent are correct. Organize the documents so the coversheet is on top and fax to the recipient (optional).
PURPOSE: Verifying the information and what is being sent is important for the confidentiality of the records.
Note: Depending on the type of documents faxed and the facility's policies and procedures, the medical assistant may need to document the activity in the patient's health record.

10

TELEPHONE TECHNIQUES

SCENARIO

Ashlynn McDowell, a recent graduate of a medical assisting program, has begun her first position as a receptionist at the Walden-Martin Family Medical (WMFM) Clinic. Ashlynn is determined to perform to the best of her abilities. However, she has never held a job in a professional office. She knows that she needs to practice all of the skills that she learned in school to be an effective receptionist.

WMFM is patient-centered care oriented and wants its patients to feel cared for and special. Ashlynn is anxious to build trust with the patients and offer them help with the problems they encounter that fall within her realm of responsibility.

WMFM recently purchased computer software that allows Ashlynn to record telephone messages on the computer, and these messages are automatically routed both to an inbox for the provider and as an entry in the patient's health record. Although the system is new to everyone in the office, Ashlynn is determined to become proficient in its use as quickly as possible.

She knows that she must speak clearly and distinctly and that she must be adept at following up. She plans to dress professionally each day so that she projects the right image to the patients. Ashlynn will strive to be the type of employee who has a willingness to learn, an ability to adapt, and a heart full of compassion for the patient. She is a team player who sincerely wants to cooperate with other staff members who might need her help.

All of the providers at WMFM are pleased that they have found such an eager person to add to their staff. They will assist and guide Ashlynn as she learns how to make the patients feel like part of the clinic family. Ashlynn's self-esteem has increased because she feels she is making a great contribution to healthcare.

While studying this chapter, think about the following questions:

- What are the features of a multiple-line telephone system?
- How can the principles of active listening be applied when communicating with patients?
- Why does tone of voice play an important role in patient perception?
- What can a medical assistant do to promote a positive image of the healthcare facility when using the telephone with patients?
- How can the medical assistant reduce patients' frustration with telephone issues?

LEARNING OBJECTIVES

1. Identify and explain the features of a multiple-line telephone system, and also explain how each can be used effectively in a healthcare facility. Also, discuss the use of cell phones.
2. Do the following related to effective use of the telephone:
   - Discuss the telephone equipment needed by a healthcare facility.
   - Summarize active listening skills.
   - Demonstrate effective and professional telephone techniques.
   - Consider the importance of tone of voice and enunciation.
3. Explain the importance of thinking ahead when managing telephone calls; also, describe the correct way to answer the telephone in the office.
4. Discuss the screening of incoming calls and list several questions to ask when handling an emergency call.
5. Place callers on hold and correctly transfer a phone call.
6. Do the following related to taking a message:
   - Document telephone messages accurately.
   - List the seven elements of a correctly handled telephone message.
   - Report relevant information concisely and accurately.
7. Discuss various types of common incoming calls and how to deal with each.
8. Discuss various types of special incoming calls and how to deal with each.
9. Discuss how the medical assistant should handle various types of difficult calls.
10. Discuss typical outgoing calls, including why knowledge of time zones and long distance calling is necessary.
11. Discuss the use of a telephone directory, and describe how answering services and automatic call routing systems are used in a healthcare facility.
12. Discuss the legal and ethical issues related to telephone techniques.

VOCABULARY

answering service A commercial service that answers telephone calls for its clients.

automatic call routing A system that distributes incoming calls to a specific group or person based on customer need; for example, the customer presses 1 for appointments, 2 for billing questions, and so on.

bilingual (bie LING gwuhl) Ability to communicate effectively in two languages.

call forwarding A telephone feature that allows calls made to one number to be forwarded to another specified number.

caller ID A feature that identifies and displays the telephone numbers of incoming calls made to a particular line.

conference call A telephone call in which a caller can speak with several people at the same time.

copayment (copay) A set dollar amount that the patient must pay for each office visit. There can be one copayment amount for a primary care provider, and a different copayment amount (usually higher) to see a specialist or to be seen in the emergency department.

emergency An unexpected, life-threatening situation that requires immediate action.

enunciation (ih nuhn see EY shuhn) The use of articulate, clear sounds when speaking.

ergonomics (ur guh NOM iks) An applied science concerned with designing and arranging things needed to do your job in an efficient and safe way.

headset A set of headphones with a microphone attached, used especially in telephone communication.

intercom A two-way communication system with a microphone and loudspeaker at each station; often a feature of business telephones.

jargon (JAHR guhn) The vocabulary of a particular profession, as opposed to common, everyday terms.

monotone (MON uh tohn) A succession of syllables, words, or sentences spoken in an unvaried key or pitch.

multiple-line telephone system A business telephone system that allows for more than one telephone line.

participating provider A physician or other healthcare provider who enters into a contract with a specific insurance company or program and by doing so agrees to abide by certain rules and regulations set forth by that particular third-party payer.

pitch The depth of a tone or sound; a distinctive quality of sound.

provider An individual or company that provides medical care and services to a patient or the public.

screen A system for examining and separating into different groups; in the healthcare facility, it means determining the severity of illness that patients experience and prioritizing appointments based on that severity.

speakerphone A telephone with a loudspeaker and a microphone; it can be used without having to pick up and hold the handset.

speed dialing A telephone function in which a selected stored number can be dialed by pressing only one key.

STAT The medical abbreviation for the Latin term *statum*, meaning immediately; at this moment.

tactful The quality of having a sense of what to do or say to maintain good relations with others or to prevent offense.

triage (tree AHZH) The process of assigning degrees of urgency to patients' conditions.

urgent An acute situation that requires immediate attention but is not life-threatening.

voice mail An electronic system that allows messages from telephone callers to be recorded and stored.

The telephone is one of the most important pieces of equipment used in a healthcare facility. It is used to communicate with patients, other healthcare organizations, and suppliers. It would be difficult to run an office without a telephone. It is often the first point of contact with patients, and this is an opportunity to make an outstanding first impression. Developing good telephone techniques will make you a valuable asset to your employer.

TELEPHONE EQUIPMENT
Multiple-Line Telephone

Familiarity with a **multiple-line telephone system** (Fig. 10.1) is a must for the medical assistant. Even the smallest healthcare facility has at least two telephone lines so that patients rarely get a busy signal when they try to contact the office. The multiple-line telephone has a button for each line, and the button flashes when a call comes in on that line. The button also flashes, although in a different rhythm, when a caller is on hold on that line; this can serve as a reminder for the medical assistant to check back with the

caller to see whether he or she would like to remain on hold or leave a message.

The multiple-line telephone also allows you to transfer calls and possibly to set up **conference calls**, which involve two or more callers. You should familiarize yourself with the multiple-line telephone system used in your healthcare practice.

Headset

Most business telephones have a handset that can be used to answer the telephone. However, the medical assistant who most frequently is responsible for answering the telephone may want to consider using a **headset** instead. Use of a headset can improve your **ergonomics** and help prevent neck strain. Also, having a headset frees your hands to use the computer or take a message.

A headset is a combination earphone and microphone that is attached to the telephone by a cord or is wireless. You can adjust the volume in the earpiece, and you may be able to adjust the volume of your voice through the microphone for callers who may have difficulty hearing. Bluetooth, a type of short-range wireless technology,

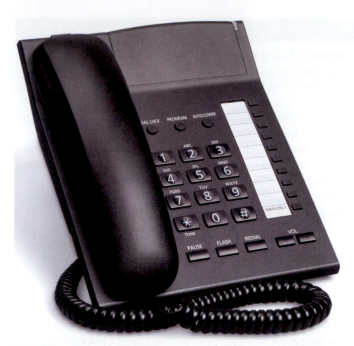

FIGURE 10.1 Multiple-line telephones allow numerous calls to come into the office at once. Each call deserves the same kind of attention and care from the medical assistant.

allows you to be more mobile while on the telephone. Because this type of headset is not as visible, people may not be aware that you are on the telephone and may start a conversation with you. You should politely indicate that you are on the telephone and you will respond to the person when you can. Some healthcare facilities have a light system that indicates to a patient that you are on the phone and you will be with them when the call is complete. Also, many headsets can be muted so that you can speak with someone without the caller hearing you.

Features

Most multiple-line business telephones have many features that allow you to perform a number of different tasks in the healthcare facility.

Speakerphone

The **speakerphone** function allows you to hear and speak to the caller without using the handset or a headset. Generally, a button on the telephone is labeled "speaker" (or is indicated with an icon), and once you push it, you can hang up the handset. This can be useful if you need to have more than two people on the call using the same phone.

You should always inform the caller that you will be putting him or her on speakerphone, and let the person know who else will be listening in. You must also be conscious of protecting patient information when using a speakerphone. The speakerphone function should not be used in areas such as the patient check-in area or anywhere a conversation can be overheard. The door or reception window should be closed so that no one just walking by can overhear the conversation.

Conference Calls

As mentioned, many multiple-line telephones allow you to set up a conference call, in which you can have multiple people on the call

from different locations. The person initiating the call calls one person, puts that person on hold, and continues the sequence until all parties are on the call. Conference calls can be used when the healthcare facility has more than one location and people from all the locations must be involved in a conversation. For example, a committee may want to discuss policies and procedures for the practice. It is a much better use of time to set up a conference call than to have many people travel to one location.

Caller ID

Caller ID allows the user to see who is calling before he or she picks up the handset to answer the telephone. The caller's telephone number and name appear on a screen, and the user can decide whether to take the call. If the user subscribes to call-waiting services, another benefit, called *call-waiting caller ID,* is often available. This function allows the user to see who is calling even when the user is already on the telephone.

Voice Mail

Voice mail affords an around-the-clock method for receiving patients' messages. Unfortunately, it can prove frustrating to those who find themselves speaking to an electronic device more often than a human being. Voice mail allows the caller to hear a recorded message that may also provide information about what to do in case of an **emergency**. Similar to an answering machine, voice mail records a caller's message, which can later be retrieved, and allows special temporary greetings when the user is away from the office. You can keep patients happy by answering voice mail messages promptly. There is also a legal necessity for getting back to patients. It can be considered abandonment if the call is not returned. This could be cause for a potential lawsuit.

CRITICAL THINKING APPLICATION   **10.1**

Ashlynn hears an employee using the speakerphone function to talk about a patient with another employee. How should she handle this situation? To whom, if anyone, should Ashlynn report this activity? What problems might be caused if this type of conversation is overheard?

Call Forwarding

Call forwarding allows the user to forward calls to another designated number, such as an **answering service**. Usually a code is entered, then the telephone number to which the calls should be forwarded. If the medical assistant is going to be busy with a patient, the calls can be forwarded to another employee until the task is completed. This prevents the user from missing important calls when away from the main telephone.

Intercom

The business telephone in the healthcare facility may also have **intercom** capabilities. This feature allows for two-way communication within the healthcare facility, but it does not require you to pick up the handset or use a headset. This type of communication is not confidential, but it can be used to notify staff members of an emergency or to ask the **provider** to come out of the exam room.

Call Hold

The multiple-line business telephone has a hold button that allows you to interrupt a call temporarily. This often is used when you have answered an incoming call and then another line rings. You can also use this feature if you need to retrieve some information or speak to someone else to get some information. It is very important to be courteous and respectful of the caller.

Speed Dialing

Speed dialing allows you to program keys on the telephone keypad to automatically call a stored telephone number by just pressing one key. For example, if the healthcare facility uses a particular laboratory for specimen testing, the telephone number for that laboratory can be programmed for the numeral 1 on the telephone keypad; then, when you want to call that laboratory, you only need to press 1 and the call will be made. Speed dialing can be a time-saver; however, all staff members must know which telephone numbers have been programmed into particular keypad numbers.

Cell Phones

Considered a luxury item only 10 years ago, cell (or cellular) phones have become commonplace. Many people no longer have a landline because of the expenses of having two phones, and the cell phone usually is the better buy for the money. Several of the more popular cell phone companies offer free long distance calls in the United States and may provide users free night and weekend minutes. Most of today's smart phones even allow users to access the internet and check email on their telephone. Cell phone companies usually offer a text messaging service, which allows the user to enter a message with cell phone keys or by voice, which then is sent directly to a cell phone number.

Many people have a personal cell phone or smart phone. It is a great way to be accessible at all times, but it also can present some issues in a healthcare facility, particularly in regard to patient confidentiality. Most cell phones have a camera that could be used to take pictures of confidential information, and that information can be transmitted quickly to someone else or put on the internet. Calls can be made or taken at inopportune times and may affect the care of patients. Most healthcare facilities have a policy that prohibits employees from having their personal cell phones with them during working hours.

We have seen an increase in the number of healthcare facilities that are supplying cell phones to their providers. The communication process is improved with the provider use of cell phones. There is ready access to patient information needed for collaboration and care coordination. The provider's cell phone number should never be given out to patients without the provider's permission.

TELEPHONE EQUIPMENT NEEDS OF A HEALTHCARE FACILITY

Number and Placement of Telephones

Few healthcare facilities can get along with just one telephone line. Two incoming lines, along with a private outgoing line with a separate number for the provider's exclusive use, is the minimum recommended number of lines.

One medical assistant can handle no more than two incoming lines; therefore, the addition of more lines may involve additional staffing. If a staff member is assigned solely to dealing with insurance and billing, a separate line and listing in the telephone directory for this service may considerably lessen the load on the main incoming lines.

Telephones should be placed where they are accessible but private. Each provider, in addition to the office manager, requires a telephone at his or her desk. A telephone should be available in the laboratory area and the clinical area, and multiple phones should be present in reception and business office areas. Many healthcare facilities also have a telephone available for patients to use. This telephone often has a separate line so that patient use does not interfere with the staff members' work.

EFFECTIVE USE OF THE TELEPHONE

Active Listening

It may seem odd to start out discussing listening instead of speaking in this chapter, but listening well while on the telephone is just as important as speaking well when it comes to communicating on the telephone. When you are on the telephone, you have fewer nonverbal cues to help you determine the message. Therefore, it is very important that you use good listening skills. When you use active listening skills, your patients realize that you think they are important and that you respect the message they are communicating to you, whether you are on the telephone or face to face.

Active Listening

- Be present in the moment.
- Focus solely on the conversation.
- Don't interrupt.
- Don't start forming your response before the person has finished speaking.
- Confirm what the speaker has said, and ask if your interpretation is correct.
- Always be respectful and professional.

Active listening involves listening to what the speaker is saying, interpreting what the message is, and restating the message to make sure that you have received the intended message. For example, you receive a telephone call from a distraught mother. Using active listening skills, you pick up on the nonverbal cues, such as her tone of voice and rate of speech, and you can tell she is upset. The mother states that her child has been very sick for the past several days, and nothing she has done has helped with the fever her child has had for 2 days. Your response should be to restate what you have heard: the child has been ill with a fever for the past 2 days, and nothing she has tried has brought the fever down. This gives the caller the opportunity to correct any misinformation or to confirm that the information is correct. If it is correct, you should follow the healthcare practice's procedures for handling this situation; most likely, you will schedule an appointment for that same day.

Developing a Pleasing Telephone Personality

Each time a medical assistant answers the telephone, he or she is representing the healthcare practice (see Procedure 10.1, p. 212). The manner in which the telephone is answered can influence the caller's impression of the whole office and whether the person wants to be seen there. When patients call the healthcare facility, they should hear a friendly yet professional voice. Just as active listening is an important skill to receive the message being sent, a pleasing telephone personality facilitates the sending of the message.

Although it may seem silly, you should always smile when you answer the telephone. The physical act of smiling affects how your words sound. It is as if your caller can hear you smile, and you have created a positive impression.

It is also important to be aware of nonverbal communication that occurs during a telephone conversation. Be aware of your tone of voice. Is it helping to send the message that you want to send? Your callers can tell if you are preoccupied and not focused on the current conversation. You should vary the **pitch** of your voice and avoid speaking in a **monotone**.

Enunciation is crucial when speaking on the telephone. You should speak very clearly and distinctly so that the caller can understand what you are saying. Many letters of the alphabet sound very similar on the telephone, such as B, P, T, and F and S. You may need to clarify with the caller by saying, "That is B as in bravo."

Nonvisual/Nonverbal Communication

- Tone of voice
- Speed of speech
- Pitch
- Volume
- Enunciation
- Pausing or hesitation

Phonetic Alphabet

A	Alpha	N	November
B	Bravo	O	Oscar
C	Charlie	P	Papa
D	Delta	Q	Quebec
E	Echo	R	Romeo
F	Foxtrot	S	Sierra
G	Golf	T	Tango
H	Hotel	U	Uniform
I	India	V	Victor
J	Juliet	W	Whiskey
K	Kilo	X	X-ray
L	Lima	Y	Yankee
M	Mike	Z	Zulu

It is important to always be courteous and **tactful**. Think about the words you will be using before actually speaking them. For those of us working in a healthcare facility, it is easy to integrate medical terminology into our conversations. However, we must be careful not to use medical **jargon** when speaking with patients because this makes the message more difficult for them to understand. For example, if you are giving a male patient preprocedural instructions, advise him that he must not eat or drink anything for 12 hours before the procedure; do not tell him he should "stay NPO" (nothing by mouth).

To create a pleasant, friendly, and professional image of the healthcare facility, you must give the caller your full attention. Do not become distracted by other things going on around you. In addition, you should never eat, chew gum, or drink when on the telephone. Use a normal volume and tone of voice, and speak directly into the mouthpiece. Be sure to speak at a moderate rate of speed because speaking too quickly makes it difficult for the caller to understand you.

CRITICAL THINKING APPLICATION   10.2

Ashlynn has a tendency to speak a little fast in her normal conversations. How will she need to adjust as she is answering phones in the healthcare facility? She also is a friendly person and enjoys talking on the phone. What precautions should she take so that this does not become an issue on the job?

MANAGING TELEPHONE CALLS

Thinking Ahead

Whether you are answering incoming calls or placing outgoing calls, it is important to be completely prepared. Before you start answering calls, make sure you have all the supplies needed to do your job. For example, for taking messages, you should have access to a computer (if your office documents telephone messages electronically) or a paper message form, in addition to working pens and a watch or clock to record the time. You should be sure to have the healthcare facility's telephone screening guidelines available. Many offices also keep a list of commonly used telephone numbers. Such a list includes poison control, other emergency numbers, community resources to which patients can be referred, and so on.

For outgoing calls, have all the information you need, such as the patient's health record, the telephone number of the person you will be calling, a list of questions, and a pad and a pen to make notes during the conversation.

Confidentiality

All communication in a healthcare facility must maintain patient confidentiality. When using the telephone, you must be aware of what is going on around you and who may be able to overhear your conversation. If patient-sensitive information will be discussed, place the call in an area where others cannot hear, especially other patients. Be careful when using a speakerphone because the sound can travel farther than you might think, and someone might overhear private medical information – this is a violation of the law, specifically the Health Insurance Portability and Accountability Act (HIPAA).

Answering Promptly

As mentioned earlier, telephone contact is often the first interaction with a patient. If the person's call is not answered promptly, this can create a negative impression before he or she even talks to someone. It is important that a call be answered within three rings. To accomplish this, you may need to do the following: (1) interrupt the call you are on by asking if you can place the person on hold for a moment; (2) answer the second call; if it is not an emergency, ask that person if you may place him or her on hold; and (3) return to the first caller.

An incoming call should never be answered with "Please hold." You should always find out the nature of the call before placing the person on hold. If it is an emergency, the second call is handled promptly, before you return to the first call. If it is not an emergency, you should always ask if you can place the person on hold and wait for an answer before pushing the hold button. If the person refuses to be placed on hold, determine the reason why and assure them that you will return to his or her call quickly.

The medical assistant who routinely answers the telephone should know how to activate emergency medical services (EMS) in his or her area. Generally, this means dialing 911. You may need to make this call for a patient who has called the healthcare facility and is now unable to contact EMS on her own. If your phone system allows it, you can set up a conference call that includes the patient, EMS, and yourself. It is important to get a telephone number where the caller can be reached, just in case you get disconnected. It also is important to keep the patient and/or caregivers on the line while contacting EMS.

Identifying the Facility

When answering incoming telephone calls, the medical assistant should identify the facility first, state his or her name, and then follow with an offer of help. For example: "Good morning, Walden-Martin Family Medical Clinic. This is Ashlynn. How may I help you?" Medical assistants must always follow the policy of the healthcare facility when answering incoming calls. Speaking slowly and smoothly, with good enunciation, ensures that your callers understand whom they have reached.

CRITICAL THINKING APPLICATION 10.3

Most offices dictate how the phone is to be answered. What should Ashlynn do if she is very uncomfortable with the way she is asked to answer the phone? Who ultimately should decide how the phone is answered?

Identifying the Caller

If the caller does not offer a name, the medical assistant should ask, "May I ask who is calling?" It can be helpful to write down the caller's name and try to use it at least three times during the conversation if it does not compromise patient confidentiality. This helps make a strong connection with the patient and assures the person that he or she has been identified correctly.

Occasionally callers refuse to identify themselves to the medical assistant and insist that they speak with the provider. You must be clear, in a professional manner, that you cannot connect the caller to the provider without knowing who the caller is. The caller may be a sales representative who knows that if she identifies herself, she will not get the opportunity to talk with the provider. When it becomes clear that the caller will not give a name but still insists on speaking with the provider, you can tell the person that the provider is busy with patients and has asked that messages be taken; if the

caller cannot leave a name for the message, then he or she may want to write a letter and mark it Personal. Most people do not want to wait for a response to a letter and will then give you their names so that a message can be taken.

Screening Incoming Calls

Most healthcare facilities expect the medical assistant answering the telephone to **screen** the calls. You must determine which calls should be routed directly to the provider, which to the **triage** area, or which to the billing office. The provider, office manager, and staff members who will be answering the telephone should work together to develop policies for screening calls.

The first step in screening calls is to determine who the caller is and the nature of the call. If the call is from a patient with a question about a statement he or she just received in the mail, the call can be transferred to the appropriate area. If the call involves determining whether a patient should be seen that day, it can be transferred to the triage area. If the caller asks to speak directly to the provider, the situation can become more complicated, and healthcare facility policies should be created to address these cases.

Healthcare facility policies often state that calls from other providers are put through immediately. If that is not possible, assure the caller that the provider will return the call as soon as possible. Some providers may also ask that calls be put through immediately for certain family members. If the provider does not want to take the calls, the medical assistant must tactfully tell the caller that the provider cannot be disturbed at this time.

Screening policies should also address how calls should be handled when the provider is out of the office. If the provider is to be out of the office for an extended period (e.g., for a conference or vacation), another provider is usually designated to handle calls. It should be explained to the patient that the provider that he or she asked for is out of the office, but another provider is taking the calls. If the call is not an emergency, take a message, and the designated provider can return the call.

If a call is an emergency, the policies for handling emergency calls apply. Many emergency calls require judgment on the part of the person answering the telephone in the medical practice. Good judgment comes from experience and proper training by the provider. It is important to know what a real emergency is, in addition to how such calls should be handled. The person answering the telephone first should determine whether the call is truly **urgent**. If so, never hang up the telephone until an ambulance reaches the patient or other help arrives. When necessary, ask another staff member to call 911 while remaining on the line with the patient. Emergency calls may include such conditions and/or symptoms as chest pain, profuse bleeding, severe allergic reactions, cessation of breathing, injuries resulting in loss of consciousness, and broken bones.

An urgent call may be an adult patient with a fever over 102° F (38.9° C), an animal bite, or an increasingly painful ear infection. Emergency calls are life-threatening, whereas an urgent call requires prompt attention but is not life-threatening. In the case of emergencies, often the provider instructs the patient to go straight to the closest hospital emergency department instead of the office. Policies and procedures manuals should indicate the action to take in emergency situations. When in doubt, always ask the office manager and/or the provider.

If the provider is in, the call may need to be transferred to him or her immediately. All offices should have a written plan of action for the times the provider is not physically present in the office. These policies should include typical questions to ask the caller to determine the validity and disposition of an emergency. Some examples of questions to ask include:

- At what telephone number can you be reached?
- Where are you located?
- What are the chief symptoms?
- When did they start?
- Has this happened before?
- Are you alone?
- Do you have transportation?

Screening Guidelines

In a facility with multiple employees, the provider may designate one individual, such as a nurse or an experienced and trained medical assistant, as the telephone screener. Every healthcare facility would be wise to have a written telephone protocol for handling urgent situations and emergencies. The protocol should state that employees are bound by the written guidelines and that unauthorized personnel may give no advice. If advice is given, it may be grounds for dismissal.

A special sheet of instructions listing specific medical emergencies (e.g., chest pain, heavy bleeding, fainting, seizure, and poisoning) should be posted by each telephone. The telephone numbers for the nearest poison control center, hospital, and ambulance should be listed.

Emergency calls should be routed to a provider immediately. Additional instructions should include what action to take if no provider is available (e.g., sending the patient to an emergency department or calling for an ambulance). Most offices have some means of constant contact with the provider, whether by pager, cell phone, or another method.

Getting the Information the Provider Needs

As the medical assistant gains experience and better knows the provider, he or she begins to have a sense of the questions the provider will have for patients who call the facility. For example, the provider is interested in how long the patient has had symptoms, what makes the symptoms better or worse, what remedies have been tried, what has worked and not worked, and other specifics about the condition. If the patient complains of painful urination, the medical assistant learns to ask about pain in the back or blood in the urine. One way to learn about questions to ask is to listen to the provider carefully as he or she questions patients about their symptoms. This can help you learn more about signs and symptoms and enable you to be a better assistant to the provider.

Remember to always be "patient with your patients." Those who call the healthcare facility for help are almost never at their best. When feeling ill, people often are short-tempered and even display poor manners. Some can be verbally abusive. Care for patients as if they were family members, and they will feel care and compassion in the medical facility.

If the provider is unavailable for only part of the day, take a message and inform the caller that the provider currently is out of the office but will return calls when he or she returns. It is important to give the caller the time frame in which the provider will be returning those calls so that the patient's time is not wasted in sitting by the phone, waiting for the call. It should be stressed that the time frame is approximate because emergencies cannot be predicted. If the caller is unavailable when the provider usually returns calls, ask what would be a convenient time and let the caller know you will try to work with that time frame.

Screening calls is an important task for medical assistants who answer the telephone. It can keep the healthcare facility running on schedule and ensure that calls that need to get to the provider do so immediately.

Placing Callers on Hold

When you are working with a multiple-line telephone, it is not uncommon for more than one call to come in at a time. If you are on one call and another line rings you should:

- Put the first call on hold
- Answer the second call
- Determine if it is an emergency or not
  - If it is an emergency, follow the emergency call procedures
  - If it is not an emergency, ask if you can place them on hold
- Return to the first call

The medical assistant should always ask before placing a caller on hold. If it has been determined through the screening process that this is a call that does not need to be put through to the provider right away, or if the call needs to be transferred to someone else in the healthcare facility and that person is not immediately available, you should ask if the caller would like to be put on hold, or if he or she would prefer to be called back. If you know that the person with whom the caller needs to speak may be busy for quite a while, inform the caller of that. The caller may still want to wait. You should check back periodically to make sure the caller still wants to remain on hold. No longer than 1 minute should pass before you check back with the caller. When you return to the call, you can use a statement such as, "Thank you for waiting. Would you like to continue to hold, or should I take a message?"

Minimizing the wait for the caller shows concern, and freeing up the telephone lines is important for other people trying to contact the healthcare facility.

Transferring a Call

During the screening process, the medical assistant may determine that the call should be transferred to the provider or to another person in the facility. Consider the following example: Ms. Fields calls your office because she has a billing question. You should ask Ms. Fields' permission and wait for a response before placing her on hold. It is also helpful to give Ms. Fields the name and extension of the person to whom you will be transferring her call (if it is not the provider); this way, if Ms. Fields' call happens to get disconnected, she will have that information when she calls back. Once you have Ms. Fields' permission to put her on hold, you should contact the person to whom the call is being transferred; in this case, that is Mr. Lewis in the billing department. Tell Mr. Lewis who is calling and the reason for the call; this allows Mr. Lewis to be prepared to help Ms. Fields when the connection is made. Mr. Lewis may ask for a moment to pull up information before you put Ms. Fields' call through.

You should stay on the line to introduce Ms. Fields to Mr. Lewis and to make sure the connection is made. If Mr. Lewis is unavailable, you should ask Ms. Fields if she would like to be connected to his voice mail. Some callers may prefer that you take a message in written form and bring it to the proper person.

Medical assistants who answer telephone calls must know who does what in the healthcare facility. An organizational chart with telephone extensions can be helpful, but it must be kept up to date so that calls can be transferred successfully.

Taking a Message

Telephone messages, whether taken in a handwritten or an electronic format, are an important part of patient care (see Procedure 10.2, p. 213). The patient relies on the medical assistant to get the message to the appropriate person. Taking messages allows information to be delivered to a provider or an appropriate person, who can make a decision (then or later), which can be communicated back to the patient without interrupting the flow of patients through the healthcare

facility. You should be sure to let the caller know when to expect a call back; for example, explain that the provider usually returns calls between 3 and 4 p.m.

Whether the message is taken in a handwritten or an electronic format, the information needed for a complete message is the same:

1. The name of the person calling
2. The name of the person to whom the call is directed
3. The caller's daytime, evening, and/or cell phone number
4. The reason for the call, including the telephone number of the caller's pharmacy if a medication is requested
5. The action to be taken
6. The date and time of the call
7. The initials of the person who took the call

Messages Taken on Paper

Many types of message pads or books are available (Fig. 10.2). Many are pressure-sensitive, making a copy of the message and serving as a telephone call log. The original is given to the person the message

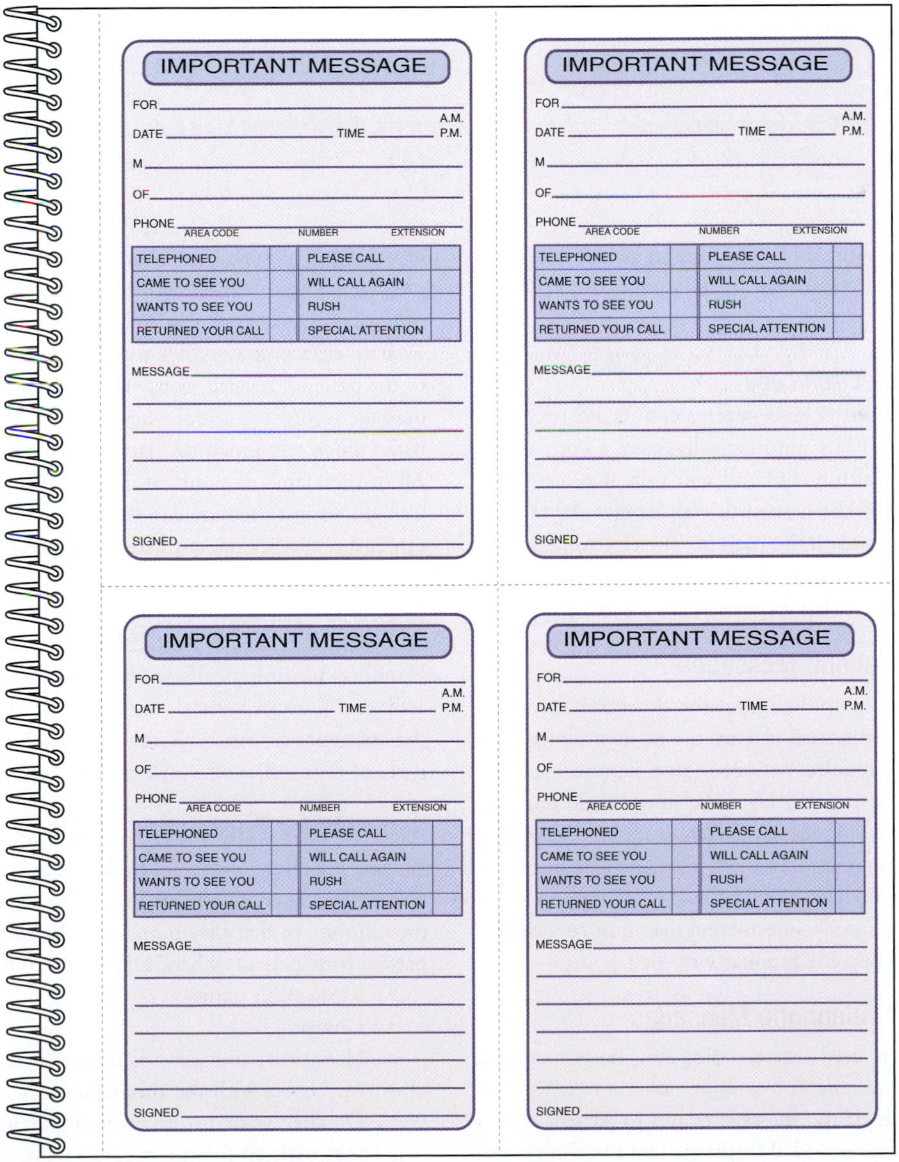

FIGURE 10.2 Telephone message forms.

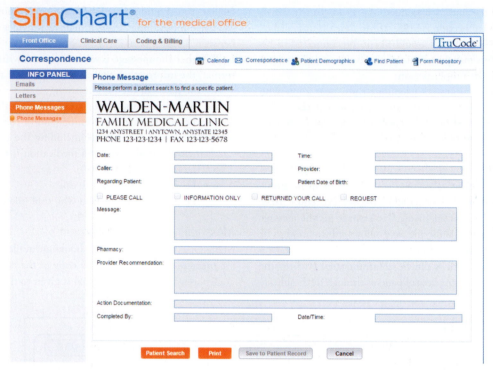

FIGURE 10.3 Telephone message screen in an electronic health record system. (Elsevier: *SimChart for the Medical Office,* St. Louis, 2015, Elsevier.)

is for, and the medical assistant will have a copy to use for follow-up. Having legible handwriting is a must when taking a manual, handwritten message.

Messages Recorded Electronically

Most electronic health record (EHR) systems can record telephone messages (Fig. 10.3). The EHR automatically saves a copy of the message to the patient's health record and sends the message to the provider, who can either call the patient directly or give the medical assistant directions to respond to the patient. The electronic system may also be able to flag a message, to indicate that it is urgent, or that it requires a call back, or that a prescription refill is requested.

Taking Action on Telephone Messages

The message process is not complete until the necessary action has been taken. If a handwritten system is used, use an identifying mark to indicate a message that requires action. If an electronic system is used, check periodically during the day to be sure you do not have to complete the response to the message, such as calling the patient back or contacting the pharmacy. For risk management purposes, the healthcare facility should have a policy on the documentation of telephone messages and the specific information that must be included. Medical assistants should become familiar with that policy.

Retaining Records of Telephone Messages

If a handwritten system is used for recording telephone messages, the healthcare facility must establish a policy on the retention of telephone message records. If the message relates to patient care, a copy of the message should be added to the patient's health record. If the health record is electronic, this may mean scanning in a copy

of the paper message and attaching it to the EHR. The copy in the message book usually is retained for the same period that the statute of limitations runs for medical professional liability cases.

If an electronic system is used, the message is automatically saved to the patient's record, along with the response to the message. The message record can show whether the patient contacted the office, if the office responded to that contact, and what the response was. All of these are key points if a medical professional liability case is brought against the provider. In addition, accurate telephone records can ensure quality patient care and customer service.

TYPICAL INCOMING CALLS

Handling incoming calls is often the responsibility of the medical assistant. You can handle many calls directly, but some will require the assistance of others. Knowing how to respond to the different types of calls will make you a valuable asset to the healthcare facility.

Requests for Prescription Refills

Patients will often call the healthcare facility when they need a prescription refilled. It could be that there were no refills left on the original prescription, or that they have used all of the refills. The information needed from patients when they request a prescription refill includes:

- Medication name
- Dosage
- How many pills are taken in a day
- Any issues with the medication
- Do they want to use a pharmacy mail-order service or will they pick up the prescription
- Pharmacy address and phone number

It is important for a medical assistant to be familiar with the common medication names and the abbreviations used in a prescription. Using the correct spelling of the medication is very important. See Appendix A for the most common medications and their spelling and Appendix B for abbreviations.

Requests for Directions

Each office should have a clear set of written directions that can be read to a caller who wants to know how to get to the office. Prepare the directions from various points in the area; for instance, one set for a patient coming from the north, and another for a patient coming from the south. Place these directions close to the telephone so that all employees can find them easily. Not all employees live close to the clinic or are familiar with the area; therefore, the written set of directions will be helpful both to staff members and to patients. Put a map on the office website and direct patients there for printable directions. Never simply suggest that callers refer to an internet map when they ask for directions.

Inquiries About Bills

A patient may ask to speak with the provider about a recent bill. Ask the caller to hold for a moment while the ledger is obtained from the computer or files. If nothing irregular is found in the ledger, return to the telephone and say, "I have your account in front of me now. Perhaps I can answer your question." Most likely the caller will have some simple inquiry (e.g., whether the insurance company has paid its portion), or the person may want to delay making a payment until the next month. Not all patients realize that the medical assistant usually makes such decisions and is the best person with whom to discuss these matters. If the healthcare facility uses an external billing service, you may need to provide the caller with that agency's telephone number. When an external billing service is used, that telephone number is often shown on the patient's statement. When necessary, post a note in the EHR or to the physical ledger card about the patient's call, such as a promise to pay on a certain date.

A patient may have questions about a statement that came in the mail. If billing matters are handled by another employee, tell the patient that the call will be transferred to the billing office. If you are responsible for billing, politely ask the patient to hold the line while you obtain the patient ledger. On returning to the line, thank the patient for waiting and explain the charges carefully. If an error has occurred, apologize and say that a corrected statement will be sent out at once. Always remember to thank the patient for calling. If patients are properly advised about charges at the time services are rendered, the number of these calls can be reduced considerably.

Inquiries About Fees

Fees vary widely in each healthcare facility, and quoting an exact fee before the provider sees the patient can be difficult. However, a good estimate should be given to patients as to what they can expect to pay, especially on the first visit. Asking a patient to just appear at the office without having any idea of the cost is unreasonable. Discuss with the provider or office manager what range should be quoted to the patient and then follow your quote with the statement that the fees vary, depending on the patient's condition and tests the provider orders. Most healthcare facilities require patients to pay the health

insurance **copayment** (or **copay**) on the day service is provided, and the caller should be informed of this. If fees are regularly discussed on the telephone, a suggested script should be included in the policies and procedures manual. Do not be evasive; have a list of fees available you can discuss with patients.

Questions About Participating Providers

Patients may call the office to inquire whether the provider is a **participating provider** with their particular insurance plan or managed care organization. A list of the insurance plans with which the provider has a contract should be readily available to the medical assistant who answers the telephone. This is important because insurance benefits vary widely for patients based on whether they see a participating provider or a nonparticipating provider. A claim may even be denied if the provider is not a provider for the patient's insurance company.

Requests for Assistance With Insurance

In the ever-changing world of health insurance, patients are often confused about their coverage, how payment is determined, and what they are actually financially responsible for when it comes to their bill from the healthcare facility. A solid understanding of the basics of health insurance, including managed care, allows you to answer patients' questions about insurance. If the question is beyond your knowledge, you should know to whom to transfer the call so that the patient can get an answer.

Radiology and Laboratory Reports

Because of the increased use of EHRs, radiology and laboratory results often are available to providers as soon as the technician has completed the test. When the patient calls for those results, a message is taken, and the provider decides whether the medical assistant can relay the results or the provider needs to speak to the patient directly.

When tests are done at a facility that is not linked to the healthcare facility's EHR, the findings usually are delivered by mail to the provider's office. If the test has been marked **STAT**, reports may be telephoned, faxed, or emailed to the provider's office and an original report delivered by mail.

It is helpful to have blank laboratory results forms available that list the various tests, with their normal values, so that you can easily and accurately document results telephoned to the healthcare facility. This can save time, and you can be assured that the test name is spelled correctly. You should repeat the results you have been given to make sure you have written them down correctly. This report must be documented in the patient's health record and sent to the provider for review.

Satisfactory Progress Reports From Patients

Providers sometimes ask patients to telephone the office to report on their condition a few days after the office visit. The medical assistant can take such calls and relay the information to the provider if the report is satisfactory. Assure the patient that you will inform the provider of the call. The report should be documented in the health record. The provider should always be immediately informed about unsatisfactory progress reports, and he or she should give instructions for the patient to follow in such situations. The provider may discuss this directly with the patient, or the medical assistant may be instructed to relay the information to the patient. All instructions given should also be documented in the health record.

Routine Reports From Hospitals and Other Sources

Routine calls may be received from hospitals and other sources reporting a patient's progress. Take the message carefully and make sure the provider sees it. The message should be placed in the patient's health record after the provider has reviewed and initialed it.

Requests for Referrals

Well-respected providers, especially primary care providers, are often asked for recommendations for referrals to other specialists. If the provider has furnished the medical assistant with a list of practitioners for this purpose, these inquiries may be handled without consulting the provider, unless the patient's insurance plan requires a written referral. However, the provider should always be informed of such requests. Referrals should also be documented in the patient's health record.

Some managed care organizations require a provider referral before a patient may see a specialist; this referral should come from the provider unless he or she has authorized automatic referrals. Most providers require the patient to come in for an office visit to discuss the referral. Afterward, a staff member calls the referral provider and notifies the office staff of the referral. This process may also be done electronically. A managed care organization may offer the option of using its website to enter the referral information and then electronically forwarding the information to the new provider. Handle these calls as quickly as possible so that the patient may make an appointment to see the referral provider.

Non-Patient-Related Calls

Not all calls concern patients. Calls may come from the accountant or the auditor or about banking procedures, office supplies, or office maintenance, most of which the medical assistant can handle or refer to the appropriate person. For some of these calls, the medical assistant may need to gather additional information and return the call.

Pharmaceutical representatives and salespeople will often call and ask to speak to the provider. A message should be taken that includes what product they want to talk to the provider about. The provider may decide to return these calls or ask that an appointment be scheduled to talk about the new product. It is also possible that the provider will ask the office manager to talk to the salesperson.

SPECIAL INCOMING CALLS

Patients Refusing to Discuss Symptoms

Occasionally patients call and want to talk with the provider about symptoms they are reluctant to discuss with a medical assistant. Patients have the right to privacy, but the provider cannot be expected to take numerous calls from patients who do not want to speak to the medical assistant. If the patient refuses to discuss any symptoms, follow the healthcare facility's procedures, which may include suggesting that the patient make an appointment with the provider to discuss the problem in person.

Unsatisfactory Progress Reports

If a patient under treatment reports that he or she is still not feeling well or that the prescription the provider wrote is not helping, do

not practice medicine illegally by giving the patient medical advice. Make detailed notes about the patient's comments and then give your notes to the provider. He or she may make a medication change or may decide that the patient should return to the office. Follow up with the patient and convey the provider's instructions.

> **CRITICAL THINKING APPLICATION   10.4**
> A patient calls the healthcare facility to report that she has been taking her prescribed antibiotic for 3 days and still isn't feeling any better. She says she might even be feeling worse than before she started taking the pills. She asks Ashlynn if she should stop taking the pills.
> - How should Ashlynn respond to this patient?
> - What actions should Ashlynn take in response to this telephone call?
> - What should Ashlynn document in the patient's record?

Requests for Test Results

When the provider orders special tests, the patient may be told to call the office in a couple of days for the results. It is ultimately the responsibility of the provider to notify the patient of test results, especially if they are abnormal. When a patient calls for the results, make sure the provider has seen them and has given permission before sharing the results with the patient. If specified in the office policy, the medical assistant can give test results to the patient. Patients do not always understand that the medical assistant cannot give out information without the provider's permission. If the results are unfavorable, the provider should be the one to inform the patient and give further instructions. This call must be handled tactfully; otherwise, the patient may feel as if the staff is concealing information.

Most providers prefer that medical assistants give only normal test results to patients. However, the medical assistant may give abnormal test results if authorized by the provider. For example, when a patient has an abnormal Pap test result, the medical assistant usually is the person who calls the patient with the result and further instructions from the provider. If the patient has any questions about the test result, she must be referred to the provider. The medical assistant needs good communication skills to relay information such as this without crossing the line of practicing medicine without a license.

The best policy for dealing with more serious abnormal test results is to schedule an appointment for the patient to see the provider. These results are best relayed in person instead of on the telephone.

Patients who call the office for test results must be appropriately identified before the results are given. Some offices use a special code that is written in the patient's health record, and knowledge of this code or password gives the person access to the information. Other offices may use the patient's date of birth or other information that is known only to the patient and has been shared with the healthcare facility. You should always use at least two different methods of identifying patients.

Medical assistants must know and follow federal regulations and the laws in their state regarding the release of any information to someone other than the patient. It is important to note that this includes information about a minor. Make sure the right individual is on the line before offering results by verifying name and date of birth. It is considered a breach of confidentiality and of the Privacy Rules of the Health Insurance Portability and Accountability Act if the patient is not identified correctly and information is released to the wrong individual.

Requests for Information From Third Parties

The patient must give permission before any member of the provider's staff can give information to third-party callers; this includes insurance companies, attorneys, relatives, neighbors, employers, and any other third party. HIPAA is very specific about the information that should be included in the release of information form. The patient must specify who can receive the information and exactly what information can be released. The release of information form also must include an expiration date. The medical assistant must carefully review the patient's form before releasing any information to third parties. Chapter 4 has more information regarding release of information.

Complaints About Care or Fees

A medical assistant may be able to offer a satisfactory explanation to a patient who complains about the care he or she received, or the charged fee. Often the patient simply does not understand a charge, and the medical assistant can provide assistance by reviewing the bill. If a patient seems angry, offer to pull the health record, research the problem, and, if needed, discuss it with the provider. Four magic words often calm the angry patient: "Let me help you." This reassures the patient that someone is willing to talk about the problem. However, if you are unable to appease the patient easily, the provider or office manager may prefer to talk directly to the patient.

When callers complain, do not attempt to blame someone else, and never argue with the patient. Find the source of the problem, and then present options to the caller as to how the situation can be resolved. Remember to treat callers in the same manner that you would wish to be treated. A complaint may seem small and insignificant to the office staff, but it may be a serious issue to the patient. Provide good customer service to patients, and complaints will be few and far between.

Calls From Staff Members' Families or Friends

Personal calls can tie up the telephone lines. Sometimes a call is necessary in emergencies, but staff members should never monopolize the telephone for personal business and conversations. Patient emergency calls could be coming through, and the lines must be clear. Keep personal calls to an absolute minimum.

HANDLING DIFFICULT CALLS

Angry Callers

No matter how efficient the medical assistant is on the telephone or how well-liked the provider might be, sooner or later, an angry caller will be on the telephone. The anger may have a legitimate cause, or the caller's irritation may have resulted from a misunderstanding. Handling such calls is a real challenge. First, take the required actions, even if it is to say that the matter will be discussed with the provider as soon as possible and that the patient will be called back later. If answers are not readily available, a friendly assurance that the situation

is important and that every attempt will be made to find the answer quickly usually calms the angry feelings.

The medical assistant may find that lowering his or her tone of voice and volume of speech may force the angry caller to do the same. This method does not always work, but it usually is true that when dealing with an angry person, calm promotes calm. Some patients may misread this method and become even angrier, thinking that their complaint is not being taken seriously. Interpersonal skills are critical when dealing with other individuals because the more skilled the medical assistant becomes, the better able he or she is to deal with multiple types of personalities.

Always avoid getting angry or defensive in response to an angry caller and try to get to the root of the real problem. Express interest and understanding, take careful notes, and follow through with the problem to the most appropriate resolution. Never "pass the buck" by saying, "That's not my job," or "I am not the person who filed that insurance claim." No matter whose fault the problem is, it is best to deal with it and find a solution instead of placing blame. It is important to respond to the patient when you said you would, even if the call is to tell him or her that you need a bit more time to work on the problem. Keeping the patient in the loop shows that you want to come up with a solution.

CRITICAL THINKING APPLICATION   **10.5**

An angry caller raises his voice at Ashlynn over an issue that happened before she began to work at the facility. She suggests that he speak with the office manager, but he refuses and continues to berate Ashlynn.

- What choices does Ashlynn have in this situation?
- Should she simply hang up on the patient?
- How can the call be handled diplomatically?

Aggressive Callers

Aggressive callers insist that they receive whatever action they feel is necessary, and they usually insist on action immediately. Treat these callers with a calm, poised attitude, but do not allow the caller's aggression to initiate inappropriate action. Reassure the caller that his or her concern is valid and will receive the full attention of the right person. Explain when the caller can expect a response from the office, and be sure to follow up with the patient.

Unauthorized Inquiry Calls

Some individuals call the provider's office requesting information to which they are not entitled. These callers must be told politely but firmly that such information cannot be provided to them because of privacy laws. Insistent callers should be referred to the office manager or provider.

Sales Calls

Sales calls often are thought of as an interruption to the provider's busy day, but some salespersons may have important information on products, equipment, or services the office uses regularly. Do not disregard salespeople, but do not allow them to monopolize time or telephone lines, either. Keep these calls quick and to the point. Most professional salespeople realize that the provider's and staff's time is extremely valuable and respect this. It may be the healthcare facility policy to give the salesperson an appointment, possibly over the lunch hour, to discuss the new product or service with the provider and/or office manager. Developing a rapport with representatives of the companies whose products the practice uses frequently may result in a discounted price and first news of sales and promotions. In turn, these professionals rarely waste the time of office personnel.

CRITICAL THINKING APPLICATION   **10.6**

Ashlynn answers the phone; the caller is a pharmaceutical representative who has been visiting the clinic for several months. She cheerfully greets him and asks if he is calling to make an appointment. He states that he wants to make an appointment with Ashlynn — for a date. How should she handle this call? What problems could arise if this were a patient and Ashlynn were to accept the date?

Callers With Difficulty Communicating

Occasionally calls come into the office from patients or family members who have difficulty with the English language. In some cases, English is not the caller's primary language, so the medical assistant must use listening skills to ensure understanding. If a certain language is predominant in the area, the healthcare facility should consider hiring a medical assistant who is **bilingual**. Some patients speak English but have a heavy accent, so you should listen carefully and ask questions to be sure you have understood the person correctly. Many resources are available to assist with translation. The healthcare facility may contract with a translator who would be available to help with telephone calls and patient visits in the office. Many online services also offer translation. If the healthcare facility has a number of patients who speak a specific language other than English, it would be helpful to have commonly used phrases available in that language, especially the phrase that would refer the patient to the specific translation service used by the healthcare facility.

Some providers may have a number of patients who are deaf or hard of hearing. These patients may use a relay system to communicate with healthcare facilities over the telephone. Some relay systems have the patient use a keyboard to enter the information to an operator, who calls the office and reads the information to you; your response is then typed back to the patient. Newer technology uses an online captioned telephone service, much like closed captioning for television. Many smart phones can use a translation app to assist the caller. You should be familiar with the way this system works so that you can engage in these conversations in a professional manner.

TYPICAL OUTGOING CALLS

Most outgoing calls in the healthcare facility are responses to incoming calls. The same rules for courtesy and diction apply to calls made from the office to patients, other individuals, and businesses.

It is helpful to plan outgoing calls in advance. For instance, if the medical assistant is placing an order for office supplies, a list should be made that includes the product, the price, the quantity needed, and a catalog page number, if applicable. Questions about the various

products ordered should be noted so that they can be asked while the sales representative is on the telephone.

Some medical assistants find it helpful to make all outgoing calls at once, when possible. This way the calls can be made one after another, and if a call back is necessary, the medical assistant is likely to still be by the telephone. Organizing calls helps increase office efficiency.

Never be rude to an individual on the telephone. Remember to treat those on the other end of the telephone as you would wish to be treated. Do not forget that you are a representative of the provider and that you must behave in a professional manner at all times.

Time Zones

When making outgoing calls, it is important to keep time zones in mind, especially when calling patients. If you are trying to contact a patient who is spending the winter somewhere else, you should place that call at an appropriate time for the patient. If you are trying to get information from an insurance company, you should call when someone is available to answer your questions. The continental United States is divided into four standard time zones: Pacific, Mountain, Central, and Eastern (Fig. 10.4). When it is noon Pacific time, it is 3 p.m. Eastern time. If you will be calling from San Francisco to a business or professional office in New York, plan to make the call no later than 1 p.m. When it is 2 p.m. on the West Coast, it is 5 p.m. on the East Coast.

Long Distance Calling

Long distance calls are simple to place, usually inexpensive, and efficient. When information is needed in a hurry, telephoning is much more expedient than written communication. Before placing a long distance call, have the correct number ready. If you do not have the number, you may access directory assistance by dialing 1, then the area code of the party you want to call, followed by 555-1212. In some areas, numbers are available by calling 1-411. Directory assistance is now an automated service in many regions, and you will be asked for the name of the city and person you are calling. Often a fee is charged for using directory assistance, so look for the telephone number using free sources whenever possible.

Some internet services, such as Skype, Jajah, or magicJack, allow the user to call long distance, and sometimes even internationally, through the computer with no long distance charges.

USING DIRECTORY ASSISTANCE

Before placing a telephone call, have the correct number ready. If you do not have the number, you may access local directory assistance by calling 411. For long distance numbers, you can access directory assistance by:

- dialing 1
- the area code of the party you want to call
- followed by 555-1212

Directory assistance is now an automated service in many regions. You will be asked for the name of the city and person you are calling. Often a fee is charged for using directory assistance, so, whenever possible, look for the telephone number using free sources.

A telephone directory would be one such free source. This directory is a list of those who have telephones, their telephone numbers and,

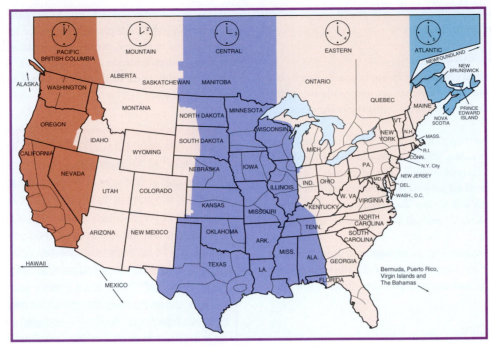

FIGURE 10.4 Time zones across the United States.

in most cases, their addresses. Yellow Pages contains listings for businesses. Directories are found on the internet and in print format.

The internet makes searching for telephone numbers much easier. Try to find telephone numbers through websites such as *www.yellowpages.com* or *www.whitepages.com,* or use a printed telephone book to avoid directory assistance charges on the monthly phone bill. A Web search for the business or provider needed may give you the information. Companies with websites usually have a "Contact Us" page that directs the user to the individual departments.

In a print telephone directory, color coding is often used to differentiate between residence listings and business listings. Governmental offices usually have their own section (commonly blue). Some print directories include ZIP code maps for the local area.

TELEPHONE SERVICES

Answering Services

If an emergency arises, patients expect to be able to contact their provider. This means that the telephone in the healthcare facility must be answered at all times, day and night, weekends and holidays. During normal office hours, the medical assistant is available to answer the telephone. After office hours, most healthcare facilities use an answering service or an answering machine that directs the caller to the answering service if there is an urgent issue.

With an answering service, a person answers the call, which can be comforting for patients. The staff at the answering service can act as a buffer for the provider after hours by screening the calls. By following the criteria given to them by the healthcare facility, they can determine whether the provider (or on-call person) should be contacted or the patient directed to the hospital emergency department, or whether a message can be taken and relayed to the healthcare facility in the morning.

It is common courtesy to call the answering service in the morning to let them know that you will be answering the calls and also to retrieve any messages taken overnight or over the weekend. You should also call the answering service when you are leaving for the day. Answering services also can be used to cover the telephone if all staff members need to be away from the telephones at the same time.

Automatic Call Routing

Many healthcare facilities have started using an **automatic call routing** system. The caller is given a menu of choices; he or she then presses a number on the telephone keypad to direct the call to the correct department. This can be an efficient way to handle a large volume of calls, but it can also be frustrating for some patients, especially elderly adults who may have trouble hearing and remembering the options. Some of the frustration can be minimized by providing a number option that connects the caller with a person (e.g., "Press 0"), who can then transfer the call to the appropriate department.

CRITICAL THINKING APPLICATION **10.7**

Ashlynn has had many complaints from patients about the new call routing system because it takes so long to "get to a human being." How can she help make modern call routing systems easier for her patients?

CLOSING COMMENTS

Patient Coaching

Today's telephone systems allow providers to educate patients while they are on hold; recordings may be played that offer health information on subjects from A to Z. These messages can be professionally recorded and/or custom designed by the provider and staff. Special events may be announced, with the option to press a certain number for more information about the event.

Legal and Ethical Issues

The guidelines for medical confidentiality apply equally to telephone conversations; therefore, take care that no one overhears sensitive information. Use discretion when mentioning the name of the caller or patient.

Do not place or receive personal phone calls during work hours. Time limitations for personal phone use should be described in the office policies and procedures manual. The telephone is a business line and should be reserved for patients and others conducting business with the office. Personal cell phones also should not be used during working hours; this takes the medical assistant's time and attention away from patient care.

Telephone message records may be brought into court as evidence; make sure all messages are complete and legible. Most offices should keep these records for at least the same period as the statute of limitations in that state.

Patient-Centered Care

When answering the telephone in a healthcare facility, the medical assistant has many opportunities to provide patient-centered care.

First and foremost, you should respect the patients' preferences. This could be using their cell phone number for returning calls or using their preferred name or nickname when talking with them. Secondly, telephone communication is a big part of coordination of care. Remaining professional in all interactions will ensure that the patient's needs will be met.

Professional Behaviors

We have talked on telephones and cell phones in our own lives, and most of us have used at least some of the special features on our phones. It is important to recognize that the way we present ourselves on the phone in our professional lives is different from the style of communication we use in our personal lives. The way we speak in our personal lives may not be appropriate in the healthcare facility. We must maintain a professional tone in communications with our patients and other contacts. For example, slang should not be used; "Hello" is not a proper way to answer a business telephone; and we must take care how we use medical terminology when on the telephone (jargon should not be used when speaking with patients). The goal is always to present a positive professional image of the healthcare facility we represent.

SUMMARY OF SCENARIO

Ashlynn is quickly becoming a part of the team at WMFM and is developing into a well-liked asset to the staff. She has learned to slow down when speaking on the phone and to adjust her volume and pitch, depending on the patient with whom she is speaking. Although she tends to be quite talkative, she is balancing just the right amount of friendly chatter with the business at hand. She does this by offering a friendly greeting to callers, getting to the point of the call, then being affable before ending the call. By expressing her concern and asking how she can be of help to the patients, Ashlynn shows them that she sincerely cares about their problems. She is careful about her tone of voice, realizing that patients may take her comments the wrong way if she does not treat them in a cordial manner.

Ashlynn takes care when she speaks to patients and others on the phone so that she does not breach confidentiality in any way. She has become comfortable with the way she is expected to answer the telephone. The pace of her speech

and the wording are now a habit. Ashlynn is determined to maintain a professional relationship with all the people related to her work environment. She is adept now at handling calls from angry patients and can maintain control with even the most aggressive callers. She leaves callers on hold for a minimum time and reassures them frequently that she is attending to their situation. By treating callers as she would want to be treated, Ashlynn reduces frustration, and she feels that the office is more efficient at handling the large volume of calls that come in each day. She shows much promise for a long and rewarding career in the medical field and is satisfied with the current track of her career. As she continues to settle into her position, she looks forward to learning more about efficiency and time management. Her positive attitude and desire to learn will only enhance her performance at work, making her a valuable employee and one worth promoting.

SUMMARY OF LEARNING OBJECTIVES

1. **Identify and explain the features of a multiple-line telephone system, and also explain how each can be used effectively in a healthcare facility. Also, discuss the use of cell phones.**

   A multiple-line telephone system has many features; most obviously, more than one telephone line comes into the office. This means that callers are less likely to get a busy signal when calling the healthcare

   facility. Additional features, such as speed dial, voice mail, and call forwarding, can increase efficiency.

   Medical assistants must understand how each feature of the telephone system works. For example, knowing when to use the speakerphone function and when not to helps protect patient confidentiality. Knowing how to use the conference call feature helps facilitate telephone

SUMMARY OF LEARNING OBJECTIVES—continued

meetings with satellite offices. Understanding how the voice mail system works is crucial to the medical assistant's work life.

Many people have a personal cell phone or a smart phone. While it is great to be accessible at all times, cell phones also present some issues in a healthcare facility, particularly in regard to patient confidentiality.

2. **Do the following related to effective use of the telephone:**
   - *Discuss the telephone equipment needed by a healthcare facility.*
   Two incoming lines is the minimum recommended number of lines for a healthcare facility. Telephones should be placed where they are accessible but private. One medical assistant can handle no more than two incoming lines; this means that the addition of more lines may involve the need for more employees.
   - *Summarize active listening skills.*
   A big part of communication is being able to listen. Honing your active listening skills also will increase your communication skills. Focus on the conversation by being present in the moment. Not only is interrupting rude, it also shows that you were not listening, truly listening, because you were coming up with your response. Part of active listening is confirming what you heard to be sure that you have received the intended message.
   - *Demonstrate effective and professional telephone techniques.*
   Medical assistants should answer the telephone promptly and professionally. A pleasing telephone personality conveys a favorable impression of the healthcare facility. Enunciate, pronouncing words clearly and distinctly. Vary the pitch of your voice, and avoid a monotonous or droning manner. Courtesy to patients and other callers is vital. First impressions are important, and a medical assistant's telephone manner sets the tone for the caller's perception of the healthcare facility. Be courteous and polite to all callers. (Refer to Procedure 10.1.)
   - *Consider the importance of tone of voice and enunciation.*
   Tone of voice can completely change the message sent. Make sure you use the correct tone of voice so that the message is not misunderstood. Enunciation also ensures that your message is not misunderstood. Communicating over the telephone has its own issues, and enunciation is crucial. Speaking clearly helps your caller to hear your message.

3. **Explain the importance of thinking ahead when managing telephone calls; also, describe the correct way to answer the telephone in the office.**
   Before you start answering calls, make sure you have all of the supplies you need to do your job. Confidentiality in a healthcare facility must always be a priority.
   Medical assistants should answer the telephone promptly and professionally. The provider's image is affected by the way telephone calls are handled. Be courteous and polite to all callers. The medical assistant should identify the facility first when picking up the phone, followed by his or her name, followed by an offer of help. If the caller does not offer a name, the medical assistant should ask who is calling.

4. **Discuss the screening of incoming calls and list several questions to ask when handling an emergency call.**
   Most healthcare facilities expect the medical assistant answering the telephone to screen the calls; this is an important task. The facility's screening policies should address how calls should be handled when the provider is out of the office, and the medical assistant should always ask before placing a caller on hold or transferring a call.
   If a phone call is an emergency, the policies for handling emergency calls apply. Ask for a phone number where the caller can be reached in case of a sudden disconnection. Ask about the chief symptoms and when they started. Find out whether the patient has had similar symptoms in the past and what happened in that situation. Determine whether the patient is alone, has transportation, or needs an ambulance. In severe cases, do not hang up the phone until the ambulance or police arrive. A special sheet of instructions listing specific medical emergencies (e.g., chest pain, heavy bleeding, seizure, fainting, poisoning) should be posted by each telephone.

5. **Place callers on hold and correctly transfer a phone call.**
   When working with a multiple-line telephone, it is important to know how to deal with more than one call at a time. When you are on a call and the other line rings, you need to place the first call on hold, answer the second call, determine whether or not it is an emergency (and follow proper protocol), and then return to the first call. During the screening process, the medical assistant may determine that the call should be transferred to the provider or to another person in the facility. Know who does what in your healthcare facility.

6. **Do the following related to taking a message:**
   - *Document telephone messages accurately.*
   When taking a telephone message, either in a handwritten or an electronic format, strive for accuracy. Be sure to get all the information the provider will need to act. Repeat any words or numbers that are not heard clearly. (Refer to Procedure 10.2.)
   - *List the seven elements of a correctly handled telephone message.*
   The seven elements of a correctly handled phone message are (1) the name of the person to whom the call should be directed; (2) the name of the person calling; (3) the caller's telephone number; (4) the reason for the call; (5) the medical assistant's description of the action to be taken; (6) the date and time of the call; and (7) the initials of the person taking the call, so that if any question arises that person can be consulted.
   - *Report relevant information concisely and accurately.*
   If a handwritten system is used for recording telephone messages, a policy must be developed on the retention of the telephone message records. Accurate records can ensure quality patient care and customer service. (Refer to Procedure 10.2.)

7. **Discuss various types of common incoming calls and how to deal with each.**
   Knowing how to respond to the different types of calls received will make you a valuable asset to the healthcare facility. Common types of incoming calls include the following: requests for directions; inquiries

Continued

SUMMARY OF LEARNING OBJECTIVES—continued

about bills; inquiries about fees; inquiries about participating providers; requests for assistance with insurance; inquiries about radiology and laboratory reports; progress reports; routine report calls from hospitals or other sources; requests for a referral; and questions about office administration matters.

8. Discuss various types of special incoming calls and how to deal with each.

If a patient refuses to discuss symptoms with a medical assistant, follow the healthcare facility's policies and procedures, which may suggest that the patient make an appointment with the provider to discuss the problem in person. Other types of special calls a medical assistant must know how to handle include unsatisfactory progress reports, requests for test results, requests for information from third parties, complaints about care or fees, and calls from a staff member's family or friends.

9. Discuss how the medical assistant should handle various types of difficult calls.

With angry callers, never return the anger. Remain calm and speak in tones that are perhaps slightly quieter than those of the caller. This often prompts the caller to lower his or her tone of voice. Offer to help the angry person and ask questions to gain control of the conversation, moving it toward resolution. Do not argue with angry callers.

Callers who have a complaint should be handled in a manner similar to that for angry callers. Remain calm and offer to help. Take a serious interest in what the caller has to say. Let the caller know that his or her concerns are important to the staff and the provider. Find the source of the problem and determine exactly what the caller wants or expects as a resolution. Always follow up on complaints and make sure they were resolved as much to the caller's satisfaction as possible.

Other types of difficult callers that medical assistants must know how to handle include aggressive callers, unauthorized inquiry calls, sales calls, and callers with difficulty communicating.

10. Discuss typical outgoing calls, including why knowledge of time zones and long distance calling is necessary.

Most outgoing calls in the healthcare facility are made in response to incoming calls. It is helpful to plan outgoing calls in advance. Organizing calls helps increase office efficiency.

The continental United States is divided into four standard time zones. Long distance calls are simple to place, usually inexpensive, and efficient. Knowledge of both concepts is important for a medical assistant handling the telephone.

11. Discuss the use of a telephone directory and describe how answering services and automatic call routing systems are used in a healthcare facility.

The primary purpose of a telephone directory is to provide lists of those who have telephones, their telephone numbers and, in most cases, their addresses. The internet makes searching for telephone numbers much easier.

Answering services are used to answer the telephone in the healthcare facility when the staff is not available. This could be during the overnight hours or during regular office hours when the staff is at lunch or in a meeting. Automatic call routing systems allow the patient to select a number from a menu to reach specific departments in the healthcare facility. The system should have an option that allows patients to choose to speak to a person if they are not sure what number to press.

12. Discuss the legal and ethical issues related to telephone techniques.

The guidelines for medical confidentiality apply equally to telephone conversations; therefore, take care that no one overhears sensitive information. Telephone records may be brought to court as evidence.

PROCEDURE 10.1   Demonstrate Professional Telephone Techniques

Task: To answer the telephone in a provider's office in a professional manner and respond to a request for action.

Scenario: Charles Johnson, DOB 3/3/1958, an established patient of Dr. Martin, has called to schedule an appointment to have his blood pressure checked. This will be a follow-up appointment that is 15 minutes long. He is requesting that the appointment be on a Friday during his lunchtime between 11:00 and 12:00.

EQUIPMENT and SUPPLIES
- Telephone
- Pen or pencil
- Appointment book or EHR with appointment scheduling abilities
- Computer
- Notepad

PROCEDURAL STEPS
1. Demonstrate telephone techniques by answering the telephone by the third ring.
   PURPOSE: To convey interest in the caller by answering promptly. This makes a positive impression on the caller.
2. Speak distinctly with a pleasant tone and expression, at a moderate rate, and with sufficient volume for the person to understand every word.
   PURPOSE: Proper enunciation will help the patient to understand.

PROCEDURE 10.1   Demonstrate Professional Telephone Techniques—*continued*

3. Identify the office and/or provider and yourself.
   PURPOSE: To assure the caller that the correct number has been reached and to identify the staff member.
4. Verify the identity of the caller, and if using an electronic health record, bring the patient's health record to the active screen of the computer.
   PURPOSE: To confirm the origin of the call.
5. Screen the call if necessary.
   PURPOSE: To determine whether the caller has an emergency and needs immediate attention or referral to a hospital emergency department.
6. Apply active listening skills to assess whether the caller is distressed or agitated and to determine the concern to be addressed.
   PURPOSE: To make sure the medical assistant hears and understands the message being sent by the patient and to show that the patient has the medical assistant's full attention.
7. Determine the needs of the caller and provide the requested information or service if possible. Provide the caller with excellent customer service. Be as helpful as possible. Check the appointment schedule and determine the first Friday that would have an open appointment between 11:00 and 12:00.
   PURPOSE: To allow the medical assistant to handle many calls and conserve the provider's and staff members' time and energy.
8. Obtain sufficient patient information to schedule the appointment, including the patient's full name, DOB, insurance information, and preferred contact method. Repeat the date and time of the appointment to ensure that the patient has the correct information.
   PURPOSE: By obtaining the correct patient information, the correct patient record will be pulled (if paper records are used) for the appointment. In an EHR the appointment will be attached to the correct patient record.
9. Terminate the call in a pleasant manner and replace the receiver gently, always allowing the caller to hang up first.
   PURPOSE: To promote good public relations, provide excellent customer service, and ensure that the caller has no further questions.

PROCEDURE 10.2   Document Telephone Messages and Report Relevant Information Concisely and Accurately

Task: To take an accurate telephone message and follow up on the requests made by the caller.

EQUIPMENT and SUPPLIES

- Telephone
- Computer
- Message pad
- Pen or pencil
- Notepad
- Health record

Scenario: Norma Washington, DOB 8/1/1944, an established patient of Dr. Martin, has called to report her blood pressure readings that she has been taking at home. Dr. Martin had made a recent change in her medication and wanted her to monitor her BP at home for 3 days and call in with the results. She has taken her blood pressure in the morning and in the evening for the past 3 days, with the following results:

Day 1: 144/92 in the am, 156/94 in the pm
Day 2: 136/84 in the am, 142/86 in the pm
Day 3: 132/80 in the am, 138/82 in the pm

PROCEDURAL STEPS

1. Demonstrate telephone techniques by answering the telephone using the guidelines in Procedure 10.1.
   PURPOSE: To answer promptly and courteously, which conveys interest in the caller and promotes good customer service.
2. Using a message pad or the computer, take the phone message (either on paper or by data entry into the computer) and obtain the following information:
   - Name of the person to whom the call is directed
   - Name of the person calling
   - Caller's telephone number
   - Reason for the call
   - Action to be taken
   - Date and time of the call
   - Initials of the person taking the call
   PURPOSE: To have accurate information, which allows the staff member or provider to address the caller's issues quickly and efficiently.
3. Apply active listening skills and repeat the information back to the caller after recording the message.
   PURPOSE: To verify that all the information was recorded accurately.
4. End the call and wait for the caller to hang up first.
5. Document the telephone call with all pertinent information in the patient's health record.
   PURPOSE: To ensure that the patient's health record is kept up to date.
6. Deliver the phone message to the appropriate person.
7. Follow up on important messages.
   PURPOSE: To make sure important issues are addressed in a timely manner.
8. If using paper messaging, keep old message books for future reference. Carbonless copies allow the facility to keep a permanent record of phone messages. If using an electronic system, the message will be saved to the patient's record automatically.
   PURPOSE: To have a permanent source of messages in case the information is needed after the paper message has been discarded. This can also serve as a telephone log.
9. File pertinent phone messages in the patient's health record. Make sure the computer record is closed after the documentation has been done.
   PURPOSE: To keep a permanent record of important information in the patient's chart.

11

SCHEDULING APPOINTMENTS AND PATIENT PROCESSING

SCENARIO

Ramona West is the medical assistant in charge of scheduling appointments and patient processing for Dr. Angela Perez. Ramona is an extremely organized person who thinks quickly and creatively. Two of her professional goals are to ensure that the healthcare facility remains on schedule throughout the day with minimal wait time for the patients, and that patient flow through the office is done in an efficient manner. She is fortunate that Dr. Perez is cooperative and time oriented, and they work well together to reach these common goals.

Ramona usually arrives at work at least 15 minutes early to begin her preparations for the day. She reviews the electronic health record for each patient to make sure test results from previous visits are available to the provider and that the medical record is complete. She pays special attention to the patients who arrive in the healthcare facility as she completes her daily tasks, remembering the importance of providing patients with good customer service. Ramona greets each patient by name and carries on a brief but cordial conversation. Patients appreciate that she goes the extra mile to remember something about them, and this promotes excellent patient relations.

Ramona leaves a little time in the morning and afternoon for emergency appointments. The healthcare facility uses an automatic call routing system to contact patients to confirm appointments in advance, which increases her show rate. She is always pleasant to the patients as they go through the check-in and checkout procedures. Her friendly, caring attitude makes her a favorite among the patients, and Dr. Perez is pleased with the relationship-building skills Ramona has developed.

While studying this chapter, think about the following questions:

- How can the medical assistant contribute to an efficient daily routine?
- How does the medical assistant contribute to keeping the daily schedule on track?
- How can the schedule be put back on track when emergencies disrupt the day?
- How does the flexibility of the medical assistant contribute to office efficiency?
- What are some ways to develop good rapport with patients?
- Why is a sign-in register a potential breach of patient confidentiality?
- What is the value of knowing some information about patients' personal lives?

LEARNING OBJECTIVES

1. Describe guidelines for establishing an appointment schedule and creating an appointment matrix.
2. Discuss the advantages of computerized appointment scheduling.
3. Discuss appointment book scheduling and explain how self-scheduling can reduce the number of calls to the healthcare facility.
4. Discuss the legality of the appointment scheduling system.
5. Discuss pros and cons of various types of appointment management systems.
6. Discuss telephone scheduling and identify critical information required for scheduling appointments for new patients.
7. Discuss scheduling appointments for established patients.
8. Discuss how the medical assistant should handle scheduling of other types of appointments.
9. Do the following related to special circumstances in scheduling:
   - Discuss several methods of dealing with patients who consistently arrive late.
   - Recognize office policies and protocols for rescheduling appointments.
   - Discuss how to deal with emergencies, provider referrals, and patients without appointments.
10. Discuss how to handle failed appointments and no-shows, in addition to methods to increase appointment show rates.
11. Discuss how to handle cancellations and delays.
12. Describe how to prepare for patients' arrivals, including patient check-in procedures.
13. Do the following related to patient reception and processing:
    - Show consideration for patients' time.
    - Properly treat patients with special needs.
    - Escort and instruct the patient.
    - Describe where health records should be placed.
14. Describe how the medical assistant should deal with challenging situations, such as talkative patients, children, angry patients, and patients' relatives and friends.

VOCABULARY

demographics Statistical data of a population. In healthcare this includes the patient's name, address, date of birth, employment, and other details.

disruption An unexpected event that throws a plan into disorder; an interruption that prevents a system or process from continuing as usual or as expected.

established patient A patient who has been treated previously by the healthcare provider within the past 3 years.

expediency (ik SPEE dee uhn see) A means of achieving a particular end, as in a situation requiring urgency or caution.

follow-up (recheck) appointment An appointment type used when a patient needs to see the provider after a condition should have been resolved or to monitor an ongoing condition, such as hypertension. Also known as a recheck appointment.

integral (IN ti gruhl) Essential; being an indispensable part of a whole.

interval Space of time between events.

matrix (MEY triks) The environment in which something is created or takes shape. A base on which to build.

no-show Failure of a patient to keep an appointment without advance notice.

Notice of Privacy Practices (NPP) A written document describing the healthcare facility's privacy practices. The patient must be provided with the NPP and sign an acknowledgment of receipt.

parameters (puh RAM it ers) Rules that control how something should be done; guidelines or boundaries.

patient portal A secure online website that gives patients 24-hour access to personal health information using a username and password.

practice management software A type of software that allows the user to enter demographic information, schedule appointments, maintain lists of insurance payers, perform billing tasks, and generate reports.

preauthorization A process required by some insurance carriers in which the provider obtains permission to perform certain procedures or services or refers a patient to a specialist.

precertification The process of determining if a procedure or service is covered by the insurance plan and what the reimbursement is for that procedure or service.

proficiency (pruh FISH uhn see) Skilled as a result of training or practice.

progress notes Documentation in the medical record to track the patient's condition and progress.

screening A system for examining and separating into different groups; in the healthcare facility, it means determining the severity of illness that patients experience and prioritizing appointments based on that severity.

triage (tree AHZH) To sort out and classify the injured; used in the military and in emergency settings to determine the priority of patients to be treated.

verification of eligibility The process of confirming health insurance coverage for the patient.

The provider's time is the most valuable asset of a medical practice. The person responsible for scheduling this time must understand the practice, be familiar with the working habits and preferences of the provider (or providers), and have clear guidelines for time management in the practice.

Appointment scheduling is the process that determines which patients the provider sees, the dates and times of appointments, and how much time is allotted to each patient based on the complaint and the provider's availability. Time management involves the realization that unforeseen interruptions and delays always occur and must be handled appropriately. In addition, the medical assistant must assign the appropriate appointment time length for the complaint, along with ensuring that the appointments are scheduled so that there are minimal gaps in the schedule. Most healthcare providers find that efficient appointment scheduling is one of the most important factors in the success of the practice. Scheduling can be done in a number of ways, and each facility must find the way that suits it best.

SCHEDULING APPOINTMENTS
Establishing the Appointment Schedule

Developing a schedule that meets the needs of both the providers and the patients is the key to keeping the office running smoothly and efficiently. The scheduling team, along with the provider, should come up with scheduling **parameters** both to meet the needs of the patients and to keep the providers' preferences and habits in mind.

Patient Needs

Consider the **demographics** of the patients when determining office hours and appointment times. The staff should answer the following questions:

- Is the office in a busy metropolitan area or a rural community?
- What type of patients are seen? Are they of a specific age or gender? Do they have common diagnoses? Is the provider a general practitioner?
- Are evening and weekend appointments needed for most of the patients served?

Knowing when the providers need to be available for patients is one of the factors in creating the patient schedule.

Provider Preferences and Habits

Consider the preferences and habits of the providers in the practice before establishing and implementing a scheduling plan. Ask the following questions:

- Does the provider become restless if the reception room is not packed with waiting patients?
- Does the provider worry if even one patient is kept waiting?
- Is the provider careful about being in the facility when patient appointments are scheduled to begin?

- Is the provider habitually late?
- Does the provider move easily from one patient to another?
- Does the provider require a "break time" after a few patients?
- Would the provider rather see fewer patients and spend more time with each one or schedule more patients each day?

All of these preferences and habits become an **integral** part of the scheduling process. Keep in mind that the provider cannot spend every moment of the day with patients. The provider also has telephone calls to make and receive, reports to examine and dictate, meetings to attend, mail to answer, and many other business responsibilities. An experienced staff can handle many but not all of these tasks.

Next, the office hours and the length of appointment time **intervals** need to be determined. Keeping in mind patients' needs and the provider's preferences and habits, decide what would be the shortest time possible for an appointment. Most healthcare facilities use 10- or 15-minute time intervals for the appointment schedule. Paper-based appointment books can be purchased with various time intervals. A computerized appointment system can also be set to the specific time interval that has been decided on. A computerized system can be customized for different providers, so that one provider could have 10-minute time slots, and another could have 15-minute time slots. If an appointment, such as a complete physical, needs longer than

15 minutes, multiple time slots are used to cover that appointment. Once the minimum time period has been set, then the appointment **matrix** can be established.

Creating the Appointment Matrix

Setting up the appointment matrix (see Procedure 11.1, p. 233) involves blocking out the times when the provider is not available to see patients (Fig. 11.1), such as:

- Lunch time
- Hospital rounds
- Conferences
- Vacation

In a paper-based appointment book, the matrix is usually established for 6 months at a time. In a computerized system the matrix can be set up indefinitely.

Establishing Guidelines for Appointment Scheduling

The first step in setting up the schedule matrix is to decide the length of the shortest office visit type. This visit type would usually be for a **follow-up** or **recheck appointment** for an established patient. Other specific appointment types should then be determined. General categories for appointment types are:

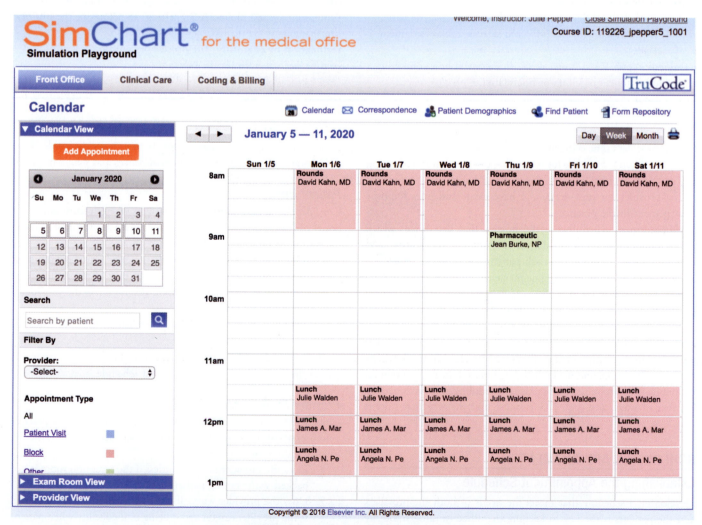

FIGURE 11.1 Schedule matrix showing provider availability.

- Follow-up or recheck
- Wellness examination
- Complete physical examination
- Urgent visit
- New patient visit
- Comprehensive visit

Each category has a specific amount of time assigned to it; for example, a follow-up or recheck appointment could be 10 to 15 minutes, and a comprehensive visit could be 30 to 40 minutes. The providers and scheduling team should work together to come up with these time periods to ensure that the office runs smoothly and efficiently. The shortest appointment time will be one line or block on the schedule. If an appointment is going to be longer than that time, multiple lines or blocks would be used. In Fig. 11.1 each line on the schedule is for 15 minutes. Hospital rounds for Dr. Julie Walden are scheduled for 1 hour, or four lines. In this example, if a patient is being seen for a recheck appointment (15 minutes), only one line would be used. If the patient were being seen for a comprehensive visit (30 minutes), two lines would be used. In a paper appointment book you may need to put arrows or a line through the additional appointment time so that another patient is not scheduled during that time (Fig. 11.2).

If it is decided that a complete physical examination should be scheduled for 30 minutes, yet the provider routinely spends 45 minutes with the patient for a complete physical, then the scheduling guidelines need to be adjusted. Well-planned scheduling and sticking to that schedule allow the provider to do more than run in and out of examination rooms with little time for the patient to talk with the provider. There will be a bit of trial and error when developing priorities for the appointment schedule.

Some providers need prompting to end the patient visit and move to the next patient. If there is a medical assistant in the examination room, he or she can help the provider remain on schedule by letting the provider know that the end of the appointment time is near. Some type of signal may be worked out, such as a hand gesture or phrase. A pager may be used when the medical assistant is not in room with the provider. When the provider's pager vibrates, he or she will know that it is time to wind things up with that patient. The clinical medical assistant and the administrative medical assistant must work together to keep the healthcare facility running smoothly and efficiently.

CRITICAL THINKING APPLICATION 11.1

- Ramona has noticed that Dr. Perez is taking a little longer with patients than normal and that she is running consistently behind schedule by approximately 5 to 15 minutes. How can Ramona help rectify this situation?
- Discuss ways of approaching the provider when he or she is the cause of the delays in the schedule. What opening remarks can the medical assistant use to start the discussion in a positive way?

Available Facilities

Another factor to keep in mind when scheduling appointments is the availability of facilities needed for a specific appointment type. Getting a patient into the office at a time when no room or equipment is available for the services needed is a waste of the patient's time. For example, suppose that a healthcare facility with two providers has only one room that can be used for minor surgery. Do not

	Monday	Tuesday	Wednesday	Thursday	Friday
8:00					
8:15					
8:30		Celia Tapia PE			
8:45		↓			
9:00	Truong Tran Recheck				
9:15					
9:30					
9:45					
10:00					

FIGURE 11.2 Blocking off time on the appointment schedule.

schedule two patients needing minor surgery for the same day and time, even if both doctors could be available. If the healthcare facility has only one electrocardiograph, do not book two electrocardiograms (ECGs) at the same time. As the medical assistant gains **proficiency** in scheduling, it becomes easier to match patient needs with the available facilities. Major equipment frequently used or a certain room with such equipment may need its own scheduling column in the appointment book or software system.

Methods of Scheduling Appointments

The two most common methods of appointment scheduling are:
- computerized scheduling
- appointment book or paper-based scheduling.

Each has advantages and disadvantages. The healthcare facility should weigh the benefits and choose the method that best suits the provider and the staff.

Computerized Scheduling

The computer has replaced the appointment book in many practices. **Practice management software** ranges from relatively simple programs that merely display available and scheduled times to more sophisticated systems that perform several other functions. Information can be entered into the computer program, such as:
- the length and type of appointment required
- the patient's day or time preferences

The computer then can select the best appointment time based on that information.

A computerized scheduling system also has the ability to search for future appointments. For example, when a patient calls and asks about a previously scheduled appointment, the system can search by his or her name to find the time and date. Computerized scheduling allows multiple users to access the schedule at the same time, minimizing the wait time for patients.

Another advantage of computerized schedules is that reports can be generated. A hard copy of the provider's daily schedule can be created showing:
- the patients' names
- telephone numbers
- the reasons for the visits

Some healthcare facilities print these out, and others use them on-screen. Healthcare facilities must have scheduling procedures to follow when the technology is down.

Appointment Book Scheduling

Office suppliers carry a variety of appointment book styles. Some appointment books show an entire week at a glance; many are color coded, with a special color used for each day of the week (Fig. 11.3). This is very helpful when the provider asks the patient to return, for instance, in 2 weeks. If Wednesdays are colored yellow, the medical assistant can flip quickly to the correct day 2 weeks later and schedule the appointment. Multiple columns may be available to correspond with the number of doctors in a group practice, and the time can be divided according to their preferences.

Self-Scheduling

Allowing patients to schedule their own appointments using the internet and the healthcare facility's website is becoming much more

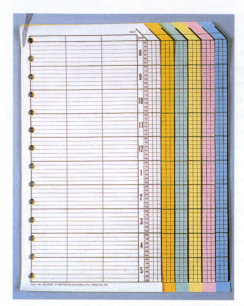

FIGURE 11.3 Color-coded appointment book pages help the medical assistant flip to the right day of the right week quickly. Appointments for multiple providers can be color-coded in the book.

common. The patient is given limited access to the schedule, seeing only the available appointment times, not the other patients who are scheduled.

Software is available that allows the patient to self-schedule through secure links to the provider's appointment book. The software or internet site for the healthcare facility should give the patient guidelines as to the amount of time needed for certain appointments or should allow only a certain length of time to be self-scheduled, such as 15 minutes. These systems will reduce the number of calls and are available to the patient 24 hours a day. Some systems also send an automatic email reminder to the patient the day before the appointment, requesting a reply to confirm. These systems are less frustrating to patients, who do not have to wait on hold to speak to the person who does scheduling for the healthcare facility. However, lengthy or complicated appointments should be scheduled through the staff.

Although this type of system for making appointments appeals to most technologically savvy people, some patients may not be comfortable using it. It does require minimal skills and internet access. Others may object to online scheduling because they do not want their names anywhere on the internet. This is a valid concern, and the facility should allow these patients to schedule over the telephone. If this system is used, some allowance must be made for patients who choose not to use it.

> **CRITICAL THINKING** APPLICATION   **11.2**
>
> The software used at WMFM can allow patients to self-schedule. Ramona has heard about patient self-scheduling and would like to try this method in the office, but Dr. Perez is concerned that her patients will miss the personal contact and is not sold on the idea. What can Ramona say to convince Dr. Perez to try this new, time-saving method of scheduling? What challenges might the use of this system bring?

Legality of the Appointment Scheduling System

Because the paper-based appointment book can be used as a legal record, it must be accurate and maintained so that it provides correct information about the patients at the healthcare facility. Patients are expected to follow the provider's orders; this includes keeping appointments. If a patient does not show up for an appointment or cancels it and does not reschedule, documentation of this fact should be placed in the patient's health record. If a patient reschedules an appointment and subsequently keeps it, there is no need to document that it was rescheduled.

Pens are permanent, and the appointment book can become illegible if a number of patients change or cancel their appointments. To make changes to an appointment book easier, pencil should be used. The information in the book includes the patient's name and a phone number where the patient can be reached. Some healthcare facilities list the reason for the appointment, but most note only the name and phone number. Listing the reason for the visit is not necessary if the medical assistant references the time needed for the appointment and blocks off that amount of time. Because the appointment book could be evidence as a legal record, it should be kept for the number of years that constitute the statute of limitations in that individual state. If the appointment book is discarded, its contents should be shredded to protect patient privacy.

Although the appointment book can be used as a legal record, actual medical records are more likely to be used in matters of litigation. Because **progress notes** are dated, a copy of the medical record shows all pertinent information about the patient's adherence to the provider's orders, including the appointments with the provider.

Computerized scheduling systems can also be used to track patient appointments. Most computerized scheduling systems will allow the user to indicate if the patient has checked in, canceled, or missed the scheduled appointment. When a patient misses or cancels an appointment, it should be documented in the electronic patient record for legal purposes.

Types of Appointment Scheduling

Different types of appointment scheduling are used to meet the various needs of the medical facility, the providers, and the patients. Some offices use a combination of methods to create the right mix of activity during the day and to ensure that the day runs smoothly and efficiently. The medical assistant should become proficient at managing appointments. The following section presents several methods of appointment scheduling.

No matter what appointment scheduling method is used, the medical assistant should make it a policy to leave some open time during each day's schedule. This is so that if a patient calls with a special problem that is not an immediate emergency, time will be available to book the patient for at least a brief visit. Mondays and Fridays generally are the most hectic days of the week. Keeping a time slot available in the morning and the afternoon specifically for emergencies also is a wise practice. A busy provider always fills these open slots, and having them in the schedule causes the least **disruption** during the day. If possible, set aside time in the morning and afternoon for a break. Even 15 minutes can give the provider time to return calls from patients, verify prescription calls, or answer questions.

Time-Specified (Stream) Scheduling

When each patient is given a specific time for an appointment, this is referred to as *time-specified* or *stream scheduling*. This method keeps a steady flow of patients moving through the office. This is the most common type of scheduling used in healthcare facilities. Studies have shown that providers can see more patients with less pressure when patient appointments are scheduled for a specific time slot. The medical assistant who is scheduling patients using this method should know the amount of time needed for each appointment type and keep time slots available for urgent visits.

Wave Scheduling

Wave scheduling is an attempt to create flexibility within each hour. Wave scheduling assumes that the actual time needed for all the patients seen will average out over the course of the day. Instead of scheduling patients at each 15-minute interval, wave scheduling has three patients in the office at the same time. They are then seen in the order of their arrival. This way, one person's late arrival does not disrupt the entire schedule.

Modified Wave Scheduling

The wave schedule can be modified in several ways. For example, one method is to have two patients scheduled to come in at 10 a.m. and a third at 10:30 a.m. This hourly cycle is repeated throughout the day. In another version, patients are scheduled to arrive at given intervals during the first half of the hour, and none are scheduled to arrive during the second half of the hour. This would allow time for urgent or walk-in patients to be seen.

Double-Booking

Booking of two patients to come in at the same time is sometimes used to work in a patient with an acute illness or injury when there are no open appointments. This works out best if one of the patients needs laboratory work or another procedure done before seeing the provider. The provider can see one of the patients while the other one is being prepared.

Open Office Hours

With the open office hours method, the facility is open at given hours, and the patients are told that they can come in at any time. This type of system is often used in an urgent care setting. Patients are then seen in the order in which they arrive, although a patient with an urgent condition may be seen ahead of those who arrived before him or her.

The open office hours system can have many disadvantages. The office may already be crowded when the provider arrives, resulting in an extremely long wait for some patients. Patients may arrive in waves throughout the day, which causes parts of the day to be very busy and other parts to be slow. This makes accomplishing other office duties difficult. Without planning, the facilities and staff can be overburdened.

CRITICAL THINKING APPLICATION 11.3

Dr. Perez would like to implement evening appointments one night each week and open the office every other Saturday morning. She feels this will better serve her patients with children who have difficulty making daytime appointments. If this is her primary goal, should other types of patients be seen during these time slots? Why or why not?

Grouping Procedures

Grouping, or categorizing, of procedures is another method of scheduling that appeals to many providers. For instance, an internist might reserve all morning appointments for complete physical examinations, or a pediatrician might keep that time for well-baby visits. A surgeon might devote 1 day each week to seeing only referral patients. Obstetricians often schedule pregnant patients on different days from gynecology patients. The providers and staff can experiment with different groupings until the plan that works best for the practice eventually becomes obvious. In applying a grouping system of appointments, the medical assistant may find it helpful to color-code the sections of the appointment book reserved for specific procedures.

Telephone Scheduling

A pleasant manner and a willingness to help are just as important on the telephone as when meeting patients face to face. This is especially true when making appointments. The telephone contact may be the patient's first impression of the facility. Often the way the appointment scheduling process is handled makes more of an impression than the convenience of the appointment time.

Be especially considerate if the time requested for an appointment is not available. Briefly explain why and offer a different date and time. Comply with the patient's wishes as much as possible, and do not show annoyance if the patient does not understand the scheduling process. Most people, however, understand the need for a well-managed office and are willing to cooperate.

Many offices offer the patient a choice when scheduling the appointment and let the patient decide which option is best for him or her. For example, the following dialog might take place during the scheduling call.

Medical assistant:	"Mrs. Thomas, Dr. Perez is available to see you in the office next Tuesday or Wednesday, January 6 or 7. Which day is better for you?"
Patient:	"I will be working on Wednesday, so I would like to come in on Tuesday."
Medical assistant:	"Do you prefer a morning or afternoon appointment?"
Patient:	"The afternoon is best for me."
Medical assistant:	"Great. Would 1:30 or 3:30 be a better time?"
Patient:	"I can be there at 1:30."
Medical assistant:	"Then Dr. Perez will see you at 1:30 next Tuesday, January 6. Thank you for calling, Mrs. Thomas. We'll see you then!"

These small courtesies allow patients to have some control of their time. Always repeat the time to reinforce the appointment and do not hesitate to ask the patient if he or she has a pen ready to jot down the time and date. While repeating the information to the patient, check the appointment book or computer screen to ensure that it was posted correctly. When you schedule appointments over the telephone, it is not possible to provide a reminder card for the appointment. Be sure to ask if the patient would like a telephone, email, or text message reminder of the appointment.

Write legibly when using an appointment book. These records could be called into court, and the medical assistant must be able to read his or her own writing if asked to testify. The patient's daytime telephone number should be recorded for every appointment scheduled. The appointment may need to be canceled or the schedule rearranged in a hurry, and many precious minutes can be saved if the telephone number is handy. Cell phone numbers also are quite useful for quickly tracking down a patient.

Scheduling Appointments for New Patients

Arranging the first appointment for a new patient requires time and attention to detail (see Procedure 11.2, p. 233). This encounter provides the first impression of the healthcare facility and may set the tone for all subsequent visits. Tact, courtesy, and professionalism are extremely important. You will need to obtain information about the *chief complaint* (why the patient needs the appointment). This information will be used to determine how much time to allow for the visit. The provider may also expect the medical assistant to give general instructions to patients being seen for specific complaints. For example, the patient may be required to be fasting for certain laboratory tests. The patient's demographic information should be collected during the conversation, including the type of insurance the patient has. Some insurance carriers restrict which providers can be used.

After the necessary information has been collected, offer the patient the first available appointment. Whenever possible, offer a choice between two dates and times. Ask the patient to arrive 15 minutes before the scheduled appointment time to complete any necessary paperwork. Also ask whether he or she knows how to get to the healthcare facility, or offer the physical address for those who use a GPS or an internet direction website (e.g., MapQuest). Tell the patient whether any special parking conveniences are available and whether the healthcare facility provides a token or parking validation.

The patient's options for the first payment should also be discussed. If payment is expected at the time of service, inform the patient. The staff should expect patient concerns about the amount of the first bill and should address this issue before the appointment so that there are no surprises or misunderstandings. Before ending the conversation, repeat the appointment date and time, and thank the patient for calling.

Some healthcare facilities mail an information packet/brochure to new patients, especially if the appointment is several days away. With the patient's permission and email address, this information can also be sent via the internet. An ideal tool to use to deliver this information is a new patient brochure (see Procedure 11.3, p. 235). This brochure can be printed with graphics and images to promote a professional impression of the healthcare facility. In addition to the brochure, the packet could include a health history form, the **Notice of Privacy Practices (NPP),** and release of information form (to obtain records from the patient's previous provider).

If another provider has referred the patient, the medical assistant may need to call the referring provider's office to obtain additional information before the patient's appointment. This information should be printed out and given to the attending provider before the patient arrives. Remember to send a thank-you note to anyone who refers a patient to the facility.

Often, the medical assistant will need to conduct **preauthorization** or **precertification** to determine whether a patient is eligible for treatment or for certain procedures. The office manager must make certain that these procedures are being done and assigns these duties to a specific person(s). More about preauthorization and precertification is included in Chapter 15.

Scheduling Appointments for Established Patients
In Person

Most return appointments for **established patients** are scheduled when the patient is leaving the healthcare facility. A good policy is to have all patients stop by the appointment desk to check out before leaving in case any information is needed from the patient or any outside scheduling must be done. The patient's health record can be reviewed to see whether the provider ordered any laboratory tests or procedures, and these can be scheduled and discussed with the patient. When making a return appointment, follow the same procedures as for scheduling any appointment by phone, offering the patient choices in the day and time slots (see Procedure 11.4, p. 236). If a certain time the patient specifically requests is not available, offer two other choices. Always give the patient an appointment card and any necessary instructions, along with a bright smile. Never forget to provide excellent customer service.

By Telephone

When scheduling an appointment over the telephone, the medical assistant usually only needs to determine when the patient must return and to find a suitable time in the schedule. Established patients do not usually need directions and parking information, unless the office has recently moved. The patient's address, telephone number, and insurance should always be verified, and any changes documented in the health record. If an email address and/or cell phone number is not on file, obtain one so as to have a quick, easy way to notify the patient of appointments and other events.

Scheduling Other Types of Appointments

The medical assistant may also schedule services other than appointments at the healthcare facility, and these will appear on the appointment schedule. This includes:

- surgeries the provider will perform at a hospital or other facility
- consultations
- outside appointments and meetings
- house calls (if the provider makes them)

The provider also must have time to get from one location to another, so driving time must be considered when arranging all appointments.

Some critical information is required when you schedule an admission to or treatments in other facilities. Always provide the facility with:

- the patient's name, address, and phone numbers (both home and cell)
- Social Security number
- insurance information
- email address
- the procedures that are to be performed
- patient's allergies

- admitting diagnosis
- provider's orders

Some facilities require a history form before admission. The patient will be required to bring a form of picture identification, such as a state driver's license, and his or her insurance card.

Inpatient Surgeries

When scheduling a surgery, provide all necessary information and state any special requests the provider may have, such as:

- the amount of blood to have available for the patient
- a specific anesthesiologist
- an assistant surgeon
- specific instruments

The facility may want the patient's insurance information and certainly will want a phone number so that the patient can be contacted before the surgery if necessary. Make sure all this information is available before placing the call.

Outpatient and Inpatient Procedure Appointments

A medical assistant is often asked to arrange laboratory or radiography appointments for patients. Before calling the facility to schedule the appointment, be sure all necessary information is available. Inform the patient of the time and place of the appointment, relay any special instructions, and then note these arrangements in the patient's health record. Some offices make a reminder call to the patient or send a reminder email or text message.

Outpatient testing is common because most providers do not have extensive x-ray or laboratory equipment in their offices. Magnetic resonance imaging (MRI), computed tomography (CT) scans, numerous x-ray evaluations, sonography, and simple blood tests all may need to be scheduled (see Procedure 11.5, p. 237). Provide the patient with the name, address, and phone number of the facility where the tests will be done.

Some patients may require a series of appointments (e.g., at weekly intervals). Try to set up these appointments on the same day each week at the same time of day. This helps reduces the risk of the patient forgetting an appointment.

In some cases, the medical assistant may be responsible for scheduling inpatient admissions or inpatient surgical procedures. This is similar to scheduling outpatient testing, but the medical assistant coordinates with a hospital rather than an outside facility, and this information should also be documented in the patient's health record.

It is often the medical assistant's responsibility to provide the patient with any special instructions for the procedure or test that is going to be performed. The patient also should be provided with written instructions. A patient undergoing general anesthesia will need to fast for approximately 12 hours before the procedure. If medications are to be taken the morning of the procedure, the patient may take them with a small sip of water. The provider will instruct the patient about which medications to take. The patient should also be instructed to leave valuables at home. If it is an outpatient procedure and the patient will be sedated in any way, the individual should be instructed to have someone drive him or her home.

Outside Visits

If the provider regularly makes house calls or visits patients in skilled nursing facilities, a special block of time must be reserved in the appointment schedule. There has been an increase in the number of providers who are making house calls again, especially if they have an elderly patient base composed of a number of people who are still living independently. The provider needs demographic information, such as addresses, room numbers, and the best route to each home or facility. Remember to allow for travel time.

There are a number of other situations that may have to be added to the schedule, sometimes without much advance warning. Handle these situations with care and courtesy.

Pharmaceutical Representatives

Representatives from drug companies are frequent visitors to healthcare facilities. They are well-trained and bring the provider valuable information on new drugs. The medical assistant is often expected to screen these visitors and turn away those whose products would not be used in that practice. If the representative or the pharmaceutical company is unknown to the office, ask for a business card and then check with the provider. The provider will decide whether to see the representative. Many healthcare facilities are limiting and even eliminating visits from pharmaceutical representatives due to the Physician Payments Sunshine Act (part of the Affordable Care Act).

Pharmaceutical representatives will often bring samples of the medications that they are going to talk to the provider about. It is important for the medical assistant to understand the policies and procedures for the handling and dispensing of the samples. Most healthcare facilities will require that these samples are kept stored in a locked cabinet or closet and are given to patients only with the provider's approval.

Specialists usually limit their visits with pharmaceutical representatives to their line of practice. The medical assistant, together with the provider, can prepare a list of the representatives with whom the provider is willing to spend time. The medical assistant can say whether the provider will be available that day and give an estimate of the waiting time or suggest a later time at which the representative may return. The representative then can decide whether to wait or return later. The pharmaceutical representative is usually quite understanding and cooperative and willing to wait patiently for a long time for just a brief visit with the provider. In turn, the medical assistant should treat the representative with courtesy, showing as much cooperation as possible.

Salespeople

Salespeople from medical, surgical, and office supply houses stop regularly at healthcare facilities. Sometimes they want to see the provider, but the office manager or the medical assistant in charge of ordering supplies can usually handle these visits.

Unsolicited salespeople can sometimes present a problem in the professional office. If the provider does not want to see such callers, the medical assistant must firmly but tactfully send them away. Suggest that they leave their literature and cards for the provider to study and say that the provider will contact them if further information is desired.

Special Circumstances
Late Patients

Every medical practice has a few patients who are habitually late for appointments. This seems to be a problem for which no cure has

been found. Emergencies and small delays can happen to anyone, but a patient who constantly arrives late can put a strain on the practice. Such patients can be booked as the last appointment of the day. Then, if closing time arrives before the patient does, the staff has no obligation to wait and other patients have not been inconvenienced. Some medical assistants tell the patient to come in 30 minutes before the scheduled appointment time. Make an effort to work with patients who have occasional difficulties arriving on time, but do not allow the schedule to be constantly disrupted by late patients.

> ### CRITICAL THINKING APPLICATION   11.4
> Seth Jones is always late for his appointments. How might Ramona approach him about this? What can Ramona do to assist Mr. Jones in arriving for appointments on time?

Rescheduling Appointments

Changes sometimes must be made to the appointment schedule. Unexpected conflicts might come up that force a patient to change the appointment time. When you reschedule an appointment, make sure the first appointment is removed from the appointment book and then set the new appointment. Otherwise, the patient will be expected in the office on 2 days, and time will be wasted with calls and follow-up, only to discover that the appointment was rescheduled. Most computerized scheduling systems will allow the medical assistant to open the appointment and change the date and time or to cut and paste the appointment into the new date and time.

Emergency Situations

Periodically, emergency or urgent calls come into the office, and an appointment needs to be scheduled. To some extent, all calls that come in go through a **screening** process to evaluate the need to see the provider, and emergencies are prioritized. Screening is an extremely important function that requires experience, knowledge of signs and symptoms, and tact.

Emergencies may involve emotional crises in addition to the more obvious physical problems. Patients with emergencies and those who are acutely ill should be seen the same day. The urgency of the call initially can be determined by having a list of questions prepared for reference. The provider should help with this list; he or she should determine what is considered an *emergency* (life-threatening) and what is *urgent* (serious but not life-threatening). The patient may need to be referred directly to a hospital emergency department, or the provider may want to see the patient that day in the office. If patients are unable to get themselves to the hospital, the medical assistant may need to contact the emergency medical services in your area. Remember to keep the patient on the phone until emergency medical technicians (EMTs) or other help arrives at the patient's location. Never place an emergency call on hold. Always obtain the name, phone number, and location at the start of the call so that the patient can be found if he or she loses consciousness or is disconnected.

Patients Without Appointments

The provider and scheduling team should come up with a policy for patients without appointments, also referred to as *walk-in patients*.

A patient who requires immediate attention most likely will be fitted into the schedule somehow. If the patient does not need immediate care, an appointment scheduled at a later time may be the answer. Be sure to follow established office policy.

Failed Appointments

Why do patients fail to keep appointments? Some are simply forgetful. Once this tendency is detected in a patient, form the habit of telephoning or emailing a reminder the day before the appointment. Automated call routing offers the patient the option of canceling an appointment and can be programmed to keep calling until the patient responds and confirms or cancels the appointment.

A patient who has been asked for payment may stay away because of an inability to pay for medical services. Do not make the mistake of classifying all such patients as "deadbeats." Many have every desire to pay, but they cannot afford to and feel embarrassed about their situation, so they avoid their appointments.

Patients may also fail to keep appointments because they are in a state of denial about their condition. For instance, if a patient recently tested positive for the human immunodeficiency virus (HIV), he or she may avoid appointments because going to see the provider forces the patient to face the reality of the disease. Take special care with such patients, and if denial is suspected, discuss this with the provider, who may want to refer the patient for counseling.

It is important to determine the reason for failed appointments and to do whatever is possible to remedy the situation. Telephone the patient to make sure no misunderstanding has occurred. If the patient's health requires ongoing care, the provider may write a letter explaining this to the patient. Send the letter by certified mail with return receipt requested. A copy of the letter needs to be added to the patient's medical record for legal protection.

For legal purposes, failed appointments need to be documented in the patient's health record and the appointment schedule. A patient may try to claim abandonment when he or she has actually been the one to miss the appointments.

No-Show Policy

Some patients may not realize the importance of keeping their appointments. The patient who does not arrive for a scheduled appointment or does not reschedule it is called a **no-show**. A busy practice must have a very specific policy on appointment no-shows and must enforce it effectively. The first time a patient fails to show, note the fact on the health record and/or ledger card. The second time, warn the patient, and if a third no-show occurs, consider dropping the patient by using the customary methods that provide legal protection for the provider. Another option, instead of dropping a patient, is to only allow the patient to schedule for same-day appointments.

The provider may wish to charge patients for not showing up for the appointment. Be understanding whenever possible, but do not let a patient take advantage of the provider's time. The office policy manual must state that patients may be charged for missed appointments, and this should be explained to new patients when their first appointment is made. Because the time slot was scheduled, and the provider was ready and available to treat the patient, it is ethical to charge the patient for missing an appointment, especially if he or she did not call to cancel or reschedule. Many providers do not press this issue, but it is an available tool if needed.

Increasing Appointment Show Rates

Everyone benefits from a full schedule of kept appointments. Appointment show rates can be increased in several ways.

Automated Call Routing

As mentioned earlier, automated call reminders can contact patients scheduled for appointments. The patient is asked to press a certain key on the phone to confirm the appointment and a different key to cancel the appointment. This same tool can be used to send messages to patients (e.g., a reminder that it is the time of year to get a flu vaccination), to introduce a new provider at the office, or to announce the availability of a new procedure. The provider can even record the call so that it sounds more personal. These systems can also be set up to send text messages to remind patients of their upcoming appointments.

Appointment Cards

Most healthcare facilities use appointment cards to remind patients of scheduled appointments and to eliminate misunderstandings about dates and times (Fig. 11.4). Make a habit of reaching for an appointment card while writing an entry in the appointment book or scheduling it on the computer. After the date and time have been written on the card, double-check with the book/computer to make sure the entries agree.

Confirmation Calls

Patients who have made appointments in advance may appreciate a confirmation call to remind them that they have a time set aside to see the provider. Always note the phone number the patient prefers the office to use for such calls. Many individuals have a home phone, cell phone, and work phone numbers; however, they may want calls from the provider to go only to their home phone. Highlight the preferred phone number in the medical record or indicate it on the computer. The office must use caution in making calls to patients because of the significance of privacy guidelines and standards. Some offices may want to prepare a release form in which the patient grants the office staff permission to contact the patient. Many providers insist that messages left on voice mail not mention the term "doctor" or "doctor's office" for confidentiality reasons. The medical assistant might say, "This is Pam at Robert Welch's office confirming your appointment tomorrow at 2 p.m. Please call us if you cannot make the appointment. Our number is 555-212-0909. Thank you!"

If the patient has signed the privacy policy and the policy states that messages from the provider's office may be left at certain numbers, the office certainly can leave messages at that number and mention that the call is from the healthcare facility. Still, it is a good idea to have an established policy on leaving messages that does not breach the patient's confidentiality.

Email Reminders

Many computer scheduling programs can send an email to patients the day before an appointment to remind them of it. This is a great timesaver for the office staff because no time is taken to perform this duty other than the original scheduling of the appointment.

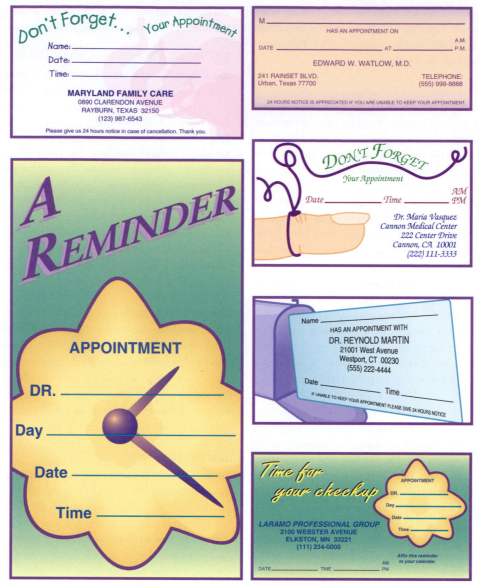

FIGURE 11.4 Examples of appointment reminder cards.

Mailed Reminders

The office staff may mail reminder letters to patients. This method is a bit time-consuming with a paper-based appointment system but worth the effort if the patients show up for their appointments. Computer scheduling systems can be set up to generate the reminder letters for scheduled appointments and also to remind patients that they are due for their annual physical or influenza vaccination.

Handling Cancellations and Delays

When the Patient Cancels

Cancellations will occur in every healthcare facility. To minimize the impact of cancellations, keep a list of patients with future appointments who would like to come in sooner. The medical assistant can begin calling those patients to try to get one of them in to fill the available opening. Each cancellation should be noted in the medical record, along with a reason for the cancellation. If the patient simply reschedules an appointment, a notation does not need to be made in the health record unless a pattern develops that might be significant to the patient's medical treatment.

When the Provider Is Delayed

Some days, the provider will be delayed in reaching the office. If you are notified before patients arrive, start calling patients with early appointments and suggest that they come later. If some patients arrive before the office learns of the delay, explain that an emergency has detained the provider. Offer them the option of rescheduling, seeing another provider, or waiting for their provider.

Show concern for the patient, but do not be overly apologetic, which might imply some degree of guilt. Most patients realize that a provider has certain priorities. The patient in the office may be inconvenienced, but it is not a "life or death" matter. If this kind of situation occurs frequently, however, consider devising a different scheduling system.

When the Provider Is Called to an Emergency

Providers are conscious of their responsibilities for responding to medical emergencies, and most patients understand if the medical assistant takes time to explain what has happened. The medical assistant may say, "Dr. Wright has been called away due to an emergency. She asked me to tell you she is very sorry to keep you waiting. There will be at least a 1-hour delay." The medical assistant should then ask the patient, "Would you like to wait? If that is inconvenient, I'll be glad to give you the first available appointment on another day. Or perhaps you'd like to have some coffee or do some shopping and return in an hour." It is also possible that another provider may be able to see the patient.

As quickly as possible, call the patients scheduled for later. In many offices, especially those of obstetricians, surgeons, and general practitioners, a whole day's appointments must be canceled. For this reason, it is particularly important to have the daytime telephone number of each patient available so that the appointment can be rescheduled. If at all possible, cancel appointments before the patient arrives in the office to find that the provider is not available. The **expediency** of the office staff in contacting patients who will be affected by an emergency is appreciated.

When the Provider Is Ill or Out of Town

Providers get sick, too, and patients scheduled to be seen during the course of the provider's recovery must be informed of this and their appointments rescheduled. They do not need to be told the nature of the illness.

When the provider is called out of town for personal or professional reasons, appointments must be canceled or rescheduled. Usually, the patient is given the name of another provider, or possibly a choice of a few, who will provide care during such absences. For security reasons, only state that the doctor is unavailable. Stating over the telephone that the provider is out of town could lead to attempted burglary or other unauthorized entry on the premises.

PATIENT PROCESSING

Patient Processing Tasks

When working at the reception desk, the medical assistant needs to screen the individuals arriving:

- *People with emergent conditions:* Individuals may be bleeding, having chest pain, or feeling very ill. It is important that the medical assistant immediately contact the **triage** nurse to see the patient. If the nurse is not available, then the medical assistant should bring the patient back to an exam room and notify the provider right away. Facilities may have procedures in place to indicate when 911 needs to be called immediately.
- *Pharmaceutical and equipment representatives:* The medical assistant should follow the facility's policies and procedures regarding when these representatives are permitted to see the providers.
- *Salespeople and visitors:* The medical assistant needs to find out the reason for the visit and then follow the facility's procedures.

The most common visitors to the facility will be patients and family members who have appointments. We will examine the tasks the medical assistant must perform when patients arrive.

Patient's Arrival

When patients arrive, two important things need to occur. First, they need to know where to go and what to do. Second, they need to be greeted as quickly as possible. Signage is helpful to indicate what patients need to do upon arrival.

Every patient has the right to expect courteous treatment in a provider's office. Regardless of the patient's economic or social status, each person who arrives should receive a cordial, friendly greeting (Fig. 11.5). A personal touch, such as greeting the patient by name, is an easy way to develop patient rapport.

Using a Patient's Name

- Use the patient's last name and title (e.g., Mrs. Crawford) unless the patient insists on the use of his or her first name or nickname.
- If you do not know the person, greet the individual and then ask for his or her name.
- Learn how to pronounce each patient's name correctly. Incorrect pronunciations may offend or irritate some people.
- Make a note of the phonetic spelling in the health record for reference. Note if the patient prefers a nickname.

The person sitting at the front reception desk should greet each patient as quickly as possible. Some experts say that a person should be greeted within 30 seconds of arriving. If this is not possible, a simple smile and eye contact will acknowledge the person. Make sure to greet the person verbally as soon as possible. If too much time elapses between the person's entrance and the greeting, the person may feel ignored or unimportant. This can impact a person's perception of the facility and, ultimately, the care provided. If the medical assistant must step away from the reception desk, it is important to check the reception area for new arrivals as soon as she or he returns.

In facilities where the receptionist is behind sliding glass windows, the environment can appear impersonal to patients. Although the closed glass windows increase patient privacy, they can also give the impression that the staff and provider are off limits to the

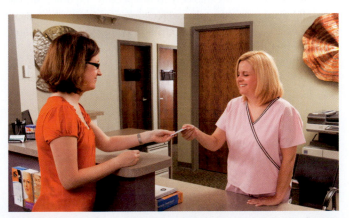

FIGURE 11.5 Greet all patients with a warm smile and assist them with forms they need to complete for the health record.

TABLE 11.1   HIPAA-Appropriate Sign-in Register

FEATURES CAUSING A HIPAA VIOLATION	FEATURES OF A HIPAA-APPROPRIATE REGISTER
• Insurance information (e.g., name, number) • Reason for visit • Demographic information (e.g., address, employer, date of birth)	• Date • Name • Arrival time • Appointment time • Appointment with • Check boxes to indicate changes (but no information can be given)

Information About Patient Information or Registration Forms

Most patient information or registration forms contain the following:
- Patient's full name and date of birth
- Responsible person's name and relationship to the patient
- Address and telephone number
- Name, address, and telephone number of contact person
- Occupation
- Place of employment
- Social Security number
- Driver's license number
- Nearest relative not living with the patient and his or her relationship
- Source of referral, if any

patients. The glass window should be open as much as possible to give the appearance of openness to others. The policies and procedures manual should indicate when the glass window should be closed.

Sign-in Register. Some facilities will have the patient sign a register. A sign-in register that promotes patients' privacy should be used (Fig. 11.6). Remember, other patients can read the prior patients' information. This is not considered a violation of the Health Insurance Portability and Accountability Act (HIPAA) privacy policy if the information disclosed is appropriately limited (Table 11.1). This is one type of incidental disclosure under HIPAA.

Infection Control in the Reception Area. It is vital for the medical assistant to take steps to protect the other patients in the reception area. The medical assistant may need to ask a few screening questions to identify patients who are ill with specific symptoms or at risk for specific diseases. These questions are set by the healthcare facility and usually recommended by the Centers for Disease Control and Prevention (CDC). Questions may include:

- "Have you traveled outside of the United States in the past 21 days?" Travel to specific countries may be included in the question. Patients who answer yes should be taken to an exam room immediately.
- "Are you coughing?" If patients are coughing, they should be encouraged to use masks. This is especially important during flu season or when other respiratory infections are prevalent. Tissues, along with waste containers and hand sanitizer, should be available for patients in the reception area.

Registration for New Patients. When someone visits the provider's office for the first time, the staff must gather information from the new patient, such as demographic and the health history information. The demographic information is usually gathered using the patient information or registration form. The patient's name should appear prominently at the top of the form, followed by other pertinent facts. The patient's personal history, medical history, and family history may be obtained by using a questionnaire.

There are many ways the healthcare facility can obtain this information. Patients may be mailed the documents a few weeks prior to the appointment or directed to complete the information using the online **patient portal**. In some facilities, patients complete this information as they wait, prior to the appointment. They may complete paper forms or provide the information using an electronic device. In some cases, the medical assistant may take the patient to a private room where he or she can ask the questions and enter the information into the electronic health record (EHR).

The medical assistant must be willing to answer any questions about the form, either in person or over the phone (Fig. 11.7). The medical assistant must then review the completed form and verify that the required information has been provided. The provider also reviews the health history information and can then add information during the patient visit.

CRITICAL THINKING APPLICATION   11.5

Often some time is needed to complete forms when a new patient arrives in the healthcare facility. How might Ramona keep the healthcare facility on schedule when new patients arrive who require health record construction and form completion? What are some ways to trim time from these activities?

In addition to collecting information from the patient, the provider must give the patient the facility's NPP document. The healthcare provider is legally obligated to give each patient a notice that explains how the health information may be used and shared. HIPAA requires that patients state in writing that they received the NPP document. The healthcare facility may ask the patient to sign a paper or an electronic document. This form is then kept in the patient's health record. If the patient refuses to sign, the provider can still use and disclose the health information as permitted by HIPAA. The refusal needs to be documented in the patient's health record.

Many times, new patients are given a brochure on the facility's policies and procedures. New patient brochures should be designed in a professional manner. The wording should be at a level that patients understand. When coaching a patient regarding the facility's policies, summarize the content of the brochure. Do not read the brochure to the patient. Use active listening skills. Make sure to address any questions the patient may have. Procedure 11.3 describes how to create the brochure and coach the patients regarding the policies.

Patient Sign-In   Date: _____

Please sign-in and notify us if:

• **New patient**   • **Phone/address change**   • **Insurance change**

No.		Patient Name print	Appt. Time	Arrival Time	Appt. with	New patient (✓)	Phone/address change (✓)	Insurance change (✓)
1		P L E A S E						
2	2							
3	3							
4	4							
5	5							
6	6							
7	7							
8	8							
9	9							
10	10							
11	11							
12	12							
13	13							
14	14							
15	15							
16	16							
17	17							
18	18							
19	19							
20	20							
21	21							
22	22							
23	23							
24	24							
25	25							

FIGURE 11.6 Sign-in sheets contain very basic information about the patient and provide information for the medical assistant about changes that need to be edited into the patient's record.

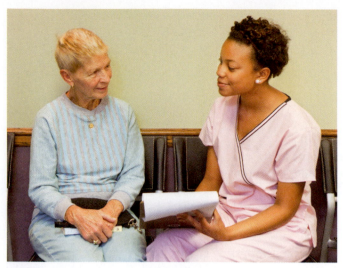

FIGURE 11.7 The medical assistant should take time to explain forms the patient does not understand and should always be willing to answer questions.

New Patient Brochure Content

The following topics should be addressed in the new patient brochure:
- Description of the practice (e.g., type of practice, mission statement)
- Location or a map of the practice
- Contact information (i.e., telephone numbers, emails, and website addresses)
- Providers' names and credentials
- Services offered
- Hours of operation
- How appointments can be scheduled
- Practice policies and procedures (e.g., payment policies, appointment cancellations, medication refills, assistance after hours)

Check-in Procedures for All Patients. During the check-in process, the medical assistant must scan or copy both sides of the patient's insurance card. The medical assistant may have to perform **verification of eligibility**. (This will be described in depth in Chapter 15.) The patient's phone number and address, along with the insurance subscriber's date of birth, should also be verified. Patients must show their insurance cards and picture identification for insurance and identity verification. These verifications take place at every patient visit for eligibility and safety reasons.

Many healthcare facilities are also scanning or copying the patient's legal photo identification. Facilities with EHRs may require a photo of the patient to be taken. The photo is uploaded to the EHR. Between the photo identification and the EHR photo, facilities are trying to reduce the amount of healthcare identity fraud. This fraud occurs when a person obtains healthcare using another person's name and insurance.

Some healthcare facilities insist that copays be collected before the office visit. Signage in the reception area often includes a statement such as "Copayments are due at the time of the appointment." Ask the patient for payment, using phrases such as "Your copay today is $15, Mrs. Crawford. Will you be writing a check or would you like to charge this visit to your Visa?" If the facility is flexible with copayment collection, the medical assistant can give the patient an option. "Mr. Thomas, would you like to pay your copay now?"

Patients With Special Needs. After a patient is checked in, the receptionist may have additional duties if the patient has special needs. Some patients arrive in wheelchairs unattended by family or friends. They may need assistance to get to the reception area. Remember to always ask patients if they need assistance before you try to assist them.

If there is a language barrier, the medical assistant may need to get translation assistance for the visit. Typical options for assistance include having a qualified translator present or using translation technology. There are many online programs that can assist with translation in many different languages. It is important for the administrative medical assistant to communicate any special needs of patients to the clinical medical assistant. In all special needs cases, it is important for you to remain professional and treat everyone with respect.

CRITICAL THINKING APPLICATION   11.6
A patient passes Ramona in the hallway as she is leaving for lunch and stops to greet her. The patient's face is familiar, but Ramona cannot recall the patient's name. Occasionally, Ramona sees a patient outside of the office (e.g., at the store). Everyone forgets someone's name on occasion.
- How might Ramona and her staff members remember names?
- What special tips or techniques can help you remember names?
- What can Ramona do the next time she sees a patient and does not remember the person's name?

Showing Consideration for Patients' Time
Patients expect to see the provider at the appointed time. There should be signage in the reception area stating that patients should let the receptionist know if they have been waiting for longer than 15 to 20 minutes. If the provider is delayed, the medical assistant should let the patients know (Fig. 11.8). The medical assistant can also offer to reschedule the appointment. Some facilities will offer patients gift cards (e.g., coffee, gas) if an error occurred in scheduling or if the patient needs to reschedule due to a long wait time. These gestures show the patients that the staff recognizes their inconvenience. It is a great customer service practice.

CRITICAL THINKING APPLICATION   11.7
Ramona offers to reschedule patient appointments if the schedule ever falls more than 15 minutes behind. If a patient becomes belligerent about the delays, how can Ramona handle the situation in a professional manner?

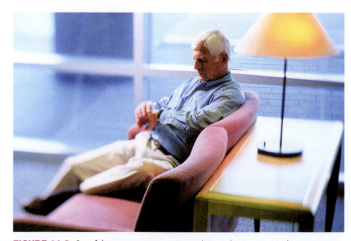

FIGURE 11.8 One of the most common patient complaints is the time spent in the reception area.

Escorting Patients to the Exam Room

In some facilities, the administrative medical assistant may escort the patient to the exam room. In other facilities the clinical medical assistant comes to the reception area and calls the name of the patient. For confidentiality, it is important to call the patient by the first and last name only. Make sure to clearly pronounce the name. If you are unsure, attempt the pronunciation and then ask the patient. Apologize for pronouncing it incorrectly. Make sure to add the pronunciation to the record for the next visit. Remember, no other information should be given in the public waiting area. When you and the patient are alone or away from the reception area, verify that the patient's date of birth matches your records. If it does not, you have the wrong patient!

Some patients may bring a family member or friend with them to an appointment. On occasion, several people may want to accompany the patient to the exam room. Based on the facility's policy, respectfully explain that the exam room has only two chairs. If the patient still insists, make every attempt to satisfy the patient's needs. Please be aware that in some cultures, it is expected that multiple people will accompany the patient to see the provider. In those situations, attempt to use a larger room if available.

Interacting With Friends and Relatives of Patients

Patients are sometimes accompanied by a relative or friend. Be cautious if they want to discuss the patient's illness. Avoid a "too casual" attitude, such as, "I'm sure there's nothing to worry about." A show of moderate concern and reassurance that "the patient is in good hands" usually takes care of the situation. Remember that health information cannot be released to anyone, including concerned friends and relatives, without the patient's consent.

It is understood that the medical assistant escorts the patient to the exam room. Ask if patients need any assistance, if it appears they might. Do not assume they need assistance – ask first and ask how you can assist them. To show respect for the patient, open doors and walk at the patient's speed.

If a urine specimen is needed, direct the patient to the restroom. Always explain how to collect the specimen and where the specimen should be placed. When you get to the exam room with the patient, instruct the patient based on the provider's wishes. If the patient needs to undress, explain what clothing items need to be removed and how to put on the gown. Make sure to indicate where the patient needs to sit. If the patient has a risk of falling, have him or her sit on the chair instead of the exam table.

If you are using an EHR, make sure to log out of the software before leaving the room and then close the door. If you need to reenter the room, always knock first out of respect for the patient. Pause before opening the door. The pause allows the patient time to prepare and time to tell you to enter.

In facilities that use paper health records, often file holders are located on the door or near the door. Place the health record in the holder in such a way that the patient's name is not visible. HIPAA considers names on health records to be incidental disclosures. It is a good practice to protect the patient's privacy. Many facilities have flags on the door to indicate the status of the patient. Adjust the flagging system so the provider knows the patient is in the room and ready to be seen.

Challenging Situations

Talkative Patients. Any professional office has problem patients. Talkative patients, for example, take up far more of the provider's time than is justified. Many times, the provider and medical assistant will devise a method to help keep everything on schedule. For instance, the medical assistant may have to page the provider after a certain time period. This alerts the provider to the time already spent with the patient. The provider can then complete the visit and move to the next patient.

CRITICAL THINKING APPLICATION   11.8

Ramona has one patient who insists on sitting close to her desk and attempting to chat the entire time she is waiting to see the provider. In addition, she comes to her appointments at least an hour early. How might Ramona subtly deal with this patient?

Children. Children frequently present special management challenges. The child may be the patient, or he or she may be accompanying the patient. Parents or guardians are responsible for their children's behavior while at the healthcare facility. If children are doing something that could be harmful, quietly speak to the parents and allow them to handle the situation. The medical assistant should not discipline the child. If the child continues to behave badly, call the parent to the exam room early. They may not be seen early, but they can wait in the exam room instead of the reception area.

In most cases (other than those that involve teens and suspected abuse situations), parents or guardians accompany the child to the exam room. Sometimes parents of older teens want to be present for the visit. Some providers find teens are more honest with their answers if parents are not present. In these situations, allowing the parent to be in the room for the interview may be helpful, but the parent can then wait in the reception area during the physical exam. This will allow the provider to ask follow-up questions, if needed, without the parent overhearing the answers. In all cases (unless indicated by state law), parental permission is required for minors to be seen.

Strategies to Use With Bad Behavior in Children

- Kneel down to the child's level and offer a book or toy.
- Lead the child away from any objects that could be broken and from other patients.
- Say to the child, "Let's come over here and play next to your dad!"

Angry Patients in the Reception Area. Every medical assistant eventually is confronted with an angry patient. The anger may simply reflect the patient's pain or fear of what the provider may discover during the exam. If possible, invite the patient into a room out of the reception area. Usually the best course is to let the patient talk out the anger. Present a calm attitude and speak in a low tone of voice. Under no circumstances should the medical assistant return the anger or become argumentative. Medical assistants must use good listening skills with angry people and must be empathetic. Notify the facility's administrator of all difficult patients or ask for help from co-workers.

There should be a policy in place for dealing with potentially dangerous individuals. Policies can include:

- Making sure that you can reach the exit if you take the patient to another room
- Having another employee close by
- Knowing under what circumstances you should contact the police or building security for assistance

Patient Checkout

When patients return to the front office for checkout, greet them with a friendly smile and call the individual by name. Form the habit of asking patients if they have any questions. Check the health record to determine when the provider wants the patient to return. Most providers note this information on the encounter form. Make the return appointment. Remember to give the patient choices on the time and day. Give the patient an appointment reminder card. If the copayment was not collected prior to the visit it may be collected during checkout.

The medical assistant can convey a sense of caring by terminating the visit cordially. Thank the patient for coming. If the patient will return for another visit, the assistant can say something such as, "We'll see you next week." If the patient will not be returning soon, a pleasant "I hope you'll be feeling better soon" is appropriate. In addition, tell patients to call the facility if they have any questions or if they need additional care. Whatever words of goodbye are chosen, all patients should leave the facility feeling that they have received top-quality care and were treated with friendliness, respect, and courtesy.

CLOSING COMMENTS

Patient Coaching

Providing patients with an information booklet about the healthcare facility can familiarize them with policies and procedures. Many providers compile an extensive booklet that even provides tips as to when the provider should be called immediately, listing symptoms and signs of emergencies.

Educating the patient about the healthcare facility's policies helps the facility run smoothly from day to day. All patients should be familiar with the policies about appointments. This leads to fewer misunderstandings and conflicts over bills that might include a charge for a missed appointment.

If the facility offers internet-based appointment scheduling or forms completion, patients must be taught how to use the system. A printed pamphlet or information sheet is helpful for providing instructions to the patient. A wise option is to have a special phone number that patients can call if they have problems with the system. For best results, choose a program that is simple to use, easy to understand, and does not breach patient confidentiality.

Legal and Ethical Issues

As mentioned earlier, the appointment schedule may be used as a legal record and could be brought by subpoena into a court of law.

Make sure all handwriting in the book is completely legible and that information is routinely collected in a consistent manner for each entry. Do not fail to note a no-show both in the patient's health record and the appointment schedule. This often is helpful when a provider must prove that the patient did not follow medical advice or that the patient contributed to his or her poor condition by missing appointments. Old appointment schedules should be kept for a time equal to that of the statute of limitations in the state where the practice is located.

A medical assistant must never offer medical advice to a patient. The patient sees the medical assistant as an extension of the provider and tends to weigh advice and comments by the medical assistant with the same validity as if they came from the provider. Provide only information the provider has approved or that is included in the healthcare facility's policies and procedures manual.

When a patient complains, listen carefully and try to resolve the problem or assure the patient that the issue will be discussed with the appropriate staff member to find a solution. If someone other than the patient asks for information about the patient, refrain from discussion unless the patient or provider has authorized the release of information.

Patient-Centered Care

Going to a healthcare facility can be intimidating and uncomfortable for many patients. It is important that the medical assistant try to put everyone at ease. Cultivate the habit of greeting each patient immediately in a friendly, self-assured manner. Establish eye contact and smile while introducing yourself to the patient.

Small talk can help put a patient at ease. Talking about the weather or an uncontroversial topic may make the patient more comfortable.

Asking personalized questions can also help. Providers and staff members sometimes make brief notes in the health record about the current events in the patient's life. On the next visit, the staff or provider can use this information to start a conversation with the patient. For instance, the patient may state she is going to Florida for a vacation. During the next visit, the provider may start off the visit by asking how her Florida trip was. Asking personalized questions will solidify the personal connection with patients. They may feel important, less intimidated, and more comfortable. It is a great way to provide excellent customer service.

Professional Behaviors

When working in scheduling and helping patients move through the healthcare facility, medical assistants have many opportunities to demonstrate professionalism. It is important to remember that we are often seeing patients when they are not at their best, so we must learn not to take all of the responses personally. When an angry patient approaches the reception desk, you should smile politely, ask how you can help the person, and respond in a soothing tone of voice. When a patient calls for an appointment and demands a day and time when the provider is not available, you should remain calm and explain why that day and time are not an option. As a medical assistant in the front office, you have the opportunity to make an amazing first impression on patients. Remember to always behave professionally.

SUMMARY OF SCENARIO

Ramona is an asset to the healthcare facility because her dedication and customer service skills help her interact with patients in a positive way. She genuinely cares about the patients and makes every effort to meet their needs while following Dr. Perez's preferences. She has found that her bright smile is a valuable aid when patients have been waiting and are growing restless.

Ramona cooperates with other staff members to get the patients seen as quickly as possible and to minimize wait time. She is flexible and can change the order of the patients seen, if needed, to maximize the use of time and facilities in the office. Because she is so cheerful and friendly, patients do not seem to mind when she asks for their cooperation. She keeps current phone numbers and cell phone information so that she can notify a patient quickly if Dr. Perez is running behind schedule. Ramona's proficiency on the computer also is an asset, and she makes frequent use of email to take care of patients' problems or to reschedule requests.

Because of the cooperation she receives from staff and patients alike, Ramona successfully runs an efficient office. She contributes to that efficiency by constantly refining her knowledge about her job. She pays attention to the times during the day that do not run as smoothly as others, evaluates the problems at those times, and then corrects them. Ramona also keeps the schedule moving by communicating with the clinical medical assistants, keeping them informed about arriving patients and those who have come early or are running late. She can quickly adjust and substitute a patient who already has arrived. Ramona has learned how to manipulate the schedule to accommodate an emergency. She knows that by making minor adjustments and keeping the waiting patients informed, the staff can handle any emergency.

All medical assistants need to develop skills in flexibility. Establishing a system that works and using it correctly makes patients and staff members more content with their experience in the healthcare facility.

SUMMARY OF LEARNING OBJECTIVES

1. **Describe guidelines for establishing an appointment schedule and creating an appointment matrix.**

   When appointments are scheduled, a medical assistant must consider (1) the patients' needs, (2) the provider's preferences and habits, and (3) the available facilities. Make every attempt to schedule a patient at his or her most convenient time; this helps prevent no-shows. The provider will outline his or her preferences, which should be a high priority to the medical assistant. However, most providers are flexible and make adjustments according to the needs of the office. The availability of facilities in the office is perhaps the most inflexible factor. If a certain room or piece of equipment is being used for one patient, it usually cannot be used for another.
   Refer to Procedure 11.1 to create an appointment matrix.

2. **Discuss the advantages of computerized appointment scheduling.**

   Computerized scheduling programs are in demand because they are easy to operate and simplify both scheduling and changing of appointments. The computer can find the first available time much faster than a person scanning an appointment book. Most programs can prepare reports and even notify patients of the impending appointment automatically by email, telephone, or text message. Web-based self-scheduling programs are becoming popular; these allow a patient to see the provider's available appointments and book his or her own date and time.

3. **Discuss appointment book scheduling and explain how self-scheduling can reduce the number of calls to the healthcare facility.**

   Office suppliers carry a variety of appointment book styles; many are color-guided.
   Self-scheduling can vastly reduce the number of calls to the office because a high number of everyday calls are requests to schedule appointments. With self-scheduling, patients can even make an appointment at midnight if they desire.

4. **Discuss the legality of the appointment scheduling system.**

   Because the paper-based appointment book can be used as a legal record, it must be accurate and maintained. Computerized scheduling systems can also be used to track appointments; missed or canceled appointments should be documented in the electronic system for legal purposes.

5. **Discuss pros and cons of various types of appointment management systems.**

   Scheduling of specific appointments is the most popular method of seeing patients. Wave and modified-wave scheduling brings two or three patients to the office at the same time, and they are seen in the order of their arrival. This type of scheduling can be modified in many ways to suit the needs of the facility. Open office hours allow patients to come to the healthcare facility when it is convenient and wait their turn to see the provider. Other scheduling methods include double-booking and grouping of like procedures.

6. **Discuss telephone scheduling and identify critical information required for scheduling appointments for new patients.**

   Extend small courtesies to patients when on the phone with them to schedule an appointment. Write legibly when using an appointment book.
   Arranging the first appointment for a new patient requires time and attention to detail. Tact, courtesy, and professionalism are all extremely important. Collect the patient's demographic data and offer the patient the first available appointment. Some healthcare facilities mail an information packet/brochure to new patients; this can also be sent via email. Often, the medical assistant will need to conduct preauthorization and precertification to determine whether a patient is eligible for treatment or for certain procedures.

Continued

SUMMARY OF LEARNING OBJECTIVES—*continued*

Refer to Procedure 11.2 to see how to schedule a new patient and to Procedure 11.3 to see how to coach patients regarding office policies and how to create a new patient brochure.

7. **Discuss scheduling appointments for established patients.**

Most return appointments for established patients are arranged when the patient is leaving the healthcare facility. Refer to Procedure 11.4. Others are reserved by telephone, and the patient's address, telephone number, and insurance should always be verified, and any changes documented in the health record.

8. **Discuss how the medical assistant should handle scheduling of other types of appointments.**

The medical assistant could be responsible for setting up other appointments, such as inpatient surgeries, outpatient and inpatient procedure appointments, outside visits, providers, pharmaceutical representatives, and salespeople. Refer to Procedure 11.5 for specific procedures on how to schedule outpatient and inpatient procedure appointments.

9. **Do the following related to special circumstances in scheduling:**

- *Discuss several methods of dealing with patients who consistently arrive late.*

  Patients who are habitually late for appointments might be told to arrive 15 minutes before the time written in the book. Some offices book these patients as the last appointment of the day, so that if they do not arrive promptly, they do not see the provider. Usually talking with the patient and gaining an understanding of why the patient arrives late improves the situation. The office can work with the patient to choose the best times that will result in a kept appointment.

- *Recognize office policies and protocols for rescheduling appointments.*

  Changes sometimes must be made in the appointment schedule. When rescheduling an appointment, make sure the first appointment is removed from the appointment book, and then set the new appointment.

- *Discuss how to deal with emergencies, provider referrals, and patients without appointments.*

  Periodically, emergency or urgent calls come into the office, and an appointment needs to be scheduled. Follow office procedures. Provider referrals and patients without appointments should also be scheduled according to office policy.

10. **Discuss how to handle failed appointments and no-shows, in addition to methods to increase appointment show rates.**

It is important to determine the reason for failed appointments and to do whatever is possible to remedy the situation. Failed appointments need to be documented. A busy practice must have a very specific policy on appointment no-shows and must enforce it effectively. Methods to increase appointment show rates include automated call routing, appointment cards, confirmation calls, email reminders, and mailed reminders.

11. **Discuss how to handle cancellations and delays.**

Cancellations will occur because of a variety of reasons (e.g., when the patient cancels, when the provider is delayed, when the provider is called to an emergency, or when the provider is ill or out of town). All situations should be handled in accordance with office policy.

12. **Describe how to prepare for patients' arrivals, including patient check-in procedures.**

Advanced preparation helps make the day go smoothly and contributes to a more relaxed atmosphere for all. Health records should be prepared for the provider, arranged sequentially. The reception desk should be in clear view of all visitors who come to the office. Use a sign-in register that promotes patients' privacy. During the patient check-in process, it is vital that the medical assistant takes steps to protect the other patients in the reception area.

13. **Do the following related to patient reception and processing:**

- *Show consideration for patients' time.*

  The medical assistant should bring the patient to the examination room for treatment or consultation as close to the appointment time as possible or explain delays.

- *Properly treat patients with special needs.*

  In all special needs cases, it is important to remain professional and treat everyone with respect.

- *Escort and instruct the patient.*

  While in the provider's office, most patients prefer to be escorted rather than simply told where to go, and this is usually the medical assistant's responsibility.

- *Describe where health records should be placed.*

  Health records should never be left in the examination room to be picked up and read by a patient. When using EHRs, it is important to remember to log out of the computer when you are ready to leave the room.

14. **Describe how the medical assistant should deal with challenging situations, such as talkative patients, children, angry patients, and patients' relatives and friends.**

For talkative patients, the patient's history could be flagged with a symbol to alert the provider. Parents are responsible for their children's behavior while at the provider's office. The medical assistant should not discipline the child. Medical assistants should use empathy and good listening skills when dealing with angry patients, and there should be a policy in place for dealing with potentially dangerous individuals. Avoid a "too casual" attitude with patients' relatives and friends; show moderate concern and empathy.

PROCEDURE 11.1   Establish the Appointment Matrix

Task: To establish the matrix of the appointment schedule.

Scenario: You have been asked to set up the schedule matrix for Dr. Julie Walden, Dr. James Martin, and Dr. Angela Perez. Block off the following times in the appointment schedule:

Dr. Julie Walden:
- Lunch: Daily from 11:30 a.m. to 12:30 p.m.
- Hospital Rounds: Mondays and Wednesdays from 8:00 a.m. to 9:00 a.m.

Dr. James Martin:
- Lunch: Daily from 12:00 p.m. to 1:00 p.m.
- Hospital Rounds: Tuesdays and Thursdays from 8:00 a.m. to 9:00 a.m.

Dr. Angela Perez:
- Lunch: Daily from 12:30 p.m. to 1:30 p.m.
- Hospital Rounds: Fridays from 8:00 a.m. to 9:00 a.m.

EQUIPMENT and SUPPLIES

- Appointment book or computer with scheduling software
- Office procedure manual (optional)
- Black pen, pencil, and highlighters
- Calendar

PROCEDURAL STEPS

1. Using the calendar, determine when the office is not open (e.g., holidays, weekends, evenings). If using the appointment book and a black pen, draw an *X* through the times the office is not open. If using the scheduling software, block the times the office is not open.
   PURPOSE: Blocking the closed times helps prevent patients from being scheduled when the office is closed.

2. Identify the times each provider is not available. If using the appointment book, write in the providers' names on each column and then draw an *X* through their unavailable times. If using the scheduling software, select each provider and block the times the provider is unavailable.
   PURPOSE: Many providers do rounds in the hospital or long-term care facilities and cannot see patients in the clinic during those times. Providers also attend meetings and conferences during the workday. These events, along with vacations and lunch times, should be blocked on their schedules.

3. Using the office procedure manual or providers' preferences, determine when each provider performs certain types of examinations. In the appointment book, indicate these examinations either by writing the examination time or by highlighting the examination times. Follow the office's procedure on indicating these examination times in the appointment book. When using scheduling software, set up the times for the examinations or use the highlighting feature if available.
   PURPOSE: Some providers perform a variety of examinations. It can be more time efficient to have the same types of examinations on the same day. For instance, a provider in a women's health department may perform both gynecologic and prenatal examinations. The provider may prefer to set aside certain days to do prenatal examinations and other days to do gynecologic examinations.

4. Using the office procedure manual or the list of providers' preferences and availability, identify other times to block on the scheduling matrix. Some providers require catch-up times and these time slots are blocked. Some medical facilities save appointment times for same-day appointments. When saving time blocks for same-day appointments, make sure to use pencil so the block indicator can be erased and the patient's information entered on the day of the appointment. For the scheduling software, block those times when patients cannot be booked and indicate the times for the same-day appointments.
   PURPOSE: Allowing appointment times to be saved for same-day appointments provides the opportunity for the provider to see a patient who needs to get in immediately and prevents the patient from being turned away or double-booked.

PROCEDURE 11.2   Schedule a New Patient

Task: To schedule a new patient for a first office visit and identify the urgency of the visit using established priorities.

Scenario: Patricia Black, a new patient, calls. She just moved to the area, and her asthma has flared up over the past 24 hours, but her albuterol inhaler is empty and she needs a new prescription for it. She states that she is doing okay, but without the albuterol she knows it will get worse within the next few days. According to your screening guidelines, she needs to be seen today, and scheduling guidelines indicate she needs a 45-minute appointment.

Continued

PROCEDURE 11.2   Schedule a New Patient—*continued*

EQUIPMENT and SUPPLIES

- Appointment book or computer with scheduling software
- Scheduling and screening guidelines
- Pencil

PROCEDURAL STEPS

1. Obtain the patient's demographic information (e.g., full name, birth date, address, and telephone number). Write this information down or enter it into the scheduling software. Verify the information.
<u>PURPOSE</u>: It is important to verify the information. If you have difficulty hearing the patient, use a system to verify the spelling (e.g., "A" as in alpha).

2. Determine whether the patient was referred by another provider.
<u>PURPOSE</u>: You may need to request additional information from the referring provider, and your provider will want to send a consultation report.

3. Determine the patient's chief complaint and when the first symptoms occurred. Use the scheduling and screening guidelines as needed.
<u>PURPOSE</u>: You must know the amount of time that will be required for the visit and how quickly the patient needs to be seen based on the chief complaint.

4. Search the appointment book or scheduling software for the first suitable appointment time and an alternate time. Offer the patient a choice of these dates and times. Be open to alternative times if the patient cannot make the initial options you gave. Provide additional appointment options as needed.
<u>PURPOSE</u>: Providing the patient with a choice of dates and times and additional options as needed helps to demonstrate sensitivity when managing appointments. It is an important customer service technique (see the following figure).

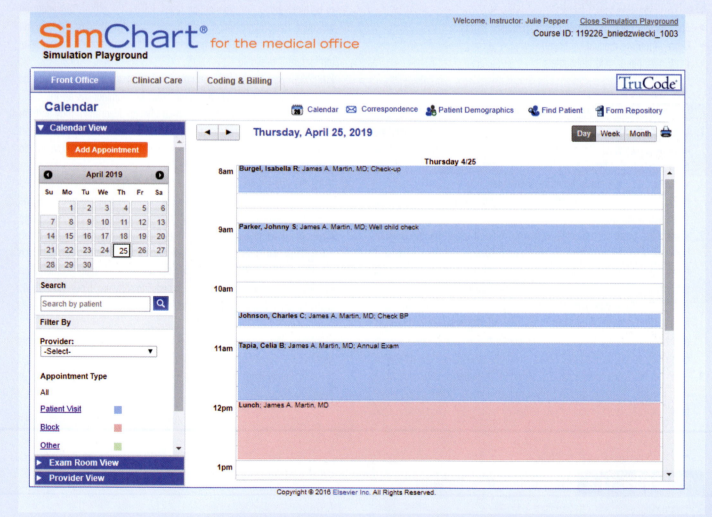

5. Enter the mutually agreeable time into the schedule. Enter the patient's name, telephone number, and add *NP* for new patient.
<u>PURPOSE</u>: The *NP* in the appointment book indicates the patient is a new patient. Having the phone number available helps increase your efficiency if you need to contact the patient.

6. Obtain the patient's insurance information. If new patients are expected to pay at the time of the visit, explain this financial arrangement when the appointment is made.
<u>PURPOSE</u>: Obtaining the patient's insurance information now ensures that the patient is seeing a provider covered by his or her insurance carrier. If

---

you explain the payment policy before the appointment, the patient can come to the appointment prepared to pay.

7. Provide the patient with directions to the healthcare facility and parking instructions if needed.

    Note: Many facilities will email or mail new-patient paperwork to the patient, who is instructed to complete the forms before the appointment and bring them to the appointment.

8. Before ending the call, ask if the patient has any questions. Reinforce the date and time of the appointment. Politely and professionally end the call, making sure to thank the patient for calling.

    PURPOSE: It is important to restate the appointment time and date to ensure the patient knows the correct information before you end the call.

    Note: For legal and safety reasons, many healthcare practices encourage patients with urgent same-day appointments to seek emergency care immediately if the condition worsens before the appointment time.

PROCEDURE 11.3 **Coach Patients Regarding Office Policies**

Tasks: Create a new patient brochure and then role-play coaching patients regarding office policies.

Scenario: You work at Walden-Martin Family Medical Clinic. Your supervisor asks you to create a new patient brochure for the clinic. The clinic information is listed below. After you complete the brochure, you coach the following patients regarding office procedures:

- Mr. Charles Johnson (he has a question regarding the payment policy)
- Ms. Monique Jones (she has a question regarding the medication refill procedure)

CLINIC INFORMATION	PROVIDERS
Walden-Martin Family Medical Clinic	Julie Walden, MD
1234 Anystreet	James Martin, MD
Anytown, Anystate 12345	Angela Perez, MD
Phone: 123-123-1234	David Kahn, MD
Fax: 123-123-5678	Jean Burke, NP

EQUIPMENT and SUPPLIES

- Computer with word processing software and printer
- Office procedure manual (optional)

PROCEDURAL STEPS

1. Using word processing software, design an informational brochure for patients that provides information about the practice and describes practice procedures. At a minimum, the information should include:
    - Description of the practice (e.g., type of practice, mission statement)
    - Location or a map of the practice
    - Contact information (i.e., telephone numbers, emails, and website addresses)
    - Providers' names and credentials
    - Services offered
    - Hours of operation
    - How appointments can be scheduled
    - Practice policies and procedures (e.g., payment policies, appointment cancellations, medication refills, assistance after hours)

    PURPOSE: Providing patients with a written brochure listing the practice's information, policies, and procedures enables patients to use it as a reference.

2. Proofread the brochure. Make revisions as needed. Print the brochure.

    PURPOSE: It is important to proofread and revise documents as needed before they go to patients.

3. Using the scenario situation for the first patient, give a brief summary of the different parts of the brochure. Use words that the patient will understand.

    PURPOSE: By discussing each part of the brochure with the potential patient, you can help explain what is stated. Summarize the information without reading the sections to the other person.

4. Ask if the patient has any questions. Actively listen to the patient's concerns. Address the patient's concerns.

    PURPOSE: By actively listening, you will be able to identify issues or confusion the patient is experiencing. It is important that the messages during the conversation are clear for both parties.

5. Using the scenario situation for the second patient, give a brief summary of the different parts of the brochure. Use words that the patient will understand.

    PURPOSE: By reviewing the brochure, you can summarize what the policies are. If the patient has an immediate question, you can answer it.

6. Ask if the patient has any questions. Actively listen to the patient's concerns. Address the patient's concerns.

    PURPOSE: By actively listening, you will be able to identify issues or confusion the patient is experiencing. It is important that the messages during the conversation are clear for both parties.

PROCEDURE 11.4	Schedule an Established Patient

Task: To manage the provider's schedule by scheduling appointments for an established patient and handling rescheduling and a no-show appointment.

Scenario: Celia Tapia has just finished seeing Dr. Martin and is checking out at your desk. You see that she needs to schedule a follow-up appointment in 2 weeks. The scheduling guidelines indicate a follow-up appointment is 15 minutes long.

EQUIPMENT and SUPPLIES

- Appointment book or computer with scheduling software
- Scheduling guidelines
- Pencil, red pen
- Reminder card
- Patient's health record

PROCEDURAL STEPS

1. Obtain the patient's name and information, purpose of the visit, the provider to be seen, and any scheduling preferences. If using the scheduling software, enter the patient's name and date of birth (DOB). Verify the correct patient is selected.
   PURPOSE: To schedule an appointment you must have the patient's information, along with the provider to be seen and the type of appointment required. Knowing any scheduling preferences or limitations will help you efficiently find an acceptable appointment time for the patient.

2. Identify the length of the appointment by using the scheduling guidelines.
   PURPOSE: Depending on the appointment type, each provider may require a different length of time for that appointment. Ensuring you schedule the appropriate amount of time will help facilitate the flow of patients on that day.

3. Search the appointment book or scheduling software for the first suitable appointment time and an alternate time. Offer the patient a choice of these dates and times. Be open to alternative times if the patient cannot make the initial options you gave. Provide additional appointment options as needed.
   PURPOSE: Providing the patient with a choice of dates and times and additional options as needed helps to demonstrate sensitivity when you are managing appointments. It is an important customer service technique (see the following figure).

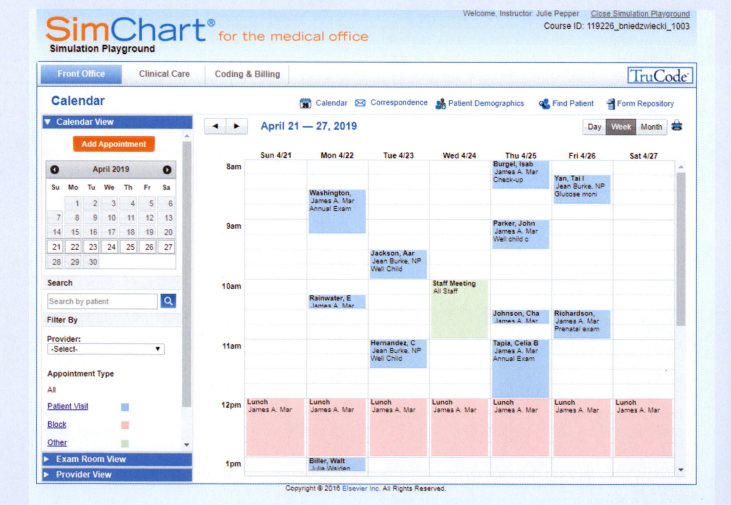

PROCEDURE 11.4 Schedule an Established Patient—*continued*

4. Using a pencil, write the patient's name and phone number in the appointment book and block out the correct amount of time. Add in any other relevant information per the facility's procedures. If using the scheduling software, create the appointment per the facility's guidelines.

PURPOSE: Adding the patient's phone number to the appointment book saves time if the patient needs to be contacted. Using pencil to write down the information in the book allows it to be erased if the patient cancels or reschedules for another time.

5. Complete the appointment reminder card and ensure the date and time on the card match the appointment time. Give the card to the patient.

PURPOSE: Using appointment reminder cards helps patients remember when their appointments are and helps reduce the number of no-show appointments.

Continuation of Scenario: Later that day, Celica Tapia calls and says she needs to reschedule her appointment for the next day at the same time.

6. When a patient calls to reschedule an appointment, follow steps 1 through 4. When the new appointment is made, make sure to erase the old appointment from the appointment log. With the scheduling software, ensure the old appointment time is removed from the schedule. Repeat the new appointment date and time to the patient.

Note: It is important to erase the old appointment so that the patient is not expected on two different days. Erasing or deleting the old appointment opens up that time for another patient.

Continuation of Scenario: Celia Tapia no-shows for her follow-up appointment.

7. In the appointment book, using a red pen, indicate the patient no-showed. Using the patient's health record, document that the patient failed to show for the follow-up examination with the provider. In an electronic system, change the appointment status to no-show and ensure that it is documented in the health record.

PURPOSE: For legal purposes, the healthcare facility must keep a record of patients who no-show for appointments. If this is indicated in the appointment book and in the health record, the practice is covered if any issues should arise. Some medical practices have procedures that include contacting the patient regarding the no-show appointment and finding out the reason. This is then also charted in the health record.

PROCEDURE 11.5 Schedule a Patient Procedure

Task: To schedule a patient for a procedure within the time frame needed by the provider, confirm with the patient, and issue all required instructions.

Scenario: Monique Jones has just completed seeing Dr. Perez and is checking out at your desk. She gives you an order from the provider that states she needs to have a magnetic resonance image (MRI) of her left ankle within a week. The radiology department in your facility performs MRIs.

EQUIPMENT and SUPPLIES

- Provider's order detailing the procedure required
- Computer with order entry software (optional)
- Name, address, and telephone number of facility where procedure will take place
- Patient's demographic and insurance information
- Patient's health record
- Procedure preparation instructions
- Telephone
- Consent form (if required for procedure)

PROCEDURAL STEPS

1. Obtain an oral or written order from the provider for the exact procedure to be performed.

PURPOSE: To schedule the procedure, you will need an order from the provider for the procedure to be performed.

2. Gather the patient's demographic and insurance information. If using an electronic health record, verify you have the correct patient.

Note: For some procedures and diagnostic tests, precertifications or preauthorizations need to be completed before the patient is scheduled. (This will be discussed in a later chapter.)

3. Determine the patient's availability within the time frame provided by the provider for the procedure (see the following figure).

PURPOSE: To make sure the patient will be able to comply with the arrangements for the test.

PURPOSE: To schedule the procedure and provide needed information.

4. Notify the patient of the arrangements and provide the information in a written format.

- Give the name, address, and telephone number of the diagnostic facility.
- Specify the date and time to report for the procedure.
- Give instructions on preparation for the test (e.g., eating restrictions, fluids, medications, enemas).

Continued

PROCEDURE 11.5 | Schedule a Patient Procedure—*continued*

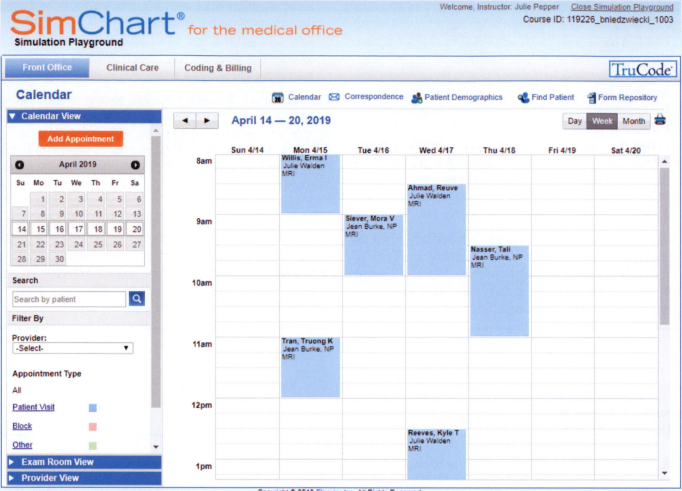

- If another facility is used, the patient will need to bring a form of picture identification and the insurance card.
- If you are not using a computerized provider order entry system, explain whether the patient needs to pick up orders or whether the order will be sent to the facility in advance.
- Ask if the patient has any questions and answer the questions.

PURPOSE: Make sure the patient understands the necessary preparations and the importance of keeping the appointment. Providing written instructions to the patient will help reinforce what was discussed and give the patient a reference for the information.

5. If a consent form is required for the procedure, ensure the provider has reviewed the form with the patient and the patient has signed the consent form. A copy of the consent form may be required by the diagnostic facility before the procedure. The consent form should be scanned and uploaded into the electronic health record or placed in the paper record.

PURPOSE: The consent form is used to make sure the patient understands the risks, benefits, and alternatives to the procedure.

6. Document the details of the scheduled procedure in the patient's health record. If applicable, create a reminder to check on the procedure results after the appointment date.

PURPOSE: Document that the procedure was scheduled. It is legally important to show that what was ordered was scheduled. Creating a reminder for yourself to check up on the results of the procedure is also important in assisting the provider.

Example: 2/27/20XX Patient scheduled for colonoscopy on 3/10/20XX 8:00 a.m. at Anytown Hospital. Patient preparation instructions given, and patient verbalized understanding.

HEALTH RECORDS

SCENARIO

Susan Beezler has just begun her career in the medical assisting profession. In the morning, she is attending medical assisting school, and in the afternoon, she works part-time for the Walden-Martin Family Medical Clinic (WMFM) as a records assistant. Susan is eager to learn about healthcare and looks forward to taking on more responsibility at the office.

Dr. David Kahn is a new provider who has recently joined WMFM. Dr. Kahn has enjoyed working with Susan and feels that her energy will be just what his patients need. He has taken a professional interest in Susan and often lets her assist him with patients when her other duties allow.

Susan knows that although she is a beginner in the office, she will gain trust from her supervisors and patients as long as she projects a teachable attitude. The office has recently converted to an electronic records system but is also still using paper records. Susan uses the information she learned in school about both types of health records. She cheerfully performs filing and even does some transcription for Dr. Kahn. The other staff members are pleased with her willingness to perform the most mundane tasks.

Susan enjoys sharing her experiences with her classmates. She is the only student currently working in the medical field, and the others ask her lots of questions about the "real world" of medical assisting. She is very careful not to breach patient confidentiality; she discusses situations only in general terms, never mentioning any patients' names.

Susan feels a great sense of pride that she is already a member of the healthcare team and able to contribute to the lives of her patients.

While studying this chapter, think about the following questions:
- What is the definition and application of subjective information?
- What is the definition and application of objective information?
- How does the HITECH act impact health records?
- How can you maintain a connection with the patient when using an EHR?
- What are the different ways to back up an EHR?
- How do you correctly destroy health records?
- How do you document in health records?
- What equipment and supplies are needed for a paper records system?
- What are the indexing rules for alphabetic and numeric filing systems?

LEARNING OBJECTIVES

1. Discuss the two types of patient records.
2. State several reasons that accurate health records are important.
3. Differentiate between subjective and objective information in creating a patient's health record.
4. Explain who owns the health record.
5. Distinguish between an electronic health record (EHR) and an electronic medical record (EMR).
6. Do the following related to healthcare legislation and EHRs:
   - Define meaningful use and relate it to the healthcare industry.
   - List the three main components of meaningful use legislation.
7. Discuss the importance of nonverbal communication with patients when an EHR system is used.
8. Discuss backup systems for the EHR, in addition to the transfer, destruction, and retention of health records as related to the EHR.
9. Discuss retention and destruction of medical records as related to paper records.
10. Describe how and when to release health record information; also, discuss health information exchanges (HIEs).
11. Identify and discuss the two methods of organizing a patient's paper medical record.
12. Discuss how to document information in an EHR and a paper health record, and how to make corrections/alterations to health records.
13. Discuss dictation and transcription.
14. Identify the filing equipment and filing supplies needed to create, store, and maintain paper health records.
15. Describe indexing rules, and how to create and organize a patient's health record.
16. Discuss the pros and cons of various filing methods and how to file patient health records.
17. Discuss the organization of files and of health-related correspondence.

VOCABULARY

age of majority The age at which the law recognizes a person to be an adult; it varies by state.

alphabetic filing Any system that arranges names or topics according to the sequence of the letters in the alphabet.

alphanumeric Describes systems made up of combinations of letters and numbers.

anthropometric (an thruh po ME trik) Pertaining to the measurement of the size and proportions of the human body.

caption A heading, title, or subtitle under which records are filed.

compliance (kuhm PLIE uhns) Meeting the standards and regulations of the practice's established policies and procedures. Can also mean cooperation.

computerized provider/physician order entry (CPOE) The process of entering medication orders or other provider instructions into the EHR.

concise (kuhn SICE) Using as few words as possible to express a message.

continuity of care The smooth continuation of care from one provider to another. This allows the patient to receive the most benefit with no interruption or duplication of care.

dictation (dik TEY shuhn) To say something aloud for another person to write down.

direct filing system A filing system in which materials can be located without consulting another source of reference.

electronic health record (EHR) An electronic record that conforms to nationally recognized standards and contains health-related information about a specific patient. It can be created, managed, and consulted by authorized clinicians and staff from more than one healthcare organization.

e-prescribing The use of electronic software to communicate with pharmacies and send prescribing information. It takes the place of writing a prescription by hand and giving it to a patient; most new or refill prescriptions can be submitted electronically, cutting down on fraud and errors.

hereditary (huh RED i ter ee) Passed from parents to offspring through the genes.

incidence (IN si duhns) How often something happens or occurs.

interface An interconnection between systems.

interoperability (in ter op er uh BIL i tee) The ability to work with other systems.

numeric filing The filing of records, correspondence, or cards by number.

objective information Data obtained through physical examination, laboratory and diagnostic testing, and by measurable information.

obliteration (ub lit uh REY shun) To remove or destroy all traces of; do away with; destroy completely.

out guides Sturdy cardboard or plastic file-sized cards used to replace a folder temporarily removed from the filing space.

parameters (puh RAM i ters) Rules that control how something should be done; guidelines or boundaries.

patient portal A secure online website that gives patients 24-hour access to personal health information using a username and password.

prognosis (prog NOH sis) The likely outcome of a disease, including the chance of recovery.

provisional diagnosis (die ug NOH sis) A temporary diagnosis made before all test results have been received.

quality control A process to ensure the reliability of test results, often using manufactured samples with known values.

retention schedule A method or plan for retaining or keeping health records and for their movement from active to inactive to closed.

reverse chronologic order The most recent item is on top, and the oldest item is last.

subjective information Data or information obtained from the patient, including the patient's feelings, perceptions, and concerns; this information is obtained through interviews or written questions.

subsequent (SUHB si kwuhnt) Occurring later or after.

tickler file A chronologic file used as a reminder that something must be dealt with on a certain date.

transcription (tran SKRIP shuhn) A typed or written copy of dictated material.

vested Granted or endowed with a particular authority, right, or property; to have a special interest in.

Health records can be found in two different formats, electronic and paper. Most healthcare facilities have switched to **electronic health records (EHRs)**. Some of the benefits of EHRs include:

- Easy storage of patient information
- Availability to multiple users at the same time
- More efficient claim submission process

The federal government has also offered financial incentives for providers to implement EHRs. Although most providers are using EHRs, there are still some who are using paper records and others who are using a combination of electronic and paper formats. When a provider is making a switch to an EHR, he or she may decide to keep the patient's previous records in the paper format and just use the electronic format moving forward. Some providers may decide to scan in the last 3 to 5 years of the paper record into the electronic record. Whatever the scenario the healthcare facility has chosen, it is important for the medical assistant to understand both systems and to be able to perform well with either one.

TYPES OF RECORDS

Paper health records have been shown to be much less efficient than an EHR. In most cases, only one person at a time can use the paper record. It is fairly common for information to be filed in the incorrect record. The entire record also can be misfiled. Gathering data for research and **quality control** is more challenging. Data are difficult to share in facilities with multiple departments or locations. The paper-based record is good for documentation of patient care, but it is not nearly as useful in other capacities.

With an EHR, multiple users can access the record at the same time. There are fewer errors because handwritten notes do not have to be interpreted. Most EHRs link the clinical information needed for billing purposes. An EHR also includes practice management capabilities that allow for patient scheduling and generation of reports needed for research and quality control.

It is important for the medical assistant to be aware of the differences between the practice management software and the EHR. You may use both during your day as a medical assistant. The EHR contains a record of patient interactions and health history. The practice management software allows the facility to operate the business side by maintaining schedules and financial information for revenue cycle management for reimbursement.

CRITICAL THINKING APPLICATION 12.1

Some of Dr. Kahn's patients are concerned that computer-based health records may not be completely private. They are worried that unauthorized individuals could access their information on the computer and do them harm. Should patients be allowed to decide whether their records are kept on computer or on paper? Why or why not?

IMPORTANCE OF ACCURATE HEALTH RECORDS

Health records are kept for five basic reasons:

- *To provide the best possible medical care for the patient.* The provider examines the patient and enters the findings in the patient's health record. These findings are clues to the diagnosis. The provider may order many types of tests to confirm the clinical findings. As the reports of these tests come in, the findings fall into place, much like the pieces of a jigsaw puzzle. With these data, the provider can prescribe treatment and form an opinion about the patient's **prognosis**. The health record provides a complete history of all the care given to the patient.
- *To provide critical information for others.* By reading through the record and discovering the methods used to treat the patient, healthcare professionals can provide **continuity of care.** Each provider knows what services have been provided and can continue the care, even from one facility to another.
  - For example, when a patient is transferred from a hospital to a skilled nursing facility, the information from the patient's hospital record helps the nursing facility staff to better care for the patient. When patients move from place to place or caregivers change, copies of the pertinent information should move with the patient to provide this continuity of care.
- *To provide legal protection for those who provided care to the patient.* A well-documented health record is excellent proof that certain procedures were performed or that medical advice was given. An accurate record is the foundation for a legal defense in cases of medical professional liability. This is one reason that writing legibly in the paper record to document exactly what happened to the patient and the provider's response are critical. Remember: If it is not documented, it did not happen.
- *To provide statistical information that is helpful to researchers.* The patient's record provides information about medications taken and the reactions to them. Health records may be used to evaluate the effectiveness of certain kinds of treatment or to determine the

incidence of a given disease. Providers often take part in drug studies that track adverse reactions and side effects. The effects of various treatments and procedures also can be tracked, and statistics gathered from patients' records. When statistical information is tracked, the patient-specific data are removed. This information may result in a new outlook on some phases of medicine and can lead to revised techniques and treatments. The statistical data from health records also are valuable in the preparation of scientific papers, books, and lectures.
- *To provide support for claims reimbursement.* This is required by most insurance companies.

CONTENTS OF THE HEALTH RECORD

The patient's health record is the most important record in a healthcare facility. For completeness, each patient's record should contain **subjective information** provided by the patient and **objective information** obtained by the provider and staff of the healthcare facility. If all entries are complete, the health record will stand the test of time. No branch of medicine is exempt from the need to keep patient health records.

Subjective Information
Personal Demographics
The patient's health record begins with routine personal data, which the patient usually supplies on the first visit when the health record is established. Most patients are required to complete a patient information form (Fig. 12.1; see Procedure 12.1, p. 264). The basic facts are:

- Patient's full name, spelled correctly
- Names of parents/guardians if the patient is a child or legally incompetent
- Patient's gender
- Date of birth (DOB)
- Marital status
- Name of spouse if married
- Home address, telephone number, and email address
- Occupation
- Name of employer
- Business address and telephone number
- Employment information for spouse
- Healthcare insurance information
- Source of referral
- Social Security number

Past Health, Family, and Social History
The past health, family, and social histories are often obtained by having the patient complete a questionnaire. The medical assistant may review the form for completeness, and he or she may need to clarify any questions or missing information with the patient before the patient is seen by the provider. The provider will also add information provided during the patient interview. The responses provide information about:

- Any past illnesses (including injuries and/or physical defects, whether congenital or acquired)
- Hospitalizations, or surgeries the patient has had (Fig. 12.2).
- Patient's daily health habits

Thank you for selecting our health care team!
To help us meet all your health care needs, please fill out this form completely in ink. If you have any questions or need assistance, please ask us - we will be happy to help.

Welcome

Patient # ____
Soc. Sec. # ____
Date ____

Patient Information (CONFIDENTIAL)

Name ____ Birth date ____ Home phone ____
Address ____ City ____ State ____ Zip ____
Check appropriate box: ☐ Minor ☐ Single ☐ Married ☐ Divorced ☐ Widowed ☐ Separated
If student, name of school/college ____ City ____ State ____ ☐ Full time ☐ Part time
Patient's or parent's employer ____ Work phone ____
Business address ____ City ____ State ____ Zip ____
Spouse or parent's name ____ Employer ____ Work phone ____
Whom may we thank for referring you? ____
Person to contact in case of emergency ____ Phone ____

Responsible Party

Name of person responsible for this account ____ Relationship to patient ____
Address ____ Home phone ____
Driver's license # ____ Birth date ____ Financial institution ____
Employer ____ Work phone ____ SSN# ____
Is this person currently a patient in our office? ☐ Yes ☐ No

Insurance Information

Name of insured ____ Relationship to patient ____
Birth date ____ Social Security # ____ Date employed ____
Name of employer ____ Union or local # ____ Work phone ____
Address of employer ____ City ____ State ____ Zip ____
Insurance company ____ Group # ____ Policy/ID # ____
Ins. co. address ____ City ____ State ____ Zip ____
How much is your deductible? ____ How much have you used? ____ Max. annual benefit ____

DO YOU HAVE ANY ADDITIONAL INSURANCE? ☐ Yes ☐ No IF YES, COMPLETE THE FOLLOWING:

Name of insured ____ Relationship to patient ____
Birth date ____ Social Security # ____ Date employed ____
Name of employer ____ Union or local # ____ Work phone ____
Address of employer ____ City ____ State ____ Zip ____
Insurance company ____ Group # ____ Policy/ID # ____
Ins. co. address ____ City ____ State ____ Zip ____
How much is your deductible? ____ How much have you used? ____ Max. annual benefit ____

I authorize release of any information concerning my (or my child's) health care, advice and treatment provided for the purpose of evaluating and administering claims for insurance benefits. I also hereby authorize payment of insurance benefits otherwise payable to me directly to the doctor.

X ____
Signature of patient or parent if minor ____ Date ____

FIGURE 12.1 The patient information form provides all of the information that the medical assistant needs to construct the patient's record.

Stickers can be used on the front of paper health records to indicate allergies, advance directives, and other information (Fig. 12.3). In an EHR, there will be alerts that may appear as a pop-up window when the record is accessed that will indicate that the patient has allergies, that immunizations are due, or that there is no advance directive on file. The alerts are helpful for the health professional because they keep important facts about the patient in the forefront of the professional's mind while he or she is treating the individual.

Past Health History. The past health history will include information about:

- previous illnesses/injuries (including childhood illnesses, such as chickenpox or measles)
- previous hospitalizations
- previous surgeries

The dates that these occurred will need to be documented, along with any complications that occurred. The provider needs to be aware of this information because it could affect the patient's current condition.

Family History. The family history includes:

- The physical condition of the various members of the patient's family
- Any illnesses or diseases individual members may have had
- Causes of death

This information is important because certain diseases may have a **hereditary** pattern. Most providers are interested in the immediate family: parents, grandparents, siblings, and children.

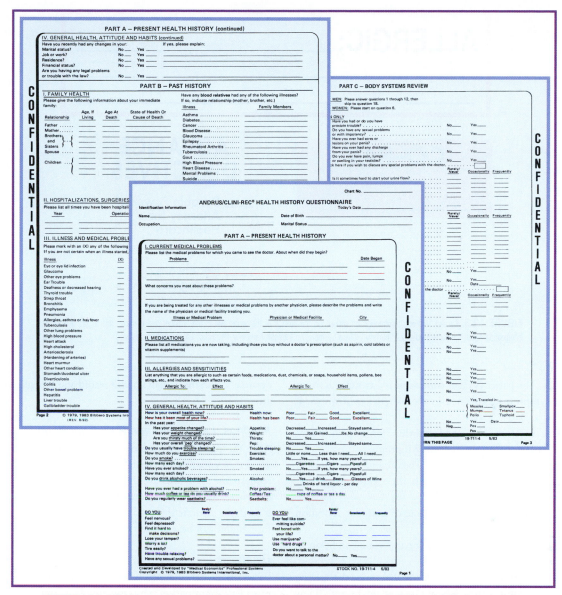

FIGURE 12.2 Self-Administered General Health History Questionnaire. Lengthy questionnaires should be completed by the patient before the individual is seen by the provider. Either mail the questionnaire to the patient in advance or ask the patient to come in early to complete the paperwork. (Courtesy Bibbero Systems, An InHealth Company, Petaluma, CA. *www.bibbero.com.*)

Social History. The social history includes information about the patient's lifestyle, such as:

- Living situation
- Marital status
- Employment
- Tobacco use
- Alcohol and drug use
- Exercise
- Nutrition

All of these factors can have an impact on a patient's overall health; they also can help highlight risk factors.

CRITICAL THINKING APPLICATION   12.2

While taking a patient's medical history, Susan asks about his social history. She asks whether he drinks alcohol. The patient immediately becomes defensive and accuses Susan of getting too personal about his affairs.

- How might Susan explain her reasons for asking these questions? What options are available if the patient refuses to discuss his social history with Susan?
- Could this opposition to questions about the social history raise suspicion in Susan's mind? What might she suspect?

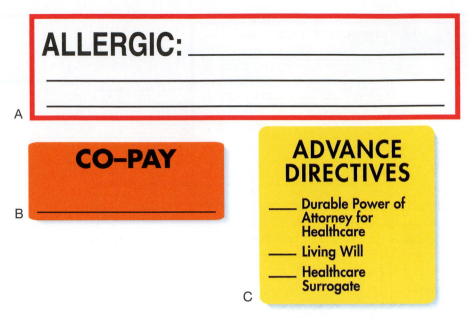

FIGURE 12.3 **Record Stickers.** Information on stickers on the outside of the record allows the provider and medical staff to see important information about the patient quickly. (Courtesy Bibbero Systems, An InHealth Company, Petaluma, CA. *www.bibbero.com.*)

Chief Complaint. The patient's chief complaint is a **concise** account of the patient's symptoms, explained in the patient's own words. It should include:

- The nature, location, frequency, and duration of pain, if any
- When the patient first noticed the symptoms
- Treatments the patient may have tried before seeing the provider and whether they have helped with the symptoms or not; when the last dose was taken
- Whether the patient has had the same or a similar condition in the past
- Other medical treatment received for the same condition in the past

Most healthcare facilities use a pain scale to determine the severity of the patient's discomfort. The medical assistant might ask, "How bad is your pain on a scale of 0 to 10, with 0 being almost no pain, and 10 being the worst pain you've ever experienced?" The pain scale or wording used in individual facilities should be documented in the office policies and procedures manual and followed by the medical assistant.

Objective Information

Objective findings, sometimes referred to as *signs,* are findings that can be observed and measured. They can include vital signs, measurements, observations made by the medical assistant, and findings from the provider's examination of the patient.

Vital Signs and Anthropometric Measurements

The medical assistant's responsibilities include:

- Taking the patient's vital signs (i.e., temperature, pulse, respirations, blood pressure, and pulse oximetry reading)
- Obtaining the person's **anthropometric** measurements (i.e., height and weight)

These measurements are documented in the patient's health record and are used by the provider in his or her assessment. If the medical assistant observes other signs, such as a rash, this would also be documented in the patient's health record and brought to the provider's attention.

Findings, Laboratory and Radiology Reports

After the provider has examined the patient, the physical findings are documented in the health record. The results of other tests or requests for these tests are then documented. If the tests were done elsewhere, the report is attached to the paper record. When an EHR is used, the separate sheet may be scanned so that it is in an electronic format and can be added to the patient's EHR.

Diagnosis

Based on all the evidence provided in the patient's past history, the provider's examination, and any supplementary tests, the provider notes his or her diagnosis of the patient's condition in the health record. If some doubt remains, this may be labeled a **provisional diagnosis**. A *differential diagnosis* is the process of weighing the probability of one disease causing the patient's illness against the probability that other diseases are causative. For example, the differential diagnosis of rhinitis, or a runny nose, could indicate allergic rhinitis (i.e., hay fever), the common cold, or even abuse of drugs or nasal decongestants.

Treatment Prescribed and Progress Notes

The provider's suggested treatment is listed after the diagnosis. Generally, instructions to the patient to return for follow-up treatment within a specific period also are noted here. If surgery or other treatment is going to be performed during the current visit, the patient must sign a consent form.

On each **subsequent** visit, when a paper record is used, the date must be entered on the record; information about the patient's condition and the results of treatment, based on the provider's observations, must be added to the health record. Notations of all medications prescribed, or instructions given, in addition to the patient's own report of how he or she is doing, should be documented in the health record. If the patient is hospitalized, the name of the hospital, the reason for admission, and the dates of admission and discharge are documented. Much of this information can be obtained from the hospital discharge summary.

The Medical Assistant's Role

It is important to ensure patient privacy when documenting in the health record. If you are interviewing the patient to obtain history information, do it where the patient's answers cannot be heard by others. If privacy is not possible, the patient should be given a form to fill out. The information can be transferred to the permanent record later. When privacy is available, the medical assistant may ask the patient questions and document the answers directly into the health record. This allows you to become better acquainted with the patient while completing the necessary records. It can also ensure that the patient understands the meaning of all of the questions.

If new patients must complete a lengthy form, there are several options:

- It can be mailed to the patient. The accompanying letter can request that it be completed and returned to the provider before the appointment.
- If the record is electronic, the patient may access his or her record through a patient portal. Using this method, the information is documented directly into the EHR system. It would then be reviewed by the medical assistant and provider during the office visit.
- Another option with an EHR is for the patient to complete a paper form, and the medical assistant enters the information into the EHR while reviewing the form with the patient.

The medical assistant may document the patient's chief complaint. The provider will question the patient in more detail. Many providers write their own entries in the record in longhand if a paper record is used. Some may document the findings directly into the computer if an electronic record is used. Others may dictate the material directly into the EHR. Another option is for a medical assistant or scribe to document the provider's findings. A final option is for the provider to use a recording device. If the material is dictated and transcribed, the provider should verify each entry. The entry must be initialed by the provider before it is entered into the patient's record. For a record to be admissible as evidence in court, the person dictating or writing the entries must be able to verify that they were true and correct at the time they were written. The best indication of this is the provider's signature or initials on the typed entry. In an EHR, the provider's electronic signature is proof of the accuracy of the entries.

Use of a Medical Scribe

A medical scribe should have an understanding of medical terminology, excellent computer skills, and a strong attention to detail. It is important that medical scribes understand that they are not obtaining the information from the patient. Their role is to document the information obtained by the provider and enter it into the EHR, per the provider's instructions.

Those healthcare facilities that have hired scribes have found that both the patients and providers are more satisfied with patient encounters. Providers are establishing a better relationship with patients because they are able to spend their time with face-to-face interaction rather than interacting with a computer.

OWNERSHIP OF THE HEALTH RECORD

Who owns the health record? Patients often assume that because the information in the health record is about them, ownership of the record is rightfully theirs. However, the owner of the physical health record is the provider or medical facility, often called the "maker," that initiated and developed the record. The patient has the right of access to the information within the record but does not own the physical record or other documents pertaining to the record. The patient has a **vested** interest and therefore has the right to demand confidentiality of all information placed in the record.

The actual paper health record should never leave the medical facility where it originated. Even the provider should refrain from taking the record from the office to the hospital or nursing facility. If information from the record is needed, copies can be made, and progress notes can be written on site and placed into the original record later. This is not an issue with an EHR because the record can be accessed by multiple users at the same time. Patients' paper records should be kept in a locked room or locked filing cabinets when the office is closed. EHRs must be protected from unauthorized access. Regulations established by the Health Insurance Portability and Accountability Act (HIPAA) state that each user must have a unique user name and password; individual access is determined by the system administrator.

Written health records must be legible. Each record should be written as if the provider and staff expect it to eventually be involved in a lawsuit; therefore, every word must be legible to an average reader years after it is written. The record can help the provider prove that he or she treated a patient in a competent manner. It can also prove that the patient was not given competent care. Every person on staff at the provider's office is responsible for writing legibly in every health record.

EHRs eliminate the issue of legibility in the record, but it is just as important to be sure that all patient care is documented in the electronic record. If care is not documented, this will leave the healthcare facility open to potential lawsuits and can affect patient care. In addition, if services are not documented, they cannot be billed to the patient or the patient's insurance company.

CRITICAL THINKING APPLICATION 12.3

On Susan's third day at work, a man comes into the office and demands to see his mother's health record. Susan accesses the record and sees that the mother has not granted permission for information to be given to her son. What should Susan do in this situation? Are there any viable reasons the son should have access to his mother's medical information?

TECHNOLOGIC TERMS IN HEALTH INFORMATION

There is some confusion regarding the acronyms *EHR* and *EMR*. These acronyms have been used interchangeably for many years. The Office of the National Coordinator for Health Information Technology (ONC) has established definitions for EHR and EMR that are easy to understand. Table 12.1 shows the definitions of EHR and EMR.

EMR is being used less and less as the federal regulations regarding electronic records have been established. There is a significant push toward having all electronic records meet the definition of an EHR. There are many advantages to having an electronic record system

TABLE 12.1 Electronic Health Record (EHR) versus Electronic Medical Record (EMR)	
ELECTRONIC HEALTH RECORD (EHR)	**ELECTRONIC MEDICAL RECORD (EMR)**
• Electronic record of health-related information about a patient • Conforms to nationally recognized interoperability standards • Can be created, managed, and consulted by authorized clinicians and staff from more than one healthcare organization	• An electronic record of health-related information about an individual • An electronic version of a paper record • Can be created, gathered, managed, and consulted by authorized clinicians and staff within a single healthcare organization

that can be accessed from more than one healthcare organization. The continuity of patient care is much more easily established when all providers have access to the same records regardless of what organization they are working for. There should be less running of duplicate tests and procedures, which will help reduce the cost of providing healthcare.

A *personal health record* (PHR) is defined by the ONC as an electronic record of health-related information about an individual that conforms to nationally recognized **interoperability** standards and that can be drawn from multiple sources, but that is managed, shared, and controlled by the individual. There are several ways that a PHR can be created. Some health insurance companies offer PHRs for those they insure; some employers offer it as a service for their employees; and some healthcare facilities offer it to their patients. It is important to remember that the patient maintains a PHR. The information from an EHR does not automatically transfer to a PHR.

Another way for patients to access their healthcare information is through a **patient portal**. Patient portals allow patients to access their actual EHRs. At any time, a patient can view progress notes, laboratory results, medications, or immunizations. Many patient portal systems also allow:

- Communication between the patient and provider
- Completion of forms online
- Requests to be made for prescription refills
- Scheduling of appointments

By establishing effective patient portals, healthcare facilities can meet some of the meaningful use requirements.

HIPAA uses the term *protected health information* (PHI), which is any information about health status, the provision of healthcare, or payment for healthcare that can be linked to an individual patient. HIPAA requires that all PHI be safeguarded. This applies to:

- EHRs
- EMRs
- PHRs
- Patient portals

THE HEALTH INFORMATION TECHNOLOGY FOR ECONOMIC AND CLINICAL HEALTH ACT (HITECH) AND MEANINGFUL USE

The HITECH Act provides financial incentives for the meaningful use of certified EHR technology to achieve health and efficiency goals. It was part of the American Recovery and Reinvestment Act to promote the adoption and meaningful use of health information technology. Remember, HIPAA was created in large part to simplify administrative processes using electronic devices. *Meaningful use* means that providers must show that they are using EHR technology in ways that can be measured significantly in quality and quantity. If providers meet the meaningful use requirements, they will qualify for incentive payments. Three main components of meaningful use can be identified:

- Use of certified EHR technology in a meaningful manner, such as **e-prescribing**
- Use of certified EHR technology for electronic exchange of health information to improve the quality of healthcare
- Use of certified EHR technology to submit clinical quality reports, procedure and diagnosis codes, surveys, and other measures

Providers can expect reductions in the amounts they are paid from Medicare and Medicaid if they are not in **compliance**. Remember, the computer system in the medical office must be more than a tool for data recall to be considered an EHR system; the provider must use the system for tasks, at a minimum, such as e-prescribing and **computerized provider/physician order entry (CPOE)**.

CRITICAL THINKING APPLICATION   12.4
Some of the patients who visit Dr. Kahn and Dr. Martin have expressed concern that electronic health records (EHRs) may not be private enough and that their health information will be "floating around on the internet." They are worried that unauthorized individuals could somehow access their information on the computer and do them harm. • How might Susan alleviate the patients' fears about their records being available on the internet? • What disadvantages with regard to confidentiality are associated with the EHR?

CAPABILITIES OF ELECTRONIC HEALTH RECORD SYSTEMS

The EHR system can perform a multitude of tasks, saving time and money in the provider's office (Fig. 12.4). The following are some of the features of a typical EHR system.

- **Specialty software.** Patient data are captured and processed into a system that is specialty-specific. The terminology and patient care treatments are compatible with the provider's specialty. However, additional features can allow the provider to include terminology from other specialties.
- **Appointment scheduler.** The appointment scheduler (Fig. 12.5) allows the staff to:
  - Track and schedule appointments
  - Create the schedule matrix

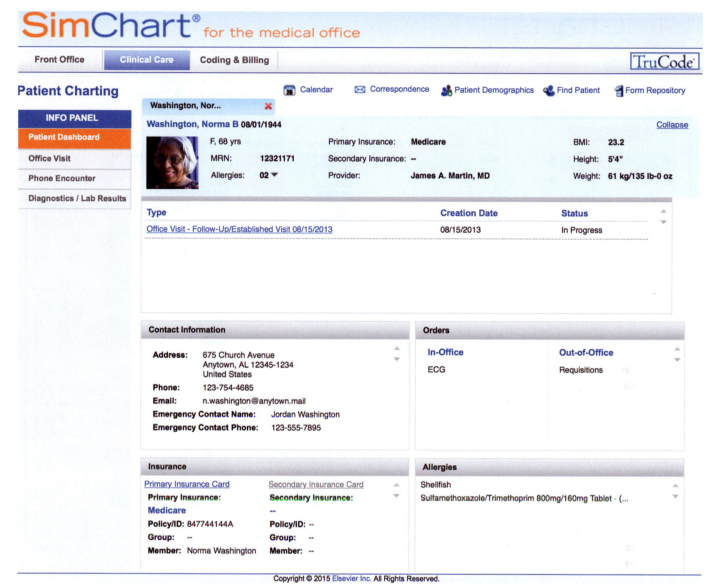

FIGURE 12.4 The electronic health record (EHR) can perform numerous tasks, in addition to displaying personal information about the patient. This allows the provider and medical assistants to interact with patients and provide better service.

- Account for recurring time blocks
  The appointments can be merged into specific types with default times so that lengthy procedures are not scheduled in short appointment blocks. The scheduler features also allow various search **parameters**; if a patient calls because he or she cannot remember the appointment time, a search can be initiated using:
- Date
- Provider's name
- Patient's name
- Keywords
- **Appointment reminder and confirmation.** The system can be programmed to automatically remind patients with a confirmation call. The staff can record the message to be sent, and patients are prompted to choose options, such as "Press one" to confirm or reschedule appointments.
- **Prescription writer.** The EHR system can produce electronic prescriptions, which can be printed and given to patients or

automatically submitted to a pharmacy. Lists can be created with the provider's most common drug choices and dosages. An allergy function can be linked to the patient's list of allergies and alert the provider of an issue. The system can also generate a patient information sheet on new prescriptions.
- **Medical billing system.** Also known as a *practice management system.* The EHR billing system can manage all of the practice's billing and accounting systems. The system also can **interface** with clearinghouses for electronic claims submission and tracking. Reports can be generated that provide accurate details of the financial state of the practice at certain intervals or whenever requested.
- **Charge capture.** The charge capture functions can store lists of billing codes, such as:
  - International Classification of Diseases (ICD)
  - Current Procedural Terminology (CPT)
  - Charges for procedures, supplies, and laboratory tests

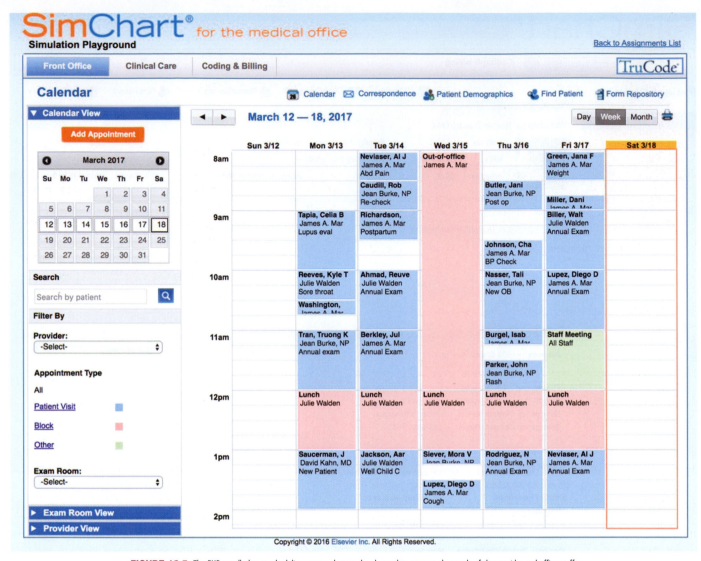

FIGURE 12.5 The EHR usually has a scheduling system that can be changed to manage the needs of the provider and office staff.

Alerts can let the user know when a certain charge does not match a diagnosis code; for instance, a blood glucose test done for a sore throat. In such cases, the software alerts the user and helps prevent errors that can lead to denial of insurance claims.

- **Eligibility verification.** EHR billing systems can perform online verification of insurance eligibility and can capture demographic data.
- **Referral management.** In the case of a referral or consultation, sharing information with another provider can be done electronically. The patient does not have to obtain copies of the record and then bring them to the new provider. This also eliminates the cost of making copies and is faster and more efficient than copying and mailing patients' records.
- **Laboratory order integration.** The laboratory order integration feature allows the user to interact with outside laboratories. The EHR can receive and post laboratory results to patients' records. Tests can be ordered from the provider's laptop, tablet, or smart phone. Results can be transmitted by fax, scan, or email and uploaded directly into the patient's record (see Procedure 12.2, p. 265).

CRITICAL THINKING APPLICATION   **12.5**

Jennifer, the office manager, has noticed that Susan seems overwhelmed in the training classes for the EHR system used by the clinic. During a break, Jennifer asks Susan whether she is having any specific problems with the training classes. She also asks for Susan's input on the system. Susan says that she just prefers clinical work and that her typing skills are a little "rusty." She is determined to do her best to learn the system and asks if she could have extra practice time.

- How might Jennifer respond to Susan's comments?
- What can Susan do to overcome her issues with the EHR system?

MAINTAINING A CONNECTION WITH THE PATIENT WHEN USING THE ELECTRONIC HEALTH RECORD

Many patients are required to choose a primary care provider (PCP) to be referred to a specialist. They also have the option of changing the PCP or specialist. The patient may decide to change providers

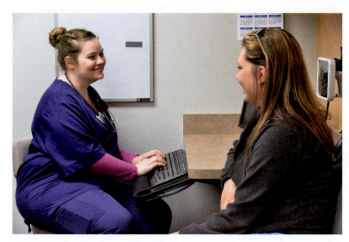

FIGURE 12.6 The medical assistant must make eye contact with the patient when using an EHR.

simply because he or she does not feel comfortable with that particular provider.

Because the change process is relatively easy, the healthcare facility should strive to provide excellent care and service to its patients. If the care begins to seem impersonal, patients may feel a strong desire to change providers. Patients are consumers of healthcare services, and they expect quality healthcare and service.

When using the EHR, the medical assistant must make sure that his or her nonverbal communication sends the right message to the patient. Eye contact is essential (Fig. 12.6). If the medical assistant constantly looks at the electronic device, the patient feels left out of the process. Make eye contact with the patient while asking questions and look at the screen only when needed to enter information. Do not shield the device from the patient's view when entering information. This can give the impression you are hiding something from the patient. Although patients may not understand anything they see on the screen, they will feel more at ease if their information is not hidden from them. Also, modify your position so that the patient feels like a part of the information process. Just as sitting in a chair across from a supervisor's desk can be intimidating, the patient may feel the same emotions sitting across from a medical assistant entering information into the EHR. Sit next to or at an angle to the patient to support the impression that those in the healthcare facility and the patient are partners in the healthcare plan.

Because patients have the right to make decisions in most aspects of their healthcare plans, offer choices wherever possible. Never expect patients to make quick decisions about their care. They may want to consult family members or give some thought to important medical decisions. The medical assistant needs to allow the patient time to think unless the patient is faced with a critical, time-sensitive decision. Providers often assume that patients will automatically follow their instructions or orders; however, some patients prefer some time to consider their options. Always follow up and make note of any wait time the patient requests, notify the provider, and enter that information into the EHR. Make sure timely communication is accomplished with the patient and that any additional orders that need to be put in place are completed. The many features of the EHR allow the medical assistant to be efficient and highly competent if he or she is willing to make an extra effort to master the EHR system.

Also, make sure patients understand all instructions given to them regarding test procedures or preparation for procedures. Most EHRs can print an instruction sheet, which the medical assistant can review with the patient. The customer service aspect of patient care is even more important when the facility uses an EHR system (see Procedure 12.3, p. 265).

> **CRITICAL THINKING** APPLICATION   **12.6**
>
> Jennifer walks behind Susan's desk and notices that she is looking at the progress notes on a patient who was recently arrested and indicted for child abuse. The case has been in the newspaper and on television consistently for several weeks. Jennifer asks Susan why she has accessed that record. Susan hesitates and then says she must have entered the wrong patient ID number. Does Susan's explanation sound convincing? Why is Jennifer concerned about Susan looking at the patient's record? Just because the individual is a patient at the clinic, does that mean any employee has the right to look at the patient's EHR?

BACKUP SYSTEMS FOR THE ELECTRONIC HEALTH RECORD

Even the best or most expensive EHR system cannot function without power. If a natural disaster occurs and the provider's office is without electricity for several days or weeks, the provider must have a backup system to protect the information contained in the EHR. HIPAA requires that the facility adopt a backup and recovery plan that includes daily offsite software backup for the EHR system. Three options are available for data preservation and backup.

- *External hard drive.* An external hard drive connects to the main computer, and with fairly simple programming it can copy the information in the EHR daily. Seven electronic folders, one for each day of the week, can hold the information from the previous day; these folders are replaced with new, updated information at designated periods. CDs and DVDs can hold daily data, and some thumb drives have enough capacity to perform this task. Once a habit of a daily backup to the external hard drive has been established, the method is relatively simple and reliable.
- *Full server backup.* The provider may want to back up the EHR system on a dedicated server, which is a large-capacity computer set aside specifically for the EHR system. With these servers, a full backup should be performed monthly. Many large medical facilities and hospitals have one or more dedicated servers for the EHR system.
- *Online backup system.* An online backup system can be used, usually for a subscription fee. Although the cost may be higher than for some other methods, online systems are easy to use because there is no external drive to carry and no CD or thumb drive to put through the process of downloading data. However, time investment is involved, because the process of contacting the company that offers the service and then downloading all the data takes several hours. Also, the initial download can take quite a while. Even so, an online system is stable and reliable.

All of these backup methods require an alternative power source in case of a disaster that interrupts electrical service. Remember that backup systems are not effective if the data are stored at the medical facility and the disaster happens at or affects that physical address. Information technology professionals usually recommend using two of the three methods for the best protection. The system must be protected from theft and unauthorized use, just like the onsite system.

Medical assistants should keep their paper health records skills sharp in case the EHR system is down for an extended period. Always have a supply of the most commonly used forms in a paper format available for use in such instances. When the EHR system comes back up, these paper forms can be scanned into the patients' EHRs.

RETENTION AND DESTRUCTION OF HEALTH RECORDS

In most medical offices, records are classified in three ways:
- *Active:* Records of patients currently receiving treatment
- *Inactive:* Records of patients whom the provider has not seen for 6 months or longer
- *Closed:* Records of patients who have died, moved away, or otherwise terminated their relationship with the provider

The process of moving a file from active to inactive status is called *purging.* An EHR system can be set up to automatically move the inactive records to another server so that processing time will not be slowed down, but the records are still readily accessible if the patient returns to the healthcare facility. Closed EHRs are also separated from the active records and are typically stored elsewhere. They may be placed on CDs or computer hard drives or maintained in inactive cloud space by the EHR vendor.

As with EHRs, paper health records are classified as active, inactive, and closed. A paper record system must have a system established for regular transfer of files from active to inactive status or possibly destruction. The expansion of records and the file space available can influence the transfer period. Records for patients currently hospitalized may be kept in a special section for quick reference and then placed in the regular active file when the patient is discharged from the hospital. In a surgical practice, the record frequently includes the specific date on which the patient is discharged from the provider's care, and the notation is made on the record, "Return prn" (from the Latin *pro re nata,* "as the occasion arises" or "when needed"). This record may safely be placed in the inactive file.

Most medical facilities use a year sticker on the file folder that indicates the last year the patient visited the clinic. If the file has a sticker showing that the patient's last visit was in 2018, and he or she presents to the clinic on January 5, 2020, a 2020 sticker should be placed over the one that indicates 2018. These stickers often are included with color-coded filing systems. The medical assistant can easily look at a group of files and see which ones need to be changed to inactive or closed status.

According to the American Medical Association (AMA) Council on Ethical and Judicial Affairs, providers have an obligation to retain patient records whether they are paper or electronic. Currently, no nationwide standard rule exists for establishing a records **retention schedule.**

Medical considerations are the primary basis for deciding how long to retain health records. For example, operative notes and chemotherapy records should always be part of the patient's health record. The laws regarding the retention of health records vary from state to state, and many governmental programs have their own guidelines for specific records retention. When no rules specify the retention of health records, the best course is to keep the records for 10 years. However, for minors, the facility should keep the records until the minor reaches the **age of majority** plus the statute of limitations. It is best to know the state requirements related to health records retention and follow those guidelines. The office policies and procedures manual should address records retention pertaining to the state where the practice exists.

The records of any patient covered by Medicare or Medicaid must be kept at least 10 years. The HIPAA Privacy Rule does not include requirements for the retention of health records. However, the rule does require that appropriate administrative, technical, and physical safeguards be applied so that the privacy of health records is maintained.

Some providers refuse to destroy or discard old records. Storage is less of an issue with EHRs because they take up much less physical space. Always refer to state laws when discarding health records.

Before old records are destroyed, patients should be given an opportunity to claim a copy of the records or have them sent to another provider. The medical facility should keep a master list of all records that have been destroyed. To legally destroy an EHR, the record, including the backup record, has to be overwritten using utility software.

RELEASING HEALTH RECORD INFORMATION

The healthcare facility must be extremely careful when releasing any type of medical information. The patient must sign a release for information to be given to any third party.

Requests for medical information should be made in writing (Fig. 12.7). HIPAA has designated that specific information must be included on the release of information form:
- Who is releasing the information
- To whom the information is being released
- What specific information is to be released
- An expiration date for the release

Accepting a faxed request for medical information or a faxed release of information from a patient is unwise. Even requests from the patient's attorney or insurance companies must be cleared by the patient for them to obtain information.

If a provider is involved in a liability suit, there will be a required exchange of information. As both parties to a lawsuit begin to prepare their cases, they enter the discovery process. Each side must disclose the pertinent facts of the case that may influence the final outcome of that case. On each occasion that information is needed from the provider, a separate request must be sent. Because the patient signs this request form, it serves as a release.

Most offices charge a fee to print or copy health records, whether it is a per-page charge or a per-record fee. If the records are sent electronically, no fee is charged. Follow the steps in the policies and procedures manual for the release of records. Some providers designate the office manager to handle requests for records releases.

Pay particular attention to records release requests involving a minor. In most cases, the parent or legal guardian is entitled to read through the patient's health records; however, according to the US Department of Health and Human Services (HHS), there are three

Central Texas Dermatology Clinic • 102 Westlake Drive • Austin, Texas 78746

AUTHORIZATION TO DISCLOSE HEALTH INFORMATION

I hereby authorize the use or disclosure of information from the medical record of:

Patient Name: _____   Date of Birth: _____

Social Security# _____   Daytime Phone: _____

I authorize the following individual or organization to disclose the above named individual's health information:

_____   Address: _____

This information may be disclosed TO and used by the following individual or organization:

_____   Address: _____

Please release the following:

____ Progress Notes   ____ Pathology Reports   ____ Lab Reports   ____ Any and all Records

____ Other Diagnostic reports (specify _____

____ Other (specify) _____

        Including Information (if applicable) pertaining to:

        ____ Mental Health   ____ Drug/Alcohol   ____ HIV/AIDS   ____ Communicable Treatment

Purpose or Need for Disclosure:

____ Continued Patient Care   ____ Personal Use

____ Attorney/Legal   ____ Insurance Claim/Application

____ Disability Determination   ____ Other(specify) _____

I understand that the information in my health record may include information relating to sexually transmitted disease, acquired immunodeficiency syndrome (AIDS), or human immunodeficiency virus (HIV). It may also include information about behavioral or mental health services, and treatment for alcohol and drug abuse.

I understand that the information released is for the specific purpose stated above. Any other use of this information without the written consent of the patient is prohibited.

I understand that I have the right to revoke this authorization at any time. I understand that if I revoke this authorization I must do so in writing and present my written revocation to the individual or organization releasing information. I understand that the revocation will not apply to information already released in response to this authorization. I understand that the revocation will not apply to my insurance company when the law provides my insurer the right to contest a claim under my policy. Unless otherwise revoked, this authorization will expire on following date, event or condition: _____

If I fail to specify an expiration date, event or condition, this authorization will expire in six months.

I understand that authorizing the disclosure of this health information is voluntary. I can refuse to sign the authorization. I need not sign this form in order to ensure treatment. I understand that I may inspect or copy the information to be used or disclosed, as provided in CFR 164.524. I understand that any disclosure of information carries with it the potential for an unauthorized re-disclosure and the information may not be protected by federal confidentiality rules. If I have questions about disclosure of my health information, I can contact Theresa Farren at 512-327-7779.

_____   _____

Signature of Patient or Legal Representative   Date

_____   _____

Relationship to Patient (If Legal Representative)   Witness

COMPLETE ONLY IF INFORMATION IS TO BE RELEASED DIRECTLY TO PATIENT:

I understand that my medical record may contain reports, test results, and notes that only a physician can interpret. I understand and have been advised that I should contact my physician regarding the entries made in my medical record to prevent my misunderstanding of the information contained in these entries. I will not hold Central Texas Dermatology liable for any misinterpretation of the information in my medical record as a result of not contacting my physician for the correct interpretation.

_____   _____

Signature of Patient or Legal Representative   Date

_____   _____

Relationship to Patient (If Legal Representative)   Witness

Dr. review/signature/date _____

Date request completed _____   # of pages copied _____

Staff Signature _____

PHI Log completed _____

FIGURE 12.7 Authorization to Release Health Records. All requests for health records should be in writing, and the request should be kept in the patient's health record.

situations in which the parent may not be legally entitled to review the records of his or her minor child:

- When the minor is the one who consents to care, and the parent is not required to also consent to care under state law
- When the minor obtains medical care at the direction of a court or a person authorized by the court
- When the minor, parent, and provider all agree that the doctor and minor patient can have a private, confidential relationship

If the provider believes that the minor might be in an abusive situation or that the parent or legal guardian may be harming the patient, the provider is required, both legally and ethically, to report the abuse.

Sometimes patients want to look at their own records. They certainly have a right to see this information, but some patients may not understand the terminology used in the record. A staff member should always remain with a patient who is looking at his or her health record. Remember, the original health record should never leave the medical facility. Always follow office policy when releasing health records.

When a release is presented to the office, provide only the records requested in the release. Do not provide information that is not requested. The patient must specify that substance abuse, mental health, or human immunodeficiency virus (HIV) records are to be released. Remember that the patient ultimately decides whether a record can be released. If any question arises about what is to be released, consult the office manager or the provider.

Health Information Exchanges

The demand for electronic health information exchange (HIE) between one healthcare facility and another, together with nationwide efforts to improve the efficiency and quality of healthcare, is creating a demand for HIEs. As more and more providers move to EHRs, it only makes sense to have a system in place that will facilitate the exchange of that information electronically to improve the timeliness of that exchange. Patient care can be improved because all providers will have access to the information needed to treat the patient.

The ONC states, There are currently three forms of HIE:

- *Directed Exchange* – The ability to send and receive secure information electronically between care providers to support coordinated care
- *Query-Based Exchange* – The ability of providers to find and/or request information on a patient from other providers, often used for unplanned care
- *Consumer-Mediated Exchange* – The ability of patients to aggregate and control the use of their health information among providers

The implementation of HIE varies from state to state. Some of the federal funding for the implementation of HIE is administered by the ONC.

ORGANIZATION OF THE HEALTH RECORD

Source-Oriented Records

The traditional patient record is a source-oriented record (SOR). Observations and data are cataloged according to their source:

- Provider (progress notes)
- Laboratory
- Radiology
- Hospital
- Consultations

Forms and progress notes are filed in **reverse chronologic order** and in separate sections of the record according to the type of form or service rendered (e.g., all laboratory reports together, all x-ray reports together, and so on). Reverse chronologic order is used so that the provider and staff members do not have to search to the bottom of the record to find a recent laboratory report or a test.

Problem-Oriented Records

The problem-oriented medical record (POR) is a departure from the traditional system of keeping patient records. The POR is a method of recording data in a problem-solving system. This system is divided into four components:

- The *database* includes the chief complaint, present illness, patient profile, review of systems, physical examination, and laboratory reports.
- The *problem list* is a numbered, titled list of every problem the patient has that requires management or workup. This may include social and demographic troubles in addition to strictly medical or surgical ones.
- The *treatment plan* includes management, additional workups needed, and therapy. Each plan is titled and numbered with respect to the problem.
- The *progress notes* include structured notes that are numbered to correspond with each problem number.

Several companies have developed file folders for organizing patient data according to the POR. The problem list (Fig. 12.8) is placed at the front of the record. Special sections are provided for current major and chronic diagnoses/health problems and for inactive major or chronic diagnoses/health problems. Progress notes usually follow the SOAP approach. SOAP is an acronym for the following:

- *S*ubjective impressions or patient reports
- *O*bjective clinical evidence or observations
- *A*ssessment or diagnosis
- *P*lans for further studies, treatment, or management

Some medical offices also use an *E* in the record to represent *evaluation*; others include *E* for *education* and *R* for *response*. The education notation shows that the patient was educated about his or her condition or given a patient information sheet. The response section is used to record an assessment of the patient's understanding of and possible compliance with the treatment plan.

The POR has the advantage of creating order and organization in the information added to a patient's health record. The records are more easily reviewed, and the likelihood of overlooking a problem is greatly reduced. The SOAP method forces a rational approach to the patient's problems and assists in forming a logical, orderly plan of patient care (Fig. 12.9). The POR is especially helpful in clinics, group practices, and hospitals, where more than one person must be able to find essential information in the record.

MASTER PROBLEM LIST

For use of this form, see AR 40-66; the proponent agency is the Office of The Surgeon General

MAJOR PROBLEMS

PROBLEM NUMBER	DATE ONSET	DATE ENTERED	PROBLEM	DATE RESOLVED
1.				
2.				
3.				
4.				
5.				
6.				
7.				
8.				
9.				
10.				
11.				
12.				

TEMPORARY (MINOR) PROBLEMS

PROBLEM LETTER	PROBLEM	DATES OF OCCURRENCES				
A.						
B.						
C.						
D.						
E.						
F.						
G.						
H.						

PATIENT'S IDENTIFICATION (Use mechanical imprint if available; for typed or written entries give: Name, SSN, Unit, Sex, Birthdate, and Duty Phone)

SUMMARY OF PROBLEMS, ALLERGIES, MEDICATIONS, SURGERIES AND TRAUMAS:

NOTE: DO NOT DISCARD FROM CHART

FIGURE 12.8 A problem list designed for a problem-oriented record (POR).

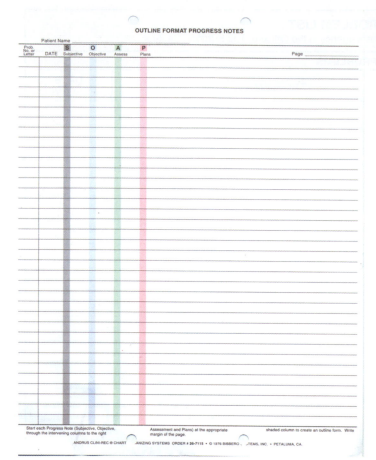

FIGURE 12.9 SOAP Progress Notes. The SOAP method keeps information organized and in a logical sequence. An actual progress note would include the provider's or medical assistant's signature or initials after each entry. (Courtesy Bibbero Systems, An InHealth Company, Petaluma, CA. *www. bibbero.com.*)

CRITICAL THINKING APPLICATION   **12.7**

Susan learned about SOAP documentation in school and is eager to use it in her new job. Dr. Kahn is seeing a patient who reports to Susan that she has had nausea and vomiting for the past 3 days. Susan obtains a weight of 132.5 pounds, temperature (T) 101.2° F tympanically, pulse (P) 94 beats/min, respiration (R) 14 breaths/min, and blood pressure (BP) 122/84 mm Hg in the right arm. What information would be documented in the Subjective field? What information would be documented in the Objective field? Who would document information in the Assessment field?

DOCUMENTING IN AN ELECTRONIC HEALTH RECORD

Documentation in an EHR involves using radio buttons, drop-down menus, and free-text boxes. The radio buttons and drop-down menus allow for standardization of the content in the EHR, and the free-text boxes allow for the documentation of the unique circumstance found with each patient (Fig. 12.10). It is important to carefully review the choices made with the radio buttons and drop-down menus. Information documented using the free-text boxes should be proofread before submitting.

DOCUMENTING IN A PAPER HEALTH RECORD

When you are documenting in a paper health record, the entry will always start with the date in the MM/DD/YYYY format. The date will be followed by the time. This may be written in standard or military time. If standard time is used, it must be followed by a.m. or p.m. (e.g., 2:00 p.m.). If military time is used, it is in a four-digit format without a colon (e.g., 1400). All entries must be written in black or blue ink, following the format designated by the healthcare facility. Documentation should be in the order in which the steps were completed. If a temperature, pulse, and respiration (TPR) measurement is done, it would be documented in the "O" or Objective section of the SOAP note starting with temperature, then pulse, and, lastly, respirations.

MAKING CORRECTIONS AND ALTERATIONS TO HEALTH RECORDS

Sometimes corrections must be made to health records. The first step is to verify the proper procedure for making corrections in the facility's policy and procedures manual. Some providers prefer a specific method for correcting errors in the health record. Erasing, using correction fluid, or any other type of **obliteration** is never acceptable. To correct a handwritten entry:

1. Draw a line through the error.
2. Insert the correction above or immediately after the error in a spot where it can be read clearly.
3. If indicated by the policies and procedures manual, write "Error" or "Err." in the margin.
4. The person making the correction should write his or her initials or signature and the date below the correction. Follow the format indicated in the policy and procedures manual (Fig. 12.11).

Errors made while using the computer are corrected in the usual way. However, an error discovered in an entry at a later date is corrected in the same manner as for a handwritten entry. This is sometimes called an *addendum*. Never attempt to alter health records without using this specific correction procedure, because this alteration of records may indicate a fraudulent attempt to cover up a mistake made by a staff member or the provider. Do not hide errors. If the error could, in any way, affect the patient's health and well-being, it must be brought to the provider's attention immediately. An EHR system will track the changes made within the record.

DICTATION AND TRANSCRIPTION

With the increased use of EHRs and voice recognition software, there is decreased need for **transcription**. If **dictation** is still done in the healthcare facility, the administrative medical assistant may find that transcribing the dictation is a job she or he will sometimes perform. Transcription can be done from handwritten notes or, more likely, from machine dictation. Smooth operation of the facility may depend on the timely, accurate performance of assigned responsibilities, such as record documentation and the preparation of special reports. Accuracy and speed are the primary requirements, along with a strong grasp of medical terminology and anatomy and physiology.

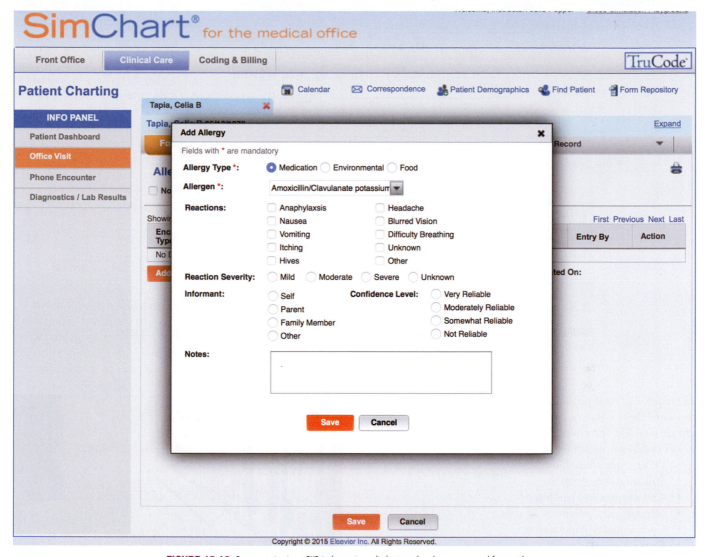

FIGURE 12.10 Documentation in an EHR is done using radio buttons, drop-down menus, and free-text boxes.

Dictation may be done using a machine transcription unit or a portable transcription unit. Many healthcare facilities now use a system that is accessed by telephone; the provider calls the system, using passwords or access codes, and records the information for the health record while speaking into the telephone. Later, employees transcribe the information into the health record. The provider must acknowledge and initial all transcripts before they are placed in the health record.

Voice Recognition Software

Some healthcare facilities use voice recognition software for transcription. When first installed, the software requires the user to say several sentences into the unit so that it "learns" to recognize the user's voice. The system can be used to dictate the following:

- Progress notes
- Letters
- Emails
- Any document in the healthcare facility that needs to be created

The provider will need to approve these documents before they are permanently attached to the patient's record. Some systems have

an authentication component that allows a type of electronic signature, such as those needed for hospital record dictation.

CREATING AN EFFICIENT PAPER HEALTH RECORDS MANAGEMENT SYSTEM

The paper health records management system should provide an easy method of retrieving information. The files should be organized in an orderly fashion. The information must be documented accurately, and corrections should be made and documented properly. The wording in the record should be easily understood and grammatically correct. An efficient method of adding documents to the record must be established so that the provider always has the most up-to-date information. Above all, the health records management system must work for the individual facility.

Filing Equipment

For years, the traditional filing system involved a vertical, four-drawer steel filing cabinet, used with manila folders with the patient's name

10/31/20XX	1:30pm T: 98.4 (TA), P62 reg, strong ^{72 error S. Beezler CMA (AAMA)}
	R: 14 reg, deep, BP: 116/72 Ⓡ arm sitting
	———————————————— Susan Beezler, CMA (AAMA)

| 10/15/20XX | 9:30am Mantoux test: 0 mm induration ^{10 error S. Beezler CMA (AAMA)} |
| | ———————————————— Susan Beezler, CMA (AAMA) |

FIGURE 12.11 Corrections to health records must be done in a legible manner and must be clearly understood. Always initial and date corrections to health records.

on the tab. The most popular system today is color coding on open horizontal shelves. Rotary, lateral, compactable, and automated files also are available. Some records are kept in card or tray files. Several factors should be considered when selecting filing equipment:

- Office space availability
- Structural considerations
- Cost of space and equipment
- Size, type, and volume of records
- Confidentiality requirements
- Retrieval speed
- Fire protection
- Cost

Drawer Files

Drawer files should be full suspension; they should roll easily, close securely, and be equipped with a locking device. The best cabinets have a center trough at the bottom of each drawer with a rod for holding divider guides. A drawback of the vertical four-drawer files is that only one person can use a file cabinet at a time. Also, filing is slower, because the drawer must be opened and closed each time a file is pulled or filed.

File cabinets are heavy and can tip over, causing serious damage or injury unless reasonable care is taken. Open only one file drawer at a time and close it when the filing has been completed. A drawer left even slightly open can injure a passerby.

Horizontal Shelf Files

Shelf files should have doors that lock to protect the contents. A popular type of shelf file has doors that slide back into the cabinet; the door from a lower shelf may be pulled out and used for workspace. Open shelf units hold files sideways and can go higher on the wall because no drawers need to be pulled out (Fig. 12.12). File retrieval is faster, because several individuals can work simultaneously.

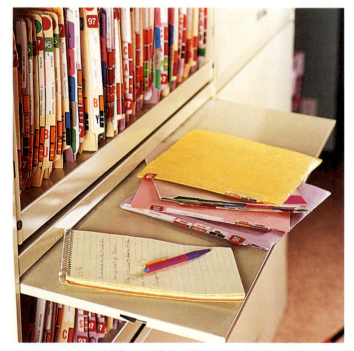

FIGURE 12.12 Open shelf filing is an efficient method, especially for color-coding filing systems. The shelf doors often can be used as workspace.

Rotary Circular Files

Rotary circular files can hold a large volume of records. They save space and clerical motion. The files revolve easily; some have push-button controls. Several people can work at one rotary file and use records at the same time. One disadvantage is that they afford less privacy and protection than files that can be closed and locked.

Compactible Files

An office with little space and a great volume of records might use compactible files, which are a variation of open shelf files. The files are mounted on tracks in the floor, and the units slide along the tracks so that access is gained to the needed records. One drawback is that not all records are available at the same time.

Automated Files

Automated files are initially very expensive, and they also require more maintenance than other types of filing equipment. They are likely to be found only in large facilities, such as clinics or hospitals. These files bring the record to the operator instead of the operator going to the record. When the operator presses a button indicating the appropriate shelf, the shelf automatically moves into position in front of the operator for record retrieval. The automated or power file is fast and can store large numbers of records in a small amount of space. However, only one person can use the unit at a time.

Card Files

Almost every office has some occasion to use a card file. This may be for patient ledgers, a patient index, a library index, an index of surgical tray setups, telephone numbers, or numerous other records. A good-quality steel box or tray is a sound investment.

Filing Supplies

Divider Guides

Each file drawer or shelf should be equipped with plenty of dividers or guides. Some authorities recommend one guide for approximately each 1½ inch of material, or every eight to 10 folders. Guides should be of good-quality heavy cardstock or strong plastic. Less-well-constructed guides soon become bent and frayed and have to be replaced. Divider guides have a protruding tab, which may be an integral part of the card or may be made of metal or plastic. The guides reduce the area of search and serve as supports for the folders. They are available in single, third, or fifth cut (i.e., one, three, or five different positions).

Out Guides

Out guides are made of heavyweight cardboard or plastic and are used to replace a folder that has been temporarily removed (Fig. 12.13). They may also have a large pocket to hold any filing that may come in while the folder is out. They should be of a distinctive color for quick detection. This makes refiling simpler and alerts the file clerk that a file is missing. Several colors may be used, each color designating the temporary location of the file. The out guide may have lines for recording information, or it may have a plastic pocket for inserting an information card.

File Folders

Most records to be filed are placed in covers or tabbed folders. The most commonly used is a general purpose, third-cut manila folder that may be expanded to ¾ of an inch. These are available with a double-thickness, reinforced tab, which greatly extends the life of the folder. Folders kept in drawers have tabs at the top; those kept on shelves have tabs at the side. Many folder styles are available for special purposes.

Hanging, or suspension, folders are made of heavy stock and hang on metal rods from side to side in a drawer. They can be used only with file cabinets equipped with suspension equipment.

Binder folders have fasteners that are used to bind papers in the folder. These offer some security for the papers, but filing the materials is time-consuming.

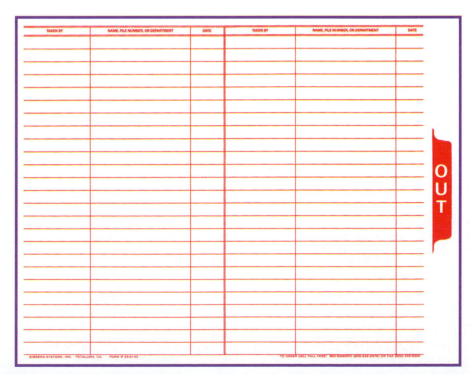

FIGURE 12.13 Out guides allow tracking of a file not in its proper location by providing information on the location of the file. (Courtesy Bibbero Systems, An InHealth Company, Petaluma, CA. *www.bibbero.com.*)

The number of papers that will fit in one folder depends on the thickness of the papers and the capacity of the folder. Near the bottom edge of most folders are one or more score marks, which should be used as the contents of the folders expand. Papers should never protrude from the folder edges, and they should always be inserted with their tops to the left. When papers start to ride up in any folder, the folder is overloaded.

Labels

The label is a necessary filing and finding device. Use labels to identify each shelf, drawer, divider guide, and folder. A label on the drawer or shelf identifies the nature of its contents. It should also indicate the range (i.e., alphabetic, numeric, or chronologic) of the material filed in that space.

The label on the divider guide identifies the range of folder headings following that divider guide up to the next divider (e.g., Ba-Bo). The label on the folder identifies the contents of that folder only, such as the following:

- Name of the patient
- Subject matter of correspondence
- Business topic

Label a folder when a new patient is seen, existing folders are full, or materials need to be transferred within the filing system.

Labels are available in almost any size, shape, or color to meet the individual needs of any facility. Visit an office supply website and review the catalogs to find the best product to meet the needs of the facility.

A narrow label applied to the front of the folder tab is the easiest to use and is satisfactory for folders kept in a drawer file. Labels for shelf filing should be identifiable from both front and back. Always type the label before separating it from the roll or protective sheet. Type the **caption** on the label in indexing order (see Procedure 12.4, p. 266).

INDEXING RULES

Indexing rules (Table 12.2) are standardized and based on current business practices. The Association of Records Managers and Administrators takes an active part in updating these rules. Some establishments adopt variations of these basic rules to accommodate their needs. In any case, the practices need to be consistent within the system:

TABLE 12.2	Applying Indexing Rules			
INDEXING RULE	**NAME**	**UNIT 1**	**UNIT 2**	**UNIT 3**
1	Robert F. Grinch	Grinch	Robert	F.
	R. Frank Grumman	Grumman	R.	Frank
2	J. Orville Smith	Smith	J.	Orville
	Jason O. Smith	Smith	Jason	O.
3	M. L. Saint-Vickery	Saint-Vickery	M.	L.
	Marie-Louise Taylor	Taylor	Marielouise	
4	Charles S. Anderson	Anderson	Charles	S.
	Anderson's Surgical Supply	Andersons	Surgical	Supply
5	Ah Hop Akee	Akee	Ah	Hop
6	Alice Delaney	Delaney	Alice	
	Chester K. DeLong	Delong	Chester	K.
7	Michael St. John	Stjohn	Michael	
8	Helen M. Maag	Maag	Helen	M.
	Frederick Mabry	Mabry	Frederick	
	James E. MacDonald	Macdonald	James	E.
9	Mrs. John L. Doe (Mary Jones)	Doe	Mary	Jones (Mrs. John L.)
10	Prof. John J. Breck	Breck	John	J. (Prof.)
	Madame Sylvia	Madame	Sylvia	
	Sister Mary Catherine	Sister	Mary	Catherine
	Theodore Wilson, MD	Wilson	Theodore (MD)	
11	Lawrence W. Jones, Jr.	Jones	Lawrence	W. (Jr.)
	Lawrence W. Jones, Sr.	Jones	Lawrence	W. (Sr.)
12	The Moore Clinic	Moore	Clinic (The)	

1. Last names are considered first in filing; then the given name (first name), second; and the middle name or initial, third. Compare the names beginning with the first letter of the name. When a letter is different in the two names, that letter determines the order of filing.
2. Initials precede a name beginning with the same letter. This illustrates the librarian's rule, "Nothing comes before something."
3. With hyphenated personal names, the hyphenated elements, whether first name, middle name, or surname, are considered to be one unit.
4. The apostrophe is disregarded in filing.
5. When you are indexing a foreign name in which you cannot distinguish between the first and last names, index each part of the name in the order in which it is written. If you can make the distinction, use the last name as the first indexing unit.
6. Names with prefixes are filed in the usual alphabetic order, with the prefix considered part of the name.
7. Abbreviated parts of a name are indexed as written if that person generally uses that form.
8. Mac and Mc are filed in their regular place in the alphabet. If the files have a great many names beginning with Mac or Mc, some offices file them as a separate letter of the alphabet for convenience.
9. The name of a married woman who has taken her husband's last name is indexed by her legal name (her husband's surname, her given name, and her middle name or maiden surname). There should be a cross-reference, such as an out guide placed where her maiden name falls directing you to her new name.
10. When followed by a complete name, titles may be used as the last filing unit if needed to distinguish the name from another, identical name. Titles without complete names are considered the first indexing unit.
11. Terms of seniority or professional or academic degrees are used only to distinguish the name from an identical name.
12. Articles (e.g., the, a) are disregarded in indexing.

FILING METHODS

The three basic filing methods used in healthcare facilities are:
- Alphabetic by name
- Numeric
- Subject

Patients' records are filed either alphabetically by name or by one of several numeric methods. Subject filing is used for business records, correspondence, and topical materials.

Alphabetic Filing

Alphabetic filing by name is the oldest, simplest, and most commonly used system. It is the system of choice for filing patients' records in most small providers' offices.

The alphabetic system of filing is traditional and simple to set up, requiring only a file cabinet or shelf, folders, and some divider guides (see Procedure 12.5, p. 267). It is a **direct filing system** in that the person filing needs to know only the name to find the desired file. Alphabetic filing does have some drawbacks:

- The correct spelling of the name must be known.
- As the number of files increases, more space is needed for each section of the alphabet. This results in periodic shifting of folders to allow for expansion.
- As the files expand, more time is required for filing or retrieving each folder because of the greater number of folders involved in the search. The time can be greatly reduced by color coding.

Numeric Filing

Practically every large clinic or hospital uses some form of **numeric filing**, combined with color and shelf filing. Management consultants differ in their recommendations; some recommend numeric filing only if more than 5000 to 10,000 records are involved. Others recommend nothing but numeric filing. Numeric filing is an *indirect filing system*, or one that requires use of an alphabetic cross-reference to find a given file. Some object to this added step and overlook the advantages of numeric filing:

- It allows unlimited expansion without periodic shifting of folders, and shelves are usually evenly filled.
- It provides additional confidentiality to the record.
- It saves time in retrieving and filing records quickly. One knows immediately that the number 978 falls between 977 and 979. By contrast, an alphabetic system, even with color coding, requires a longer search to locate the exact spot.

Several types of numeric filing systems can be used:

- In a straight, or consecutive, numeric system, patients are given consecutive numbers as they first start using the practice. This is the simplest numeric system and works well for files of up to 10,000 records. It is time-consuming, and the chance for error is greater when documents with five or more digits are filed. Filing activity is greatest at the end of the numeric series.
- In a terminal digit system, patients also are assigned consecutive numbers, but the digits in the number usually are separated into groups of twos or threes and are read in groups from right to left instead of from left to right. The records are filed backward in groups. For example, all files ending in 00 are grouped together first, then those ending in 01, and so on. Next the files are grouped by their middle digits so that the 00 22s come before the 01 22s. Finally, the files are arranged by their first digits, so that 01 00 22 precedes 02 00 22.
- Middle-digit filing begins with the middle digits, followed by the first digits, and finally by the terminal digits. Numeric filing requires more training, but once the system has been mastered, fewer errors occur than with alphabetic filing.

CRITICAL THINKING APPLICATION   **12.8**
Susan is unsure whether alphabetic or numeric filing is best in the healthcare facility. What are some advantages and disadvantages of each method?

Subject Filing

Subject filing can be either alphabetic or **alphanumeric** (e.g., A 1-3, B 1-1, B 1-2, and so on) and is used for general correspondence. The main difficulty with subject filing is indexing, or classifying; that is, deciding where to file a document. Many papers require *cross-referencing*. An example would be if you had a subject folder for

Laboratory Supplies and the same organization provides you with your General Medical Supplies; there should be a notation in the Laboratory Supplies folder stating, "See Also General Medical Supplies," and vice versa. All correspondence dealing with a particular subject is filed together. The papers in the folders are filed chronologically with the most recent on top. The subject headings are placed on the tabs of the folders and filed alphabetically.

Color-Coding

When a color-coding system is used, both filing and finding files is easier, and misfiling of folders is kept to a minimum. The use of color visually restricts the area of search for a specific record. A misfiled record is easily spotted even from a distance of several feet. In color coding, a specific color is selected to identify each letter of the alphabet. Any selection of colors may be used, and the division of the alphabet is determined by one's own needs. However, studies have shown that the frequency with which different letters occur varies widely.

Alphabetic Color-Coding

As medicine continues to consolidate into larger facilities with more patients in one system, the filing of patients' records becomes more complicated, and color coding becomes more useful. Several color-coding systems use two sets of 13 colors: one set for letters A to M, and a second set of the same colors on a different background for letters N to Z.

Many ready-made systems are available for use. Self-adhesive, colored letter blocks with either two or three letters in the specific colors are supplied in rolls. The color blocks with the appropriate letter are placed on the index tab of the folder, along with the patient's full name. The letters are in pairs so that they can be seen from either side of the record. Strong, easily differentiated colors are used, creating a band of color in the files that makes spotting out-of-place folders easy (Fig. 12.14).

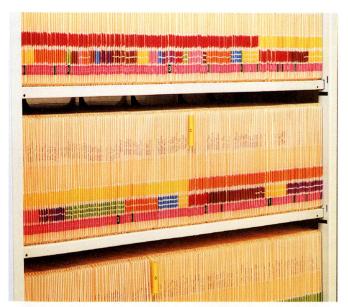

FIGURE 12.14 With color-coding of patients' records, a misplaced file is easily spotted. (Courtesy Bibbero Systems, An InHealth Company, Petaluma, CA. *www.bibbero.com*.)

Numeric Color-Coding

Color coding is also used in numeric filing. Numbers 0 through 9 are each assigned a different color. In a terminal digit filing system, the colors for the last two numbers are affixed to the tab. If the number 1 is red and 5 is yellow, all files with numbers ending in 15 have a red and yellow band. Usually a predetermined section of the number is color coded.

Other Color-Coding Applications

Color can work in many other ways for the efficient healthcare facility. Small tabs in a variety of colors can be used to identify certain types of insured patients and other specific information. For example, a red tab over the edge of the folder may identify a patient on Medicare; a blue tab may identify a Medicaid patient; a green tab may identify a workers' compensation patient; matching tabs may be attached to the insured's ledger card; research cases may be identified by a special color tab; and brightly colored labels on the outside of a patient's record can indicate certain health conditions, such as drug allergies. In a partnership practice, a different color folder or label may identify each provider's patients. Color also can be used to differentiate dates: one color for each month or year.

The use of color in filing is limited only by the imagination. One word of caution: Every person in the facility who uses the files must know the key to the coding, and the key should also be written in the facility's policy and procedures manual.

ORGANIZATION OF FILES

Providers find studying a disorganized patient record very difficult. Some systematic method must be followed in placing items in the patient folder. From the filing standpoint, it should be emphasized that when a patient record is not in actual use, it should be in only one place – the filing cabinet or on the shelf. Many precious hours can be wasted searching for misplaced or lost records that were carelessly left unfiled.

The patient's full name, in indexing order, should be typed on a label and the label attached to the folder tab. A strip of transparent tape can be placed on the label to prevent smudging. The patient's full name should also be typed on each sheet in the folder. Some types of records common to the healthcare setting, other than patient records, are health-related correspondence, general correspondence, practice management files, miscellaneous files, and tickler or follow-up files.

Health-Related Correspondence

Correspondence pertaining to patients' health should be filed in the patient's health record. Other medical correspondence should be filed in a subject file.

General Correspondence

The provider's office operates as both a business and a professional service. Correspondence of a general nature pertaining to the operation of the office is part of the business side of the practice. Usually, a special drawer or shelf is set aside for the general correspondence.

The correspondence is indexed according to subject matter or the names of the correspondents. The guides in a subject file may appear in one, two, or three positions, depending on the number of headings, subheadings, and subdivisions.

Practice Management Files

Of course, the most active financial record is the patient ledger. In facilities that still use a manual system, this is a card or vertical tray file, and the accounts are arranged alphabetically by name. At least two divisions are used: active accounts and paid accounts.

Miscellaneous Files

Papers that do not warrant an individual folder are placed in a miscellaneous folder. In that folder, all papers relating to one subject or with one correspondent are kept together in chronologic order, with the most recent on top, and then filed alphabetically with other miscellaneous material. Related materials may be stapled together. Never use paper clips for this purpose. When as many as five papers accumulate with one correspondent or subject, a separate folder should be prepared. Other business files include records of income and expenses, financial statements, income and payroll tax records, canceled checks, and insurance policies. These papers may be filed chronologically.

Tickler or Follow-Up Files

The most frequently used follow-up method is a **tickler file**, so called because it tickles the memory that something needs to be done or followed up on a particular date. The tickler file is always in a chronologic arrangement. In its simplest form, it consists of notations on the daily calendar. If information, such as an x-ray report or a laboratory report, is expected about a patient with an appointment to come in, the medical assistant might make a note on the calendar or tickler file a day ahead to check on whether the report has arrived.

The tickler file can be a part of a computerized health record system or could be as simple as an email sent to oneself. Many people put reminders on their cell phones using an application (app) specially designed for memos and reminders. The tickler file could also be a card file: 12 guides, one for each month, are placed at the front of the cabinet, container, or other object used to hold the folders. Notations of actions to be taken are placed behind the guides for specific days of the current month. Notations for future months are placed behind the guide for that month. To be effective, the tickler file must be checked first thing each day.

The tickler file can be used in many ways. It is a useful reminder of recurring events, such as payments, meetings, and so forth. On the last day of each month, all the notations from behind the next month's guide are distributed among the daily numbered guides, and the guide for the month just completed is placed at the back of the file.

Transitory or Temporary File

Many papers are kept longer than necessary because no arrangement is made for separating those with a limited usefulness. This situation can be prevented by having a transitory or temporary file. For example, if a medical assistant writes a letter requesting a reprint of the new patient brochure, the file copy is placed in the transitory folder until the reprint is received. When the reprint is received, the file copy is destroyed. The transitory file is used for materials with no permanent value. The paper may be marked with a "T" and then destroyed when the action is completed.

CLOSING COMMENTS

Just as in every aspect of the medical profession, advances in health records management are occurring rapidly, allowing providers and other caregivers to perform their duties more efficiently and accurately. A medical assistant must constantly be willing to learn and to adapt to changes arising from legislation and technologic advances. Computers have become generally accepted as a means of recording health information.

A primary goal of all healthcare facilities is to provide efficient, high-quality patient care. The EHR system can help the staff reach that goal. In the future, every provider's office, hospital, pharmacy, and healthcare facility may be able to access information in minutes, which will improve patient care and save lives. Stay abreast of news and articles related to EHR systems. The healthcare industry is one of constant growth and learning, and today's information technology provides the medical assistant with endless opportunities to make that growth rewarding and applicable to her or his current position.

Legal and Ethical Issues

The authority to release information from the health record lies solely with the patient unless such a release is required by law through a subpoena duces tecum. Ownership of the record often is a subject of controversy. The record belongs to the provider; the information belongs to the patient.

Remember that the EHR system contains information that is confidential at all times. The patient must authorize the release of health information in electronic form, just as if it were a piece of paper. EHR systems must:

- Maintain the security and confidentiality of data
- Be easily retrievable
- Have safeguards against the loss of information
- Protect patients' rights to confidentiality and privacy
- Require identification and authentication for access

By supporting these requirements, the medical facility remains in compliance with applicable laws and gains the trust of patients, who are reassured that their health information is secure and safe.

Patient-Centered Care

Patients worry about the security of their information, particularly about who can access it. Lawsuits are often filed when patients discover that an unauthorized person has accessed their protected health information. The medical assistant should listen to a patient's concerns and explain the safety procedures that apply to the EHR in language the patient can understand. Some facilities prepare a brochure to

---

CRITICAL THINKING APPLICATION   **12.9**

Susan is responsible for checking the tickler file daily. What types of documents and duties might she find inside these files?

explain the conversion process to the patient and the advantages of the EHR system.

The medical assistant should expect hesitation and even reluctance from patients who are concerned about the privacy of their health information. Patients are concerned about lack of control over who views their records. Be prepared to answer their questions about the safety of their records as related to the EHR. The medical assistant must know how the EHR is protected and what security measures are in place to be able to reassure the patients that their records are protected at all times.

Professional Behaviors

Once the medical assistant has been trained on the EHR system and has had the opportunity to use it for a time, daily use should become second nature. In fact, it may be difficult to imagine a workday without the system! By being open to change and willing to learn, the medical assistant can set a good example for all employees and will be more receptive to the process of change. Be encouraging to other staff members while training on the system, and if technology comes easily to you, share your knowledge with others and assist wherever possible. Do not expect to master the system in a week; instead, realize that a new system has a learning curve and be patient with and receptive to the educational process. Keep technical support phone numbers handy and feel free to use them whenever a new or complicated issue arises. Work as a team, and if possible, help others who might find learning the system more of a struggle. Above all, while getting used to the new technology, make sure your attitude is one of enthusiasm, interest, and curiosity.

SUMMARY OF SCENARIO

Susan looks forward to attending her medical assisting classes each day and works diligently to perform to the best of her ability in the classroom. She strives to do well on each procedure check-off and each examination she completes. Her instructors provide excellent feedback and appreciate her contributions to the class.

Susan has the attitude that everything she is allowed to do in the healthcare facility is a learning tool. She regularly asks for additional responsibilities and is always ready to assist a co-worker. Dr. Kahn has recognized that she has the desire to learn, and he gives her many opportunities to glean more knowledge through the everyday activities in the office.

Although she is new to the medical profession, Susan learns quickly and thinks logically. She knows the rules and regulations on patient confidentiality and is always careful about the information she provides to those who request it. She is never hesitant about asking her office manager for guidance if she is unsure about any aspect of her duties. Susan is understanding and respectful when patients are concerned about their privacy. Her confidence and warm personality play a role in the trust she earns from the patients at the clinic.

Susan is willing to admit when she has made an error and has sought advice from Dr. Kahn and her office manager when an error needed correction. Although filing is not one of her favorite duties, she can be counted on to do her best while completing this important task. She realizes that filing is critical because the documents in the patient's health record direct the care provided to the patient. An abnormal laboratory report that is missing can make a crucial difference in the patient's care. She takes pride in her work, and she is efficient and accurate where health records are concerned. When she is faced with a new task, she considers it a learning experience and asks for help if she is not completely sure about the way to handle a situation.

Susan's co-workers are supportive and always willing to help her as she learns to be the best medical assistant she can be. Her future as a professional medical assistant certainly holds opportunity and chances for advancement. Just as important, patients trust her. She has alleviated patients' concerns about EHRs by taking the time to explain privacy policies and exactly what information will be accessible to third parties. This trust also gives patients the confidence to reveal personal information and to know that it will be held in the strictest confidence, not just by Susan, but by each employee in the provider's office.

SUMMARY OF LEARNING OBJECTIVES

1. **Discuss the two types of patient records.**

   The two major types of patient records are the paper health record and the electronic health record (EHR). The EHR is much more efficient than the paper record, and most healthcare facilities have switched to EHRs for a number of reasons.

2. **State several reasons that accurate health records are important.**

   Health records must be accurate primarily so that the correct care can be given to the patient. The record also helps ensure continuity of care between providers so that no lapse in treatment occurs. The

   record serves as indication and proof in court that certain treatments and procedures were performed on the patient; therefore, it can be excellent legal support if it is well maintained and accurate. Health records also aid researchers with statistical information.

3. **Differentiate between subjective and objective information in creating a patient's health record.**

   Subjective information is provided by the patient, whereas objective information is provided by the provider. Examples of subjective information include the patient's address, Social Security number, insurance information, and description of what he or she is experiencing. Objective information is obtained through the provider's questions and observations made during the examination.

Refer to Procedure 12.1 to see how to create a patient's health record and register a new patient in practice management software.

4. **Explain who owns the health record.**

The provider owns the physical health record, but the patient controls the information contained in it.

5. **Distinguish between an electronic health record (EHR) and an electronic medical record (EMR).**

The EHR is an electronic record of health-related information about an individual that conforms to nationally recognized interoperability standards and that can be created, managed, and consulted by authorized clinicians and staff from more than one healthcare organization. The EMR is an electronic record of health-related information about an individual that can be created, gathered, managed, and consulted by authorized clinicians and staff within one healthcare organization.

6. **Do the following related to healthcare legislation and EHRs:**
   - *Define meaningful use and relate it to the healthcare industry.*
     Meaningful use, defined simply, means that providers must show that they are using EHR technology in ways that can be measured significantly in quality and quantity. If providers meet the meaningful use requirements, they will qualify for incentive payments.
   - *List the three main components of meaningful use legislation.*
     The three main components of meaningful use are (1) use of certified EHR in a meaningful manner, such as e-prescribing; (2) use of certified EHR technology for electronic exchange of health information to improve the quality of health care; and (3) use of certified EHR technology to submit clinical quality reports, procedure and diagnosis codes, surveys, and other measures.

7. **Discuss the importance of nonverbal communication with patients when an EHR system is used.**

Eye contact is critical when an EHR system is used with patients. Body language must indicate that the medical assistant is open to and listening to the patient's concerns, not just concentrating on data entry. Providers and medical assistants alike may have to relearn how to interact with patients in a natural way while using the laptop or tablet in the examination room. Realize that during the implementation period, processing and serving patients may take longer because the staff is using new technology. Most patients are understanding about this if the medical assistant explains that a new system is in place and asks for patience. Because patients are not always technologically savvy, most will be supportive and interested in the EHR system.

8. **Discuss backup systems for the EHR, in addition to the transfer, destruction, and retention of health records as related to the EHR.**

The provider must have a backup system for the EHR in case a medical office is without power for a significant amount of time. The EHR systems can be set to automatically back up the information at specified times during the day. This means that a minimum amount of data would be lost if the power went out. Options include external hard drive, full server backup, and online backup systems. In most medical offices, records are classified in three ways: active, inactive, and closed. The process of moving a file from active to inactive is called *purging*. Providers have an obligation to retain patient records. The records of any patient covered by Medicare or Medicaid must be kept at least 10 years.

9. **Discuss retention and destruction of medical records as related to paper records.**

As with EHRs, paper health records are classified as active, inactive, or closed. Large healthcare facilities may find it advisable to convert their paper health records to microfilm.

10. **Describe how and when to release health record information; also, discuss health information exchanges (HIEs).**

The healthcare facility must be extremely careful when releasing any type of medical information; the patient must sign a release for information to be given to any third party. Requests for medical information should be made in writing. Pay particular attention to records release requests involving a minor.

There are currently three kinds of HIE — directed exchange, query-based exchange, and consumer-mediated exchange — and the implementation of HIE varies from state to state.

11. **Identify and discuss the two methods of organizing a patient's paper medical record.**

The source-oriented medical record (SOMR) categorizes the content by its source, such as provider, laboratory, radiology, hospital, and consultation. Within each source category the content is arranged in reverse chronologic order so that the most recent content is viewed first.

The problem-oriented medical record (POMR) categorizes each of the patient's problems and elaborates on the findings and treatment plans for all concerns. Detailed progress notes are kept for each individual problem. This method addresses each of the patient's concerns separately, whereas a source-oriented record may address all problems and concerns at one time, usually covering one to three patient concerns per office visit. The POMR helps ensure that individual problems are all addressed.

12. **Discuss how to document information in an EHR and a paper health record, and how to make corrections/alterations to health records.**

Documenting information in an EHR involves using radio buttons, drop-down menus, and free-text boxes. When you are documenting in a paper health record, the entry will always start with the date in the MM/DD/YYYY format. All entries must be written in black or blue ink and follow the format designated by the healthcare facility.

To create a handwritten correction to a health record, a line should be drawn through the error, the correction inserted above or immediately after, and the person making the correction should write his or her initials or signature and the date below the correction. Errors made while using an EHR are corrected in the usual way; however, an error discovered in an entry at a later date is corrected in the same manner as for a handwritten entry.

Continued

SUMMARY OF LEARNING OBJECTIVES—continued

13. **Discuss dictation and transcription.**

    With the increased use of EHRs and voice recognition software, there is decreased need for transcription. Transcription can be done from handwritten notes, or more likely from machine dictation. Accuracy and speed are important. Some healthcare offices use voice recognition software for transcription.

14. **Identify the filing equipment and filing supplies needed to create, store, and maintain paper health records.**

    Several types of equipment and supplies are needed to manage patients' records. Office space availability; structural considerations; cost of space and equipment; size, type, and volume of medical records; confidentiality requirements; retrieval speed; fire protection; and cost should all be considered when choosing filing equipment. Filing equipment includes drawer files, horizontal shelf files, rotary circular files, compactible files, automated files, and card files. Filing supplies include divider guides, out guides, file folders, and labels.

15. **Describe indexing rules, and how to create and organize a patient's health record.**

    Five basic steps are involved in document filing: (1) The papers are conditioned, which is the preparatory stage for filing. (2) The documents are released, which means they are ready to be filed because they have been reviewed or read and some type of mark has been placed on the document to indicate this. (3) The documents are indexed, which involves deciding where each document should be filed and coding it with some type of mark on the paper indicating

    that decision. (4) Sorting involves placing the files in filing sequence. (5) The actual filing and storing of the documents are the last step. Refer to Table 12.2 for indexing rules. Refer to Procedure 12.4 for information on creating and organizing a paper health record.

16. **Discuss the pros and cons of various filing methods and how to file patient health records.**

    Both the alphabetic and numeric filing systems have advantages and disadvantages. Perhaps most important is the staff's preference. Some find it easier to retrieve files that are in standard alphabetic order, whereas others prefer a numeric system. The numeric system is more confidential than an alphabetic system. Some staff members prefer a combination of the two, called the alphanumeric system. Both effectively keep health records in good order and allow the medical assistant to spot a misfiled record quickly.

    Refer to Procedure 12.5 to see how to file patient health records.

17. **Discuss the organization of files and of health-related correspondence.**

    When a patient record is not in actual use, it should only be in the filing cabinet or on the shelf. Health-related correspondence, including general correspondence, should be filed appropriately. Practice management files are usually divided into active and paid accounts. Papers that do not warrant an individual folder are placed in the miscellaneous folder. Follow-up files are frequently called "tickler files." Transitory (i.e., temporary) files can be helpful for material with no permanent value.

| PROCEDURE 12.1 | Register a New Patient in the Practice Management Software |

Task: Register a new patient in the practice management software, prepare a Notice of Privacy Practices (NPP) form and a Disclosure Authorization form for the new patient, and document this in the electronic health record (EHR).

Scenario: The patient received both documents and signed the Disclosure Authorization form.

EQUIPMENT and SUPPLIES

- Computer with SimChart for the Medical Office or practice management and EHR software
- Completed patient registration form
- Scanner

PROCEDURAL STEPS

1. Obtain the new patient's completed registration form. Log into the practice management software.

   PURPOSE: The registration form will provide the information needed to create the new record in the practice management system.

2. Using the patient's last and first names and date of birth, search the database for the patient.

   PURPOSE: To help ensure the integrity of the practice management and EHR systems, a search for the new patient's name must always be done before registering that person. This prevents a double record from

   being created if the patient had been entered into the database at an earlier time.

3. If the database does not contain the patient's name, add a new patient and enter the patient's demographics from the completed registration form.

   PURPOSE: This will create the patient's record in the practice management system.

4. Verify that the information entered is correct and that all fields are completed before saving the data.

   PURPOSE: Errors during the registration process can affect the communication with the patient (e.g., if a wrong address or email is entered) or can affect billing (e.g., if the incorrect insurance information is added). Accuracy is extremely important when entering the patient's information.

   Note: The software will generate a health record number for the patient.

5. Using the EHR software, prepare and print a copy of the NPP and a Disclosure Authorization form for the new patient. The Disclosure Authorization form should indicate the disclosure will be to the patient's insurance company.

PROCEDURE 12.1 Register a New Patient in the Practice Management Software—*continued*

PURPOSE: Before the medical office can release patient information to the insurance company, the patient has to give consent in writing.

6. Using the EHR, document that the patient received a copy of the NPP and signed the Disclosure Authorization form. Scan the Disclosure Authorization form and upload it into the EHR.

PURPOSE: Documentation in the health record provides a legal record of what was done or communicated to the patient.

7. Log out of the software upon completion of the procedure.
PURPOSE: Logging into and out of the software helps to protect the integrity of the data saved in the software and prevents unauthorized people from viewing the information.

PROCEDURE 12.2 Upload Documents to the Electronic Health Record

Task: Scan paper records and upload digital files to the EHR.

Scenario: A new patient brings in a laboratory report and a radiology report that he would like to have added to his EHR. You need to scan in the original documents and upload them to the EHR.

EQUIPMENT and SUPPLIES

- Scanner
- Computer with SimChart for the Medical Office or EHR software
- Patient's laboratory and radiology reports

PROCEDURAL STEPS

1. Obtain the patient's name and date of birth if not on the reports.
PURPOSE: You will need the patient's name and date of birth to find the patient's EHR.
2. Using a scanner that is connected to the computer, scan each document, creating an individual digital image for each.
PURPOSE: The reports should be scanned separately and not combined to create one file. Each type of report must be uploaded separately to the correct location in the EHR.
3. Locate the file of the two scanned images in the computer drive. Open the files to ensure the images are clear.

PURPOSE: When you are scanning and uploading documents to the EHR, it is crucial that the image of the document is clear and can be easily read by the provider. If the image is blurred, rescan the document.

4. In the EHR, search for the patient, using the patient's last and first names. Verify the patient's date of birth.
PURPOSE: Before you begin uploading to or documenting in the EHR, it is critical to verify that the correct record is opened.
5. Locate the window to upload diagnostic/laboratory results and add a new result. Enter the date of the test. Select the correct type of result. Browse for the image file of the laboratory file and attach it. Save the information. Select the option to add a new result and repeat the steps to upload the second report. Verify that both documents were uploaded correctly.
PURPOSE: Errors during the upload may affect the ability to see the files. Verifying at the time of the upload will help you ensure that providers can see the results in the future.

PROCEDURE 12.3 Protect the Integrity of the Medical Record

Task: Protect the integrity of the medical record.

Scenario: You are mentoring a medical assistant student, who is in practicum. You notice the student routinely does not sign out of the electronic health record before leaving the desk. The facility's policy is to sign out or lock the computer before leaving it.

Directions: Role-play the scenario with a peer, who plays the student. You, the medical assistant, must explain to the "student" the facility's policy. Also address the hazards of not protecting the medical record. If the student does not change this behavior, you will need to address the situation with the department supervisor.

PROCEDURAL STEPS

1. Professionally and respectfully discuss the situation with the student.
2. Inform the student about the facility's policy and the hazards of not protecting the electronic health record.
PURPOSE: It is important that the student be knowledgeable about the policies and the hazards of not protecting the EHR.
3. Provide the student with strategies to protect the electronic health record.
4. Inform the student what will occur if he or she does not protect the electronic record.

PROCEDURE 12.4   Create and Organize a Patient's Paper Health Record

Task: Create a paper health record for a new patient. Organize health record documents in a paper health record.

EQUIPMENT and SUPPLIES

- End tab file folder
- Completed patient registration form
- Divider sheets with different color labels (4)
- Progress note sheet (1)
- Name label
- Color-coding labels (first two letters of last name and first letter of first name)
- Year label
- Allergy label
- Black pen or computer with word processing software to process labels
- Health record documents (i.e., prior records, laboratory reports)
- Hole puncher

PROCEDURAL STEPS

1. Obtain the patient's first and last names.
   PURPOSE: To customize the record for the patient, the first and last names will be required.

2. Neatly write or word-process the patient's name on the name label. Left justify the last name, followed by a comma, the first name, middle initial, and a period (e.g., Smith, Mary J.).
   PURPOSE: The label should be easy to read. The last name always comes before the first name.

3. Adhere the name label to the bottom left side of the record tab. When you hold the record by the main fold in your left hand, the writing should be easy to read. (For directional purposes, assume the record main fold is on the left and the tab is at the bottom.)
   PURPOSE: Placing the labels in correct position will make it easier to find the information needed.

4. Put the color-coding labels on the bottom right edge of the folder. Start by placing the first letter of the last name at the farthest right edge. Working left, place the second letter of the last name, then the first letter of the first name, and lastly the year label. The year label should be close to the name label.
   PURPOSE: When the folders are in the file cabinet, they are sorted by the colored labels, starting with the top label (first letter of the last name), followed by the second and remaining labels.

5. Place the allergy label on the front of the record. If allergies are known, clearly write the allergy on the label in red ink.
   PURPOSE: Allergies need to be clearly identified on medical records.

6. Place the divider labels on the record divider sheets if they come separately. Ensure the labels on the divider sheets are staggered so they do not overlap. Print the name of the section on the front and back of the label. The print should be easy to read when the record is held by the main fold. (Suggested names for dividers: Progress Notes, Laboratory, Correspondence, and Miscellaneous.)
   PURPOSE: Placing divider labels on the divider sheets in a staggered pattern allows the provider to easily see all sections of the health record.

7. Using the prongs on the left-hand side of the record, secure the registration form.
   PURPOSE: The registration form should be in an easy-to-find location in the record.

8. Using the prongs on the right-hand side of the record, secure the index dividers with a progress note sheet under the progress note tab.
   PURPOSE: The provider will need the progress note sheet to document data regarding the visit.

Scenario: The patient authorized his or her prior provider to send health records to your agency. You need to organize these records within the paper health record.

9. Verify the name and the date of birth on the health record, and ensure they match the information on the health record.
   PURPOSE: Before you organize and file documents in a patient's health record, it is critical to ensure the health record is for the correct patient.

10. Open the prongs on the right side of the record, and carefully remove the record to the point at which the documents need to be inserted. For the documents being inserted, punch holes in the proper location. Insert the papers into the record, and then reassemble the remaining part of the record. Continue to do this until all the documents are filed within the health record.
    PURPOSE: Documents need to be placed in the correct location in the record so the provider can easily find information.

PROCEDURE 12.5   File Patient Health Records

Task: File patient health records using two different filing systems: the alphabetic system and the numeric system.

Scenario: The agency uses the alphabetic system. You need to file health records in the correct location.

EQUIPMENT and SUPPLIES

- Paper health records using the alphabetic filing system
- Paper health records using the numeric filing system
- File boxes or file cabinet

PROCEDURAL STEPS

1. Using alphabetic guidelines, place the records to be filed in alphabetic order.
   PURPOSE: Placing the records in alphabetic order before filing in the box or cabinet will make the filing process more efficient.
2. Using the file box or file cabinet, locate the correct spot for the first file.
   PURPOSE: It is important that you place the record in the correct spot so that others can locate the record.

3. Place the health record in the correct location. Continue these filing steps until all the health records are filed.
4. Using numeric guidelines, place the records to be filed in numeric order.
   PURPOSE: Placing the records in numeric order before filing in the box or cabinet will make the filing process more efficient.
5. Using the file box or file cabinet, locate the correct spot for the first file.
   PURPOSE: It is important that you place the record in the correct spot so that others can locate the record.
6. Place the health record in the correct location. Continue these filing steps until all the health records are filed.

13

DAILY OPERATIONS AND SAFETY

SCENARIO

Marie Van Bakel, a certified medical assistant (CMA), is a new medical assistant at Walden-Martin Family Medical (WMFM) Clinic. She was hired to work with the family medicine providers. This is Marie's first job as a new graduate from a medical assisting program. She is excited to work in family medicine. This was the same specialty she worked in during her medical assisting practicum. Because this is a small healthcare facility, Marie's responsibilities are different from what they would be in a larger facility. She and the administrative medical assistant, Catherine, are the only staff members in the office at the start of the

day. The providers make hospital rounds at that time. The providers and the rest of the medical assistants come in later.

Marie and Catherine need to open the office and prepare for the patients. Marie is also responsible for the inventory of clinical supplies and administrative and clinical equipment. During Marie's interview, Dr. Walden expressed her concern about the lack of procedures for ordering and maintaining inventory. She would like Marie to develop those procedures. Having little exposure to supplies and ordering during her practicum, Marie realizes she needs to learn about these procedures.

While studying this chapter, think about the following questions:
- What are the opening and closing duties for the medical assistant?
- How is inventory performed on equipment and supplies?
- What should be considered when ordering supplies?
- How does a medical assistant use correct body mechanics when working with supplies and equipment?
- How does a medical assistant evaluate the work environment?
- How does a medical assistant respond to facility-related emergencies?

LEARNING OBJECTIVES

1. Explain tasks for the medical assistant to handle when opening and closing the healthcare facility.
2. List the steps involved in completing an inventory and perform an equipment inventory with documentation.
3. Explain the purpose of routine maintenance of administrative and clinical equipment and perform routine maintenance of equipment.
4. Discuss warranties, service calls, and purchasing equipment.
5. Discuss inventory management, inventory management control systems, and ordering supplies.
6. Identify the principles of body mechanics and perform a supply inventory with documentation while using proper body mechanics.
7. Evaluate the work environment to identify unsafe working conditions.
8. Identify critical elements of an emergency response plan to use in the event of a natural disaster or other emergency and participate in a mock exposure event.
9. Demonstrate the proper use of a fire extinguisher.
10. Recognize the physical and emotional effects on persons involved in an emergency situation.

VOCABULARY

accounts payable Money owed by a company to other companies for services and goods; pertains to paying the facility's bills.

answering service A commercial service that answers telephone calls for its clients.

backordered An order placed for an item that is temporarily out of stock and will be sent at a later time.

billable service Assistance (i.e., service) that is provided by a healthcare provider and can be billed to the insurance company or patient.

buying cycle How often an item is purchased; this depends on how frequently the item is used and the storage space available for it.

crash cart Emergency medications and equipment (e.g., oxygen, intravenous [IV] and airway supplies) stored in a cart and ready for an emergency.

de-escalating Reducing the level or intensity; bringing down a person's anger or elevated emotions.

depreciate To diminish in value (e.g., the value of an item) over a period of time; a concept used for tax purposes.

discrepancy A lack of similarity between what is stated and what is found; for instance, the computer inventory count is different than the physical count.

disinfect To destroy or render pathogenic organisms inactive; this does not include spores, tuberculosis bacilli, and certain viruses.

VOCABULARY—*continued*

fire doors Doors made of fire-resistant materials; they close manually or automatically during a fire to prevent it from spreading.

initiative The ability to start a task and independently complete it.

inventory A detailed list of equipment and supplies owned and stored; the process of counting the supplies in stock.

invoices Billing statements that list the amount owed for goods or services purchased.

packing slip A document that accompanies purchased merchandise and shows what is in the box or package.

progress notes Documentation in the paper health record that can be used to track the patient's condition and progress.

purchase order (PO) number A unique number assigned by the ordering facility that allows the facility to track or reference the order.

quality control A process to ensure the reliability of test results, often using manufactured samples with known values.

restock The process of replacing the supplies that were used.

sanitize The process of cleaning equipment and instruments with detergent and water in order to remove debris and reduce the number of microorganisms.

sterilize The process of removing all microorganisms.

vendors Companies that sell supplies, equipment, or services to other companies or individuals.

workplace emergencies Unforeseen situations that threaten the employees and visitors; they can disrupt the services provided.

In the ambulatory healthcare facility, the medical assistant has opening tasks to accomplish to prepare the department for patients. At the end of the day, after the last patient leaves, the medical assistant has duties to close the department for the night. Besides these daily duties, the equipment and supply inventory are managed by the medical assistant. Having adequate supplies available to use for patients is critical to the functioning of the department. These topics are addressed in this chapter.

In addition, the medical assistant must be knowledgeable about environmental safety and security. This chapter discusses workplace violence, evaluating the environment, emergency response plans, and the effects of stress. Keeping the work environment safe is an important role for every employee.

OPENING AND CLOSING THE HEALTHCARE FACILITY

Employees who are responsible for opening the ambulatory healthcare facility must arrive before the patients in the morning. These employees must prepare for the day. Preparation time will vary based on the size of the practice and the number of patients on the schedule.

In smaller facilities, a few reliable employees are given keys to unlock the doors and deactivate the alarm system. In larger facilities, employees must use the locked employee entrances. Employees can unlock the doors by entering unique codes into a keypad or by using unique keycards. Both systems are developed to monitor who enters the building. Usually security, custodial, or supervisory personnel are responsible for deactivating the alarm system in larger facilities. Staff members then open the main patient doors at a set time.

Opening Tasks for the Medical Assistant

The clinical medical assistant assists the provider with patient treatments and procedures (e.g., injections, wound care, and diagnostic tests). The administrative medical assistant works in the reception area. In larger facilities, both types of medical assistants have opening duties. If the healthcare facility is small, then the medical assistant may be required to perform both administrative and clinical tasks. Often this is called performing "front office" and "back office" activities.

It is important for the clinical medical assistant to prepare the clinical equipment and exam rooms for patient visits. An unprepared area can cause delays in patient care. Facility opening tasks for the clinical medical assistant include the following:

- Prepare the exam rooms by turning on the lights, ensuring supplies are stocked, and making sure the rooms have been cleaned appropriately and are safe for patients.
- Ensure prescription pads (if used) are stored outside of the exam rooms, in a locked cabinet. Prescription pads should never be accessible to patients. Some patients or staff might take the pads and try to forge a prescription, which is illegal.
- Unlock supply cabinets (with the exception of the narcotics cabinet, which remains locked).
- Ensure restrooms have adequate supplies for patients (e.g., urine specimen containers, cleansing towelettes).
- Perform **quality control** tests on laboratory equipment and complete refrigerator and freezer temperature logs.

In addition to these tasks, the clinical medical assistant must follow up on outstanding patient issues from the prior day. The medical assistant also needs to handle new diagnostic test reports (e.g., x-ray reports). For agencies using paper health records, this would require the following:

- Obtaining the patient's paper health record
- Attaching the diagnostic report to the record
- Giving the health record and report to the provider to review

For facilities with electronic health records (EHRs), this process is completed using the electronic messaging system in the software.

Often medical assistants notify patients of normal test results and document the notification in the health record. No test result can be given to the patient unless the provider has authorized its release or the facility's procedures allow it. The medical assistant must follow the facility's procedures when notifying the patient of the results.

Opening tasks for the administrative medical assistant include the following:

- Check the voice mail or answering service messages. The answering service may email or fax messages to the facility. All messages need to be addressed and documented in the patient's health record.

- Update the voice mail message.
- Switch the phone, so patients can reach the facility instead of the answering service.
- Turn on computers, copy machines, and other office equipment.
- Prepare the reception area for patients.
- Print schedules of the day's appointments. A schedule is kept for the paper health record preparation. Other copies are given to the clinical medical assistants, providers, and the medical laboratory. In some facilities, the EHR allows staff to reference the schedule using the software, thus eliminating the printed schedule.

In addition to these duties, the administrative medical assistant must compile any remaining required paperwork for the day's visits. Usually this is done the prior afternoon. A few patient visits may be added to the schedule that need to be completed. For healthcare facilities with EHRs, required patient education literature (e.g., well-child visit documents) and preprinted paper screening forms may be prepared.

For facilities with paper health records, the medical assistant must do the following:
- Pull the paper health records, using a copy of the appointment schedule.
  - Verify that the correct record was pulled for each patient.
  - Check off the patient's name on the copy of the appointment schedule.
- Review each record.
  - Have all recently received documents (e.g., laboratory reports, radiograph readings) been placed correctly and permanently attached to the record?
  - Are documents (e.g., laboratory reports) missing that are needed for the visit?
  - Is there enough space available in the progress notes for the provider to write in the record? If not, place additional progress notes pages in the record.
- Arrange the health records in the order in which the patients will be arriving. The record for the first visit of the day should be on top. Larger facilities may alphabetize the health records.

CRITICAL THINKING APPLICATION   **13.1**

When opening the family medicine office, what jobs does Marie, the clinical medical assistant, need to do to prepare for the day? What jobs does Catherine, the administrative medical assistant, need to do to prepare for the day?

Closing Tasks for the Medical Assistant

At the end of the day, the medical assistant needs to help with the closing duties. The clinical medical assistant must ensure that all the patients have left by checking the exam and treatment rooms. The clinical medical assistant will complete the following closing duties:
- **Restock** the rooms and organize any reading materials.
- **Disinfect** the exam table, writing table, counters, computer keyboards, and chairs (i.e., surfaces that are made of plastic, metal, or wood).

- Secure (put away) confidential documents.
- Turn off computers and other devices.
- **Sanitize**, disinfect, or **sterilize** equipment and instruments.
- Lock supply and medication cabinets.
- Verify and count the narcotic medications stock, following the facility's procedure.

The administrative medical assistant will complete the following closing duties:
- Prepare the patient records and documents for the next day.
- Turn off the computers, copy machine, and other office equipment.
- Switch phones to voice mail or the answering service.
- Follow office procedures for handling money at the end of the day.
- Secure (put away) any confidential documents.
- Clean up the reception area (neatly arrange the magazines, disinfect toys, and remove garbage and unsolicited advertisements). Turn off the lights, television, stereo, and other devices.

With time being short in the morning, it is important to take care of as much as possible the evening before you leave.

Depending on the facility, the medical assistant may be responsible for turning off the lights, activating the alarms, and locking the doors. In larger facilities, the custodial or security staff handles these responsibilities.

Daily and Monthly Duties

Medical facilities either employ custodial staff or hire cleaning services. This cleaning takes place after hours each day. Larger facilities that employ custodial staff will have the staff clean high-traffic areas several times a day. These areas include the restrooms and the entrances. During wet weather, it is critical that the floors are kept dry to prevent people from slipping and falling.

The medical assistant also is responsible for cleaning and organizing the reception area and exam rooms. During slow times, medical assistants are expected to do extra duties, including restocking medical and office supplies, forms, and patient literature. The cabinets and drawers need to be straightened and reorganized. Medications and supplies that have expiration dates need to be checked monthly. The **crash cart** and other emergency supplies need to be inventoried monthly and after each use (Fig. 13.1). Many facilities use a master list of crash cart supplies with expiration dates. This helps ensure that all supplies are in the crash cart and expiring supplies and medications can be easily identified.

It is important that the healthcare facility be clean and organized. By taking the **initiative** to perform those tasks during quiet times, you will be considered a more valuable employee. Supervisors and providers value employees who look for additional activities that can be done during quiet times.

CRITICAL THINKING APPLICATION   **13.2**

The office uses a local cleaning service to clean the facility's rooms. The staff members arrive after hours and are gone by the time Catherine and Marie open the office in the morning. Over the past month, Marie has noticed that the rooms do not look as clean as they should. Should she address this concern? If so, with whom should she discuss it?

EQUIPMENT AND SUPPLIES

Another medical assistant duty is to manage the equipment and supplies in the medical office. In smaller facilities, this may involve ordering and maintaining an inventory control system. In larger facilities, purchasing department employees are hired for such roles.

Equipment

In a healthcare facility, administrative and clinical equipment are used. The medical assistant needs to know how to operate, maintain, and handle issues with the equipment. For financial and tax purposes, the purchase cost and age of each item need to be recorded. The process of gathering and creating a list of the equipment in the facility is called managing **inventory**.

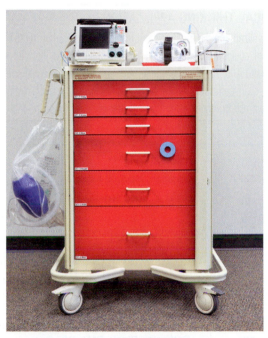

FIGURE 13.1 Crash carts must be inventoried monthly or after each use to ensure that medication and supplies have not expired and all the required supplies are available for an emergency.

Equipment Inventory

For all clinical and administrative equipment, records need to be maintained. These records are used to replace equipment lost in a disaster or theft. The healthcare facility's accountant also uses the information when preparing tax paperwork. For instance, records should be maintained for the following items:

- Small equipment (e.g., thermometers, glucose monitors), which is deducted as an expense for the year in which it was purchased.
- Large office equipment (e.g., computer hardware, calculators, and copiers), which depreciates over 5 years.
- Office furniture items (e.g., desks, files, safes, exam tables), which depreciate over 7 years.

The equipment inventory also is used by supervisors to identify equipment that needs to be replaced. Preplanning equipment purchases is a financial strategy for the practice. It allows the practice to be prepared and to plan for future investments.

CRITICAL THINKING APPLICATION   **13.3**

Marie needs to learn more about managing inventory. She reviews her medical assistant textbook and reads articles online. She decides to start by creating an inventory list of the equipment in the medical office. What are some advantages of having an updated list of administrative and clinical equipment?

When you are creating an equipment inventory list, it is helpful to use spreadsheet software (Fig. 13.2). In some situations, you may have inventory forms that you can complete (see Procedure 13.1, p. 286). For all equipment, document the following information:

- Equipment name, manufacturer, and serial number
- Purchase date, cost, and supplier
- Warranty information (e.g., start and end date, warranty coverage)
- Location of the equipment (optional)
- Unique facility number given to that piece of equipment (optional)

Equipment Name	Manufacturer / Serial Number	Location / Facility Number	Purchase Date / Supplier	Cost	Warranty Information
Laser Printer	HP / HP3598XA	Medical Assistant Desk / LP59483	08/01/20XX / Best Office Supplies	$325	Parts and labor expires 07/31/20XX
AT2 Plus ECG / Spirometry	Schiller / WA4893X	Treatment Room / ES00012	05/02/20XX / Medical Equipment Supplies	$2987	Parts and labor expires 05/01/20XX

FIGURE 13.2 An equipment inventory list can be created in a spreadsheet and provides useful information about the administrative and clinical equipment in the facility.

The owner's or operation manual and warranty information should be kept at a central location and available to users. Many operation manuals are available online. The manuals are used to do the following:

- Problem-solve performance issues
- Identify service schedules and routine maintenance
- Identify parts or supplies needed for the operation of the machine

The medical assistant is responsible for monitoring equipment safety and proper functioning. Routine maintenance helps to ensure the best performance of the equipment. Potential issues should not be overlooked. Actions should be taken to prevent injury to staff or patients and costly damage to the equipment. The medical assistant should do the following:

- Check electrical cords on equipment for damage
- Address any suspected overheating issues
- Investigate any unusual noise or change in performance
- Clean and maintain equipment routinely in accordance with the operation manual

Routine maintenance varies with the equipment. Copiers and printers may entail changing toner or cartridges. For clinical equipment, maintenance may include changing filters or batteries.

It is important to keep track of routine maintenance. Making a schedule as a reminder for routine maintenance can be helpful. Many facilities use logs to track routine maintenance and service calls (Fig. 13.3). Information commonly found on the routine maintenance log includes:

- Equipment name, serial number, location of machine, and facility's unique equipment number (if applicable)
- Manufacturer's name
- Date of purchase
- Warranty information (e.g., start and end date, warranty coverage)
- Service provider contact information, such as telephone number
- Date and time and description of maintenance activities performed
- Signature of person performing maintenance

Procedure 13.2 on p. 286 explains the steps involved in creating a maintenance log, performing the maintenance, and then documenting the maintenance.

CRITICAL THINKING APPLICATION   13.4

Marie realized that the facility did not have maintenance logs for the various pieces of equipment. She decided to start making logs, but she realized there were a lot of logs she would have to make. How could she create logs in a time-efficient manner? For a small office, describe options that she could use to organize the logs so they are easy to locate and use.

Maintenance Log

Equipment Name: **Laser Printer**   Serial #: **HP3598XA**   Location: **Medical Assistant Desk**

Facility #: **LP59483**   Manufacturer: **HP**   Purchased: **08/01/20XX**

Warranty Information: **Parts and labor expires 07/31/20XX**

Freqency of Inspections: **Every 6 months**

Service Provider: **Best Office Supplies**

Date	Time	Maintenance Activities	Signature
12/15/20XX	0956	Replaced toner cartridge	Marie Van Bakel, CMA (AAMA)
02/11/20XX	1235	Service call: Office Repair Company – to fix stray ink marks on copies	Catherine Black, RMA

Maintenance Log

Equipment Name: **AT2 Plus ECG/Spirometry**   Serial #: **WA4893X**   Location: **Treatment Room**

Facility #: **ES00012**   Manufacturer: **Schiller**   Purchased: **05/02/20XX**

Freqency of Inspections: **Every 12 months**

Warranty information: **Parts and labor expires 05/01/20XX**

Service Provider: **Medical Equipment Suppliers**

Date	Time	Maintenance Activities	Signature
10/23/20XX	1123	Replaced battery	Marie Van Bakel, CMA (AAMA)
05/02/20XX	1445	No tracing, cleaned stylus with alcohol	Marie Van Bakel, CMA (AAMA)

FIGURE 13.3 Equipment maintenance logs are used by the staff and outside repair agencies to track maintenance activities.

Service Calls and Warranties

When equipment is purchased, a warranty is given for a period of time. The warranty is the manufacturer's guarantee. If the piece of equipment needs to be repaired or has a defective part, the manufacturer will pay for the cost of the repair. In some cases, the item may be replaced. Warranty language includes details on what is covered. Some warranties are not honored if someone other than a "recognized" serviceperson attempts to fix the machine. Extended warranties lengthen the protection time and can be purchased for some equipment.

For complex or expensive equipment, the healthcare facility may contract with a service provider for repairs and routine service checks. This assistance is necessary for some equipment. It also helps to extend the lifetime of those machines. For repairs on other equipment, it might be necessary to ship or bring the machine to the repair service. Usually the cost for onsite repairs is more than if the machine is taken or shipped to the service provider for repairs. One of the main concerns when a piece of equipment breaks down is the effect on the healthcare facility. Some service providers will also loan equipment to facilities while the repairs take place. This service greatly lessens the burden on the practice.

Purchasing Equipment

The process of purchasing equipment can vary depending on the size of the organization. Large agencies have purchasing departments. The staff researches the need and identifies the best equipment to purchase. The medical assistant may be involved with the process in smaller practices.

Many factors are considered when equipment is being replaced:
- Age of the equipment and the availability of parts
- Frequency and cost of repairs
- Utilization of the machine and whether new features will lead to extra billable services

---

CRITICAL THINKING APPLICATION   **13.5**

Currently, the providers are using an offsite radiology service. They are contemplating creating a small radiology room where they could take x-rays. How could Marie assist the providers with their plans for a potential purchase of x-ray equipment?

Leasing medical equipment is becoming a popular option for smaller facilities. The healthcare facility pays a fee to lease an item, such as monitoring equipment, diagnostic testing equipment, computer systems, and exam tables. The fee is less than what it would cost to purchase the item. The lease fees are tax deductible and allow the healthcare facility to provide extra billable services.

The medical assistant may help identify potential new equipment models to purchase or lease. Using the internet and contacting the company's salespeople are two ways to get additional information. Some salespeople will meet with the staff and demonstrate the product. In addition to research, the medical assistant may need to explain the usage of the machine and the frequency of repair checks. Usually the supervisor or provider has the final say as to whether the purchase should occur.

Supplies

Many supplies are required to run the medical office and treat patients. Supplies include administrative items (e.g., pens, paper, envelopes, and paperclips) and clinical items (e.g., bandages, vaccines, medications, slings, and splints). The medical assistant must make sure there are enough supplies to treat patients. A lack of supplies can greatly affect the services provided to patients. It can be expensive for the healthcare facility because of last-minute ordering at higher prices. On the other hand, overstocking supplies can be a financial waste to the facility. Many supplies have expiration dates and cannot be used beyond that date. Having adequate amounts of supplies in inventory is crucial.

Inventory Management

Inventory management involves ordering, tracking inventory, and identifying the quantity of product to purchase. The goal of inventory management is to have adequate supplies on hand. It is important not to have too much stock that will expire or take a long time to use.

The medical assistant in charge of ordering and managing supplies must keep a record on each item in inventory. The record can be a manual entry written in a notebook or on index cards. It can be computerized in a spreadsheet or inventory control system software. For each inventory item, the medical assistant must record the following:
- Item details: item name, size, quantity, item number, supplier's name, and cost (Fig. 13.4).
- *Quantity to reorder*: amount of supplies that need to be ordered. This amount reflects the product used during the **buying cycle**.
  - For instance, the healthcare facility's buying cycle for 2 × 2 nonsterile gauze (100 per pack) is 1 month. The facility typically goes through 25 packs in 1 month. This would be the quantity used during the buying cycle. It would also be the quantity to reorder each time (see Fig. 13.4).
- *Reorder point*: point at which low inventory requires the product to be ordered.
  - For instance, when the inventory of 2 × 2 nonsterile gauze packs gets depleted to 5 packs, the medical assistant must reorder (see Fig. 13.4). Five is the reorder point or the quantity that triggers an order to be placed to replenish the inventory. The reorder point for medical and administrative supplies can be different for each item because of the usage rate and the time it takes to receive the item after it is ordered.

How to Calculate the Reorder Point

The reorder point can be calculated based on the number used per day and the number of days it takes to order and receive the product.

For instance, the practice uses 0.5 pack of 2 × 2 nonsterile gauze per day. It takes 4 days to receive the order from the medical supply company. The medical practice may also want 6 extra days' worth of supplies on hand to prevent issues related to running out of the item. Here is how you would figure out the reorder point:

Stock to cover order time: 0.5 pack per day × 4 days to receive order = 2 packs

Extra stock: 6 days × 0.5 pack per day = 3 packs

Reorder point: 2 packs (stock to cover order time) + 3 packs (6-day supply) = 5 packs

Item Name	Size	Quantity	Item Number	Supplier's Name	Reorder Point	Quantity to Reorder	Cost	Stock Available	Order (✓)
Nonsterile gauze sponges, 8 ply	2"x 2"	100/pkg	NG0022	Midwest Medical	5	25	$2.31/pkg		
Sterile gauze sponges, 12 ply, 2/pkg	2"x 2"	25 pkg/box	NG0042	Midwest Medical	4	20	$3.99/box		

FIGURE 13.4 A supply inventory list shows details of items in the inventory. For efficiency, use two extra columns ("Stock Available" and "Order") as shown. This list can be duplicated and used whenever an inventory is performed.

Inventory Control Systems

An inventory control system helps to make inventory management work well. Large medical facilities use computerized inventory control systems. These systems monitor usage and inventory in stock. They also identify items that need to be ordered. Smaller facilities may use simple computerized or manual systems.

Weight-Based Inventory Systems

The weight-based system uses separate bins for each type of product. Each bin is connected to a scale. The weight of each type of product is entered into the software. The software monitors the weight of each bin. When an item is removed from a bin, the software reduces the inventory count.

For example, the weight of a 3 mL syringe (i.e., 15 grams) is entered into the software. The bin is filled with 30 syringes and attached to the scale. Using the weight of the bin, the software registers 30 syringes in inventory. An employer removes two syringes, and the weight drops 30 grams. The software drops the total syringes to 28.

This type of inventory system reduces the risk of errors and also provides up-to-date inventory information, without requiring employees to count supplies.

To help create an efficient computerized system, many medical facilities use bar codes to track inventory, for insurance, and for patient billing for supplies (Fig. 13.5). With this system, each item has a unique bar code. The bar code is scanned with a bar code reader when items are added or taken from inventory. Software monitors the inventory quantity. For bar codes to work successfully, the staff must be diligent in scanning the bar codes when taking a product from stock. Bar code inventory control systems work successfully in large and small healthcare facilities.

Several manual systems can be used to identify supplies that need to be ordered. The following are some of the more common methods used in medical facilities:

- When staff identify a product that needs to be ordered, the item is written in a log. This process is like making a list of what you need at the grocery store. The person responsible for ordering supplies then prepares the order based on the information in the log.

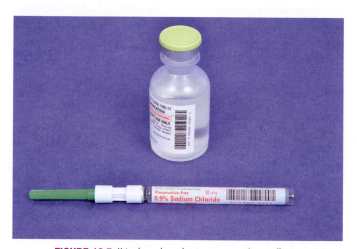

FIGURE 13.5 Using bar codes makes inventory control more efficient.

- Another system includes using product identification slips, which contain the name of the product. The slips or cards are attached to the product or a box/package of items. When the product is used, the slip is put in a special location, such as a box or plastic pocket. The medical assistant uses the slips in the box or pocket to prepare the supply order.
- The two-bin system consists of having a main bin for each item in inventory and then a backup bin for each item. When the main bin is emptied, the backup bin is used, and the product is reordered.
- The medical assistant responsible for ordering performs a hand count of the items in stock to identify what needs to be ordered. This system is explained in the next section.

CRITICAL THINKING APPLICATION   13.6

Marie decided to implement a manual system for inventory. Of the manual systems discussed, which method might work best in the small facility? Discuss your answer.

Taking Inventory

Inventory (counting supplies) must be taken at specific times. Many businesses that use automated inventory control systems hand count their inventory at least once a year. Usually this is done around the close of the business year. These companies compare their hand counts to the computer counts and identify **discrepancies**. The discrepancies are followed up on. The manual inventory procedure provides the company with information on the actual number of items in stock. With this information, the financial value of the inventory can be calculated and used for financial reports and taxes at the close of the business year.

For medical offices that do not implement inventory control systems, performing inventory or counting the items in stock is important before each buying cycle.

One of the most frequent errors when performing inventory is to report a different quantity than what is on the supply inventory list. For instance, a medical assistant counts nonsterile sponges. Each package should be counted as 1 and not as 100 each. For example, in Fig. 13.4, if there were 6 packages of nonsterile gauze sponges left in the supply cabinet, it should be noted that the stock available was 6 packages. It should not be indicated as 600 sponges, or 600 each. Counting each item in a box or package when the product is inventoried by box or package creates conflict and confusion when looking at the reorder point.

The medical assistant should use a supply inventory list to be most efficient when counting supplies (Fig. 13.6). The supply inventory list shows all the items in stock. The medical assistant can mark down the inventory counts for each item on the document (see Procedure 13.3, p. 287). If the supply inventory list is not available, then the medical assistant needs to write down the item number, size, quantity (e.g., 100/box), manufacturer, and any other identifying information. This process takes a lot more time. Using abbreviations can be helpful.

Common Inventory and Purchase Abbreviations

BTL: Bottle
BX: Box
CS: Case
EA: Each
PKG: Package

PO: Purchase Order
PPD: Prepaid
PYMT: Payment
QTY: Quantity

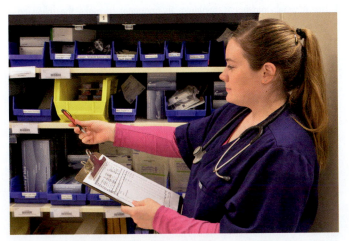

FIGURE 13.6 A medical assistant performing an inventory.

When you perform an inventory, work in a systematic manner. Start with one supply cabinet, working from top to bottom, before moving on to another cabinet. All stock areas should be inventoried before the supply order is prepared.

Price Consideration When Ordering Supplies

When you order supplies, price comparison shopping is important. The healthcare facility must balance the time it takes against the money saved. Some medical offices compare prices only on more expensive items or items that are used in vast quantities. They may compare prices every 6 to 12 months. When you compare prices, consider the following:

- Shipping and handling charges
- Quality and amount (e.g., 10 per box), as these must be the same among products
- Quantity discounts or price breaks for buying a certain amount

---

Quantity Discounts

Quantity discounts or price breaks save money. The more of an item purchased when you order, the cheaper the product becomes, as this example shows:

Quantity 1 to 5, $1.50 per each item
Quantity 6 to 15, $1.25 per each item

If the medical assistant purchased a quantity of 6, the price per each would be cheaper than if 4 were purchased. Before ordering extra product, consider the following:

- Storage space
- How quickly the item will be used
- Shelf life (or expiration date) of the item
- Buying too much just to get a price break may not be in the best interest of the healthcare facility.

Some medical facilities join group purchasing organizations (GPOs). These organizations combine orders from many different medical facilities. Combining orders results in volume discounts from specific **vendors**. GPOs typically purchase both supplies and medications. Physician buying groups (PBGs) offer providers potential cost-saving pricing for vaccines. The drawback is that the provider must exclusively use the vaccines from the contracted manufacturers.

CRITICAL THINKING APPLICATION 13.7

Currently the facility orders its clinical supplies from two vendors. Marie would like to do some cost comparisons to get the best deals on supplies. She does not have a lot of time to spend on the research. How might she approach this situation? Where should she start first? What might be a long-term goal for her?

Ordering Supplies

If the facility is not part of a buying group, the medical assistant might need to order supplies. It is important to select just a few vendors if possible. The medical assistant can use the following:

- Supplier's printed catalog, though it may only be printed a few times a year and may not provide accurate item availability and pricing.
- Supplier's website store, which would have the most accurate prices, sale prices, and available stock

Many vendors require the creation of an account before ordering. Some medical facilities use **purchase order (PO) numbers**, giving each order a unique reference number. This PO number should be included on the order sheets, added to the online information, or provided during the phone order. Vendors add the PO number to the order's documentation (i.e., **packing slip** and statement). This way both parties can use it as a reference if questions come up. The healthcare facility uses the purchase order number to track the order.

Creating an Account for Purchasing

When creating an account for purchasing supplies, consider these points:

- Use the facility's information (address, fax number, and phone number)
- Be prepared to give the provider's license number when ordering medications and needles
- Fax the provider's license number, if required, before ordering
- Provide a copy of the provider's Drug Enforcement Administration (DEA) registration if narcotics are being ordered; narcotics require special tracking documentation and thus a high level of authorization when they are purchased

---

Payment terms may vary among vendors. Payment methods may include credit card, check, money order, or a line of credit. Typically, the line of credit is good for 30 to 60 days. **Invoices** are sent to the facility and should be paid after the purchases have been received. Orders can typically be placed via fax, mail, phone, or online. If the medical assistant is faxing or mailing the order, the vendor usually requires the order to be placed on the vendor's order sheet. The medical assistant should keep a copy of the phoned-in, mailed, or faxed order or a printout of the online order to verify that the order was filled correctly.

Receiving the Order

Orders can arrive via the mail, a national delivery service (e.g., FedEx, United Parcel Service [UPS]), or a local delivery service. The delivery person may require a signature from an employee. This signature is used to track who received the delivery.

The medical assistant must check the delivery as soon as possible. Some medications, such as vaccines, are shipped in a cold environment and must remain at a cold temperature. These medications need to be placed in the refrigerator or freezer immediately upon arrival. Storage information for medications can be found in the package

insert or on the manufacturer's website. If the medication warms up too much, it may be adversely affected. For instance, vaccines that get too warm can have reduced potency. This means they may not protect patients against the disease.

Vaccine Storage Guidelines

For All Vaccines

- Unpack vaccines immediately.
- Each type of vaccine should be placed in its own tray, which allows for airflow. Place newer vaccines behind older vaccines. Keep vaccine vials in their original boxes to prevent light exposure.

For Refrigerated Vaccines

- The ideal temperature for refrigerated vaccines is 36° F to 46° F.
- Do not store vaccines next to the wall, top shelf, door, or floor of the refrigerator.
- Do not put food or beverages in the vaccine storage refrigerator. Place bottles of water in the crisper bins to maintain the temperature.
- Make sure the door is closed.

For Frozen Vaccines

- Ideal temperature for refrigerated vaccines: −58° F to 5° F.
- Leave 2 to 3 inches between the vaccine and the freezer wall.
- Use water bottles to help maintain the temperature.
- Make sure the door is closed.

Temperature Monitoring Equipment

The CDC recommends temperature monitoring equipment (Digital Data Loggers [DDL]) for all vaccine storage units. All vaccine storage units (e.g., refrigerators, freezers, transport containers) must have a temperature monitoring device. Simple thermometers can show the minimum and maximum temperatures since the last reset. A DDL records a temperature at least every 30 minutes and provides the most accurate storage temperatures. The CDC recommends keeping the digital data from the DDLs for 3 years. These data may need to be shown to demonstrate compliance when the facility is involved with vaccination programs.

Check Temperature

Use a simple maximum/minimum thermometer to make the following inspections:

- Check and log temperatures twice a day (see Fig. 13.7).
- Check the current temperature.
- Check the minimum and maximum temperatures. This represents the coldest and warmest temperatures that occurred since you last checked it.
- Reset the thermometer if needed.
- If the temperature is outside the range, contact the vaccine manufacturer and report the total amount of time the temperature was outside the range.

From Resources on Proper Vaccine Storage and Handling. *https://www.cdc.gov/vaccines/hcp/admin/storage/index.html*; and Vaccine Storage & Handling Toolkit. *https://www.cdc.gov/vaccines/hcp/admin/storage/toolkit/storage-handling-toolkit.pdf*. Accessed March 10, 2019.

		Refrigerator Temperature			Freezer Temperature			
Date	Time	Max	Min	Current	Max	Min	Current	Initials
10/11/xx	0750	40° F	37° F	39° F	3° F	–13° F	–12° F	MVB
10/11/xx	1722	38° F	35° F	38° F	–8° F	–28° F	–19° F	BMN
10/12/xx	0752	42° F	36° F	39° F	–13° F	–23° F	–18° F	MVB
10/13/xx	0748	47° F	38° F	38° F	–8° F	–27° F	–22° F	MVB

FIGURE 13.7 Example of a temperature log. (Adapted from CDC: Vaccine storage and handling: recommendations and guidelines. *http://www.cdc.gov/vaccines/recs/storage/default.htm.* Accessed March 10, 2019.)

CRITICAL THINKING APPLICATION   13.8

Using the information in the Vaccine Storage Guidelines box and Fig. 13.7, answer the following questions:

- Did all the refrigerator temperatures fall within the required range? Explain.
- Did all the freezer temperatures fall within the required range? Explain.
- If a temperature was outside the required range, what should be done?
- Were the temperatures checked twice daily?

When an order arrives, remove the packing slip from the box. Compare the items in the package to the packing slip (Fig. 13.8). Check off all items received. Some vendors may indicate items that are **backordered** and will be arriving later. Note any discrepancies or differences on the packing slip. Any items that are damaged should be noted on the packing slip. The copy of the original order should be compared against the packing slip, and any differences should be noted. Any discrepancies or damaged items should be addressed with the supply company as soon as possible.

The packing slip should be attached to the copy of the order once the supplies have been reviewed. When the complete order has been received, the copy of the order with the packing slips attached should be filed if the order was prepaid. If a line of credit was used, the copy of the order with the attached packing slips is placed in the **accounts payable** folder to wait for the invoice's arrival. The person responsible for paying the healthcare facility's bills will match the invoice with the copy of the order, ensuring everything is in order before paying the bill.

The items received should be put away as soon as possible, and the boxes should be discarded. When you are putting supplies away, it is important to rotate stock. This means the new stock should go in the back and the older stock needs to be moved forward so it can be used first. Any items with expiration dates should be placed so that the items expiring first are in front, so they are used first. For

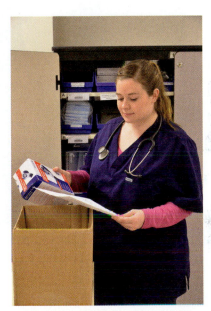

FIGURE 13.8 Comparing the packing slip to the contents in the box is an important step in receiving supplies.

stock without expiration dates, consider the saying "first in, first out" (FIFO), which means when new stock comes in, it is placed behind the older stock. The older stock needs to be used first. If you are removing expired stock, remember to subtract the quantity from the inventory system.

SAFETY AND SECURITY

Body Mechanics

The Occupational Safety and Health Act (OSH Act) of 1970 is enforced by the Occupational Safety and Health Administration (OSHA). It requires that employers provide a workplace that is free from serious recognized hazards. Employers must comply with OSH Act standards. In the healthcare environment, most injuries are sprains, strains, and tears. Back injuries are one of the most common injuries.

They can result from microtrauma related to repetitive activity over time or from one traumatic experience. Reasons for back injuries include the following:

- Improper lifting or lifting items too heavy for the back to support
- Reaching, twisting, or bending when lifting
- Bad body mechanics when lifting, pushing, pulling, or carrying items
- Poor footing or constrained posture

Proper body mechanics entails using the appropriate muscles and body movements to maintain correct posture and body alignment. Proper body mechanics will increase coordination and endurance. The risk of strain and injury to the body decreases. Medical assistants need to protect themselves from bodily harm while lifting, reaching, and carrying heavy objects (Figs. 13.9 and 13.10). Using proper body mechanics is important to prevent injuries. (See Procedure 13.3 on p. 287, which explains how to use correct body mechanics when performing a supply inventory.)

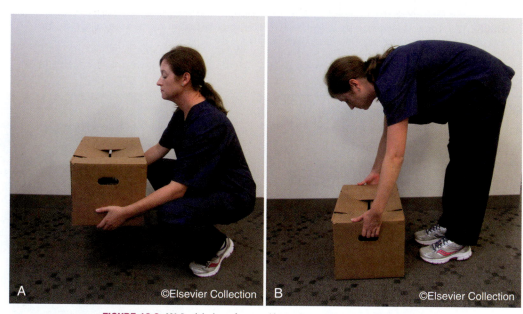

FIGURE 13.9 **(A)** Bend the knees for proper lifting technique. **(B)** Improper lifting technique.

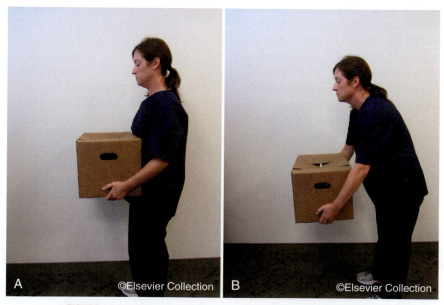

FIGURE 13.10 **(A)** Carrying an item close to the body. **(B)** Improper carrying technique.

Principles of Proper Body Mechanics

- To lift an object, maintain a wide, stable base with your feet. Your feet should be shoulder-width apart, and you should have good footing. Bend at the knees, keeping your back straight. Lift smoothly, using the major muscles in your arms and legs. Use the same technique when putting the item down. Bending over to lift or to set down a heavy object increases your risk of injury.
- When lifting and carrying heavy items, keep the item directly in front of you to avoid rotating your spine.
- Keep your movements smooth. Jerky or uncoordinated movements increase the risk for injury.
- When reaching for an object, your feet should face the object. Twisting or turning with a heavy load can cause injury.
- Prevent reaching and straining to get an object. Clear away barriers, and use a firm and level surface (e.g., a step stool) to get close to the object. Avoid standing on tiptoes.
- Get help if the item is too heavy to lift by yourself.
- Store heavy objects at waist level or below.

Providing a Safe Environment

Security and safety are important to the well-being of the ambulatory care staff, patients, and visitors. The healthcare facility can draw unwanted attention from those seeking drugs and money. Having plans in place that can be implemented when security is in question is critical for all.

Ways to Keep Safe

- Stay alert for suspicious people.
- Listen to your instincts if a situation or person makes you feel strange or on edge.
- Try to alert another employee if a situation occurs. Many agencies have code words for emergency situations.
- Use emergency alarms when needed. Many will notify the local police department.
- Keep yourself at a distance from the person (e.g., try to separate yourself from the person by a desk or another piece of furniture).
- Position yourself so you are the closest to the door.
- Discuss the situation with the provider or supervisor if you are uncomfortable rooming a patient.
- Follow the facility's safety procedures.

Medical facilities can be a target for those wanting to steal money, narcotic medications, and prescription pads. The staff should implement measures to limit the amount of money available in the building. Cash and checks from patients should be deposited daily to limit the quantities of money in the facility. Cash drawers should be stored out of the sight of patients and visitors. As mentioned earlier, prescription pads should remain out of the view and reach of patients. Narcotic

medications, if present in the healthcare facility, should always be in a double-locked cabinet with the keys hidden. Depending on the type of clinic, some will post signs stating there are no narcotic medications on site.

Many facilities have chosen to keep the employee entrance doors locked during business hours. The doors require either a key card or unique code to enter the building. In high-crime areas, low-staffed clinics, or rural clinics, the doors to the patient care areas are also locked. This prevents the unauthorized entry of people to the patient care areas in the back, thereby increasing the security.

CRITICAL THINKING APPLICATION 13.9

Over the past 6 months, crime and break-ins have increased in the local area around the clinic. Many people believe the healthcare facility has a supply of narcotic medications in stock, which is *not* true. What strategies can the staff implement to increase the security of the healthcare facility?

Workplace Violence

Stories of workplace violence are becoming more common. Healthcare employees face an increased risk of work-related assaults, primarily from patients and visitors. In the *Guidelines for Preventing Workplace Violence for Healthcare and Social Service Workers*, published by OSHA (available at *https://www.osha.gov/Publications/osha3148.pdf*), increased risk factors for violence in healthcare include the following:

- Working with patients or family members who have a history of violence, abuse alcohol or other substances, are gang members, or carry firearms or other weapons
- Poorly designed work environments, including inadequately lit hallways, rooms, parking lots, and other areas, which can limit vision of potential situations and interfere with escape plans
- Lack of emergency communication (e.g., alarms, healthcare facility's emergency procedures) and training of employees
- Working in neighborhoods with high crime rates
- High employee turnover
- Long waits for patients in overcrowded, uncomfortable reception areas
- Unrestricted areas, allowing public access to the major areas of the building
- A perception that violence is tolerated, and the police will not be called

OSHA encourages healthcare employees to take "universal precautions for violence." This means that violence should be expected. Violence can be avoided or lessened by respecting others, protecting the dignity of others, and through teamwork to prevent violence. Medical assistants should report patient incidents or at-risk patient behaviors and situations to the manager.

Healthcare facilities should have violence prevention programs in place. Management and employees should work together to identify hazards and plan preventive strategies. According to OSHA, strategies to secure the workplace environment include:

- Physical barriers (e.g., locked doors, enclosures, bullet-proof windows, security guards)
- Bright, effective lighting and accessible exits
- Closed-circuit video (inside and outside of the building)

- **De-escalating** areas for patients and visitors
- Secure work area for those working alone; panic buttons
- Name badges to identify employees

All employees should be trained to handle workplace violence and facility lockdown procedures. Lockdown is used when it is safer to stay where you are. This procedure is employed when there is a dangerous person in the building or in the area:

- Lock or barricade the doors. If the person is in the area, lock windows and pull shades.
- Keep away from the windows and doors.
- If the person is in the building, silence cell phones. Contact 911 immediately and hide in a locked room.

Evaluating the Work Environment

It is important to safeguard both the patients and the employees from injuries in the healthcare facility. The medical assistant should continually evaluate the environment for safety. From a flipped-over rug to a burned-out light in the stairway, safety risks can lead to falls and injuries. This section explains how to evaluate the work environment for unsafe working conditions. By fixing or correcting issues, the environment becomes safer for all.

Remember that for all injuries that occur to patients, visitors, and employees, an incident report form must be completed. Incident report forms are discussed in Chapter 4.

Preventing Falls and Injuries

Accidents can be expensive for the healthcare facility, because costs can range from losses of employee workdays to lawsuits. Preventing accidents is therefore critical. In the healthcare facility, there are many areas that can be prone to slips, trips, and falls. In the winter months, depending on the facility's geographic location, slips and falls can be common because of snow and ice. The healthcare facility should have employees who oversee the sidewalks for patients and visitors. Inside the facility, high-risk situations for accidents include the following:

- *Water or trash on floors*: Standing water on floors should be cleaned up. Signage should be used to indicate wet floors. Paper wrappings, covers, and other items should not be tossed on the floor during procedures, due to an increased risk of injury.
- *Dim lighting*: Burned-out light bulbs should be replaced. All stairwells should have adequate lighting.
- *Flooring and rugs*: Rugs and mats need to be smooth and flat. Flooring that is old and pulling up needs to be replaced. Carpeting with holes can catch a shoe heel, causing the person to trip and fall.
- *Cords, cables, and other objects in walkways*: Electrical cords, computer cables, boxes, and other potential tripping hazards should never be in the walkway. Hallways and **fire doors** need to be clear of debris. Unused wheelchairs and walkers should be collapsed if possible and moved out of the way.
- *Heavy objects placed on high shelves*: These items can fall and injure someone. Reaching for a heavy object can also cause injury. Store heavier items on lower shelves so they do not have to be lifted any higher than necessary.
- *Using unsafe objects to stand on*: A chair or box could collapse or move when a person stands on it. Use a stable stepstool to reach for things.

Preventing Electrical Issues and Fires

Malfunctioning equipment can also cause accidents. Any equipment that is not functioning or does not sound normal should not be used until it can be serviced and checked out. The medical assistant should follow the facility's procedure in this situation. Usually, the supervisor is notified if equipment is malfunctioning.

The medical assistant can help prevent injuries and fires in many ways:

- Check electrical cords and plugs for cracks, fraying, or other damage.
- Ensure power strips are not overloaded.
- Do not use electricity near water.
- Turn off equipment that appears to be overheating or malfunctioning.
- Store potentially flammable chemicals and supplies according to the manufacturers' guidelines.
- Keep combustibles (e.g., paper, cardboard, cloth, flammable chemicals) away from heat sources.

Many fires are started by smoking materials. It is important to have adequate No Smoking signs at the facility's doors. Deep, nontip ashtrays should be outside the doors, so visitors have an adequate place to dispose of smoking materials.

Cautery equipment and lasers are commonly used in healthcare. Cautery equipment, by design, gets hot. Inappropriate use can cause fires. Lasers can cause health issues (e.g., burns and blindness) and fires. All staff members using or assisting with lasers should take a safety class. Signage should be on the door where the laser is being used. Water should be available if needed. Oxygen, other gases, and combustible chemicals should not be in the room when laser equipment is used.

Procedure 13.4 on p. 287 describes how to evaluate the environment for unsafe working conditions. Remember that when issues are found, it is important to fix them. If you cannot fix the unsafe condition, let your supervisor know immediately. Delays can increase the risk of others being injured.

Emergency Response Plan

A variety of emergency situations can occur and impact the healthcare facility. Each facility should have a plan to respond to the situations. An emergency response plan addresses possible **workplace emergencies**. This document guides the staff on handling emergencies and may protect the business. The occurrence of natural disasters may vary around the country. The emergency response plan should cover only potential emergencies seen at the facility and in the community (Table 13.1). Table 13.2 provides the critical elements that at the minimum must be in the emergency response plan.

Having a plan is the first step. The employer also needs to train new staff on the procedures. Yearly refresher courses and mock drills help employees remain current on these procedures. The employer should document employee participation at the training sessions.

Evacuation Procedures

Evacuation procedures involve exit routes and procedures for moving employees, patients, and visitors to safe locations. Floor maps with evacuation exit routes and emergency equipment locations should be posted throughout the facility (Fig. 13.11). It is recommended that at least two routes should be identified, which provides a backup route in case the primary route is blocked. Exit routes must follow these conventions:

- Be clearly marked and well lit
- Be wide enough to accommodate several people
- Not pass areas where flammable products (e.g., oxygen tanks, chemicals) are stored
- Be clear of debris and obstructions at all times

Some employees must assist those who need help evacuating. According to the Americans with Disabilities Act (ADA), safety requirements are needed for people in multistory buildings who need access to wheelchairs. *Areas of rescue assistance* are safe places where people in wheelchairs or those who cannot do stairs can await help in emergency situations. Typically, these areas are stairwells that have alarms that communicate with emergency personnel. Evacuation chairs can be used to move people down the stairs.

Evacuation is done by priority, either by location or by people. Evacuation priority by location includes:

1. People in immediate danger
2. People located on the floor where the emergency is occurring
3. People on the floors immediately above and below the floor with the situation
4. People on the rest of the floors

Evacuation priority by people means the people nearest the emergency leave first, followed by the ambulatory people, and last the nonambulatory people. As people evacuate by priority, it is important that appointed staff remain behind to verify that everyone is out. All rooms, including restrooms, need to be checked.

Evacuation procedures vary based on the emergency (see Procedure 13.5, p. 288). There are five types of evacuations:

- *Shelter-in-place evacuation*: A shelter-in-place is an interior room with no windows. In cases of tornados and other severe storms, employees, patients, and visitors should evacuate to shelter-in-place locations. Typically, these locations should be on the lowest level possible. Shelter-in-place locations are also used when a contaminant (e.g., chemical) is released into the environment.
- *Local evacuation*: Involves moving one or more people out of immediate danger (e.g., evacuating a patient from an exam room where a chemical spill occurred).
- *Horizontal evacuation*: Involves evacuating people off the same floor as the emergency situation.

TABLE 13.1   Potential Emergencies

EVENT	TYPE	EXAMPLES
Natural	Geological hazards	Tsunami, volcano, landslide, and earthquake
	Meteorological hazards	Flood, tornado, hurricane, and ice
	Biological hazards	Foodborne illnesses and communicable disease
Human caused	Accidental events	Hazardous spill, fire, and transportation incident (aircraft, vehicle)
	Intentional events	Robbery, lost person, bomb threat, terrorism, and weapons
	Technology-caused events	Telecommunication, electrical power, water, and cyber security issues

TABLE 13.2   Critical Elements of an Emergency Response Plan

CRITICAL ELEMENTS	INCLUDES
Methods to report a fire and other emergencies	• How to alert employees of the emergency (e.g., alarms, overhead paging system) • How to alert law enforcement and the fire department
Evacuation policy and procedure	• Evacuation conditions • Clear chain of command and designated person to order the evacuation and to account for employees (may be called an evacuation warden) • Patient sign-in sheets or schedules that are used to account for patients. • Evacuation procedures, including routes and meeting locations; maps should be posted
Critical shutdown procedures	• Names of specific employees who must perform certain procedures before leaving • Critical shutdown procedures (describe what needs to be done); examples include turning off the water, gas, electricity, and oxygen (if piped into the exam rooms)
Emergency escape/exit routes and procedures	• Floor plan, workplace map, safe areas, and procedures
Rescue and medical duties	• Names of workers who need to perform rescue and medical duties
Whom to contact for additional information	• Names, titles, and contact information of internal and external people who can provide additional information on emergency response plans (internal people would be management and other employees; external people might be community leaders and specialists)

From How to Plan for Workplace Emergencies and Evacuations. *https://www.osha.gov/Publications/osha3088.html.* Accessed January 10, 2019.

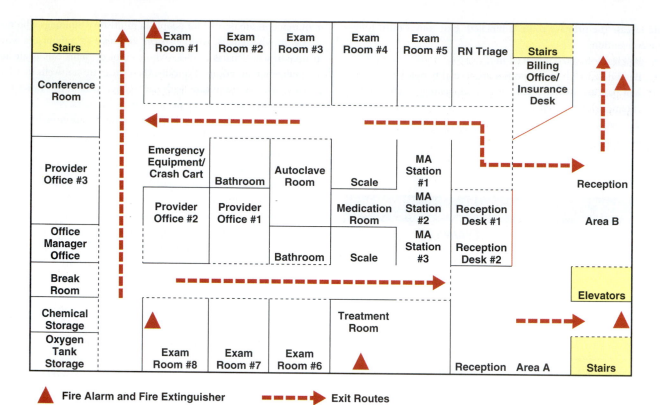

FIGURE 13.11 A floor map with exit routes and emergency equipment indicated.

Legend: ▲ Fire Alarm and Fire Extinguisher   ----► Exit Routes

---

- *Vertical evacuation*: Involves evacuating people who are located on the floors above and below the situation.
- *Building evacuation*: Involves evacuating everyone from the building to a safe location outside the building.

Fire Response

A medical assistant should be aware of the healthcare facility's fire response procedures. It is important to know how to activate the alarms, evacuate people, and use a fire extinguisher for small fires. Fire response actions include the following:

- A wall-mounted fire extinguisher, manual pull station (alarm), warning alarms, smoke alarms, and automatic sprinkler systems should be located throughout the facility per state code. An employee should be assigned to routinely check this equipment and replace it as needed.
- If you smell smoke or suspect a fire, think of the acronym *RACE*:
  - *Rescue* individuals threatened by the fire.
  - *Activate* the alarm if you discover the fire or respond if you hear the alarm.
  - *Confine* the fire by closing doors and fire doors to slow the spread of the fire.
  - *Extinguish* only small fires; otherwise *evacuate* individuals from the area.
- Do not use elevators if a fire is suspected. This will reduce the risk of entrapment.
- If a fire is suspected, immediately disconnect oxygen supplies, or turn off oxygen tanks to prevent an explosion.
- Use the correct type of extinguisher for the fire (Table 13.3).
- For small fires, use the *PASS procedure* as you operate a fire extinguisher (see Procedure 13.6, p. 289).

TABLE 13.3   Uses of Fire Extinguishers

LABELED CLASS	USED FOR
A	Water extinguisher: used on *ordinary combustibles* (e.g., paper, wood, rubber, cloth, and many plastics)
B	Carbon dioxide (CO_2) extinguisher: used on flammable liquids; fires in oils and grease
C	Dry chemical extinguisher: used on electrical equipment; fires in wiring, fuse boxes, computers, and other electrical sources
ABC	Multipurpose dry chemical extinguisher. Used on ordinary combustibles, flammable liquids, or electrical equipment
D	Fires involving combustible metals: may be found in the medical laboratory
K	Fires involving combustible cooking oils and fats: found in the kitchen

- *Pull* the pin.
- *Aim* the nozzle or hose at the base of the fire.
- *Squeeze* the handle to release the extinguishing agent.
- *Sweep* the nozzle or hose from side to side at the base of the fire until the fire is out. *Evacuate if you are not successful or doubt your ability to put out the fire.*

New Fire Extinguisher Technology

A new type of fire extinguisher, the Eliminator, changes the way fire extinguishers are used (Fig. 13.12A). This new fire extinguisher has an ergonomically designed handle and spray hose. Most fire extinguishers need to be serviced and maintained to keep them operable. This extinguisher allows facilities to maintain it easier and cheaper than other extinguishers. When using the Eliminator, a person must follow "TPASS" (Fig. 13.12B):

T: Twist the lock to break the seal.
P: Push the level down. This will pressure the extinguisher.
A: Aim the valve nozzle at the base of the fire.
S: Squeeze the valve level.
S: Sweep the valve nozzle from side to side to put out the fire.

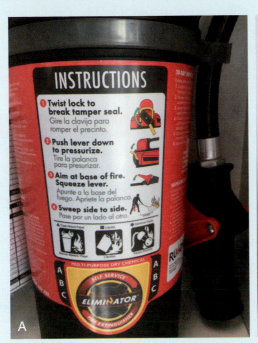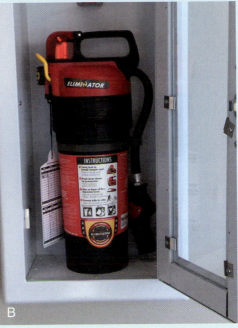

FIGURE 13.12 (A) The Eliminator is a new type of fire extinguisher. **(B)** Users must follow "TPASS" when using the Eliminator.

CRITICAL THINKING APPLICATION   **13.10**

One morning when the weather was stormy, Marie and Catherine were discussing the facility's emergency policy and procedures. How would you respond to a tornado warning and the need to evacuate to a shelter-in-place? How would you respond if you found a wastebasket on fire in the facility?

Effects of Stress

When a person is involved in an emergency, this can cause physical and emotional symptoms, including:

- Shock, disbelief, irritability, crying, sadness, and anger
- Fear, anxiety, a feeling of numbness, a feeling of powerlessness, and difficulty making decisions
- High blood pressure, high blood glucose levels, back pain, and stomach problems
- Loss of interest in normal activities, trouble concentrating
- Nightmares, sleep problems, and tension

The term *general adaptation syndrome* (GAS) is used to describe the long- and short-term effects of stress on the body. GAS was originally described by Hans Selye. He felt the syndrome impacted the nervous and the endocrine systems. The stages include the following:

- *Stage 1 – Alarm reaction*: This is the immediate reaction to the stressor. The "fight or flight" response occurs. The body releases the hormones cortisol, adrenaline, and noradrenaline. This provides energy, preparing the body for physical activities. This stage can impact the immune system, causing the person to be more susceptible to illness.
- *Stage 2 – Adaptation stage*: If the stressor continues, the individual's body adapts to the stressor.
- *Stage 3 – Exhaustion stage*: At this point, the body's resistance has been diminished by the continued stress. The body is more susceptible to disease.

CRITICAL THINKING APPLICATION   **13.11**

Ella Rainwater had an appointment to see Dr. Martin. Marie was rooming Ms. Rainwater and had to obtain her medical history. The patient reported that she was going through a divorce and was having issues with sleeping. She said that she cannot concentrate on her job and finds herself crying throughout the day. She cannot think and is not interested in socializing any more. Based on what you learned in this chapter, what might be occurring with Ms. Rainwater?

CLOSING COMMENTS

Patient Coaching

In the ambulatory healthcare environment, many types of supplies are available. A medical assistant may be tempted to give patients supplies to use at home for the ordered treatments, such as wound care. Many healthcare facilities do not allow this for a variety of reasons, including financial considerations. If supplies are given to patients, the low inventory may impact the care of other patients.

The medical assistant should coach the patient on what supplies are needed for the treatments prescribed. Making a list of supplies, along with specific details and where to purchase the items, is helpful for patients.

Legal and Ethical Issues

The medical assistant has important tasks to prepare and monitor the equipment in the healthcare facility. As mentioned in this chapter, quality control procedures are done on equipment to ensure the accuracy of test results. The medical assistant must accurately complete the quality control procedures and document the results daily or as indicated by the facility's policies and procedures. The lack of precision with quality control can lead to issues with the accuracy of test results that will impact patient care.

Besides quality control, the medical assistant is responsible for ensuring the medications that must remain cold or frozen are at the proper temperatures. This responsibility begins when the shipment of medications arrives. It is critical to open these packages very soon after delivery and to place the medications in the refrigerator or freezer. The medical assistant is also responsible for monitoring to make sure the medications remain at the proper temperature. The refrigerator and freezer temperature log must be completed as directed. Any issues with the temperature must be addressed immediately. It is unethical for the medical assistant not to address the problem when medications become too warm. This can impact the quality of the medication and ultimately the patient.

Patient-Centered Care

Safety is a concern for both patients and healthcare professionals. The medical assistant should be alert for potential situations that could turn violent. Treating patients and family members with respect, listening to their concerns, and following through with promises are especially important when working in healthcare. A person who feels respected and listened to is less likely to get angry to the point of violence.

Professional Behaviors

The medical assistant has many important duties to help the healthcare facility operate. From managing inventory to safety procedures, these duties are important to the success of the facility. Keeping the right amount of supplies in stock so providers can treat patients also requires paying attention to details.

The medical assistant also needs to be knowledgeable about the emergency policies and procedures of the healthcare facility. During an emergency is not the time to read the procedure on what to do! It is important for the medical assistant to be calm, cool, and composed during these times. This will help others around you to remain calm.

SUMMARY OF SCENARIO

Marie has started to implement an inventory management process that is helping her identify when to reorder and how much to reorder. She initially started by hand-counting the inventory, and then she identified how much was used each buying cycle. It took a few months for her to identify trends. She found certain times of the year affected the quantity of products used. For instance, providers tend to use more casting products in the winter and summer months, which means Marie will need to increase her stock of those items during these times of the year. Marie knows that the more she learns, the more efficient she can become when managing inventory. She has already helped the facility save money by identifying cheaper vendors for commonly used expensive items. Marie loves her new job and the variety of responsibilities she has. She looks forward to continual learning.

SUMMARY OF LEARNING OBJECTIVES

1. **Explain tasks for the medical assistant to handle when opening and closing the healthcare facility.**
   Facility opening tasks for the clinical medical assistant include the following:
   - Prepare the exam rooms by turning on the lights, ensuring supplies are stocked, and making sure the rooms have been cleaned appropriately and are safe for patients.
   - Ensure prescription pads (if used) are stored outside the exam rooms, in a locked cabinet.
   - Unlock supply cabinets.
   - Ensure restrooms have adequate supplies.
   - Perform quality control tests on laboratory equipment and complete refrigerator and freezer temperature logs.
   - Follow up on outstanding patient issues from the prior day.
   - Handle new diagnostic test reports.
   Opening tasks for the administrative medical assistant include the following:
   - Check the voice mail or **answering service** messages.
   - Update the voice mail message. Switch the phone, so patients can reach the facility instead of the answering service.

- Turn on computers, copy machines, and other office equipment.
- Prepare the reception area for patients.
- Print schedules of the day's appointments.
- Compile any remaining required paperwork for the day's visits.

2. **List the steps involved with completing an inventory and perform an equipment inventory with documentation.**

The steps involved with completing an inventory include:

- Gather information on the supplies to be inventoried, including name, size, quantity, item number, supplier's name, cost, reorder point, and quantity to reorder.
- Create a supply inventory list.
- Inventory the supplies by counting the number of items.
- Document the count on the supply inventory list.
- Neatly replace the supplies, making sure the older supplies are in front of the new supplies.

Procedure 13.1 discusses the steps involved with performing an equipment inventory with documentation.

3. **Explain the purpose of routine maintenance of administrative and clinical equipment and perform routine maintenance of equipment.**

The medical assistant is responsible for monitoring equipment safety and proper functioning. Routine maintenance helps to ensure the best performance of the equipment. Potential issues should not be overlooked. Actions should be taken to prevent injury to staff or patients and costly damage to the equipment.

Procedure 13.2 discusses the steps involved when performing routine maintenance of equipment.

4. **Discuss warranties, service calls, and purchasing equipment.**

When equipment is purchased, a warranty is given for a period of time. The warranty is the manufacturer's guarantee. If the piece of equipment needs to be repaired or has a defective part, the manufacturer will pay for the cost of the repair.

For complex or expensive equipment, the healthcare facility may contract with a service provider for repairs and routine service checks. This assistance is necessary for some equipment. It also helps to extend the lifetime of those machines. For repairs on other equipment, it might be necessary to ship or bring the machine to the repair service.

The process of purchasing equipment can vary depending on the size of the organization. Large agencies have purchasing departments. The staff researches the need and identifies the best equipment to purchase. The medical assistant may be involved with the process in smaller practices.

5. **Discuss inventory management, inventory management control systems, and ordering supplies.**

Inventory management involves ordering, tracking inventory, and identifying the quantity of product to purchase. The goal of inventory management is to have adequate supplies on hand. It is important not to have too much stock that will expire or take a long time to use. The medical assistant in charge of ordering and managing supplies must keep a record on each item in inventory.

An inventory control system helps to make inventory management work well. Large medical facilities use computerized inventory control systems. These systems monitor usage and inventory in stock. They also identify items that need to be ordered. Smaller facilities may use simple computerized or manual systems.

To order supplies, the medical assistant can use the supplier's printed catalog or supplier's website store. Payment terms may vary among vendors. Orders can arrive via the mail, a national delivery service, or a local delivery service. Be sure to put away the items as soon as possible after they are received.

6. **Identify the principles of body mechanics and perform a supply inventory with documentation while using proper body mechanics.**

Principles of body mechanics include:

- To lift an object, maintain a wide, stable base with your feet. Your feet should be shoulder-width apart, and you should have good footing. Bend at the knees, keeping your back straight. Lift smoothly, using the major muscles in your arms and legs. Use the same technique when putting the item down.
- When lifting and carrying heavy items, keep the item directly in front of you to avoid rotating your spine.
- Keep your movements smooth.
- When reaching for an object, your feet should face the object.
- Avoid reaching and straining to get an object. Clear away barriers, and use a firm and level surface (e.g., a stepstool) to get close to the object.
- Get help if the item is too heavy to lift by yourself.

Procedure 13.3 discusses the steps involved when performing a supply inventory with documentation. This procedure also describes how to use proper body mechanics when performing inventory procedures.

7. **Evaluate the work environment to identify unsafe working conditions.**

Procedure 13.4 describes the steps involved in evaluating the work environment.

8. **Identify critical elements of an emergency response plan to use in the event of a natural disaster or other emergency and participate in a mock exposure event.**

Table 13.2 presents the critical elements that must be in an emergency response plan. These elements include:

- Methods to report a fire and other emergencies
- Evacuation policy and procedure
- Critical shutdown procedures
- Emergency escape/exit routes and procedures
- Rescue and medical duties
- Whom to contact for additional information

Procedure 13.5 describes a mock exposure scenario and the steps involved in responding to an exposure event.

9. **Demonstrate the proper use of a fire extinguisher.**

Procedure 13.6 describes the steps involved in using a fire extinguisher.

Continued

SUMMARY OF LEARNING OBJECTIVES—*continued*

10. **Recognize the physical and emotional effects on persons involved in an emergency situation.**

    The term *general adaptation syndrome* (GAS) is used to describe the long- and short-term effects of stress on the body. The stages include the following:

    - *Stage 1 — Alarm reaction*: This is the immediate reaction to the stressor. The body releases the hormones cortisol, adrenaline,

    and noradrenaline. This provides energy, preparing the body for physical activities.

    - *Stage 2 — Adaptation stage*: If the stressor continues, the individual's body adapts to the stressor.
    - *Stage 3 — Exhaustion stage*: At this point, the body's resistance has been diminished by the continued stress. The body is more susceptible to disease.

PROCEDURE 13.1   Perform an Equipment Inventory With Documentation

Tasks: Perform an equipment inventory. Document the inventory on the equipment inventory form.

EQUIPMENT and SUPPLIES

- Pens
- Administrative or clinical equipment
- Purchase information (e.g., date, cost, and supplier) and warranty information (e.g., start and end date, warranty coverage)
- Equipment inventory form

PROCEDURAL STEPS

1. For the equipment to be inventoried, gather the following information for each piece of equipment:
   - Name of equipment, manufacturer, and serial number
   - Location and facility number (if applicable)
   - Purchase date, cost, supplier, and warranty information

PURPOSE: It is important to have the essential information required when creating the spreadsheet.

2. Complete an equipment inventory form by adding the gathered information for each item inventoried (see Fig. 13.2).

   PURPOSE: Creating an equipment inventory list on the computer will help you organize the information. It will also help you maintain the information easily.

3. Review the document created. Make any necessary revisions.

   PURPOSE: It is important to proofread your work to ensure it is accurate.

PROCEDURE 13.2   Perform Routine Maintenance of Equipment

Tasks: Perform routine maintenance of administrative or clinical equipment. Document the maintenance on the log.

EQUIPMENT and SUPPLIES

- Maintenance log(s)
- Administrative or clinical equipment (e.g., oral thermometers)
- Supplies for routine maintenance (e.g., battery)
- Operation manual, if needed
- Pens
- Information regarding the equipment (i.e., name, serial number, location, facility number, manufacturer, purchase date, warranty information, frequency of inspections, and service provider)

PROCEDURAL STEPS

1. Gather information on the piece of equipment identified for routine maintenance, including name, serial number, location, facility number, manufacturer, purchase date, warranty information, frequency of inspections, and service provider.

PURPOSE: It is important to have the essential information required when completing the log.

2. Fill in the equipment details on the log (see Fig. 13.3).

   PURPOSE: Adding the equipment details helps identify the machine. It provides a quick reference to useful information that the service provider might request. The form serves as a log for documenting the maintenance activities performed.

3. To perform the maintenance activities, gather the required supplies. If you are not familiar with the procedure or the required supplies, refer to the operation manual.

   PURPOSE: You need to be familiar with the supplies and the procedure before you start the maintenance.

4. Perform the maintenance activities as directed in the operation manual. Take any required safety precautions necessary to protect yourself and others.

PROCEDURE 13.2 | Perform Routine Maintenance of Equipment—*continued*

PURPOSE: Following the outlined procedure in the operation manual will help you successfully complete the maintenance without injuring yourself and others or damaging the machine.

5. Clean up the work area.
   PURPOSE: It is important to clean up after yourself.

6. Using a pen, document the date, time, and the maintenance activity performed, and include your signature on the log.
   PURPOSE: The log, indicating the activities performed, will serve as a communication tool for future reference and services needed on that piece of equipment.

PROCEDURE 13.3 | Perform a Supply Inventory With Documentation While Using Proper Body Mechanics

Tasks: Perform a supply inventory using correct body mechanics. Document the inventory on the supply inventory form.

EQUIPMENT and SUPPLIES

- Pens
- Administrative or clinical supplies to be inventoried
- Purchase information (e.g., item number, cost, and supplier) for supplies in inventory
- Reorder point and quantity to reorder for each item in inventory
- Supply inventory form

PROCEDURAL STEPS

1. For the supplies in inventory, gather the following information for each item:
   - Name, size, quantity (e.g., purchased individually, 100 per box)
   - Item number, supplier's name, cost
   - Reorder point and quantity to reorder
   PURPOSE: This information is required as you create the inventory form.

2. For each supply item, enter information on the inventory form. Make sure the appropriate entry is in the right location (see Fig. 13.4).
   Note: The "Stock Available" column will be empty for now.
   PURPOSE: Creating a supply inventory list will help you organize the information and maintain the information easily.

3. Review the document. Make any necessary revisions.
   PURPOSE: Make sure the document is correct, so errors do not impact the inventory process.

4. Using the supply inventory list, inventory the supplies in the department. Identify how the supply should be counted (e.g., individually, by the box), and count the number of items in stock.
   PURPOSE: Identifying the correct quantity by which the item is inventoried enables you to increase the accuracy of the inventory. Counting an item

by "each" when it comes as a package can cause confusion when you try to identify what needs to be ordered.

5. Add the number in the appropriate row under the "Stock Available" header.
   PURPOSE: Making sure you add the number to the right column and row will keep your inventory form accurate.

6. Compare the reorder point number to the stock available number. If the stock available number is at or below the reorder point, indicate that the item needs to be reordered by checking the appropriate column.
   PURPOSE: Identify the supplies that need to be ordered.

7. Make sure the supplies are neatly arranged. The older stock should be in front of the newer stock.
   PURPOSE: It is important to clean up your workspace. The oldest stock must be moved to the front to ensure it is used first.

8. Repeat steps 5 through 7 until all supplies have been inventoried.

9. Use proper body mechanics when lifting and moving supplies by maintaining a wide, stable base with your feet. Your feet should be shoulder-width apart, and you should have good footing. Bend at the knees, keeping your back straight. Lift smoothly with the major muscles in your arms and legs. Use the same technique when putting the item down.
   PURPOSE: Correct body mechanics will reduce your risk for injury when carrying or lifting heavy objects. See Figs. 13.9 and 13.10 for proper body mechanics when lifting boxes.

10. Use proper body mechanics when reaching for an object. Clear away barriers and use a stepstool if needed. Your feet should face the object. Avoid twisting or turning with a heavy load.
    PURPOSE: Straining when reaching or standing on tiptoes can increase your risk for injury.

PROCEDURE 13.4 | Evaluate the Work Environment

Tasks: Evaluate the work environment and identify unsafe working conditions.

EQUIPMENT and SUPPLIES

- Work environment evaluation form
- Pen

PROCEDURAL STEPS

1. Observe the environment for slipping, tripping, or fall risks. Document your findings to the following questions:

Continued

PROCEDURE 13.4   Evaluate the Work Environment—*continued*

- Is the lighting appropriate? Are any lights burned out? Are any areas dim?
- Is the flooring or carpeting ripped or pulled up? If rugs/mats are present, are they folded?
- Is water on the floor? Is signage present warning of the water?
- Are items cluttering the hallway, making walking difficult?
- Are cords, cables, and other items in the walkway?
- Is trash on the floor?
- Are heavy items on high shelves? Is a sturdy stepstool available?

PURPOSE: When the floor is cluttered or the flooring is damaged, the risk of falls increases.

2. Observe the environment for safety and security issues. Document your findings to the following questions:
   - Are rooms available that can be locked and used during workplace violence? Is there limited visibility from the hallway into the room?
   - Are there areas in the building with limited visibility?
   - If the building is accessible to the public, are there any safe zones or areas for staff?
   - Are the emergency call lights in the exam rooms and bathrooms functioning?
   - Are the oxygen tanks (if available) checked per the facility's policy?

PURPOSE: Having a safe area in a building is important during a workplace violence situation.

3. Observe the environment for fire risks and electrical issues. Document your findings to the following questions:
   - Are electrical cords and plugs free from cracks, fraying, or other damage?
   - Are power strips overloaded?
   - Is electricity being used near a water source?
   - Are flammable chemicals and supplies stored according to manufacturers' guidelines?

- Are combustibles (e.g., paper, cardboard, cloth, flammable chemicals) away from heat sources?

PURPOSE: The risk of fires increases when cords are damaged or power strips are overloaded. Safe storage of chemicals is important to reduce the fire risk.

4. Observe the environment for fire containment and evacuation strategies. Document your findings to the following questions:
   - Are building diagrams posted on walls? Are exit routes indicated? Are two or more exit routes indicated on the map? Are fire alarms and fire extinguishers indicated?
   - Are exit routes uncluttered?
   - Are exit signs visible and lit?
   - Are fire doors unlocked and able to be closed in an emergency?
   - Are interior rooms available for severe storms?
   - Are smoke detectors located throughout the building? Are fire alarms available?
   - Are fire extinguishers available and checked routinely (per the facility's policy)?
   - Are flammable products (e.g., oxygen tanks, chemicals) stored along the exit routes?

PURPOSE: Two or more exit routes should be available. Flammable products should not be stored in the location of the exit routes. Closed fire doors will help contain the fire.

5. Based on your observations, summarize your findings. If risks are present, create a list of issues that need to be addressed. Describe what needs to be done for each risk.

PURPOSE: Creating a list of issues that need to be addressed is important in a professional setting.

PROCEDURE 13.5   Participate in a Mock Exposure Event

Tasks: Demonstrate self-awareness in an emergency situation. Participate in a mock exposure event and document specific steps taken. Recognize the physical and emotional effects on individuals involved in an emergency situation.

Scenario: You and Beth are in the autoclave room, and two chemicals spill, creating toxic fumes. Beth is having trouble breathing. The following staff, patients, and visitors are present in the clinic:

Rooms	Staff and Reception Areas
1 – Teen and his mother	Reception Area A – Four people waiting
2 – Older woman in a wheelchair	Reception Area B – Five people waiting
3 – Mother with three little children	**Staff**
4 – Adult female	Tim – In MA station 3
5 – Empty	Rose – At the insurance desk
6 – An older couple	Dave and Patty – At the receptionist desk
7 – Adult male	Julie Walden, MD – In provider office 1
8 – Empty	Angela Perez, MD – In room 3
Procedure room – Empty	Jean Burke, NP – In room 7

PROCEDURE 13.5   Participate in a Mock Exposure Event—*continued*

EQUIPMENT and SUPPLIES

- Paper
- Pen
- Floor map (see Fig. 13.11)
- Computer with internet access

PROCEDURAL STEPS

1. Using the scenario, describe how you would handle the emergency exposure situation with Beth.
   - Identify four steps a medical assistant could take to demonstrate self-awareness while responding to this emergency situation.
   - Describe exposure control mechanisms or how you might limit the exposure to other people once you remove Beth from the room.

   PURPOSE: It is important to be self-aware of how you would respond in emergency situations. Exposure control mechanisms are ways to limit the exposure to other people. How might you contain the situation? How might you prevent others from being impacted by the exposure?

2. Scenario continues: Dr. Walden alerted the staff to evacuate the building. The outdoor safe meeting location is at the back of the parking lot. Document the steps to handle the exposure event and evacuation from the building:
   - Describe what each staff member and provider should do to help with the evacuation procedure and notify 911.
   - Describe the steps (evacuations) in the order that they should occur.
   - Describe how the staff may ensure all individuals are out of the building.

   PURPOSE: It is important to know which individuals need to be evacuated first, second, etc. Employees should work with individuals in their area unless they have an appointed duty. Making sure all individuals are out of the building is important before the staff leaves the area.

3. Dr. Walden is in charge during the emergency. Describe what her responsibilities include.

   PURPOSE: The evacuation warden's name is listed in the emergency response plan. This person is in charge of the evacuation.

4. Dave took the patient registry. Describe why the patient registry is important.

   PURPOSE: The patient registry lists the patients that have checked in for appointments. It is important to take this document during evacuations.

5. Scenario continues: Two weeks after the event, Beth confides to you that she is not doing well. She recovered from the exposure, but since the event she has had difficulty sleeping. She is anxious when she goes into the autoclave room. She is having trouble concentrating on her job. She mentioned she has had two nightmares of emergencies occurring in the department in which she gets injured.
   - Describe what might be occurring with Beth and the symptoms that relate to it.
   - Discuss what you might encourage her to do about the situation.

   PURPOSE: It is not uncommon after an emergency that individuals involved experience issues related to the emergency.

6. Research the physical and emotional effects of stress on the body. Identify four physical effects and four emotional effects of stress on persons involved in an emergency situation. Cite your resources.

7. Describe how the physical and emotional effects of stress would be different for Beth, you, the providers, and the other employees present.

8. Describe how a medical assistant could limit the physical and emotional effects of stress on each person/group: Beth, the providers, the other employees present in the facility, and yourself.

PROCEDURE 13.6   Use a Fire Extinguisher

Tasks: Select the correct fire extinguisher and demonstrate its use.

Scenarios:
a. You are working in the medical laboratory, and an electrical fire starts.
b. You are working in the clinic, and a fire starts in a wastebasket.
c. You are working in the medical laboratory, and a chemical fire starts (combustible metal fire).

EQUIPMENT and SUPPLIES

- Fire extinguisher

PROCEDURAL STEPS

1. Using the scenarios, identify the type of fire extinguisher required to put out each fire.

   PURPOSE: The correct fire extinguisher must be used to put out the fire. Using the wrong extinguisher can make the fire worse.

2. Hold the extinguisher by the handle with the hose or nozzle pointing away from you. Pull out the pin that is located below the trigger.

   PURPOSE: Pulling the pin allows the extinguisher to be used.

3. Stand about 10 feet from the fire. Aim the extinguisher hose or nozzle at the base of the fire. Keep the extinguisher in an upright position as you work.

   PURPOSE: The most efficient method of putting out fires is to work at the base of the fire.

4. Squeeze the trigger slowly and evenly.

   PURPOSE: Squeezing slowly allows the discharge to come out in a steady flow.

5. Sweep from side to side until the fire is out.

   PURPOSE: As the fire nearest to you is put out, you can move closer to the rest of the fire.

14

PRINCIPLES OF PHARMACOLOGY

SCENARIO

Gabe Garcia, CMA (AAMA), has worked for Walden-Martin Family Medical (WMFM) Clinic for 3 years. He was hired right after he completed his medical assistant program. Gabe was asked to be Mark Allen's mentor for practicum. Mark has just completed all of his medical assistant courses at the local college and now needs 160 hours of practicum. He is excited to be working with Gabe.

Gabe works with several of the WMFM Clinic providers. He spends 1 to 2 hours a day working with prescription refills. Gabe also rooms patients, obtains their vital signs and history, and assist with injections. Mark will have a lot of great experiences with Gabe.

While studying this chapter, think about the following questions:
1. What are the sources and uses of drugs?
2. What is pharmacokinetics?
3. How does drug legislation affect the medical assistant practice?
4. What are the four names of a drug?
5. What information is contained in the different sections of the drug reference information?
6. How does a medical assistant prepare prescriptions for the provider to sign?

LEARNING OBJECTIVES

1. Describe the sources and uses of drugs.
2. Describe pharmacokinetics, including absorption, distribution, metabolism, and excretion.
3. Discuss drug action, including the factors that influence drug action, the therapeutic effects of drugs, and adverse reactions to drugs.
4. Explain drug legislation that is important in the ambulatory care setting. Also, discuss dietary supplements.
5. Describe the four types of drug names.
6. Describe various methods to access drug reference information.
7. Identify the classifications of medications, including the indications for use, desired effects, side effects, and adverse reactions.
8. Discuss the terminology used in drug reference information, including describing the differences among biologic half-life, onset, peak, and duration.
9. Discuss types of medication orders.
10. List the four parts of a prescription and the information required for all prescriptions; prepare prescriptions using prescription refill procedures; and define commonly approved abbreviations.
11. Describe common requirements for scheduled substances.
12. Discuss over-the-counter (OTC) medications and herbal supplements.

VOCABULARY

addiction A disease that occurs when a person cannot stop or limit the use of a drug, even after negative consequences have been experienced.

analgesic (an ahl JEE zik) A drug that reduces or eliminates pain.

antiarrhythmic (an tee ah RITH mik) A drug that prevents or alleviates heart arrhythmias.

antibiotic (an ti bie OT ik) A drug that destroys or inhibits the growth of bacteria.

anticoagulant (an tee koe AG yuh lant) A substance (i.e., medication or chemical) that prevents the clotting of blood.

anticonvulsant (an tee kahn VUL sahnt) A drug used to prevent or treat seizures.

antihistamine (an tee HIS tah meen) A drug that counteracts the effects of histamine.

anti-inflammatory (an tee in FLAM ah tor ee) A medication that prevents or reduces inflammation.

antimalarial (an tee mah LAR ee ahl) A drug used to treat or prevent malaria.

antiseptic (an ti SEP tik) A substance that inhibits the growth of microorganisms on living tissue (e.g., alcohol and povidone-iodine solution [Betadine]).

form Physical characteristics of a medication (e.g., tablet and suspension).

metabolites (muh TAB uh lites) Byproducts of drug metabolism

National Provider Identifier (NPI) An identifier assigned by the Centers for Medicare and Medicaid Services (CMS) that classifies the healthcare provider by license and medical specialties.

psychiatrists Medical doctors who have been specially trained to diagnose and treat patients with mental, emotional, and behavioral conditions.

reconciling Comparing a document with another document to ensure that they are consistent.

side effects Unpleasant effects of a drug in addition to the desired or therapeutic effect.

therapeutic range Is reached when the blood concentration of a medication is high enough for the therapeutic effect to occur.

toxicity Harmful and deadly effects of a medication that can develop due to the buildup of medication or byproducts in the body.

Pharmacology is the study of the properties, actions, and uses of drugs. A *drug* is a chemical substance used to cure, treat, prevent, or diagnose disease. In the ambulatory care setting, medical assistants deal with medication, from history taking to administering medications. Medical assistants must have a general understanding of the classification of drugs. They need to know how to pronounce the medication names. They must know how to give medications, typical **side effects**, and the dose to give. New medications are continually being developed and released for patient treatment. Thus, medical assistants must stay updated on medications.

PHARMACOLOGY BASICS

Medications have been around for a long time. The first medications came from natural products found in our ancestors' living environment. Today, with advancing technology, most medications are created in a laboratory setting. These sources and others will be explained along with the uses of medications.

In addition, a basic description of how medication enters, moves through, and exits the body will be given. This knowledge will help the medical assistant identify patients who may be at risk for medication issues because of their age or a disease process.

Sources of Drugs

Drugs are either created from natural sources or made synthetically in a laboratory. Plants, animals, minerals, and microbiologic sources are natural sources of drugs.

Natural Sources of Drugs

Plants are the oldest source of drugs. Our ancestors found that different plants helped with different symptoms. Leaves, bark, stems, roots, and fruits have been used in medicinal preparations through the years. Some examples of medicinal plant sources include:

- Digitalis, an **antiarrhythmic** medication, comes from the purple foxglove flower.
- Nicotine comes from tobacco leaves.
- Quinidine, an **antimalarial** medication, comes from the bark of the cinchona tree.

Animals are also a source of medications. Natural substances are extracted from animal tissues and organs. Heparin, an **anticoagulant**, comes from pig intestines. Lanolin is found in topical preparations used to protect the skin. It comes from the sebaceous glands of sheep.

Other medications are developed with lactose and gelatin, which are from animals.

Minerals and microbiologic substances are other natural sources of medications. Examples of minerals include:

- Iron is used to treat iron-deficiency anemia.
- Iodine is an **antiseptic**.
- Zinc is used as a supplement and is found in topical pastes for wounds.

One microbiologic source is *Penicillium chrysogenum*. This is a fungus that creates penicillin.

Synthetic Sources of Drugs

Many medications originated in nature but have been recreated in the laboratory setting. For instance, insulin initially came from cattle and pigs. Many people developed allergies to the insulin. Now synthetic insulin is widely used. Biotechnology and genetic engineering techniques are continually being used to create new medications. With the help of technologic advances, individualized medications are also being produced. (Individualized medications will be discussed later in the chapter.) Synthetic medications are cheaper to produce because they are created in mass volumes. The quality of synthetic medications can also be controlled.

Uses of Drugs

When studying medications, it is important to identify the uses of drugs. Why are they being prescribed? What do they do in the body? Some medications may have more than one use. There are eight common uses of drugs:

- *Prevention*: Drugs used to prevent diseases. Example: vaccines are given, and the body creates antibodies to protect against specific diseases.
- *Treatment*: Drugs that relieve the symptoms while the body fights off the disease. Example: acetaminophen brings down a fever (*antipyretic*), while the body fights off a viral infection.
- *Diagnosis*: Drugs used to diagnose or monitor a condition. Example: contrast medium (radiopaque dye) is given to highlight organs on x-rays.
- *Cure*: Drugs that eliminate the disease. Example: amoxicillin, an **antibiotic**, is used to cure strep throat.
- *Contraceptive*: Drugs used to prevent pregnancy. Example: Depo-Provera is a contraceptive injectable medication.

- *Health maintenance*: Medications used to maintain or enhance health. Examples: vitamins and minerals.
- *Palliative*: Drugs that do not cure or treat the disease but improve the quality of life. Example: Morphine, an **analgesic**, is commonly used by patients with cancer.
- *Replacement*: Drugs used to increase the blood levels of naturally occurring substances in the body. Example: levothyroxine is used for patients with hypothyroidism.

CRITICAL THINKING APPLICATION   14.1

Gabe and Mark are discussing the basics of pharmacology and the eight common uses of medications. Gabe asks Mark which use would include taking an **antihistamine** for allergy symptoms. How would you answer this question?

Pharmacokinetics

Pharmacokinetics is the study of drug absorption, distribution, metabolism, and excretion in the body. Through pharmacokinetics, we understand when a medication starts to work in the body. We know how it moves through the body and what organs metabolize and excrete the drug from the body. Some of the patients you will be working with will have greater risks of side effects and **toxicity**. Understanding the basics of pharmacokinetics will help you identify those at greater risk for problems.

Absorption

Drugs can be administered in many ways. *Route* is the means by which a drug enters the body. Where a drug enters the body is considered the *site of administration*. *Absorption* is the movement of drug from the site of administration to the bloodstream. The following are commonly used routes:

- *Oral* (po): Medications taken by mouth.
- *Sublingual* (SL): Placed under the tongue to dissolve; absorbs quickly into the bloodstream.
- *Buccal*: Placed between the cheek and the gums dissolve and absorb quickly.
- *Intramuscular* (IM): Injected into the muscle. The greater the number of blood vessels in the muscle, the quicker the absorption.
- *Subcutaneous* (subcut): Injected just below the skin; moves into the capillaries or the lymphatic vessels and is brought to the bloodstream. This process is slower than the absorption of intramuscular drugs.
- *Intravenous* (IV): Injected directly in the bloodstream and has the fastest absorption rate.

The rate of absorption is influenced by the following factors:

- *Route*: Oral medications need to pass through the gastrointestinal (GI) tract. This takes time. IV medications are directly administered into the bloodstream and have virtually no absorption time. They start working faster than drugs given by other routes.
- *Blood flow to the absorption area*: Medication given by the sublingual and buccal routes is absorbed quickly into the bloodstream. These sites are rich with blood vessels. IM medications absorb quicker than subcut medications. The muscle tissue has more blood vessels than the subcutaneous tissue.
- *Ability of the medication to be absorbed*: Liquid medications are easier to absorb than solid medications. Solid medications need to be broken down before they absorb. Acidic medications are absorbed in the stomach. Base (or alkaline) medications are absorbed in the intestines.
- *Conditions at the site of the absorption*: Some medications must be taken with food, which can slow the absorption of the medication. Typically, medications taken on an empty stomach can be absorbed faster. The intestines provide more surface area than the stomach for the absorption of medications.

Distribution

Once the drug is absorbed into the blood, it rapidly circulates through the body (unless it has to go through the liver). During this time, the drug is brought to the body tissues. The movement of absorbed drug from the blood to the body tissues is called *distribution*. The speed of the drug's movement from the blood to the tissues varies greatly. Some drugs bind with proteins in the blood and move slowly into tissues. Some drugs accumulate in certain tissues. These tissues act as *reservoirs*, slowly releasing the drug into the bloodstream and keeping the blood levels from decreasing too rapidly. This process prolongs the effect of the drug. Circulation issues (e.g., peripheral artery disease) can also slow the distribution of medication.

For the medication to move into certain organs, it must be able to pass through the tissues. The blood-brain barrier allows only certain fat-soluble medications to pass into the cerebrospinal fluid and the brain. In comparison, the placental membrane allows most drugs to pass through from the mother to the baby in utero. This is why only certain medications are prescribed during pregnancy.

Routes Impact the Dose

Oral medications are absorbed in the stomach or in the intestines. The blood containing the absorbed digestive nutrients and drugs passes through the hepatic portal vein and the liver before it circulates to the rest of the body. In the liver, some of the drugs are chemically altered. Some of the active drug is lost during this first pass through the liver. This reduces the amount of drug in the circulating blood that can be used.

For instance, a person is having an allergic reaction and needs Benadryl. If the drug is to be taken orally, the person takes 50 mg. If it is to be given intravenously, 10 mg may be given. This is because all 10 mg gets into the bloodstream, whereas some of the 50 mg is lost as it passes through the liver before circulating through the body. It is important for a medical assistant to realize that doses (e.g., 10 mg) may vary based on the route used to give the medication.

Metabolism

Metabolism is a series of chemical processes whereby enzymes change drugs in the body. Metabolism is necessary so that medications can be cleared from the body. Active forms of drugs may be converted into water-soluble compounds, which are eventually excreted. Prodrugs can be changed into active forms of drugs.

Prodrugs

Prodrugs are medications that are administered in an inactive form. Through the normal metabolic processes, the medication is changed into an active form of a drug. The liver and the intestines are sites that can convert prodrugs to active forms of drugs. For instance, sulfasalazine (Azulfidine) is an **anti-inflammatory** drug that is used to treat ulcerative colitis. It is also a prodrug, since it is ingested in an inactive form. Bacteria in the colon change the drug into an active drug that is used by the body.

Most drug metabolism occurs in the liver. Younger children, older adults, and those with liver disease may have issues metabolizing medications. These populations could be at risk for drug toxicity. To prevent toxicity, the dose of medication is adjusted for at-risk populations.

Excretion

Excretion is the movement of **metabolites** out of the body. Most drugs are excreted through the large intestine and kidneys. The large intestine excretes the undigested drug products in the stool. The kidneys excrete metabolites in the urine. CLIA-waived urine drug screening test can detect certain metabolites.

Drugs can also be excreted in breast milk. This is critical information to have when a mother is breastfeeding her baby. As with pregnancy, only a limited number of drugs are safe with breastfeeding. Most drug references indicate if medications pass into the breast milk. Other ways drugs can be excreted are through sweat, exhaled air, and saliva.

Young children, older adults, and those with kidney disease are at risk for the buildup of metabolic drug byproducts in the body. These populations are at greater risk for symptoms of toxicity.

Drug Action

Drugs are chemicals that can cause changes in the cells. There are four main drug actions:

- *Depressing*: Slows down the cell's activity. For example, narcotic medications reduce the activity in the brain's respiratory center. This action slows the respiration rate.
- *Stimulating*: Increases the cell's activity. For instance, caffeine increases brain activity.
- *Destroying*: Kills cells or disrupts parts of cells. For example, chemotherapy medications destroy cancer cells.
- *Replacing substances*: Substances required by the body can be given as medications. For instance, patients with type 1 diabetes mellitus take insulin.

Factors Influencing Drug Action

One might think that a drug works the same for everyone. This is not so. Personal characteristics can cause minor differences in how a drug works from one person to another. Many factors influence drug action:

- *Age*: Infants and older adults have problems metabolizing and excreting medications. Their liver and kidneys are less effective. This can lead to possible drug accumulation and toxicity.
- *Body size*: A person's size affects the amount of drug needed. Children's dosages are calculated based on body weight. Thinner people require less medication than heavier people.
- *Gender*: Women have a higher proportion of body fat. Hormonal differences can affect metabolism. Women can react differently to some medications compared to men.
- *Genetics*: Genetic makeup can affect how a person responds to drugs. (This is discussed in more depth in the Pharmacogenomics section.)
- *Diseases:* Poor circulation, liver disease, and kidney disease can alter drug action.
- *Diet*: Certain foods can affect a drug's action. For instance, milk products can diminish the effects of tetracycline, an antibiotic.
- *Drug dosage, route, and timing of administration*: The greater the amount of drug taken, the greater the effect will be. The route will also affect drug action. Drugs absorb, distribute, and metabolize differently based on the administration route. Some drugs work better when taken with food, whereas others do not.
- *Mental state*: People with positive attitudes tend to do better than those with negative attitudes.
- *Environmental temperature*: In hot weather, heat relaxes blood vessels. This can speed up the distribution of medication, thus speeding up the drug's action.

Pharmacogenomics. Most medications are dosed as "one size fits all." Each person's genetic makeup affects how that person responds to medications. *Pharmacogenomics* or *pharmacogenetics* is the study of how genetic factors influence a person's metabolic response to a specific medication. Pharmacogenomics testing usually requires a small blood or saliva sample. The sample is analyzed to determine if a specific medication will be an effective treatment for a particular individual. Testing can determine the best dose of medication and if the person could have serious *adverse reactions* (unexpected or life-threatening reaction) from the medication. A different test is required for each medication. Pharmacogenomics is largely used in cancer treatments, but it is becoming more common in other areas of medicine.

Therapeutic Effects

Medications can have local or systemic effects. Medication effects that are seen at the site of administration are *local effects*. Medication effects that are seen throughout the body are *systemic effects*. Each medication has one or more *therapeutic effect* or desired effect. This is the intended action of the medication. For instance, the therapeutic effect of a pain reliever is to reduce pain.

Sometimes multiple doses are needed to achieve the therapeutic effect. Other times just one dose of medication can achieve the therapeutic effect. For some medications, the provider may prescribe a higher initial dose, called a *loading dose*. This helps to quickly increase the medication level in the blood. A loading dose helps the person achieve the **therapeutic range** sooner. A *maintenance dose* is the amount of medication needed to keep the blood levels within the therapeutic range. If the blood levels go beyond the therapeutic range, the person can experience signs and symptoms of toxicity. This is considered a *toxic dose* of medication. A *lethal dose* is the amount of medication that could kill a person.

TABLE 14.1   Common Adverse Reactions

ADVERSE REACTIONS	DESCRIPTION
Allergy	Drug allergy occurs when a person develops antibodies against a specific drug. When the drug is taken, the antibodies attack the antigens from the drug. Tissues are damaged during this process, and histamines are released. Histamines cause the allergic reactions.
Anaphylaxis	Extreme hypersensitivity to a specific drug (antigen) can cause life-threatening symptoms, including swelling of the mouth and airway, difficulty breathing, wheezing, loss of consciousness, and death.
Idiosyncrasy	A peculiar response to a certain drug. For instance, Benadryl causes drowsiness. When it is given to children, they often get extremely agitated.
Cumulative effect	For medications taken routinely, often the prior dose is not completely metabolized and excreted before the next dose is given. This can lead to a buildup of medication or byproducts that can produce toxic effects.
Toxicity	The harmful and possibly deadly effects of the medication that can develop due to the buildup of medication or byproducts in the body. People with liver or kidney disease, young children, older adults, and those who overdose are at risk for toxicity.
Drug interactions	When two or more drugs are taken, sometimes a drug-drug interaction can occur. The interactions can be helpful or harmful. Three types of drug interactions can occur: • *Antagonism*: One drug reduces or blocks the effect of another drug. Example: Naloxone is given for narcotic overdosage. • *Synergism*: The combined effect of two drugs used together is greater than the sum of each drug's effect (e.g., 1 + 1 > 2). Example of a harmful interaction: Alcohol has a synergistic effect on antidepressants. • *Potentiation*: A type of synergism; one drug increases the effect of the second drug. With L-dopa and carbidopa, one drug has no effect but increases the effect of the other drug (e.g., 0 + 1 > 1).
Tolerance	The need for a larger dose to get the same therapeutic or desired effect. Tolerance can be seen when taking narcotic pain medications and **anticonvulsants**.
Drug dependence	Strong psychological or physical need to take a certain drug. Withdrawal symptoms can be experienced when a person stops using a drug. Drug dependence can occur with or without **addiction**.

CRITICAL THINKING APPLICATION   14.2

Gabe and Mark are discussing therapeutic effect and loading dose. Gabe shares that patients sometimes get confused on how much medication to take when they are given two amounts, a loading dose and the regular amount. How might a healthcare professional instruct a patient who needs to take a loading dose?

Adverse Reactions

Most of the time when a medication is correctly administered, the therapeutic effect occurs. However, sometimes issues arise, and the person has problems with the medication. The person can experience an unexpected or life-threatening reaction, which is called an *adverse reaction*. Table 14.1 lists common adverse reactions.

Many experts and drug reference information will include side effects with adverse reactions. They may divide these into mild, moderate, and severe reactions. The side effects usually fall into the mild category. Severe adverse reactions are those that can cause disability, hospitalization, death, or birth defects.

Other reference information separates adverse reactions/events and side effects. Adverse reactions or events would be those that are life-threatening and may cause disability or birth defects. Side effects would be unpleasant effects of the drug, in addition to the desired

or therapeutic effect. They can be harmless or may cause injury. The most common side effects include symptoms of gastrointestinal (GI) distress, such as nausea, vomiting, constipation, and diarrhea.

DRUG LEGISLATION AND THE AMBULATORY CARE SETTING

In the ambulatory care environment, medications can be prescribed, administered, and dispensed.

- *Prescribe* means to order a medication as a treatment for a condition. Doctors (MDs [including **psychiatrists**], DOs, and dentists) and advanced practice professionals, including physician assistants (PAs), nurse practitioners (NPs), and certified nurse midwives (CNMs), can prescribe medications. State prescribing laws can vary for advanced practice professionals.
- *Administer* means to give a prescribed dose of medication to a patient. Medical assistants, nurses, and providers can administer medications. State laws related to medication administration by medical assistants can vary.
- *Dispense* means to give a supply of medication that the patient will take at a later time. In most scenarios, pharmacists dispense medications.

Federal and state legislation governs these three activities. The following sections will discuss these laws, the agencies responsible for overseeing the laws, and the laws' effect on medical assistants.

> **CRITICAL THINKING APPLICATION**   **14.3**
>
> At WMFM Clinic, pharmaceutical representatives drop off sample medications that are given to patients. Usually, the provider will give a few days' worth of samples to a patient to ensure the patient is tolerating the medication. If the patient has no issues, then he or she gets the prescription filled. Mark sees the provider bag up a few samples and attach directions to the bag. The provider gives the bag to Gabe and asks him to give it to the patient. Mark asks Gabe, "Who is dispensing the medication?" How would you answer this question?

Food, Drug, and Cosmetic Act

The Food, Drug, and Cosmetic Act of 1938 is enforced by the Food and Drug Administration (FDA). The FDA is a federal agency in the Department of Health and Human Services (HHS). The FDA is responsible for the safety, effectiveness, security, and quality of drugs, cosmetics, and food. Some of the areas overseen by the FDA include:

- *Foods*: Dietary supplements, bottled water, food additives, infant formula, and other food products
- *Drugs*: Prescription drugs (brand name and generic) and nonprescription (over-the-counter) drugs
- *Biologics*: Vaccines, blood, and blood products
- *Medical devices*: Medical equipment (from simple [tongue depressor] to complex [heart pacemaker]), dental devices, and surgical implants

> ## Dietary Supplements
>
> Dietary supplements are oral products that contain a "dietary ingredient." This ingredient can include a vitamin, mineral, amino acid, herb, or another substance that can supplement a person's diet. Dietary supplements come in many forms, including tablets, powders, energy bars, and liquids. Federal law does not require a dietary supplement to be proven safe, nor must any claims for it be proven truthful before the product appears on the market. The Food and Drug Administration (FDA) monitors the safety of such products after they are on the market.
>
> The function of dietary supplements is to provide nutrients that are not obtained in the foods we eat and drink. Some examples of uses of dietary supplements include:
>
> - Calcium and vitamin D for bone health and low vitamin D levels
> - Folic acid in pregnancy to prevent spina bifida
> - Iron for low iron levels
> - Fiber for constipation
>
> Before starting a dietary supplement, it is important to talk with the provider. Some medications may interact with dietary supplements. Some dietary supplements may work against medications. For instance, taking vitamin K promotes blood clotting, and Coumadin (warfarin) delays blood clotting.

Manufacturers must submit applications for new products to the FDA. Manufacturers must provide adequate data to show the safety and effectiveness of the product. The FDA must determine if drugs, devices, and products are safe and effective. Once this is determined, then the product is released to the general public.

The FDA monitors the safety of products released to the market. The FDA Adverse Event Reporting System (FAERS) is a computerized database that helps the FDA monitor drugs. It contains reports of adverse events reported to the FDA. MedWatch is the FDA's reporting program. It provides information on products overseen by the FDA. MedWatch is available to healthcare professionals (*www.fda.gov/safety/medwatch/*).

If the FDA determines a medication is unsafe, it will recall the medication. The medical assistant should remove any recalled medications from the stock and sample cabinets. (*Sample medications* come from pharmaceutical companies and are used for patients.) Concerned patients may contact their providers. The provider will determine what action to take for each patient.

Controlled Substances Act

The Controlled Substances Act (CSA), Title II of the Comprehensive Drug Abuse Prevention and Control Act of 1970, is a federal law. The Drug Enforcement Agency (DEA) is a federal law enforcement agency under the US Department of Justice. The DEA enforces the CSA. The DEA oversees the manufacturing, importation, possession, use, and distribution of illegal and legal controlled substances.

Under the CSA, controlled substances are divided into five schedules. These schedules are arranged from the greatest to the least abuse potential (Table 14.2). State statutes also address procedures related to scheduled medications. It is important for the medical assistant to know the schedule of commonly ordered medications. Some controlled substance prescriptions are handled differently. This will be discussed later in the chapter.

Compliance With the Controlled Substance Act

Providers prescribing controlled substances need a DEA registration number. Each provider has a unique number. The DEA number is good for 3 years. The medical assistant may need to assist the provider in renewing or obtaining a DEA number. This can be done at the DEA website at *www.deadiversion.usdoj.gov*. Additional state requirements may need to be met before a provider can prescribe controlled substances.

Controlled substances have a paper trail. This record starts with the manufacturer and ends when the medication is dispensed or administered. In some healthcare facilities, the in-house pharmacy handles the controlled substances that are administered. The provider gives the medical assistant a prescription for a patient. The medical assistant gives the pharmacist the prescription and, in return, gets the medication. (Please note that some state laws do not allow medical assistants to administer controlled substances.) With this scenario, the pharmacist is responsible for managing the paperwork for the controlled substances.

In healthcare facilities without pharmacies, providers must take the responsibility of ordering controlled substances from the manufacturer. The medical assistant must help the provider comply with the Controlled Substance Act. The following sections will discuss common compliance activities.

TABLE 14.2   Schedule of Controlled Substances

SCHEDULE	PSYCHOLOGICAL AND PHYSICAL DEPENDENCE	EXAMPLES
I	Highest potential for abuse; drugs with no currently accepted medical purpose.	Heroin, lysergic acid diethylamide (LSD), ecstasy
II/IIN (C–II)	High level of abuse; can lead to severe psychological or physical dependence	Schedule II narcotics: oxycodone (OxyContin, Percocet), fentanyl (Duragesic), codeine, morphine Schedule IIN stimulants: amphetamine (Adderall), methamphetamine (Desoxyn), methylphenidate (Concerta, Ritalin LA)
III/III N (C–III)	Moderate to low physical dependence or high psychological dependence	Schedule III narcotics: acetaminophen with codeine (Tylenol #2 or #3), buprenorphine (Suboxone) Schedule IIIN non-narcotics: ketamine, anabolic steroids (e.g., Depo-Testosterone)
IV (C–IV)	Low potential for abuse relative to substances in Schedule III	Schedule IV substances: alprazolam (Xanax), clonazepam (Klonopin), diazepam (Valium), lorazepam (Ativan)
V (C–V)	Lowest potential for abuse relative to substances listed in Schedule IV; contains limited quantities of certain narcotics	Schedule V substances: Robitussin AC, ezogabine (Potiga)

Storage. All controlled substances must be adequately safeguarded. They need to be kept in a locked cabinet or safe of substantial construction. Keys should be placed in a locked area accessible only to authorized persons. Controlled substances should be kept in their original containers.

Storage of Medications

- Store controlled substances in a different location than non-narcotic medications.
- Refer to package inserts for specific storage information.
- Store medications in a cool, dry location. Keep medications away from light, heat, or moisture.
- For refrigerated and frozen medications, keep temperature logs to ensure the appropriate temperature range is maintained.
- Medications with different lot numbers or expiration dates should not be combined or repackaged.
- Keep *stock medications* (purchased by department) separated from *sample medications* (given by pharmaceutical manufacturers for patients).
- Keep medications out of exam rooms. Lock medication cabinets at the end of the day.
- For information on vaccine storage, refer to Chapter 13.

Inventory Records. It is important to keep an ongoing log of controlled substances received from manufacturers and administered to patients. Medications are tracked by the manufacturer, lot number, and expiration date. This information is found on the package. When a patient needs a controlled substance, the medical assistant must complete the log. The log typically requires:

- The medication information (name, dose, lot number, and expiration date)
- The ordering provider's name
- Information on the patient receiving the medication (name, date of birth, address, health record number, etc.)
- The name or initials of the healthcare professional administering the medication

The log must be kept separate from the patient's health record. The medication must also be documented in the patient's health record after it is administered.

Periodic **reconciling** of the log with the actual inventory count is important to identify missing medications. An inventory of all controlled substances must be done at least annually, unless required more often by law. Some states have special requirements for the inventory. It is important for the medical assistant to be knowledgeable about the special state requirements. The controlled substance inventory and log records need to be kept for 2 years. The records may be inspected by individuals authorized by the state attorney general.

Drug Destruction

Expired controlled substances are returned to the place from where they were received. For example, controlled substances that were sent by the manufacturer must be returned to the manufacturer, along with the required paperwork.

Sometimes a controlled substance must be destroyed in the healthcare facility. Examples of such situations are:

- Only part of the medication is used for the patient, and the extra amount must be destroyed.
- The patient refuses the medication after it has been opened and prepared.

- The medication is accidentally contaminated before it can be administered.

In these situations the controlled substance must be destroyed in the presence of two authorized persons (e.g., medical assistants, nurses). An entry on the waste log must be made. This information must include the date; the drug's name, strength, and quantity; the reason for destruction, and the signatures of both persons.

Discarding Medications in the Healthcare Facility

Discard medication that is expired, contaminated, unlabeled, or opened and not used. Some healthcare facilities have medication discarding programs to prevent medications from entering the city's water supply. Remember, if the medication is a controlled substance, two authorized employees must sign a waste log before the medication is discarded. Both employees must witness the disposal.

To discard medication, follow these steps if the facility has no other procedures in place:

- Return expired controlled substances to the place from which they were received (e.g., manufacturer), accompanied by the proper paperwork.
- Flush liquids down the sink.
- Flush pills down the toilet.
- Mix powdered medications with water and flush them down the toilet.
- Flush fluid from syringes down the sink and discard the syringe in a biohazard sharps container.

Theft and Diversion Reporting

Diversion of controlled substances means using the medication for personal reasons. If a medical assistant identifies that controlled substances are missing, it is important to notify the provider and supervisor. Many states and the DEA require any theft or loss to be reported to them within a given period of time. A report must be completed and filed by the deadline.

Medical Assistant's Role in Preventing Drug Abuse. By following these guidelines, the medical assistant can help prevent drug abuse.

- Carefully monitor patients who repeatedly call for prescription refills of controlled substances. Be aware that some patients will give *aliases* (false names).
- Request health records from other facilities for patients who report previous prescriptions for scheduled drugs.
- If the facility uses paper prescription pads, keep blank pads in a locked cabinet. They should be stored away from patient treatment areas.
- Never use prescription pads for notepads. Never use preprinted or presigned forms.
- Secure computers used for electronic health record (EHR) documentation to prevent patient access to prescription generation.
- Keep only a limited supply of controlled substances on hand.
- Keep accurate, complete records of controlled substances administered. Patients' records should contain information on prescribed and administered controlled substances.

DRUG NAMES

A single drug may have up to four names: chemical, generic, official, and brand. The drug is known by its chemical name until it receives FDA approval. The medical assistant should be familiar with the brand and generic names of common medications.

- *Chemical name:* Represents the drug's exact chemical formula. For example, the chemical name of ibuprofen is 2-(4-isobutylphenyl) propanoic acid.
- *Generic name:* Assigned by the US Adopted Names (USAN) Council. Similar medications are given similar-sounding generic names. All drugs need to have the generic name on the packaging. For example, ibuprofen is a generic name.
- *Official name:* Used to list the medication in the United States Pharmacopeia and the National Formulary (USP–NF). This book provides the standards (strength, purity, etc.) for drugs in the United States. In many cases, the official name is the same as the generic name. For example, ibuprofen is also the drug's official name.
- *Brand name:* Also called the *trade name*. The manufacturer assigns and registers the medication name. No other company can use that name. Usually the brand name begins with a capital letter and is followed by the registered sign (®). For example, brand names of ibuprofen include Advil and Motrin.

Generic Versus Brand Medications

If you ever walk through the pain medication aisle at a local store, you will see many bottles of ibuprofen products. Generally, the more expensive products are name brands, and less expensive products are generic products.

The company that initially created the medication will market it using a brand name. That company has sole rights to manufacture the medication until the patent expires. During this time, it is not uncommon for the price to be higher. The manufacturer may have spent years developing the medication before it went to market. Once the patent expires, other companies may create their own version of the medication. Some will market the medication under a brand name and others will use generic names.

When a company creates a medication, the company determines the appearance of the medication (e.g., color, size, and shape). It also comes up with the inactive ingredients or additives. This might be a color, sweetener, flavor, fillers, binders, and so on. For the active ingredient, the medication (i.e., ibuprofen), the company must comply with the FDA's regulations. The active ingredient must be of the same quality, purity, and amount as any other FDA-approved ibuprofen product of the same strength.

Most people do not notice a difference between generic and brand name medications. Other people do notice a difference. Their bodies may react to the inactive ingredients differently. This can affect their treatment for certain conditions. The provider can indicate if a generic medication can be used for prescriptions. This is important to keep in mind if you are assisting a provider by preparing prescriptions.

CRITICAL THINKING APPLICATION   14.4

Mark and Gabe are working with Janine Butler, a patient being seen for hypertension. While they are reviewing Janine's current medication list, she asks them what the difference is between generic and brand name medications. How might you answer this question?

DRUG REFERENCE INFORMATION

A medical assistant is obligated to become familiar with the drugs that are most frequently prescribed in the department. It is essential to know their indications, adverse reactions, administration routes, dosage, and storage. Using drug reference information can help the medical assistant learn about drugs. In the ambulatory care environment, drug reference information is available in both print and digital form.

With each drug (including drug samples and stock medications), the manufacturer includes a package insert. The package insert provides information about the medication, side effects, administration techniques, dosages, storage, and so on.

Drug handbooks provide condensed, more common information on the drugs. Many of these books are organized by the generic names of drugs.

An old classic, the *Physician's Desk Reference* (PDR), was a very large book that contained a comprehensive collection of package insert information. After publishing the 2017 version (the 71st edition), the company stopped printing the PDR. The drug reference information is available through its digital online products (*Prescribers' Digital Reference* [PDR]), its app, and other products that integrate with electronic health records. More information can be found on the website (*www.pdr.net*).

The digital drug reference information has a huge advantage over print information. Digital information can be updated more quickly and easily than the print information. The market for digital drug information has grown over the years. Digital drug reference information is available online, through apps, and with electronic health records.

- Online drug reference information is available from many sites. It is important for the medical assistant to use reliable websites. Government websites (e.g., *medlineplus.gov* and *www.fda.gov*) contain updated, reliable information. Sites that patients use may contain older information and can include medications that are not available in the United States.
- When selecting an app for drug reference information, be sure it is routinely updated. Read the reviews, and research the company providing the information. Only use reputable apps for drug reference information.
- Many electronic health record software programs incorporate drug reference information. This makes it easy for healthcare professionals to look up drug information.

Drug Classification

Drugs are grouped by classification or class. It is important for a medical assistant to be aware of the class of drugs. Oftentimes patients will ask what a specific medication is for, and the medical assistant

can provide that information. Table 14.3 provides a list of classifications of medications with descriptions.

Drug Terminology

Regardless of how drug reference information is obtained, it is important for the medical assistant to understand the terminology. The following terminology is typically found in drug reference information.

- *Names:* Usually the generic name is listed with the trade names. Some references may indicate if the trade name found is in the United States or Canada.
- *Description:* Describes the medication and its general use.
- *Boxed warning:* Also referred to as a *black box warning*. It addresses serious or life-threatening risks. This information also appears on the drug's label.
- *Dosage:* Specifies the route, dose, and timing of the medication; usually corresponds to an indication (disease or condition). May provide information on doses for different age ranges. *Maximum dosage* indicates the greatest amount of medication a person should have within a 24-hour period.
- *Indication:* Conditions or diseases for which the drug is used.
- *Dosage considerations:* Indicates recommended changes in dosages for special populations (e.g., patients with hepatic impairment, renal impairment).
- *How supplied:* Lists the **form** (e.g., chewable tablets, capsules) and the strength (e.g., 250 mg)
- *Administration:* Provides information on how the medication should be administered. Includes important administration techniques, such as information on shaking the medication, if it needs to be taken with food, and so on.
- *Contraindications:* Reasons or conditions that make administration of the drug improper or undesirable. For example, aspirin is contraindicated in patients with GI bleeding.
- *Precautions:* Indicates necessary actions or special care that needs to be taken when the patient is on the medication. May include information on laboratory tests, special populations (children and geriatric), pregnancy, breastfeeding, and so on.
- *Adverse reactions:* Also called *side effects* in some information. This section describes known undesirable experiences associated with the medication. Reactions may be divided into severe (life-threatening, serious reactions), moderate, and mild.
- *Interactions:* Includes medications, foods, and beverages that interact with the medication. These products may either increase or reduce the medication level in the blood. They may also increase the risk of adverse reactions if taken together with the drug.
- *Action:* How the drug provides therapeutic results in the body, or the use of the drug.
- *Pharmacokinetics:* Provides information on the absorption, distribution, metabolism, and excretion of the medication. Information on when the drug is at its highest level in the body or when the drug starts working may be included. Important terms for understanding the pharmacokinetics of a drug include:
  - *Biologic half-life:* The time it takes half of the drug to be metabolized or eliminated by normal biologic processes.
  - *Onset:* The time it takes for the drug to produce a response.

TABLE 14.3   Examples of Medication Classifications

CLASSIFICATION	DESCRIPTION	CLASSIFICATION	DESCRIPTION
Analgesic	Relieves pain	Contraceptive	Inhibits conception (prevents pregnancy)
Anesthetic	Produces local or general anesthesia	Corticosteroid	Reduces inflammation
Antacid	Neutralizes stomach acid	Decongestant	Relieves nasal and sinus congestion
Anti-Alzheimer	Treats dementia (Alzheimer)	Diuretic	Increases urinary output and lowers blood pressure
Antianxiety	Reduces anxiety and tension	Electrolyte	Maintains normal electrolyte level and proper functioning of the body systems
Antiarrhythmic	Treats heart arrhythmias		
Antibiotic	Treats bacterial infections	Erectile dysfunction agent	Facilitates an erection
Anticholinergic	Reduces smooth muscle spasms	Expectorant	Thins bronchial secretions, making it easier to cough up mucus
Anticoagulant	Decreases blood clotting ability		
Anticonvulsant	Reduces the frequency and severity of seizures	Hematopoietic	Promotes blood cell production
Antidepressant	Treats depression	Hemostatic	Clots blood
Antiemetic	Reduces nausea and vomiting	Hormone replacement	Replaces hormones or compensates for hormone deficiencies
Antifungal	Treats fungal infections		
Antigout	Reduces the uric acid in the body	Laxative	Promotes stools
Antihistamine	Relieves allergies by blocking the histamine action	Leukotriene receptor antagonist	Blocks the action of substances that cause asthma and allergic rhinitis
Antihyperglycemic	Reduces blood glucose level	Miotic	Drains excessive fluid from the eye, used for glaucoma
Antihypertensive	Lowers blood pressure		
Anti-inflammatory	Reduces inflammation	Muscle relaxant	Reduces pain
Antimigraine	Treats or prevents migraine headaches	Mydriatic	Dilates the pupil, used for ophthalmic procedures
Antineoplastic	Slows or stops the growth of cancer cells		
Antiplatelet	Prevents the function of platelets (formation of clots)	Osteoporosis agent	Promotes bone mineral density, used to treat osteoporosis
Antipsychotic	Alters the chemical actions in the brain	Proton-pump inhibitor	Reduces the acid produced in the stomach
Antitussive	Suppresses coughs	Sedative-hypnotic	Slows brain activity, allowing sleep
Antiviral	Treats viral infections	Stimulant	Stimulates the brain and body, makes the person more alert
Bronchodilator	Relaxes the smooth muscles of the bronchi		
Cholesterol-lowering agent	Reduces low-density lipoprotein and triglycerides in the blood while increasing the high-density lipoprotein	Tumor necrosis factor (TNF) inhibitor	Blocks the action of TNF, preventing inflammation in autoimmune disorders

- *Peak*: The time it takes for the drug to reach its greatest effective concentration in the blood.
- *Duration*: The time during which the drug is present in the blood at great enough levels to produce a response.

Pregnancy and Lactation Labeling Rule

In 2015 the Pregnancy and Lactation Labeling Rule (PLLR) replaced the pregnancy risk letter categories (e.g., A, B, C, D, and X) with more comprehensive information. The goal is to provide the provider and patient with pregnancy and lactation information. This information can be used when discussing the risks versus the benefits of a medication. The FDA created the new system to help with patient-specific counseling and informed decision making for pregnant and breastfeeding mothers who need medication therapies. The system consists of three subcategories with detailed information about the following:

- *Pregnancy*: Includes information on the risks during pregnancy for the mother and baby, in addition to data on the risk of adverse developmental outcomes.
- *Lactation*: Includes information on the presence of the drug in breast milk, the effects on a breast-fed child, and the impact on milk production.
- *Females and males of reproductive potential*: Includes information about when pregnancy testing or contraception is required during drug therapy and data that suggest drug-associated fertility effects.

Table 14.4 provides drug information on the top 50 commonly prescribed medications. Please use drug reference information for additional information on these products.

CRITICAL THINKING APPLICATION   14.5
Gabe mentions to Mark that he learned that the FDA had changed the pregnancy risk categories. Mark had not heard about this. Gabe further explains why. Describe how the changes provide more information to providers and patients.

TYPES OF MEDICATION ORDERS

A *medication order* refers to directions given by a provider for a specific medication to be administered to a patient. The medical assistant receives the information from the provider. The provider must give this information:

- Patient's name and health record number or date of birth (DOB) (e.g., Noemi Rodriguez DOB 11/04/1971)
- Medication name, dose, and route (e.g., Tylenol 1 g po)

The provider can give the order over the phone or in person. This type of order is called a *verbal order*. It is important for the medical assistant to write down the order and read it back to the provider. This process ensures the order was heard and recorded correctly. The provider can also give the medical assistant a *written order*. Usually, these are written on a prescription pad or in an electronic message. A written order only needs clarification from the provider if the medical assistant cannot read the order or has a question.

Text continued on p. 306

TABLE 14.4   Information on Commonly Prescribed Medications

GENERIC NAME	BRAND/TRADE NAME(S)	CLASS/ SCHEDULE	MEDICATION INFORMATION
hydrocodone/ acetaminophen (APAP)	Vicodin, Norco, Lortab	Analgesics (narcotic [opioids]) C–II	*Indication*: moderate to severe pain *Desired effects/action*: changes the way the brain and nervous system respond to pain *Side effects*: GI intolerance, difficulty urinating, anxiety, fuzzy thinking *Adverse reaction*: slowed breathing, chest tightness
oxycodone/ acetaminophen (APAP)	Percocet, Oxycet, Roxicet	Analgesics (narcotic [opioids]) C–II	*Indication*: moderate to severe pain *Desired effects/action*: changes the way the brain and nervous system respond to pain *Side effects*: GI intolerance, flushing, headache, mood changes *Adverse reaction*: slowed breathing, angina, hypersensitivity, seizures
tramadol	Ultram, Conzip	Analgesics (narcotic [opioids]) C–II	*Indication*: moderate to severe pain *Desired effects/action*: changes the way the brain and nervous system respond to pain *Side effects*: GI intolerance, difficulty sleeping, change in mood, dry mouth *Adverse reaction*: hallucinations, agitation, hypersensitivity, arrhythmias
memantine	Namenda	Anti-Alzheimer	*Indication*: Alzheimer disease *Desired effects/action*: reduces the brain chemicals that cause the dementia *Side effects*: GI intolerance, edema, weight loss, dizziness, anxiety, aggression *Adverse reaction*: angina, seizures, hypertension

TABLE 14.4   Information on Commonly Prescribed Medications—*continued*

GENERIC NAME	BRAND/TRADE NAME(S)	CLASS/ SCHEDULE	MEDICATION INFORMATION
alprazolam	Xanax	Antianxiety (benzodiazepines) C–IV	*Indication:* anxiety and panic disorders *Desired effects/action:* decreases abnormal excitement in the brain *Side effects:* drowsiness, headache, dizziness, GI intolerance, dry mouth, weight changes *Adverse reaction:* seizures, jaundice, depression, memory problems
clonazepam	Klonopin	Antianxiety (benzodiazepines) C–IV	*Indication:* seizures, panic attacks *Desired effects/action:* decreases abnormal excitement in the brain *Side effects:* drowsiness, coordination problems, joint pain, blurred vision, changes in sex drive *Adverse reaction:* hypersensitivity
diazepam	Valium	Antianxiety (benzodiazepines) C–IV	*Indication:* relieves anxiety, muscle spasms, and seizures *Desired effects/action:* produces a calming effect *Side effects:* GI intolerance, weakness, tiredness, drowsiness, dry mouth *Adverse reaction:* restlessness, frequent urination, blurred vision
digoxin	Lanoxin, Digitek, Cardoxin	Antiarrhythmics	*Indication:* congestive heart failure (CHF), atrial fibrillation *Desired effects/action:* helps the heart work better, controls heart rate *Side effects:* dizziness, drowsiness, visual changes (blurred, yellow), arrhythmias *Adverse reaction:* swelling of hands and feet, unusual weight gain, difficulty breathing *Assessment:* take apical pulse, hold if <60 in adults, <70 in children, and <90 in infants
cephalexin	Keflex	Antibiotics (cephalosporin)	*Indication:* bacterial infections (e.g., urinary tract, ear, and pneumonia) *Desired effects/action:* stops bacteria growth *Side effects:* GI intolerance, agitation, confusion, headache *Adverse reaction:* hypersensitivity, watery or bloody stools, hallucinations
azithromycin	Zithromax, Zithromax Z-Paks, Zmak	Antibiotics (macrolide)	*Indication:* bacterial infections (e.g., sexually transmitted infections, bronchitis, and pneumonia) *Desired effects/action:* stops bacteria growth *Side effects:* GI intolerance, headache *Adverse reaction:* hypersensitivity, mouth sores, arrhythmias, jaundice, dark-colored urine
amoxicillin	Amoxil, Moxtag	Antibiotics (penicillin)	*Indication:* bacterial infections (e.g., pneumonia, gonorrhea, ear, and throat) *Desired effects/action:* stops bacteria growth *Side effects:* GI intolerance *Adverse reaction:* hypersensitivity, seizures, jaundice
warfarin	Coumadin	Anticoagulants	*Indication:* prevents blood clots from forming *Desired effects/action:* decreases clotting ability of the blood *Side effects:* GI intolerance, loss of hair, chills *Adverse reaction:* hypersensitivity, infection, angina, jaundice, bleeding
gabapentin	Neurontin, Horizant	Anticonvulsants	*Indication:* seizures, postherpetic neuralgia, restless legs syndrome (RLS) *Desired effects/action:* decreases abnormal excitement in the brain; reduces seizures *Side effects:* drowsiness, blurred vision, anxiety, memory problems, weakness, GI intolerance *Adverse reaction:* hypersensitivity, seizures

Continued

TABLE 14.4   Information on Commonly Prescribed Medications—*continued*

GENERIC NAME	BRAND/TRADE NAME(S)	CLASS/ SCHEDULE	MEDICATION INFORMATION
duloxetine	Cymbalta	Antidepressant (selective serotonin and norepinephrine reuptake inhibitors [SNRIs])	*Indication:* major depressive disorder, generalized anxiety disorder, diabetic peripheral neuropathy, fibromyalgia, chronic pain *Desired effects/action:* increases the amounts of serotonin and norepinephrine in the brain; helps to maintain mental balance and stop pain signals in the brain *Side effects:* orthostatic hypotension *Adverse reaction:* suicidal thoughts, hepatotoxicity, seizures, glaucoma, hyponatremia
citalopram	Celexa	Antidepressant (selective serotonin reuptake inhibitors [SSRIs])	*Indication:* depression *Desired effects/action:* increases the amount of serotonin in the brain; helps to maintain mental balance *Side effects:* GI intolerance, frequent urination, weakness, joint pain, weight loss *Adverse reaction:* angina, shortness of breath, arrhythmias, hallucinations, coma, hypersensitivity, confusion, seizures, suicidal thoughts
escitalopram	Lexapro	Antidepressant (selective serotonin reuptake inhibitors [SSRIs])	*Indication:* depression, generalized anxiety disorder (GAD) *Desired effects/action:* increases the amount of serotonin in the brain; helps to maintain mental balance *Side effects:* GI intolerance, increased sweating, change in sex drive, flulike symptoms *Adverse reaction:* unusual excitement, hallucinations, confusion, arrhythmias, severe muscle stiffness, suicidal thoughts
sertraline	Zoloft	Antidepressant (selective serotonin reuptake inhibitors [SSRIs])	*Indication:* depression, obsessive-compulsive disorder (OCD), panic attacks, posttraumatic stress disorder (PTSD) *Desired effects/action:* increases the amount of serotonin in the brain; helps to maintain mental balance *Side effects:* GI intolerance, weight changes, difficulty falling asleep, change in sex drive, excessive sweating *Adverse reaction:* seizures, abnormal bleeding, arrhythmias, hypersensitivity, suicidal thoughts
trazodone	Oleptro	Antidepressant (serotonin modulators)	*Indication:* depression *Desired effects/action:* increases the amount of serotonin; helps to maintain mental balance *Side effects:* GI intolerance, weakness, headache, confusion, sweating, decreased coordination *Adverse reaction:* angina, fainting, seizures, coma, arrhythmias, suicidal thoughts
promethazine	Promethegan	Antihistamines	*Indication:* allergies, allergic conjunctivitis, anaphylaxis, sedation for procedures, motion sickness *Desired effects/action:* blocks histamine action *Side effects:* drowsiness, difficulty sleeping, ringing in ears, blurred vision, GI intolerance *Adverse reaction:* wheezing, slowed breathing, sweating, stiff muscles, decreased alertness
metformin	Glucophage, Fortamet, Glumetza, Riomet	Antihyperglycemics	*Indication:* type 2 diabetes mellitus *Desired effects/action:* reduces glucose absorption and increases body's response to insulin; controls the blood glucose level *Side effects:* GI intolerance, metallic taste in the mouth, flushing of the skin, nail changes *Adverse reaction:* angina, rash

TABLE 14.4   Information on Commonly Prescribed Medications—*continued*

GENERIC NAME	BRAND/TRADE NAME(S)	CLASS/ SCHEDULE	MEDICATION INFORMATION
valsartan	Diovan	Antihypertensive (angiotensin II receptor antagonists)	*Indication:* hypertension, heart failure, postmyocardial infarction (MI) *Desired effects/action:* prevents vasoconstriction, which lowers the blood pressure *Side effects:* headache, dizziness, flu symptoms, GI intolerance, blurred vision, mild itching *Adverse reaction:* hyperkalemia, arrhythmias
losartan	Cozaar	Antihypertensive (angiotensin II receptor antagonists)	*Indication:* hypertension, heart failure *Desired effects/action:* lowers the blood pressure *Side effects:* headache, dizziness, diarrhea, muscle cramps and pain, nasal congestion, cough, upper respiratory infections, sinusitis *Adverse reaction:* chest pain, difficulty swallowing, hoarseness
benazepril	Lotensin	Antihypertensive (angiotensin-converting enzyme [ACE] inhibitors)	*Indication:* hypertension *Desired effects/action:* causes vasodilation, lowering the blood pressure *Side effects:* cough, drowsiness, headache *Adverse reaction:* jaundice, difficulty breathing, lightheadedness, swelling, hoarseness
lisinopril	(no brand names)	Antihypertensive (angiotensin-converting enzyme [ACE] inhibitors)	*Indication:* hypertension, heart failure *Desired effects/action:* causes vasodilation, lowering the blood pressure *Side effects:* cough, dizziness, tiredness, GI intolerance, rash *Adverse reaction:* angina, lightheadedness, difficulty swallowing, hypersensitivity
atenolol	Tenormin	Antihypertensive (beta blockers)	*Indication:* hypertension, angina *Desired effects/action:* relaxes blood vessels and slows the heart rate, thus improving blood flow and decreasing blood pressure *Side effects:* dizziness, tiredness, depression, GI intolerance *Adverse reaction:* shortness of breath, swelling of legs and hands, weight gain, fainting
metoprolol	Lopressor	Antihypertensive (beta blockers)	*Indication:* hypertension, angina *Desired effects/action:* relaxes blood vessels and slows the heart rate, thus improving blood flow and decreasing blood pressure *Side effects:* dizziness, tiredness, depression, GI intolerance *Adverse reaction:* hypersensitivity, weight gain, arrhythmias
carvedilol	Coreg	Antihypertensive (beta blockers)	*Indication:* heart failure, hypertension *Desired effects/action:* relaxes blood vessels and slows the heart rate, thus improving blood flow and decreasing blood pressure *Side effects:* hyperglycemia, tiredness, weakness, dizziness, visual changes, joint pain, difficulty sleeping *Adverse reaction:* shortness of breath, swelling of arms and legs, arrhythmias
amlodipine	Norvasc	Antihypertensive (calcium channel blockers)	*Indication:* hypertension, angina *Desired effects/action:* relaxes the vessels so the heart does not have to pump as hard *Side effects:* GI intolerance, headache, swelling of legs and arms, tiredness, flushing *Adverse reaction:* more frequent or severe angina, fainting, arrhythmias
ibuprofen	Advil, Motrin, Midol	Anti-inflammatory drugs (nonsteroidal [NSAIDs])	*Indication for use:* osteoarthritis, rheumatoid arthritis, fever, pain *Desired effects/action:* stops the body's production of substances that causes pain, fever, and inflammation *Side effects:* GI intolerance, ringing in the ear *Adverse reaction:* weight gain, hypersensitivity, hoarseness, jaundice, bloody urine, stiff neck

Continued

TABLE 14.4   Information on Commonly Prescribed Medications—*continued*

GENERIC NAME	BRAND/TRADE NAME(S)	CLASS/ SCHEDULE	MEDICATION INFORMATION
clopidogrel	Plavix	Antiplatelets	*Indication:* used to prevent clots after a stroke, heart attack, or severe angina *Desired effects/action:* prevents platelets from collecting and forming clots *Side effects:* excessive tiredness, GI intolerance, nosebleed, dizziness *Adverse reaction:* hypersensitivity, bloody and tarry stools, coffee grounds–looking emesis, blood in urine, visual changes
aripiprazole	Abilify	Antipsychotics (atypical)	*Indication:* schizophrenia, bipolar disorder, major depressive disorder, Tourette disorder *Desired effects/action:* changes the actions of chemicals in the brain *Side effects:* GI intolerance, insomnia, headache, anxiety, trouble swallowing *Adverse reaction:* suicidal thoughts, stroke, compulsive behaviors, orthostatic hypotension, tardive dyskinesia
quetiapine	Seroquel	Antipsychotics (atypical)	*Indication:* schizophrenia, bipolar disorder *Desired effects/action:* changes the activity of certain substances in the brain *Side effects:* drowsiness, pain in joints, weakness, GI intolerance, difficulty concentrating and speaking *Adverse reaction:* seizures, visual changes, uncontrollable movements, arrhythmias
tiotropium	Spiriva	Bronchodilators	*Indication:* chronic obstructive pulmonary disease (COPD) *Desired effects/action:* prevents bronchospasms *Side effects:* dry mouth, GI intolerance, nosebleed, muscle pain, cold symptoms *Adverse reaction:* hypersensitivity reaction, paradoxical bronchospasm, glaucoma, urinary retention
albuterol	Ventolin HFA, Proventil HFA, Proair	Bronchodilators	*Indication:* bronchospasm (e.g., asthma) *Desired effects/action:* relaxes bronchial muscles and increases air flow to lungs *Side effects:* headache, dizziness, insomnia, cough, sore throat, nausea, vomiting, dry mouth *Adverse reaction:* paradoxical bronchospasm, cardiovascular effects, hypersensitivity, hypokalemia
atorvastatin	Lipitor	Cholesterol-lowering agent	*Indication:* hyperlipidemia, hypertriglyceridemia *Desired effects/action:* slows production of cholesterol in the body; decreases LDH and triglycerides; increases HDL *Side effects:* GI intolerance, joint pain, memory loss, confusion *Adverse reaction:* muscle pain, lack of energy, angina, weakness, hypersensitivity, dark-colored urine, jaundice
rosuvastatin	Crestor	Cholesterol-lowering agent	*Indication:* hyperlipidemia, hypertriglyceridemia *Desired effects/action:* slows production of cholesterol in the body; reduces LDH and triglycerides; increases HDL *Side effects:* headache, depression, muscle and joint pain, insomnia, GI intolerance *Adverse reaction:* muscle damage leading to acute renal failure and liver damage
simvastatin	Zocor	Cholesterol-lowering agent	*Indication:* hyperlipidemia, hypertriglyceridemia *Desired effects/action:* slows production of cholesterol in the body; reduces LDH and triglycerides; increases HDL *Side effects:* GI intolerance, memory loss, confusion, headache *Adverse reaction:* muscle pain, dark red urine, lack of energy, jaundice, hypersensitivity

TABLE 14.4	Information on Commonly Prescribed Medications—*continued*		
GENERIC NAME	**BRAND/TRADE NAME(S)**	**CLASS/ SCHEDULE**	**MEDICATION INFORMATION**
methylprednisolone	Medrol	Corticosteroid (oral)	*Indication:* arthritis, certain cancers, allergies, asthma *Desired effects/action:* relieves inflammation symptoms *Side effects:* GI intolerance, increased hair growth, insomnia, acne *Adverse reaction:* swollen face and legs, visual problems, infection, black or tarry stool
fluticasone	Flonase nasal spray, Flovent HFA, Flovent Diskus	Corticosteroid (nasal and inhaled)	*Indication:* hay fever, allergies (nasal spray); asthma (inhaled) *Desired effects/action:* reduces inflammation and allergy reaction *Side effects:* headache, dryness in mouth, hoarseness or deepened voice *Adverse reaction:* reduced bone marrow density, immunosuppression, adrenal suppression, glaucoma, cataracts, hypersensitivity in individuals with milk allergy (Diskus)
furosemide	Lasix	Diuretics	*Indication:* hypertension *Desired effects/action:* causes the kidneys to increase the excretion of water and salt *Side effects:* frequent urination, blurred vision, headache, constipation, diarrhea *Adverse reaction:* ringing in the ears, loss of hearing, blisters, jaundice, hypersensitivity
hydrochlorothiazide (HCTZ)	Microzide, Oretic	Diuretics	*Indication:* hypertension *Desired effects/action:* causes the kidneys to increase the excretion of water and salt *Side effects:* frequent urination, diarrhea, loss of appetite, headache, hair loss *Adverse reaction:* joint pain, unusual bleeding, hypersensitivity, visual change
potassium	K-Tab, Klor-Con, K-Dur, Micro-K	Electrolyte	*Indication:* mineral supplement needed for certain diseases and medications (e.g., diuretic) *Desired effects/action:* proper functioning of the body systems *Side effects:* GI intolerance *Adverse reaction:* confusion, listlessness, gray skin, black stools
levothyroxine	Synthroid, Levothroid, Levoxyl	Hormone replacement (thyroid hormone)	*Indication:* hypothyroidism, pituitary TSH suppression *Desired effects/action:* replacement hormone; regulates body's energy and metabolism *Side effects:* reversible hair loss, dry skin, GI intolerance, headache, nervousness *Adverse reaction:* cardiac arrhythmias, angina, myocardial infarction, heart failure
montelukast	Singulair	Leukotriene receptor antagonists	*Indication:* asthma, exercise-induced bronchospasms *Desired effects/action:* blocks the action of substances that cause asthma and allergic rhinitis *Side effects:* headache, dizziness, heartburn, stomach pain, tiredness *Adverse reaction:* hypersensitivity, numbness in arms and legs, swelling of the sinuses
carisoprodol	Soma	Muscle relaxant C–IV	*Indication:* painful musculoskeletal conditions (e.g., strains, sprains, muscle injuries) *Desired effects/action:* reduces pain *Side effects:* drowsiness, clumsiness, tachycardia, GI intolerance *Adverse reaction:* difficulty breathing, fever, weakness, burning in the eyes, seizures
cyclobenzaprine	Flexeril	Muscle relaxant	*Indication:* painful musculoskeletal conditions (e.g., strains, sprains, muscle injuries) *Desired effects/action:* works on the brain and nervous system to allow muscle relaxation *Side effects:* GI intolerance, extreme tiredness, dry mouth *Adverse reaction:* hypersensitivity, angina

Continued

TABLE 14.4   Information on Commonly Prescribed Medications—*continued*

GENERIC NAME	BRAND/TRADE NAME(S)	CLASS/ SCHEDULE	MEDICATION INFORMATION
esomeprazole	Nexium	Proton-pump inhibitors	*Indication:* gastroesophageal reflex disease (GERD), erosive esophagitis, *Helicobacter pylori* ulcers *Desired effects/action:* reduces the amount of stomach acid *Side effects:* headache, drowsiness, dry mouth, GI intolerance *Adverse reaction:* acute interstitial nephritis, *C. difficile*, bone fracture, systemic lupus erythematosus, cyanocobalamin (vitamin B_{12}) deficiency, hypomagnesemia
omeprazole	Prilosec	Proton-pump inhibitors	*Indication:* gastroesophageal reflux disease (GERD), ulcers, *H. pylori* *Desired effects/action:* reduces stomach acid *Side effects:* GI intolerance, headache *Adverse reaction:* hypersensitivity, dizziness, arrhythmias, muscle spasm
zolpidem	Ambien, Edluar, Zolpimist	Sedative – hypnotics C–IV	*Indication:* insomnia *Desired effects/action:* slows activity in the brain, allowing sleep *Side effects:* drowsiness, headache, dizziness, drugged feeling, unsteady walking, GI intolerance *Adverse reaction:* jaundice, hypersensitivity, light-colored stools, angina, blurred vision
methylphenidate	Concerta, Ritalin LA	Stimulants C–II	*Indication:* attention deficit hyperactivity disorder (ADHD), narcolepsy *Desired effects/action:* changes certain substances in the brain, allowing a person to concentrate and focus *Side effects:* nervousness, difficulty falling asleep, GI intolerance, restlessness, muscle tightness *Adverse reaction:* angina, arrhythmias, seizure, blurred vision

In addition to describing how medication orders are given to the medical assistant, they can be described by the type of order. The following are five types of medication orders.

- *Routine order*: Medication taken at a regular interval until it is canceled or expired. (Most non-narcotic routine orders expire in 12 months.) Examples: "Vitamin B_{12} 100 mcg IM monthly" and "Synthroid 75 mcg qam po."
- *Standing order*: Order applies to all patients who meet specific criteria. For departments, usually all providers agree collectively on standing orders and sign the order. Example: "For patients 18 years and older, with no allergy to acetaminophen and who have a temperature of 103°F or higher: give acetaminophen 650 mg po × 1 dose."
- *PRN order*: Medication that is given on an "as needed" basis for specific signs and symptoms. (It is important to indicate these symptoms when documenting the administered medication in the patient's health record.) Example: "Acetaminophen 325 mg, 2 tabs po q 4–6 hr prn pain."
- *Single order* or *one-time order*: Medication is administered one time. Example: "Acetaminophen 650 mg po × 1 dose."
- *Stat order*: Medication is administered one time right now. Example: "EpiPen 0.3 mg IM stat."

Prescriptions

A *prescription* is a written order by a provider to the pharmacist. It tells the pharmacist what medication and how much should be dispensed to the patient. There are four parts to a prescription: superscription, inscription, signature, and subscription. Fig. 14.1 describes the four parts of a prescription.

Medical Assistant's Role

In some ambulatory care facilities, medical assistants prepare prescriptions for providers to sign. Some such scenarios may include:

- A patient may request refills while the medical assistant is rooming the patient. The medical assistant may prepare the prescriptions, so the provider just needs to sign for the refills.
- A patient may call the department and request a refill on a medication. Using a medication refill protocol, the medical assistant needs to see if the patient can get a refill (Fig. 14.2). If the patient can, then the medical assistant prepares the prescription and has the provider sign it.

The prescription must be written in ink or be computer-generated. A medical assistant can prepare prescriptions for the provider to sign. The provider is responsible for ensuring the prescription meets federal and state laws and regulations. All prescriptions need to include this information:

- Date of issue (when it was written)
- Patient information (name and address are required; date of birth is helpful)
- Provider's full name and address
- Drug name (e.g., amoxicillin)
- Drug strength (e.g., 500 mg)

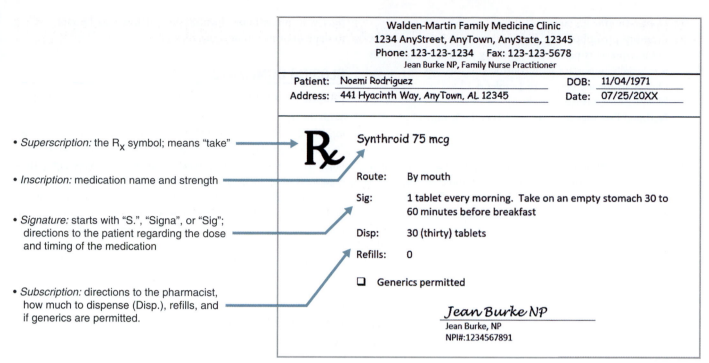

- *Superscription:* the R$_x$ symbol; means "take"

- *Inscription:* medication name and strength

- *Signature:* starts with "S.", "Signa", or "Sig"; directions to the patient regarding the dose and timing of the medication

- *Subscription:* directions to the pharmacist, how much to dispense (Disp.), refills, and if generics are permitted.

Walden-Martin Family Medicine Clinic
1234 AnyStreet, AnyTown, AnyState, 12345
Phone: 123-123-1234   Fax: 123-123-5678
Jean Burke NP, Family Nurse Practitioner

| Patient: | Noemi Rodriguez | DOB: | 11/04/1971 |
| Address: | 441 Hyacinth Way, AnyTown, AL 12345 | Date: | 07/25/20XX |

R$_x$ Synthroid 75 mcg

Route: By mouth

Sig: 1 tablet every morning. Take on an empty stomach 30 to 60 minutes before breakfast

Disp: 30 (thirty) tablets

Refills: 0

☐ Generics permitted

Jean Burke NP
Jean Burke, NP
NPI#:1234567891

FIGURE 14.1 Parts of a prescription.

Prescription Refill Protocol
Walden-Martin Family Medical Clinic

Description: A Certified Medical Assistant (CMA) can refill current hypertensive medications that fall within the guidelines of this protocol.

Step 1	Step 2	
For medications to be refilled, the following points need to be addressed.	Qualifying Medications	Prescription Refill
• Has the person seen the provider within the last year? • Is the prescription for a hypertensive, hyperlipidemia, or hyperthyroidism medication, a current prescription? • Is the person free of concerns or complications due to the medication? • Is it time for a refill? (The medical assistant must verify that it is time for a refill.) If the answers to the above questions are all YES, then proceed to Step 2. If any of the answers to the above questions are NO, then schedule the person for an appointment with the provider	amlodipine amlodipine/benazepril atenolol atenolol/Chlorthalidone benazepril captopril diltiazem enalapril felodipine fosinopril irbesartan isradiprine lisinopril losartan nifedipine quinapril ramipril	Extend the current prescription for 6 months. Instruct patient that in 6 months: • A visit to the provider will be required • Blood pressure reading will be required • Lab work may be required

FIGURE 14.2 Example of a prescription refill protocol. The medical assistant uses a protocol to determine what action to take with prescription refill requests.

- Dosage form (e.g., tablets)
- Quantity prescribed (e.g., 14 [fourteen]) – writing out the number prevents people from altering the prescription. This is especially important with controlled substances.
- Directions for use (e.g., take 1 tablet q 12 hr)
- Number of refills (e.g., Refills 0)
- **National Provider Identifier (NPI)** and signature of provider (a manual signature is required for controlled substances)
- Indicate if a generic is acceptable

If an electronic prescription is sent to the pharmacy and a paper copy is given to the patient, the copy should indicate that it is a copy ("Copy only – not valid for dispensing"). Procedure 14.1 on p. 313 indicates how to prepare prescriptions using a prescription refill procedure. Only facility-approved abbreviations should be used when preparing prescriptions and documenting in the patients' health records. Table 14.5 provides commonly approved abbreviations.

Once the prescriptions are prepared, they need to be given to the provider to sign. Either the provider or the medical assistant needs to document the refills in the patient's health record. The facility's policy will indicate who is responsible for the documentation.

Controlled Substance Prescriptions

For security reasons, the provider's DEA number should be used only on controlled substance prescriptions. It is not appropriate for the number to appear on non-narcotic prescriptions. The NPI is a national number that is unique to the provider. This number is found on prescriptions and may be used for tracking or treatment identification purposes.

The medical assistant needs to be aware of the special requirements for controlled substances. It is important for the medical assistant to stay updated on which frequently prescribed medications are controlled substances. Table 14.6 describes common requirements for scheduled substances.

CRITICAL THINKING APPLICATION   **14.6**

Mark and Gabe are working on prescription refills. A patient who just started taking a schedule 2 medication calls in for a refill. He says he was not happy that there were no refills on his original prescription. How might Gabe handle this type of call? What could he say to help the patient understand the situation?

OVER-THE-COUNTER MEDICATIONS AND HERBAL SUPPLEMENTS

Over-the-counter (OTC) medications and herbal supplements can affect medication treatment. It is important for the medical assistant to obtain a list of current prescription, OTC medications, and herbal supplements (Tables 14.7 and 14.8). Some patients may hesitate or may not want to share this information. They may not realize that OTC medications and herbal supplements can interfere with prescription medications. It is important for medical assistants to be professional and respectful when dealing with these situations. If they explain that sometimes the OTC medications and herbal supplements

react with prescription medications, patients may be more willing to share information on what they take.

CLOSING COMMENTS

Patient Coaching

With the frequency of opioid abuse, prescribing guidelines are changing. The Centers for Disease Control and Prevention (CDC) published "Guideline for Prescribing Opioids for Chronic Pain" (available at *https://www.cdc.gov/drugoverdose/pdf/Guidelines_Factsheet-a.pdf*). These guidelines help support providers who are working with patients with chronic pain. The medical assistant may need to coach patients on home care treatments. Opioids are not first-line or routine therapy for chronic pain. The medical assistant may need to coach the patient on the importance of using nonpharmacologic therapy and nonopioid pharmacologic therapy for chronic pain. For patients who receive opioid prescriptions, frequent follow-up is needed for the provider to evaluate the benefit and risk of the drug.

Legal and Ethical Issues

The magnitude of opioid abuse has increased dramatically, and it is currently considered a crisis. According to the CDC, in 2017 more than 70,230 people died from a drug overdose in the United States. About 67.8% of these deaths involved prescription or illicit opioid use. Many ambulatory care facilities have adopted procedures for specific controlled substance prescriptions. Before patients can get these prescriptions, they need to have a urine drug test. The urine drug test helps a provider assess what drugs the patient has taken. The provider expects the results to show the drug prescribed, but he or she also checks for other prescribed controlled substances and illicit drugs. In many cases, if the drug test shows evidence of illicit drug use or prescription-controlled substances not prescribed by the provider, the patient is referred for substance abuse counseling and treatment.

Patient-Centered Care

Many healthcare facilities require that patients receive a printout of their current medications at the end of each visit. When patients are taking a number of medications, it is important for the medical assistant to encourage these patients to carry a current medications list in their wallet or purse. This can be helpful in an emergency or when the patient needs to see a different provider.

Professional Behaviors

When working with prescription refills, it is important for the medical assistant to process the refill in a timely fashion. If the medical assistant procrastinates and does not process the refill, the patient may not have the medication when she or he needs it. Some medications need to be taken on a daily basis. If a dose is skipped, the patient may have serious consequences.

It is also important that the medical assistant honors what that patient was told. If the patient is told that the medication will be sent to a pharmacy by a specific time, it is important for the medical assistant to ensure this is done. If the medication is held up for some reason, the medical assistant should notify the patient about the delay.

TABLE 14.5   Commonly Approved Abbreviations

TYPE	ABBREVIATIONS	MEANING	TYPE	ABBREVIATIONS	MEANING
Routes and medication forms	subcut	subcutaneous		prn	as needed
	ID	intradermal		qh	every hour
	IM	intramuscular		q(2,3,4,6,8)h	every (2, 3, 4, 6, 8) hours
	IV	intravenous			(q2h = every 2 hours)
	NAS	nasal		qid	four times a day
	po, PO	by mouth		tid	three times a day
	tinct	tincture		bid	twice a day
	ung.	ointment		qam	every morning
	sol., soln	solution		stat, STAT	immediately
	cap	capsule	**Medications**	ASA	aspirin
	tab(s)	tablet(s)		APAP	acetaminophen
Measurements	C	Celsius		Fe	iron
	F	Fahrenheit		K	potassium
	m	meter		MOM	milk of magnesia
	cm	centimeter		NS	normal saline
	mm	millimeter		NSAID	nonsteroidal anti-inflammatory drug
	kg	kilogram		OTC	over-the-counter (drugs)
	g	gram		PPD	purified protein derivative (tuberculin skin test)
	mg	milligram			
	mcg	microgram			
	L	liter	**Miscellaneous**	$\overline{aa}$	of each (used in prescriptions)
	mL	milliliter		aq	water
	gr	grain		$\overline{c}$	with
	gtt(s)	drop(s)		med	medicine
	lb	pound		NKA	no known allergies
	fl oz	fluid ounce		NKDA	no known drug allergies
	oz	ounce		NPO	nothing by mouth
	pt	pint		Pt, pt	patient
	qt	quart		qs	quantity sufficient
	Tbs, tbsp	tablespoon		Rx	take
	tsp	teaspoon		Sig	give the following directions
Timing	ac	before meals		$\overline{s}$	without
	pc	after meals		VO	verbal order
	ad lib	as desired		x	times
	d	day			
	AM, a.m.	morning			
	PM, p.m.	afternoon			
	noc, noct	night			
	h, hr	hour			
	min	minute			
	$\overline{p}$	after			

TABLE 14.6   Special Requirements for Controlled Substances

SCHEDULE	PRESCRIPTION SPECIFICS
I	Not currently used for medical purposes.
II/IIN (C–II)	Written prescription manually signed by the provider or an electronic prescription that meets all DEA requirements for electronic prescriptions for controlled substances. No refills. In some cases, the prescription can be faxed to the pharmacy. The medication cannot be dispensed until the original prescription is given to the pharmacy.
III/III N and IV (C–III, C–IV)	Call-in prescriptions, written prescriptions, and electronic prescriptions are allowed. Faxed prescriptions must be manually signed by the provider prior to faxing. Prescription good for 6 months. No more than five refills are allowed.
V (C–V)	Phoned prescriptions, written prescriptions, e-prescriptions, and faxed prescriptions allowed. Prescription is good for 12 months (e.g., non-narcotic prescriptions). Refill quantity is up to the provider.

TABLE 14.7   Common Over-the-Counter (OTC) Medications

MEDICATION: GENERIC NAME (BRAND/TRADE NAME)	CLASSIFICATION	INDICATION AND DESIRED EFFECT	ADVERSE REACTION(S)	DRUG INTERACTION(S)
aspirin ibuprofen (Advil, Motrin) naproxen (Aleve, Naprosyn)	Analgesics (nonsteroidal anti-inflammatory drugs [NSAIDs])	Inflammation and pain relief	GI bleeding, compromised renal function, tinnitus, diarrhea, and nausea	Antihypertensives, hyperglycemics, sulfa antibiotics, diuretics
acetaminophen (Tylenol)	Analgesic, antipyretic	Relief of pain and fever	Liver damage	Warfarin
pseudoephedrine (Sudafed)	Decongestant	Relief of nasal congestion caused by colds, allergies, and hay fever	Hypertension, vasospasm, arrhythmia, cerebrovascular accident	Antidepressant – monoamine oxidase inhibitors (MAOIs)
diphenhydramine (Benadryl)	Antihistamine	Cough, cold, allergy, and insomnia	Drowsiness, confusion, hallucinations, delirium	Acetaminophen with oxycodone, alprazolam, amitriptyline, metoprolol
dextromethorphan (Benylin and many DM cough and cold formulas)	Antitussive	Suppression of cough reflex	Dizziness, lethargy, nausea	Antidepressant – monoamine oxidase inhibitors (MAOIs)

TABLE 14.8   Commonly Used Herbal Supplements

NAME	USES	SIDE EFFECTS AND CAUTIONS
Acai	Weight loss and antiaging; antioxidant	Little scientific information about the safety of acai; no scientific evidence to support use for any health-related purpose; might affect magnetic resonance imaging (MRI) results.
Aloe vera	Aloe gel is used for burns, frostbite, psoriasis, and cold sores. It can also be taken orally for osteoarthritis, bowel diseases, and fever.	Topical use of aloe gel is likely to be safe. More studies are needed to determine the safety of oral preparations. People with diabetes should be cautioned against using aloe, as it may lower blood glucose levels.

TABLE 14.8   Commonly Used Herbal Supplements—*continued*

NAME	USES	SIDE EFFECTS AND CAUTIONS
Black cohosh	Relieve symptoms of menopause; treat menstrual irregularities and premenstrual syndrome; induce labor.	Headaches, gastric complaints, heaviness in the legs, weight problems; safety unknown for pregnant women or those with breast cancer.
Echinacea	Treat or prevent colds, flu, and other infections; believed to stimulate the immune system.	Most studies indicate echinacea does not appear to prevent colds or other infections; some people experience allergic reactions, including rashes, increased asthma, and anaphylaxis; gastrointestinal (GI) side effects.
Flaxseed	Flaxseed and flaxseed oil are used for constipation, diabetes, high cholesterol levels, cancer, and other conditions.	Few reported side effects; contains soluble fiber and is an effective laxative; both flaxseed and flaxseed oil can cause diarrhea. It is not recommended during pregnancy.
Garlic	Treat high cholesterol, heart disease, hypertension; prevent certain types of cancer, including stomach and colon cancer.	Some evidence indicates garlic can slightly lower blood cholesterol levels and may slow development of atherosclerosis; side effects include breath and body odor, heartburn, GI upset, and allergic reactions; acts as a mild anticoagulant (similar to aspirin); may increase the risk of bleeding; interferes with effectiveness of saquinavir, a drug used to treat human immunodeficiency virus (HIV) infection.
Ginger	Alleviate nausea associated with postoperative state, motion sickness, chemotherapy, and pregnancy; used for rheumatoid arthritis, osteoarthritis, and joint and muscle pain.	Short-term use can safely relieve pregnancy-related nausea and vomiting; also, may help with chemotherapy nausea and vomiting. Side effects most often reported are gas, bloating, heartburn, and nausea.
Asian ginseng	Support overall health and boost immune system; improve mental and physical performance; treat erectile dysfunction, hepatitis C, and menopause symptoms; lower blood glucose and control blood pressure.	Limited information available, more studies needed. May affect blood glucose levels and blood pressure; thus, patients should discuss this with their provider. May interact with certain medications, such as anticoagulants.
Ginkgo biloba	No conclusive evidence that it helps any health condition.	Side effects may include headache, stomach upset, and allergic skin reactions. Ginkgo may increase the risk of bleeding with pregnancy and in those on anticoagulants.
Green tea	Improve mental alertness, relieve digestive symptoms and headaches, promote weight loss; may have protective effects against heart disease and cancer.	Safe in moderate amounts; possible complications include liver problems with concentrated green tea extracts but not when used as a beverage. A specific green tea extract ointment is a prescription drug used for treating genital warts.
St. John's wort	Treat mental disorders and nerve pain; kidney and lung diseases, insomnia and wounds.	Some scientific evidence shows it helps treat mild to moderate depression; not effective in treating major depression. Side effects include photophobia (increased sensitivity to sunlight), anxiety, dry mouth, dizziness, GI symptoms, fatigue, headache, and sexual dysfunction. Can cause life-threatening reactions with certain medications. Drugs that can be affected include the following: • Antidepressants • Birth control pills • Cyclosporine (prevents rejection of transplants) • Digoxin (heart medication) • Some HIV and cancer medications • Warfarin and related anticoagulants

Modified from the National Center for Complementary and Alternative Medicine. *https://nccih.nih.gov/health/herbsataglance.htm.* Accessed September 23, 2018.

SUMMARY OF SCENARIO

Mark is enjoying working with Gabe. He is amazed at how much Gabe knows about medications that the providers commonly prescribe. Mark feels that he will never be as fluent with the medications as Gabe is. He even mentioned this to Gabe. His mentor laughed and said he felt the same way during his own practicum. Over the years, he has used drug reference materials to help him learn about medications. He has made it a practice to look up medications

he does not know. This helped him become more fluent. He assured Mark that if he was willing to read up on medications, he, too, will become fluent with them.

Mark is looking forward to administering medications with Gabe. Now that he understands how to use the drug reference materials, he will be working hard to learn the medications he encounters.

SUMMARY OF LEARNING OBJECTIVES

1. **Describe the sources and uses of drugs.**

   Drugs are either created from natural sources or made synthetically in a laboratory. Plants, animals, minerals, and microbiologic sources are natural sources of drugs. There are eight common uses of drugs: prevention, treatment, diagnosis, cure, contraceptive, health maintenance, palliative, and replacement.

2. **Describe pharmacokinetics, including absorption, distribution, metabolism, and excretion.**

   Pharmacokinetics is the study of drug absorption, distribution, metabolism, and excretion in the body. Absorption is the movement of drug from the site of administration to the bloodstream. The movement of absorbed drug from the blood to the body tissues is called *distribution*. Metabolism is a series of chemical processes whereby enzymes change drugs in the body. Excretion is the movement of the metabolites out of the body.

3. **Discuss drug action, including the factors that influence drug action, the therapeutic effects of drugs, and adverse reactions to drugs.**

   Drugs are chemicals that can cause changes in the cells. Four main drug actions are depressing, stimulating, destroying, and replacing substances. This chapter discussed the factors that influenced drug action, including age, body size, gender, genetics, diseases, diet, drug dosage, route, timing of administration, mental state, and environmental temperature. Each medication has one or more therapeutic effects or desired effects. This is the intended action of the medication. The person can experience an unexpected or life-threatening reaction, which is called an *adverse reaction*. Table 14.1 lists common adverse reactions.

4. **Explain drug legislation that is important in the ambulatory care setting. Also, discuss dietary supplements.**

   The Food, Drug, and Cosmetic Act is enforced by the Food and Drug Administration (FDA). The FDA is responsible for the safety, effectiveness, security, and quality of drugs, cosmetics, and food. The Controlled Substances Act (CSA), Title II of the Comprehensive Drug Abuse Prevention and Control Act of 1970, is a federal law. The DEA enforces the CSA. The DEA oversees the manufacturing, importation, possession, use, and distribution of illegal and legal controlled substances.

   Dietary supplements are oral products that contain a "dietary ingredient." This ingredient can include a vitamin, mineral, amino acid, herb, or another substance that can supplement a person's diet. The FDA monitors the safety of such products after they are on the market.

5. **Describe the four types of drug names.**

   The four types of drug names are:
   - *Chemical name*: Represents the drug's exact chemical formula.
   - *Generic name*: Assigned by the US Adopted Names (USAN) Council.
   - *Official name*: Used to list the medication in the United States Pharmacopeia and the National Formulary (USP–NF).
   - *Brand name*: Also called the *trade name*, used by one manufacturer.

6. **Describe various methods to access drug reference information.**

   Print drug references include package inserts and drug handbooks. Digital drug references include apps, products integrated with electronic health records, and online websites.

7. **Identify the classifications of medications, including the indications for use, desired effects, side effects, and adverse reactions.**

   Table 14.3 provides a list of classifications of medications with descriptions. Table 14.4 lists commonly prescribed medications and information on each, including the generic name, brand/trade name, class, schedule, indication, desired action, side effects, and adverse reactions.

8. **Discuss the terminology used in drug reference information, including describing the differences among biologic half-life, onset, peak, and duration.**

   The following terminology is typically found in drug reference information:
   - *Names:* Usually the generic name is listed with the trade names.
   - *Description:* Describes the medication and its general use.
   - *Boxed warning:* Addresses serious or life-threatening risks.
   - *Dosage:* Specifies the route, dose, and timing of the medication.
   - *Indication:* Conditions or diseases for which the drug is used.
   - *Dosage considerations:* Indicates recommended changes in dosages for special populations.
   - *How supplied:* Lists the form and the strength.
   - *Administration:* Provides information on how the medication should be administered.
   - *Contraindications:* Lists reasons or conditions that make administration of the drug improper or undesirable.

SUMMARY OF LEARNING OBJECTIVES—*continued*

- *Precautions*: Indicates necessary actions or special care that needs to be taken when the patient is on the medication.
- *Adverse reactions*: Also called *side effects* in some information. This section describes known undesirable experiences associated with the medication. Reactions may be divided into severe (life-threatening, serious reactions), moderate, and mild.
- *Interactions*: Includes medications, foods, and beverages that interact with the medication. These products may either increase or decrease the medication levels in the blood.
- *Action*: How the drug provides therapeutic results in the body, or the use of the drug.
- *Pharmacokinetics*: Provides information on the absorption, distribution, metabolism, and excretion of the medication.

The differences among biologic half-life, onset, peak, and duration:
- *Biologic half-life*: Time it takes half of the drug to be metabolized or eliminated by normal biologic processes
- *Onset*: The time it takes for the drug to produce a response
- *Peak*: The time it takes for the drug to reach its greatest effective concentration in the blood
- *Duration*: The time during which the drug is present in the blood at great enough levels to produce a response

9. **Discuss types of medication orders.**
   The provider can give the order over the phone or in person; this type of order is called a *verbal order*. The provider can also give the medical assistant a *written order* by using a prescription pad or in an electronic message. Besides describing medication orders by how they are given to the medical assistant, they can also be described by the type of order. Five types of medication orders are:
   - *Routine order*: Medication is taken at a regular interval until it is canceled or expired.
   - *Standing order*: Order applies to all patients who meet specific criteria.
   - *PRN order*: Medication is given on an "as needed" basis for specific signs and symptoms.
   - *Single order* or *one-time order*: Medication is administered one time.
   - *Stat order*: Medication is administered one time right now.

10. **List the four parts of a prescription and the information required for all prescriptions; prepare prescriptions using prescription refill procedures; and define commonly approved abbreviations.**
    There are four parts to a prescription: superscription, inscription, signature, and subscription. Fig. 14.1 describes the four parts of a prescription. All prescriptions need to include the date of issue; patient information; provider's full name and address; drug name, strength, and dosage form; quantity prescribed; directions for use; number of refills; NPI; and if a generic is acceptable.
    Procedure 14.1 describes how to prepare prescriptions using a prescription refill procedure.
    Table 14.5 provides commonly approved abbreviations regarding route, medication form, measurements, timing, and medications.

11. **Describe common requirements for scheduled substances.**
    - *Schedule I*: Not used.
    - *Schedule II*: Written prescription manually signed by the provider or an electronic prescription that meets all DEA requirements for electronic prescriptions for controlled substances. No refills.
    - *Schedules III and IV*: Call-in prescriptions, written prescriptions, and electronic prescriptions are allowed. Faxed prescriptions must be manually signed by the provider prior to faxing. Prescription good for 6 months. No more than five refills are allowed.
    - *Schedule V*: Phoned prescriptions, written prescriptions, e-prescriptions, and faxed prescriptions allowed. Prescription is good for 12 months (e.g., non-narcotic prescriptions). Refill quantity is up to the provider.
    Also refer to Table 14.6.

12. **Discuss over-the-counter (OTC) medications and herbal supplements.**
    Tables 14.7 and 14.8 provide information on the common OTC medications and herbal supplements.

PROCEDURE 14.1   Prepare a Prescription

Tasks: Prepare a prescription using a prescription refill protocol. Use approved abbreviations.

Scenario: You received a call from Noemi Rodriguez (DOB 11/04/1971). She is requesting refills on three of her prescriptions from Jean Burke, NP. She saw Jean Burke 10 months ago. Noemi has NKA. She is doing well with the prescriptions and has no concerns. You determine it is time for refills. Her prescriptions include Coumadin 5 mg, 1 tablet orally daily; Tenormin 50 mg, 1 tablet orally daily; and Plendil 5 mg, 1 tablet orally daily.

EQUIPMENT and SUPPLIES
- SimChart for the Medical Office (SCMO) or paper prescriptions and pen
- Prescription refill protocol (see Fig. 14.2)
- Drug reference book or online resource

PROCEDURAL STEPS
1. Using the scenario, look up the generic medication names using the drug reference book or online resource.
   PURPOSE: Generic names are typically used in the healthcare facility, though patients may give the brand name.

Continued

PROCEDURE 14.1   Prepare a Prescription—*continued*

2. Read the prescription refill protocol. Compare the generic names to the list of medications given. Identify medications that meet the protocol.
   PURPOSE: All the criteria need to be met for the medical assistant to prepare prescriptions using the prescription refill protocol.
3. Prepare prescriptions for refill according to the protocol using SCMO or paper prescriptions.
   a. Using SCMO: Search for the patient. Verify the date of birth before selecting the patient. On the INFO PANEL, select Phone Encounter. Complete the fields on the Create New Encounter window and save. Check the box beside the No Known Allergy statement on the allergy screen and save. Select Order Entry from the Record dropdown list and select Add in the Out-of-office section (see the following figures).

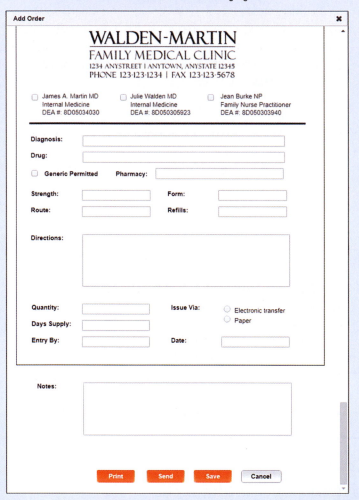

b. Using paper prescriptions: Add in the patient's complete name, date of birth, and address.
   PURPOSE: Most agencies using electronic health records require medical assistants to update the allergy screen when preparing refills. Prescriptions require the patient's name and address. If the DOB is available, add this to the prescription. An electronic health record will automatically add this information when it sends the prescription to the pharmacy.
4. Using the information in the scenario, complete the prescription information on either the paper prescription or in the SCMO fields. Use only approved abbreviations.
   PURPOSE: All information is required on the prescription for it to be accepted by the pharmacist and filled for the patient.
5. Complete any additional prescriptions as needed by the prescription refill protocol.
   PURPOSE: The patient requested refills on the medications indicated. Any medications that can be refilled should have prescriptions prepared for the provider.
6. Review the prescriptions for any errors. Void the prescription and redo if needed.
   PURPOSE: It is important to prepare accurate prescriptions. Any errors need to be fixed before giving the prescriptions to the provider.
   Note: After the provider signs the prescriptions and depending on the facility's policy, the medical assistant may need to document the refill in the health record. This cannot be done until the provider approves the prescriptions.

HEALTH INSURANCE ESSENTIALS

15

SCENARIO

Jon Bimmell, a registered medical assistant (RMA), has worked for Walden-Martin Family Medical Clinic (WMFM) for 3 years. Jon started with WMFM as a receptionist. Donna Potter, the office manager, recognized that Jon was very detail oriented, so, 2 years ago, she asked him to take charge of the health insurance policies and procedures manual for the practice.

Jon also trains all new medical assistants on how to verify patient health insurance coverage and eligibility. Because Jon has learned quite a bit about health insurance, he can answer most of the patients' questions about their coverage, benefits and/or the exclusions of their policies. He knows where to direct patients who have more complicated questions and how to follow up – one of the most important duties of a professional medical assistant. He has a great attitude about assisting patients with insurance questions and does not hesitate to call the insurance company on the patient's behalf.

He provides patients with exceptional customer service. When patients call him for assistance, he responds within 24 hours (often within 1 hour) with answers to their questions or a resource to help them. Jon is willing to help any staff member with other duties when necessary and prides himself on being a patient advocate. He is an enthusiastic team player who puts patients first.

While studying this chapter, think about the following questions:
- How important is the verification of services and benefits for reimbursement?
- How are private health insurance plans and government health insurance plans different?
- Why is it important to verify eligibility and preauthorize services before the patient appointment is scheduled?
- When and why is preauthorization necessary for patients who have a managed care health plan?
- Why is it important to educate patients on their health insurance benefits?

LEARNING OBJECTIVES

1. Discuss the purpose of health insurance and discuss the concept of cost-sharing.
2. List and discuss various government health insurance plans.
3. Summarize private health insurance plans.
4. Review traditional (fee-for-service) health insurance plans.
5. Differentiate among the different types of managed care models.
6. Outline managed care requirements for patient referral, obtain a referral with documentation, and discuss utilization management.
7. Describe the process for preauthorization and how to obtain preauthorization, including documentation.
8. Discuss participating provider contracts, including contracted fee schedules.
9. Interpret information on a health insurance identification (ID) card.
10. Explain the importance of verifying eligibility and be able to verify eligibility for services, including documentation.
11. Describe other types of insurance, including disability, life, long-term care, and liability insurance.
12. Discuss the Affordable Care Act's effect on patient healthcare access.

VOCABULARY

beneficiary A designated person who receives funds from an insurance policy.

capitation (ka pi TAY shun) A payment arrangement for healthcare providers.

claim A formal request for payment from an insurance company for services provided.

explanation of benefits (EOB) A document sent by the insurance company to the provider and the patient explaining the allowed charge amount, the amount reimbursed for services, and the patient's financial responsibilities.

fee schedule A list of fixed fees for services.

gatekeeper The primary care provider, who is in charge of a patient's treatment. Additional treatment, such as referrals to a specialist, must be approved by the gatekeeper.

health insurance exchange An online marketplace where people can compare and buy individual health insurance plans. State health insurance exchanges were established as part of the Affordable Care Act.

indigent (IN di jent) Poor, needy, impoverished.

online insurance Web portal An online service provided by various insurance companies that allows providers to look up a patient's insurance benefits, eligibility, claims status, and explanation of benefits.

policy A written agreement between two parties in which one party (the insurance company) agrees to pay another party (the patient) if certain specified circumstances occur.

preauthorization A process required by some insurance carriers in which the provider obtains permission to perform certain procedures or services.

premium The amount paid or to be paid by the policyholder for coverage under the contract, usually in periodic installments.

preexisting condition A health problem that was present before new health insurance coverage started.

provider network An approved list of physicians, hospitals, and other providers.

Qualified Medicare Beneficiaries (QMBs) Low-income Medicare patients who qualify for Medicaid for their secondary insurance.

referral An order from a primary care provider for the patient to see a specialist or to get certain medical services.

resource-based relative value system (RBRVS) A system used to determine how much providers should be paid for services provided. It is used by Medicare and many other health insurance companies.

third-party administrator (TPA) An organization that processes claims and provides administrative services for another organization. Often used by self-funded plans.

utilization management A decision-making process used by managed care organizations to manage healthcare costs. It involves case-by-case assessments of the appropriateness of care.

waiting period The length of time a patient waits for disability insurance to pay after the date of injury.

Insurance is something that is purchased to help protect against loss or harm from specified circumstances. Using automobile insurance as an example, the specified circumstances are those related to a car accident. The insurance could pay for damage done to your vehicle or other vehicles. It could also pay for medical expenses for anyone injured in the accident. With health insurance, the specified circumstances are those related to the policyholder's health. This insurance would pay for hospital expenses, provider expenses, and certain supplies and equipment.

A **policy** is purchased with a **premium** or payment. The premium can be paid by an individual, an employer, or a combination of employer contribution and individual (employee) contribution.

The policy is considered a legal contract and will stay in force as long as the premium is being paid. The policy will specify exactly what services are covered. The more services that are covered, the higher the premium cost. The person responsible for the payment of the premium is referred to as a *subscriber*.

Most policies require the patient to pay a portion of the healthcare expenses. This is referred to as *cost-sharing*, which includes the following:

- *Deductible*: A set dollar amount that the policyholder must pay before the insurance company starts to pay for services. It can be as low as $100 and as high as $5,000. The higher the deductible, the lower the premium.
- *Co-insurance*: After the deductible has been met, the policyholder may need to pay a certain percentage of the bill and the insurance company pays the rest. A typical split is 80/20 – the insurance company pays 80%, and the policyholder pays 20%.
- *Copayment*: A set dollar amount that the policyholder must pay for each office visit. Copayments may differ for different types of office visits. For example, there can be one copayment amount for a primary care provider and a different copayment amount (usually higher) to see a specialist or to be seen in the emergency department.

The policy will specify the dollar amounts for the deductible, co-insurance, and copayment. The premium is not usually considered part of cost-sharing.

In order for the insurance carrier to pay for services, a **claim** must be submitted. The claim is reviewed by the insurance company to determine if the services provided are covered under the policy. It is important for a medical assistant to be familiar with the different types of insurance so that claims can be submitted accurately. This will result in faster payment for the healthcare facility.

BENEFITS

The federal government requires all health plans to cover essential health benefits. There are 10 categories of essential health benefits:

- Ambulatory patient services
- Hospitalization
- Mental health and substance use disorder services
- Prescription drugs
- Preventive and wellness services and chronic disease management
- Emergency services
- Maternity and newborn care
- Rehabilitative and habilitative services and devices
- Laboratory services
- Pediatric services, including oral and vision care

In addition to the essential health benefits, an insurance policy may cover other services. For a group policy, an employer can pick and choose the benefits it wants for employees, such as vision or dental coverage. Medical assistants should contact an insurance company to determine if certain services are covered under a patient's policy.

HEALTH INSURANCE PLANS

There are two types of health insurance plans in the United States:

- Government health insurance plans
- Private health insurance plans

Health insurance plans typically cover health services and procedures that are deemed medically necessary. *Medically necessary* services are those that are necessary to improve the patient's current health. Most insurance policies do not cover elective procedures. *Elective procedures* are medical procedures that are not deemed medically necessary, such as a facelift or another cosmetic procedure. The Affordable Care Act (ACA) states that health insurance plans must cover preventive care. *Preventive care* includes services provided to help prevent certain illnesses or that lead to an early diagnosis. Insurance companies must cover preventive care services and cannot impose cost-sharing for those services.

Preventive Care Services

- Alcohol misuse screening
- Blood pressure screening
- Cholesterol screening
- Colorectal cancer screening
- Depression screening
- Diabetes (type 2) screening
- Diet counseling
- Hepatitis B and C screening
- Human immunodeficiency virus (HIV) screening
- Immunization vaccines
- Lung cancer screening
- Obesity screening and counseling
- Tobacco use screening
- Sexually transmitted infection (STI) prevention counseling

Government Health Insurance Plans

Government health insurance plans provide coverage with reduced or no monthly premiums for the **indigent**, the elderly, the military,

and government employees. There are a number of different plans, but patients need to qualify by:

- Age
- Income
- Government occupation
- Health condition

A patient who is age 65 or older can qualify for *Medicare*. A low-income patient may be eligible for *Medicaid*. Dependents of military personnel are covered by *TRICARE*. Surviving spouses and dependent children of veterans who died in the line of duty are covered by the *Civilian Health and Medical Program of the Veterans Administration* (CHAMPVA). Employees who are injured or become ill due to work-related issues are covered under *workers' compensation insurance*.

Medicare

Medicare is a federal health insurance program that provides healthcare coverage for individuals who are age 65 or older; people who are disabled; and patients who have been diagnosed with end-stage renal disease (ESRD). Medicare refers to those covered by Medicare as *beneficiaries*. Medicare currently is the world's largest insurance program. In 2017 there were more than 58 million beneficiaries. The Medicare program is administered by the Centers for Medicare and Medicaid Services (CMS), a division of the Department of Health and Human Services (HHS). Laws enacted by Congress regulate the Medicare program.

The Medicare plan is divided into four parts (Table 15.1):

- Part A covers inpatient hospital charges. It is financed with special contributions deducted from employed individuals' salaries, with matching contributions from their employers. Due to these contributions and regular Social Security contributions, there is no monthly premium for Part A.
- Part B covers ambulatory care, including primary care and specialists. Beneficiaries are required to pay a monthly premium. Beneficiaries can visit any specialist without a referral.

TABLE 15.1 Comparing Medicare Plans

	COVERED SERVICES	MONTHLY PREMIUM	DEDUCTIBLE
Part A	Inpatient hospital care, skilled nursing facilities, home health care, and hospice services	$0	$1,340 deductible for each benefit period (2018); Days 1–60: $0 co-insurance for each benefit period; Days 61–90: $335 co-insurance per day of each benefit period; Day 91 and beyond: $670 co-insurance per each "lifetime reserve day" after day 90 for each benefit period (up to 60 days over a lifetime)
Part B	Outpatient hospital care, durable medical equipment, provider's services, and other medical services	$134	$183 (2018), plus 20% co-insurance for all medical services
Part C	Expanded inpatient hospital and outpatient hospital care benefits	Varies by plan	Varies by plan
Part D	Prescription drugs	Varies by income	Varies by plan

From Medicare: Medicare Costs at a Glance. *https://www.medicare.gov/your-medicare-costs/costs-at-a-glance/costs-at-glance.html.* Accessed July 29, 2018.

- Part C is an option for Medicare-qualified patients to turn their Part A and Part B benefits into a private plan that can offer some additional benefits. The private plan must cover everything that would be covered under Part A and Part B.
- Part D is a prescription drug program offered to Medicare-qualified individuals that requires an additional monthly premium.

Basic medical coverage for Medicare Part B is 80% of the allowed amount after the deductible. This means that patients are responsible for the remaining 20%. The allowed amount is determined using a **resource-based relative value scale (RBRVS)**. Some patients choose to purchase a private supplemental health insurance policy to help cover the 20%. These policies can also pay for services not covered by Medicare. These supplemental health insurance plans are known as *Medigap* policies. Federal regulations now require Medicare supplement policies to be uniform to avoid confusion for the purchaser.

CRITICAL THINKING APPLICATION   **15.1**

Jana Green is a Medicare patient who has Part A and Part B coverage. Will Medicare cover her office visit with a cardiologist? What percent of the bill will she be responsible for?

The fee schedule for Medicare Part B is determined using the RBRVS. This system consists of three parts:
- Provider work
- Charge-based professional liability expenses
- Charge-based overhead

The provider work component includes the degree of effort and time needed by a provider to perform a particular service or procedure. The professional liability and overhead components are computed by the CMS.

The RBRVS fee schedule is designed to provide nationally uniform payments to healthcare providers. Payments are adjusted to reflect the differences in practice costs across geographic areas. The fee schedule includes a conversion factor, which is a single national number applied to all services paid under the fee schedule. Conversion factors are set by Congress and changed annually, at the request of the CMS.

Depending on the contract between the provider and the insurance carrier (especially Medicare, Medicaid, and other government programs), the provider writes off the difference between the RBRVS schedule and his or her fee.

Contracts between the provider of service and the insurance company vary greatly, depending on the insurance. It is important for the medical assistant to know the contract terms for each insurance company. As insurance payments are received, the medical assistant should examine the **explanation of benefits (EOB)** closely to ensure that all benefits have been reimbursed correctly.

Medicaid

Medicaid is the government program that provides medical care for the indigent. This program is funded by both federal and state governments to provide medical care for people meeting specific eligibility criteria. All states and the District of Columbia have Medicaid programs, but program specifics vary by state. A person eligible for

Medicaid in one state may not be eligible in another state, and covered medical services may differ.

The federal government provides funding to each state for Medicaid programs. To receive this funding, each state is required to cover certain services. The individual states decide what additional services will be covered.

Mandatory Medicaid Benefits

In order to receive federal funds for Medicaid, each state Medicaid plan must cover the following services:
- Inpatient hospital services
- Outpatient hospital services
- Nursing facility services
- Early and periodic screening, diagnostic, and treatment (EPSDT) services
- Home health services
- Physician services
- Rural health clinic service
- Federally qualified health center services
- Laboratory and x-ray services
- Family planning services
- Nurse midwife services
- Certified pediatric and family nurse practitioner services
- Freestanding birth center services
- Transportation to medical care
- Tobacco cessation counseling for pregnant women

From Medicaid: List of Medicaid Benefits. *https://www.medicaid.gov/medicaid/benefits/list-of-benefits/index.html.* Accessed July 29, 2018.

An ambulatory care facility has the right to limit the number of Medicaid patients it accepts into the practice. The medical office cannot pick and choose which Medicaid patients they are willing to see. There can be no discrimination based on age, gender, race, religious preference, or national origin. The Medicaid **fee schedule** is the lowest of all insurance companies, and it may not be in the medical office's financial interest to accept a large number of Medicaid patients. A provider who accepts Medicaid patients automatically agrees to accept Medicaid's allowed amount as payment in full for covered services. Some patients who are eligible for Medicaid are required to pay a copayment. The provider can collect the copayment from the patient but cannot bill for any amount over the allowed amount.

Eligibility for benefits is determined by the respective states, but most Medicaid recipients also are some or all of the following:
- Low-income families
- Qualified pregnant women and children
- Recipients of Temporary Assistance for Needy Families (TANF)
- Individuals who receive Supplemental Security Income (SSI)
- Individuals who receive certain types of federal and state aid
- Individuals who are **Qualified Medicare Beneficiaries (QMBs)** – Medicaid pays for Medicare Part B premiums, deductibles, and co-insurance for qualified low-income elderly individuals
- Individuals in institutions or receiving long-term care in nursing facilities and intermediate-care facilities

Government Managed Care Plans

In an effort to reduce costs and increase the delivery of efficient care, Medicare and many Medicaid programs offer their members the option to join a managed care plan. These managed care plans must cover all services that would be covered under Medicare or Medicaid. The identification cards will look just like the ones issued to people not on Medicare or Medicaid. The government managed care plan may have a copayment that the patient would be responsible for.

Children's Health Insurance Program

The Children's Health Insurance Program (CHIP) is a state-funded program for children whose family income is above the Medicaid qualifying income limits. Although Medicaid does not typically have a premium, CHIP does. The premiums are typically 5% of the family monthly income. State CHIP programs cover:

- routine checkups
- immunizations
- doctor visits
- prescriptions
- dental care and vision care
- inpatient and outpatient hospital care
- laboratory tests and x-ray services
- emergency services

CHIP programs are similar to managed care plans in that care is covered only through the designated network of providers. There are smaller copayments for medical services for CHIP patients.

TRICARE

TRICARE is the comprehensive healthcare program for uniformed service members and retirees and their families. Members of the National Guard/Reserve and their families can also be covered under TRICARE.

The TRICARE program is managed by the military in partnership with civilian hospitals and clinics. It is designed to:
- expand access to health care
- ensure high-quality care
- promote medical readiness

All military hospitals and clinics are part of the TRICARE program and offer high-quality health care at a low cost. TRICARE offers two types of plans:
- TRICARE Prime
- TRICARE Select

Review Table 15.2 for a comparison of the TRICARE plans.

Civilian Health and Medical Program of the Veterans Administration

CHAMPVA, a health benefits program similar to TRICARE, provides coverage for the families of veterans who were permanently disabled or killed in the line of duty. The Department of Veterans Affairs (VA) shares the cost of certain healthcare services and supplies with eligible beneficiaries.

Workers' Compensation

Workers' compensation is an insurance plan for individuals who are injured on the job or become ill due to job-related circumstances. An example of a job-related illness would be mesothelioma caused by inhaling asbestos. The insurance plan covers:

- medical care and rehabilitation benefits
- weekly income replacement benefits
- death benefits to dependents

The provider accepts the workers' compensation reimbursements as payment in full and does not bill the patient. Time limitations are set for the prompt reporting of workers' compensation cases. The employee is obligated to promptly notify the employer. The employer must then notify the insurance company and refer the employee to a healthcare provider.

All 50 states have passed workers' compensation laws to protect workers against the loss of wages and the cost of medical care resulting from an occupational accident or disease, as long as the employee was not proven negligent. State laws differ regarding employees who are included, and the benefits provided by workers' compensation insurance. Federal and state legislatures require employers to maintain workers' compensation coverage to meet minimum standards, covering most employees, for work-related illnesses and injuries. The purpose of workers' compensation laws is to provide prompt medical care to an injured or ill worker so that the person may be restored to health and return to full earning capacity in as short a time as possible.

Private Health Insurance Plans

Health insurance plans that are available from commercial insurance companies are considered private plans. The majority of people are part of an employer group plan. Those that are not eligible for an employer plan can purchase insurance on their own. This is referred to as an *individual health insurance plan*. Most private plans use managed care to reduce the costs of delivering quality health care.

Employer Group Plans

Many businesses offer a *group policy*, a private health insurance plan purchased by an employer for a group of employees. These plans can cover the employee, his or her spouse (i.e., domestic partner), and their children. Typically, an employer pays a certain percentage of the premium for full-time employees. This makes the cost of the insurance plan more affordable for the employee. Part-time employees can be part of the group policy, but most employers do not pay a part of the premium for part-time employees. Employers also determine the health insurance benefits under the group policy. Health insurance monthly premiums and benefits can vary from employer to employer. For example, the health insurance plan for Employer A covers chiropractic care, but the health insurance plan for Employer B does not. The premium for a group policy is usually lower than that for an individual plan because of the large pool of employees. The insurance company will receive premiums from a larger number of people, and just a few of them will need a lot of services. The employees' share of the premium is often paid through payroll deductions.

Self-Funded Group Health Plans

Many large companies or organizations have enough employees that they can fund their own insurance program. This is called a *self-funded plan*. Technically, a self-funded plan does not fit the true definition of insurance. The employer pays employee healthcare costs from the funds collected from employee monthly premiums. Usually, the costs of benefits and premiums for self-funded plans are similar to those for group plans. Self-funded plans tend to work best for companies that are large enough to offer good benefit coverage and reasonable

TABLE 15.2   Comparing TRICARE Plans

ACTIVE DUTY FAMILY MEMBERS

	TRICARE PRIME	TRICARE SELECT
Annual deductible	None	$150/individual or $300/family for E-5 and above; $50/$100 for E-4 and below
Annual enrollment fee	None	None currently; 1/1/2020 $150/individual or $300/family
Civilian outpatient visit	No cost	Primary Care – $21 Specialty – $31
Civilian inpatient admission	No cost	$18.60 a day ($25 minimum)
Civilian inpatient mental health	No cost	$18.60 a day ($25 minimum)
Civilian inpatient skilled nursing facility care	$0 per diem charge per admission; no separate copayment/cost-share for separately billed professional charges	$18.60 a day ($25 minimum)

RETIREES (UNDER 65), THEIR FAMILY MEMBERS, AND OTHERS

	TRICARE PRIME	TRICARE SELECT
Annual deductible	None	$150/individual or $300/family
Annual enrollment fee	$289.08/individual or $578.16/family	None
Civilian copays	None	20% of negotiated fee
Outpatient emergency care mental health visit	$12 per visit	$20 Primary $30 Specialty
Civilian inpatient cost-share	$11 a day ($25 minimum) charge per admission	Lesser of $250 a day or 25% of negotiated charges plus 20% of negotiated professional fees
Civilian inpatient skilled nursing facility care	$11 a day ($25 minimum) charge per admission	$250 per diem copayment or 20% cost-share of total charges for institutional care, whichever is less, plus 20% cost-share of separately billed professional charges

From TRICARE: Health Plan Costs. *https://tricare.mil/Costs/HealthPlanCosts.* Accessed July 29, 2018.

premium rates and are able to pay large claims for expensive medical services. Often a **third-party administrator (TPA)** handles paperwork and claim payments for a self-insured group.

Self-funded health care is an arrangement in which an employer provides health or disability benefits to employees with its own funds. This is different from fully insured plans, in which the employer contracts with an insurance company to cover the employees and dependents. In self-funded health care, the employer assumes the direct risk for payment of the claims for benefits. The terms of eligibility and coverage are stated in the insurance plan document, which includes provisions similar to those found in a typical group health insurance policy.

Individual Health Insurance Plans

An individual health insurance plan is one that is not offered by an employer or another group. An individual policy can cover just one person or a family. These policies can be purchased through a **health insurance exchange** or directly from an insurance company. Premiums for an individual plan are generally higher than for a group plan.

HEALTH INSURANCE MODELS

There are basically two different models of health insurance today:
- Traditional health insurance
- Managed care organizations

You can find these options in both employer group plans and individual plans.

Traditional Health Insurance

Traditional health insurance plans pay for all or a share of the cost of covered services, regardless of which provider, hospital, or other licensed healthcare provider is used. Because providers are paid for each office visit, test, procedure, or other service they deliver, traditional insurance plans are often called *fee-for-service plans*. This was the first type of health insurance. Traditional health insurance plans provide the most flexibility for the patient but are also the costliest option.

Policyholders of fee-for-service plans and their dependents choose when and where to get healthcare services. When the policy is purchased, the subscriber is often given a fee schedule, which explains the benefit payment amounts. Benefits are usually paid to the insured, unless that person has authorized payment to be made directly to the provider. This is referred to as *assignment of benefits*.

The fee schedule amounts can be determined by a process called *usual, customary, and reasonable* (UCR). UCR is the amount paid for a medical service in a geographic area based on what providers in the area usually charge for the same of similar service.

Managed Care Organizations

Managed care organizations (MCOs) are health insurance companies whose goal is to provide quality, cost-effective care to its members. MCOs negotiate reduced rates with contracted providers and hospitals. In return, the managed care plan increases the provider's patient load. Many MCOs require the patient to choose a *primary care provider* (PCP), who coordinates the patient's care. Managed care plans can also require **referrals** for their patients to be treated by a specialist, thus limiting patient access to more expensive care. The **preauthorization** process can further control patient care costs. Medical care, testing, or medication therapy is provided only when it is justified to the health insurance plan. It is important that medical assistants be familiar with the various models of managed care to fully understand their effects on healthcare costs.

Models of Managed Care Organizations

Patient care is coordinated through a network of providers and hospitals. There are different types of managed care plans, such as health maintenance organizations (HMOs), preferred provider organizations (PPOs), and exclusive provider organizations (EPOs). They provide health care in return for scheduled payments and coordinate health care through a defined network of PCPs, hospitals, and other providers.

Health Maintenance Organization. HMOs are health plans that are regulated by HMO laws, which require them to include preventive care as part of their benefits package. The goal of the HMO health

insurance plan is to reduce the cost of health care while still providing quality health care. HMO plans typically have the lowest monthly premiums among other health insurance plans. The patient's out-of-pocket expenses are also very low. Patients are not required to pay a deductible or co-insurance.

Patients are required to select a PCP, who acts as the **gatekeeper** to more specialized care. The insurance plan will not pay for services that are not included in its **provider network**; patients are 100% financially responsible for medical expenses incurred outside the HMO network of providers. For example, patients wanting to visit the dermatologist for eczema must visit their PCP first; they would be fully responsible financially if they made an appointment with a dermatologist directly. The PCP can either treat the patient or refer him or her to the specialist.

PCPs receive financial incentives when they reduce the cost of patient care. In the earlier example, prescribing medicine to the patient is more cost-effective than referring the patient to the specialist. HMOs always require:

- referrals from the PCP to specialists
- precertification and preauthorization for hospital admissions, outpatient procedures, and treatments (Fig. 15.1).

HMOs can be set up using several different models. The payment structure can be different for each of those models (Table 15.3).

CRITICAL THINKING APPLICATION   15.2

Noemi Rodriguez, a patient, calls to make an appointment with the endocrinologist because she is having trouble managing her diabetes. She tells Jon over the phone when she is making the appointment that she has Aetna HMO. Will Jon be able to schedule Ms. Rodriguez's appointment with the endocrinologist? Why or why not? What would she need to make an appointment?

Preferred Provider Organization. A PPO is a managed care network that contracts with a group of providers. The providers agree on a predetermined list of charges for all services, including those for both normal and complex procedures. The PPO model of managed health care uses the fee-for-service concept that many providers prefer. Typically, the patient's financial responsibilities represent, on average, 20% to 25% of the allowed charge, but this depends on the patient's

TABLE 15.3   Health Maintenance Organization (HMO) Models

MODEL	STRUCTURE	PAYMENT STRUCTURE
Independent practice association (IPA)	General or family practice provider or provider group that practices independently and may contract with several HMOs. Can see patients outside of the HMO.	**Capitation** or fee-for-service
Staff	One or more providers hired by an HMO. Providers see only HMO patients.	Salaried
Group	Multispecialty group with or without a primary care provider (PCP; i.e., gatekeeper); may contract with several HMOs.	Capitation or fee-for-service
Network	HMOs contract with multiple provider groups. Those providers can see patients outside of the HMO. Provides wider geographic coverage for members.	Capitation or fee-for-service

Preauthorization Request Form

**TO BE COMPLETED BY
PRIMARY CARE PHYSICIAN
OR OUTSIDE PROVIDER**

☐ Medicare ☑ Blue Cross/Blue Shield ☐ Tricare ☐ Health Net
☐ Medicaid ☐ Aetna ☐ Cigna ☐ Other
Group No.: 54098XX

Name: (First, Middle Initial, Last) Louann Campbell   Date: 7-14-20XX
☐ Male ☑ Female   Birthdate: 4-7-1952   Home Telephone Number: (555) 450-1666
Address: 2516 Encina Avenue, Woodland Hills, XY 12345-0439
Primary Care Physician: Gerald Practon, MD
Referring Physician: Gerald Practon, MD
Referred to: Raymond Skeleton, MD   Office Telephone number: (555) 486-9002
Address: 4567 Broad Avenue, Woodland Hills, XY 12345
Diagnosis Code: M54.5   Diagnosis: Low back pain
Diagnosis Code: M51.27   Diagnosis: Sciatica
Treatment Plan: Orthopedic consultation and evaluation of lumbar spine; R/O herniated disc L4-5
Authorization requested for: ☐ Consult only ☐ Treatment Only ☐ Consult/Treatment
☑ Consult/Procedure/Surgery ☐ Diagnostic Tests
Procedure Code: 99244   Description: New patient consultation
Procedure Code: Description:
Place of service: ☑ Office ☐ Outpatient ☑ Inpatient ☐ Other   Number of visits: 1
Facility: Length of stay:
List of potential future consultants (i.e., anesthetists, surgical assistants, or medical/surgical):
Physician's Signature: *Gerald Practon, MD*

TO BE COMPLETED BY PRIMARY CARE PHYSICIAN
PCP Recommendations: See above   PCP Initials: GP
Date eligibility checked: 7-14-20XX   Effective Date: 1-15-20XX

TO BE COMPLETED BY UTILIZATION MANAGEMENT
Authorized: Auth. No.   Not Authorized:
Deferred: Modified:
Effective Date: Expiration Date:

FIGURE 15.1 Preauthorization Request Form.

health insurance policy. A provider who joins a PPO does not need to change the manner of providing care and continues to treat and bill patients on a fee-for-service basis. When a patient covered under a PPO plan comes for treatment, the provider treats the patient and bills the PPO. Patients do not need to visit their PCP to obtain a referral to a specialist for more specialized care. And, they typically have more control over healthcare choices.

PPOs provide their subscribers with a list of participating providers and healthcare facilities from which they can access in-network health care at PPO reduced rates. Rates are quite often lower than those charged to non-PPO patients. This gives the patient more choices for providers. If the patient chooses to see a provider that is not in the PPO network, the deductible, co-insurance, and copayments will be higher.

Although patients have the option to visit a specialist when they feel the need, they are still required to obtain preauthorization for more expensive services, such as diagnostic imaging.

CRITICAL THINKING APPLICATION   **15.3**

Diego Lupez calls Jon; he is upset because he received a patient statement with a balance owing. He tells Jon that he has full-coverage insurance through his employer, and he does not know why he has a balance. What information can Jon share with Mr. Lupez to explain his financial responsibility?

Exclusive Provider Organization. An EPO combines features of an HMO (e.g., an enrolled group or population, PCPs, and an authorization system) and a PPO (e.g., flexible benefit design and fee-for-service payments). Patients with EPO coverage will not be covered for services outside the designated network of providers (unless there is an emergency), but they may not need to obtain a referral for specialized care. Unlike HMO members, EPO plan members are not required to choose a PCP.

Table 15.4 compares the different types of managed care plans.

TABLE 15.4   Managed Care Plans

PLAN	PROVIDERS	ACCESS TO SPECIALIZED CARE	DEDUCTIBLE, CO-INSURANCE, COPAYMENT
Health maintenance organization (HMO)	Must see only HMO providers and choose a primary care provider (PCP).	Referral required for specialized care.	Usually no deductible or co-insurance. Copayments required for office visits and prescriptions.
Preferred provider organization (PPO)	No PCP required. There is a network of providers, but out-of-network providers can be seen.	No referral required. Preauthorization needed for expensive services.	Lower deductible and co-insurance if an in-network provider is used. Copayments required for office visits and prescriptions.
Exclusive provider organization (EPO)	Must see network providers. No PCP required.	No referral needed.	Usually no deductible or co-insurance. Copayments required for office visits and prescriptions.

Referrals

Patients seeking specialized care must first visit their assigned PCP to obtain a referral to a specialist or for more specialized therapy or care. Patients with HMO plans can only obtain a referral to the specialist by visiting their assigned PCP. HMOs will measure how many patients are referred to specialists by individual PCPs. Approval or denial of a referral can take anywhere from a few minutes to a few days. There are three types of referrals:

- A *regular referral,* which usually takes 3 to 10 working days for review and approval. This type of referral is used when the provider believes that the patient must see a specialist to continue treatment.
- An *urgent referral,* which usually takes about 24 hours for approval. This type of referral is used when an urgent but not life-threatening situation occurs.
- A *STAT referral,* which can be approved online when it is submitted to the utilization review department through the provider's Web portal. A STAT referral is used in an emergency situation as indicated by the provider.

A *regular referral* is the most common type and can be inconvenient for the patient. With most managed care plans, preauthorization needs to be obtained for a referral. Remember this cardinal rule: never tell the patient the referral has been approved unless you have a hard copy of the authorization. A referral is authorized after the approval has been received. When a referral is approved, the PCP's office and the patient should receive a copy of the authorization. Always review the authorization thoroughly and confirm details, such as approved diagnosis and procedure codes and the exact period of time the authorization lasts. The patient will receive a letter with an authorization number and details regarding the approved services. The patient must bring the authorization to the specialist's office on the date of his or her appointment.

Utilization Management/Utilization Review

Utilization management is a form of patient care review by healthcare professionals who do not provide the care but are employed by health insurance companies. It is a necessary component of managed care to control costs. A *utilization review committee* reviews individual cases to ensure that medical care services are medically necessary.

For this committee to function properly, having the correct diagnosis code is critical. This committee also reviews all provider referrals and cases of emergency department visits and urgent care. For referrals, the committee reviews the referral and either approves or denies it, so it is important to submit accurate documentation. The medical assistant should contact the utilization review department directly; it should never be left to the patient to contact this department.

Precertification/Preauthorization

In an effort to control costs, many MCOs require precertification for certain procedures and services. Precertification is the process of proving to the insurance company that the service is medically necessary. The insurance company, in turn, will determine if it is a covered service and what the reimbursement will be. Precertification must be done before the procedure or service is performed.

To obtain precertification, the medical assistant:

- calls the provider services phone number on the back of the patient's health insurance ID card.
- provides the insurance company with procedures and/or services requested and the diagnoses.
- documents the outcome of the call in the patient's health record, including the precertification number.

Precertification does not guarantee payment of services. The process ensures that both the healthcare provider and the patient are informed both of the amount that the insurance company will pay and also the amount that the patient will have to pay.

Each insurance company has its own precertification requirements. Almost every MCO requires precertification, but medical assistants must confirm this by contacting the insurance company. Successful medical billers are diligent in obtaining precertification.

The precertification and preauthorization processes are very similar. The insurance company is contacted after the primary care provider recommends the procedure or service. In fact, many health insurance companies use the terms precertification and preauthorization interchangeably. However, precertification specifically determines whether the procedure is medically necessary, and preauthorization gives the provider approval to render the medical service. Precertification and preauthorization can be requested through an insurance company's online Web portal.

Precertification/Preauthorization Examples

1. Dr. David Kahn is the primary care provider (PCP) for Janine Butler, who has heartburn that has not improved with medication.
2. Because Ms. Butler's condition is not improving, Dr. Kahn requests preauthorization for her to see Dr. Eduard Hamilton, a gastrointestinal (GI) specialist. Ms. Butler is insured by a managed care organization (MCO).
3. The MCO authorizes Ms. Butler to see Dr. Hamilton; this authorization is sent to Ms. Butler, Dr. Kahn, and Dr. Hamilton. When Ms. Butler receives the authorization, she schedules an appointment with Dr. Hamilton.
4. After evaluating Ms. Butler, Dr. Hamilton orders an esophageal **endoscopy**. However, Ms. Butler is concerned about her financial responsibility. Therefore, Dr. Hamilton's office requests precertification for the endoscopy on Ms. Butler's behalf.
5. The MCO notifies Dr. Hamilton that the plan would reimburse a total of $1,500, and Ms. Butler would be financially responsible for $400. The precertification is sent both to Dr. Hamilton and Ms. Butler, who agree to its financial terms and schedule the procedure.

PARTICIPATING PROVIDER CONTRACTS

With all government health plans and most private health plans, healthcare providers must become *participating providers* (PARs). These providers are contracted with the insurance plan and have agreed to accept the contracted fee schedule as payment in full. Healthcare providers can apply to become PARs through a process called *credentialing*. Credentialing is the process of confirming the healthcare provider's qualifications, including the healthcare provider's license to practice medicine, affiliated organizations, and his or her education and professional background.

Once the healthcare provider is credentialed, the health insurance plan issues a contract to become an in-network PAR. The contract includes a fee schedule that the health insurance company will use to reimburse the provider for health services provided. By signing the contract, the provider agrees to accept the health insurance plan's fee schedule, even if it is lower than the provider's fee schedule.

Contracted Fee Schedules

Payment for services is typically made after the health services are provided. Once the service has been provided to the patient, the healthcare provider must submit a health insurance claim, which includes the diagnosis and procedure codes, in addition to the total charges. Although the healthcare provider establishes his or her own fee schedule, health insurance plans maintain their own rates at which they reimburse. When the provider becomes a participating provider, he or she agrees to the insurance plan's fee schedule and will not collect more than that amount.

When setting up a fee schedule a healthcare provider considers three things:
• Time
• Expertise
• Services

In every case, healthcare providers must place an estimate on the value of these services. Fees for medical procedures and services differ from office to office based on the type of practice. An office visit with a family practice provider may cost less than an office visit with a specialist. In the past, most providers worked on a fee-for-service basis; that is, patients were charged for the provider's service based on each individual service performed.

In recent years, health insurance plans, particularly government plans and managed healthcare organizations, have greatly influenced what healthcare providers can be reimbursed by establishing the allowable charge. The *allowable charge* is the maximum dollar amount that the insurance plan will pay for a procedure or service. The patient cannot be charged for the amount above the allowable charge if the provider and/or the healthcare facility is a PAR.

THE MEDICAL ASSISTANT'S ROLE

A medical assistant can be involved in many different tasks related to health insurance. Being familiar with the technology and forms that are used will make you more efficient at your job.

Health Insurance Identification Card

When a patient is enrolled in a health insurance plan, he or she will be issued a health insurance ID card that supplies the following information:

• Health insurance company
• Health plan type
• Subscriber identification number
• Co-pay amounts
• Health plan name
• Subscriber's name and covered dependents
• Policy group number
• Health plan contact phone numbers

The medical assistant must be able to identify all of the information provided on the health insurance identification card. To ensure that the person with the insurance card is actually the person named on the card, the medical assistant also should ask to see a photo ID. This information needs to be entered into the practice management software for accurate billing. The medical assistant will also be responsible for scanning in an image of the health insurance identification card. Both sides of the card should be scanned, because there is important information, usually instructions for preauthorization, on the back side of the card. Review Fig. 15.2 for a sampling of different ID cards for common insurance companies.

Verifying Eligibility

Verification of eligibility is the process of confirming health insurance coverage for the patient. When you are scheduling an appointment, health insurance information should be collected (unless it is an emergency situation). If the healthcare facility is not part of the patient's network of providers, the individual should be informed of this. The patient can then decide if he or she still wants to schedule an appointment. The medical assistant should also verify the *effective date,* or date the insurance coverage began, and confirm that the patient will be covered on the date the medical services are provided. The medical assistant should make it a practice to review each insurer's

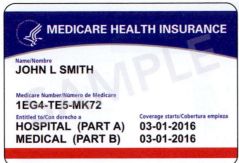

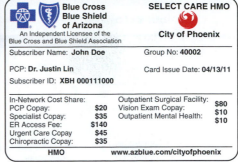

Medicare: The Medicare card uses the patient's social security number as the ID number. The card also details the plan coverages, in this case Part A and Part B.

HMO ID Card: Notice the Health Insurance Plan and the HMO Plan are both listed. Common copayments are also listed.
HMO members are required to choose PCP which is designated on their health ID card.

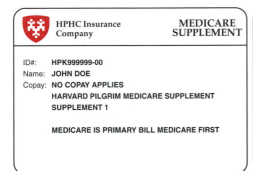

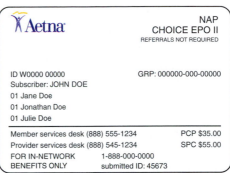

Medicare Secondary Insurance: The ID card states that it is a supplement to Medicare, thus Medicare should be billed as the primary. The ID number does not match the Medicare card.

EPO Plan ID Card: Members are not required to choose a PCP, but can only use their benefits for in-network providers and facilities. Notice the ID number stays the same for the insured and all family members listed.

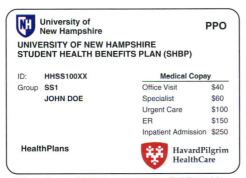

PPO plan ID card: PPO patients have the most flexibility to visit whichever provider, primary care or specialist they choose. Notice the medical copays are slightly higher than HMO copayments.

FIGURE 15.2 A variety of different health insurance identification cards.

online insurance Web portal, which can verify insurance eligibility, benefits, and exclusions, prior to the patient's appointment. If the online insurance Web portal is not available, the medical assistant should contact the provider services desk; the phone number should be listed on the patient's health insurance ID card.

CRITICAL THINKING APPLICATION   **15.4**

Robert Caudill, an elderly patient, calls to make an appointment but is unsure what his benefits are. How can Jon find out what benefits Mr. Caudill qualifies for? Is it appropriate for Jon to educate Mr. Caudill on his health insurance benefits? Why or why not?

In the recent past, the medical assistant would have to call the health insurance company to verify eligibility for each and every patient. Each call to the health insurance company automated system would take at least 5 minutes, and the medical assistant would not have access to all of the patient's benefit information unless he or she spoke to a member services agent, which would take even more time. Today, most privately sponsored health insurance plans offer online insurance provider portals, which allow for quick and easy verification of eligibility (Fig. 15.3). The healthcare facility will have to apply for access to the online Web portal. Once it has been approved, a patient's benefits can be looked up in their entirety in seconds instead of minutes. Information on a patient's benefit plan can be uploaded to the electronic health record (EHR) very quickly; this process reduces the use of paper in the healthcare facility.

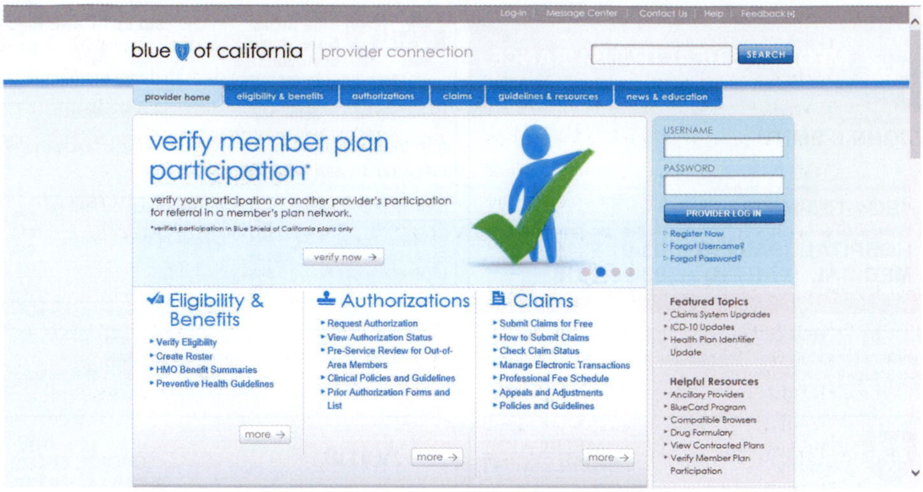

FIGURE 15.3 A provider's Web portal for online health insurance. (From Fordney MT: *Insurance handbook for the medical office,* ed 14, St Louis, 2017, Elsevier.)

OTHER TYPES OF INSURANCE

When you work in a healthcare facility, the most common type of insurance you will see is health insurance. However, there are other types of insurance that can require the involvement of a healthcare provider. These other types of insurance will be discussed below.

Disability Insurance

Disability insurance is a type of insurance that provides income replacement if the patient has a disability that is not work related. The disability means that the employee is unable to perform his or her work functions or duties. It could involve either short-term disability or long-term disability benefits. Both provide 40% to 70% of the individual's predisability income. Many employers offer a disability policy to their employees. Generally, the employee pays the monthly premium. These policies can also be purchased by an individual.

Short-term disability means that a person is unable to work for 9 to 52 weeks. Long-term disability policies pick up when short-term benefits are exhausted. Long-term disability coverage will pay out until the patient returns to work or for the number of years specified in the policy. Some policies will pay out until the patient reaches the age of 65 and then is eligible for Social Security benefits. There may be a **waiting period** before benefits can be paid. Sick time can be used for the waiting period days.

Weekly or monthly cash benefits are provided to employed policyholders who become unable to work as a result of an accident or illness. The accident or illness must not be related to work, because that would be covered under workers' compensation. Payments are made directly to the insured and are intended to replace lost income resulting from an illness or other disability. Disability payments are not intended for payment of specific medical bills, and a disability insurance policy should not be confused with a regular health insurance plan.

The medical office may be involved in the examination of the patient to determine the level of disability and when the disability ends. There are forms that must be completed by a healthcare provider and then submitted to the insurance carrier.

Life Insurance

Life insurance provides payment of a specified amount, upon the insured's death, either to his or her estate or to a designated **beneficiary**. Annuity life insurance policies provide monthly cash benefits if the policyholder becomes permanently and totally disabled. Sometimes the proceeds from life insurance are used to meet the expenses of the insured person's last illness.

The healthcare facility may be required to complete physical examination forms when a patient is applying for life insurance. If there is an annuity policy, the healthcare provider may have to determine if there is a permanent disability and submit documentation.

Long-Term Care Insurance

Long-term care insurance is a relatively new type of insurance that covers a broad range of maintenance and health services for chronically ill, disabled, or developmentally delayed individuals. Medical services may be provided on an inpatient basis (e.g., at a rehabilitation facility, nursing home, or mental hospital), on an outpatient basis, or at home.

Liability Insurance

Liability insurance covers losses to a third party caused by the insured. There are many types of liability insurance, including automobile, business, and homeowners' policies. Liability policies often include benefits for:

- medical expenses resulting from traumatic injuries
- lost wages
- sometimes pain and suffering

All liability insurance policies are payable to victims injured by the insured person's home or car, without regard to the insured person's actual legal liability for the accident.

THE AFFORDABLE CARE ACT

In the early 2000s it became clear that a large number of Americans lacked basic health insurance. **Preexisting conditions** made it difficult for Americans who did not work full time or were self-employed to obtain health insurance. In addition, the health insurance market was discriminating against young adults 18 years or older, who may not have been qualified to receive health benefits because they could not find full-time employment.

In 2010 the Patient Protection and Affordable Care Act, known as the *Affordable Care Act* (also Obamacare), was enacted. It increased the quality, availability, and affordability of private and public health insurance for more than 44 million uninsured Americans. The legislation included new qualifying regulations, taxes, mandates, and subsidies. The federal mandate not only has opened opportunities for more Americans to obtain affordable health insurance, but also works to reduce overall healthcare spending in the long run. The following are other patient protections and provisions under the Affordable Care.

- Insurance companies are prohibited from dropping patient health coverage if the individual gets sick or makes an unintentional mistake on the health insurance application.
- Preexisting conditions and gender discrimination were eliminated, so patients cannot be charged more based on their health status or gender.
  - Young adults can remain on their parent's or guardian's insurance policy until age 26.
  - *Health insurance marketplaces* were created, where low- to middle-income Americans can compare plans and lower their costs on healthcare coverage.
  - States expanded Medicaid coverage to 15.9 million Americans to include those who qualify for cost assistance through the marketplace.
  - Individuals seeking health insurance can apply only during the open enrollment period, which is established by each state.

With more Americans having health insurance, the number of office visits to providers across the country is expected to increase. Thus, efficient health insurance management policies should be instituted to meet the new demand for services.

CLOSING COMMENTS

Health insurance and benefits coverage can be confusing to the patient. Medical assistants should educate themselves on the specific details of all plans accepted at the healthcare facility. Managed care has often been criticized in the media for its cost-saving practices. Extra efforts made by medical assistants to overcome these challenges and educate their patients on how to use their health insurance plans will improve the quality of care delivered to their patients. Providers and healthcare facilities need to evaluate their ability to accept the fee schedule of insurance plans they are contracted with, especially since Medicaid's fee schedule is the lowest in the industry.

Patient Coaching

It is important for patients to understand how their insurance works. Many people, especially elderly individuals, believe that if they have

health insurance, all charges for their healthcare will be covered. The responsibilities of a medical assistant include keeping the patient informed of his or her financial responsibilities and answering questions about the person's benefits and exclusions. Often healthcare facilities provide their patients with informational brochures that explain how health insurance and reimbursement work and provide definitions of some of the more common terms used in the insurance claims process. If patients are well advised and comfortable with insurance facts before treatment begins, the medical experience will go more smoothly, and collection of their financial responsibilities will be easier. The medical assistant must practice good communication skills, patience, and tact when discussing reimbursement and financial responsibilities issues with patients.

Legal and Ethical Issues

Verification of eligibility is a process that is important not only to ensure the insurance plan is valid at the time of service, but also to ensure the patient's identity. Falsifying one's identity to use someone else's health insurance benefits is a common fraudulent practice. The only way to prevent this type of health insurance fraud is to diligently verify all patients when they schedule appointments with the healthcare facility. A state-issued ID should be presented with the patient's health insurance ID to verify identity. If medical assistants suspect fraud, they should report it to the health insurance plan immediately and the patient should be informed that he or she cannot be seen by the medical professional until issues relating to the health insurance are resolved.

Professional Behaviors

Patients can be confused or angered when insurance companies deny authorization of services or referrals. Although these decisions are made by insurance companies, many times the blame is put on the medical front office assistants. In situations such as these, it is important for medical assistants to stay calm and listen to the patient's concerns. In most cases, the patient will come to realize that there is nothing the medical assistant can do, but the patient may need to express frustration. Once the patient has calmed down, the medical assistant can then recommend options, such as paying cash or making payment arrangements; the medical assistant can also bring the patient's attention to his or her insurance member services hotline. Compassionately assure patients that their health is most important and that you will do what you can, so they can receive the appropriate medical treatment.

If the patient continues to escalate the situation and/or becomes belligerent, excuse yourself from the discussion and ask either an office manager or another medical assistant to step in. A medical assistant should never return anger and/or frustration to the patient. Remember, the patient may be mentally compromised and frustrated from extensive health care problems, so don't exacerbate the situation by releasing your own anger. If the patient's health is made the primary concern, the healthcare facility can work with the insurance company, so the patient can receive appropriate medical care.

SUMMARY OF SCENARIO

Although he was initially nervous about explaining fees to patients and asking for payment, Jon has become more comfortable in doing this aspect of his job, because he now understands the business aspect of the practice. Patients understand that providers must charge for their services and have become accustomed to copayments and co-insurance amounts. Many times, these fees are collected in advance, before the patient sees the provider. This practice saves time on checkout, and most patients believe that the copay is a small cost compared with the entire fee that providers charge to manage their care in one office visit.

Jon has noticed that the usual, customary, and reasonable fees that Dr. Kahn, a member of the practice, charges his patients directly affect the reimbursements that are paid by various insurance and managed care companies. Jon has attended several health insurance billing seminars sponsored by Medicare and Blue Cross/Blue Shield, and he believes that this extra training has resulted in a reduction in health insurance claim rejections at WMFM.

SUMMARY OF LEARNING OBJECTIVES

1. **Discuss the purpose of health insurance and discuss the concept of cost-sharing.**

   Insurance is something that is purchased to help protect against loss or harm from specified circumstances. A premium can be paid by an individual, an employer, or a combination of employer contribution and individual (employee) contribution. Most policies require the patient to pay a portion of the healthcare expenses, which is known as *cost-sharing*, and includes deductibles, co-insurance, and copayments.

2. **List and discuss various government health insurance plans.**

   Government health insurance plans include Medicare, Medicaid, TRICARE, CHAMPVA, CHIP, and workers' compensation. The elderly, disabled, military, indigent, and those injured at work may qualify for one of these programs. Because these programs are sponsored by the government, participating providers (PARs) must accept a lower fee schedule for reimbursements.

3. **Summarize private health insurance plans.**

   Private health insurance plans, also known as commercial insurance plans, are for-profit organizations. As such, health insurance companies make annual changes to the participating provider contract to negotiate lower payments. Most privately sponsored plans use managed care to reduce the costs of delivering quality healthcare.

   Self-funded healthcare, or self-insurance, is an arrangement in which an employer provides health or disability benefits to employees with its own funds. This is different from fully insured plans, in which the employer contracts with an insurance company to cover the employees and dependents. In self-funded healthcare, the employer assumes the direct risk for payment of the claims for benefits.

4. **Review traditional (fee-for-service) health insurance plans.**

   Traditional health insurance plans pay for all or a share of the cost of covered services. These services are also known as *fee-for-service* and were the first type of health insurance. Policyholders of fee-for-service plans and their dependents choose when and where to get healthcare services. Fee schedule amounts can be determined by a process called *usual, customary, and reasonable* (UCR).

5. **Differentiate among the different types of managed care models.**

   Managed care is a broad term used to describe a variety of healthcare plans developed to provide healthcare services at lower costs. It is important for the medical assistant to be familiar with various plan types such as the health maintenance organization (HMO), preferred provider organization (PPO), and exclusive provider organization (EPO) and to understand the policies of each one.

6. **Outline managed care requirements for patient referral, obtain a referral with documentation, and discuss utilization management.**

   Obtaining preauthorization for making referrals must be done according to the guidelines of the individual insurance companies. If the medical assistant is uncertain about the procedure, he or she should always refer to the insurance plan's policies and procedures manual.

   Utilization management is a form of patient care review by healthcare professionals who do not provide the care but are employed by health insurance companies. The medical assistant should contact the utilization review department directly; it should never be left to the patient to contact this department.

7. **Describe the process for preauthorization and how to obtain pre-authorization, including documentation.**

   Managed care plans, including HMOs, PPOs, and EPOs, require preauthorization for medical services such as surgery, expensive medical tests, and medication therapy. Preauthorization may be requested by calling the health insurance plan, which should be documented in the patient's electronic health record (EHR).

   Many insurance companies require preauthorization, usually within 24 hours, if a patient is to be hospitalized or undergo certain medical procedures. Insurance claims for payment will be denied if proper preauthorization is not obtained.

8. **Discuss participating provider contracts, including contracted fee schedules.**

   With all government health plans and most private health plans, healthcare providers must become participating providers. Credentialing is the process of confirming the healthcare provider's qualifications. Payment

SUMMARY OF LEARNING OBJECTIVES—*continued*

for services is typically made after the health services are provided. When setting up a fee schedule, a healthcare provider should consider time, expertise, and services.

9. **Interpret information on a health insurance identification (ID) card.**

    As proof of health insurance coverage, patients are issued a health insurance ID card with the health plan name, patient's name, subscriber ID, and health plan contact information (see Fig. 15.2).

10. **Explain the importance of verifying eligibility and be able to verify eligibility for services, including documentation.**

    It is important to verify insurance benefits before you provide services to patients. Verifying benefits is necessary to ensure that the patient is covered by insurance and to determine what benefits will be paid for routine and special procedures and services. Verification protects the provider and the patient against unexpected medical care costs.

    Many problems for both the patient and the medical office can be prevented if the medical assistant develops and follows a procedure for verifying insurance benefits before services are provided. This procedure includes gathering as much information as possible about the demographics of the patient and his or her insurance coverage. A pragmatic and tactful discussion with all new patients to explain the facility's established policy on insurance claims processing

and the collection of fees not covered by the patient's policy will pay off.

11. **Describe other types of insurance, including disability, life, long-term care, and liability insurance.**

    Disability insurance is a type of insurance that provides income replacement if the patient has a disability that is not work related. Life insurance provides a payment of a specified amount, upon the insured's death, either to his or her estate or to a designated beneficiary. Long-term care insurance covers a broad range of maintenance and health services for chronically ill, disabled, or developmentally delayed individuals. Liability insurance covers losses to a third party caused by the insured.

12. **Discuss the Affordable Care Act's effect on patient healthcare access.**

    In 2010, the Patient Protection and Affordable Care Act was enacted (it is also known as the *Affordable Care Act,* or Obamacare). It increased the quality, availability, and affordability of private and public health insurance for more than 44 million uninsured Americans. The legislation included new qualifying regulations, taxes, mandates, and subsidies. The federal mandate not only opens opportunities for more Americans to obtain affordable health insurance, but also works to reduce overall healthcare spending in the long run.

DIAGNOSTIC CODING ESSENTIALS

SCENARIO

Mike Simeone, a recent medical assistant graduate, excelled in his diagnostic coding course. Recently, he found an entry-level coding position at the Walden-Martin Family Medical Clinic (WMFM).

Mike is a little nervous but also excited about starting ICD-10-CM coding. Mike has used encoder software in some of his classes, which helped him determine the most specific and accurate code. Mike noticed that the new

software update in the medical office has the most recent ICD-10-CM codes.

Mike has had some previous experience working in health records, which gives him a strong understanding of the importance of accurate, quality documentation. He knows where to look to find diagnostic statements in providers' orders, treatment plans, progress notes, surgical reports, and other medical reports.

While studying this chapter, think about the following questions:

- How do the format, layout, and conventions of the ICD-10-CM manual help the medical assistant search for the most accurate and specific diagnostic code?
- Why is the quality of health record documentation critical to diagnostic coding?

- Why does the medical assistant need to know the steps for performing diagnostic coding?

LEARNING OBJECTIVES

1. Describe the historical use of the International Classification of Disease (ICD) in the United States and describe how diagnostic coding is related to medical necessity.
2. Identify the structure and format of the *International Classification of Diseases, 10th Revision, Clinical Modification* (ICD-10-CM).
3. Describe how to use the Alphabetic Index to select main terms, essential modifiers, and the appropriate code (or codes) and code ranges.
4. Do the following related to the Tabular List:
   - Explain how to use the Tabular List to select main terms, essential modifiers, and the appropriate code (or codes) or code ranges.
   - Summarize coding conventions as defined in the ICD-10-CM coding manual.
5. Review the Official Coding Guidelines to assign the most accurate ICD-10-CM diagnostic code.
6. Explain how to abstract the diagnostic statement from a patient's health record.
7. Describe how to use the most current diagnostic codes and perform diagnostic coding.
8. Identify how encoder software can help the coder assign the most accurate diagnostic codes.
9. Explain the importance of coding guidelines for accuracy, discuss special rules and considerations that apply to the code selection process, and maximize third-party reimbursement.
10. Review medical coding ethical standards.

VOCABULARY

abstract Collecting important information from the health record.
cataract (KAT ur ackt) Progressive loss of transparency of the lens of the eye.
chronic Developing slowly and lasting for a long time, generally 3 or more months.
contraindicate (kon truh IN di kayt) To specify that an agent or procedure should not be used.
dementia (di MEN shah) A mental disorder in which the individual experiences a progressive loss of memory, personality

alterations, confusion, loss of touch with reality, and stupor (seeming unawareness of, and disconnection with, one's surroundings).
diagnosis (die ag NOH sis) Determining the cause of a condition, illness, disease, injury, or congenital defect.
diagnostic statement Information about a patient's diagnosis or diagnoses that has been taken from the medical documentation.
encoder Software that will apply diagnostic or procedure codes to medical conditions or procedures.

encounter form A document used to capture the services/procedures and diagnoses for a patient visit. The fees for the services/procedures are usually included on the encounter form.

epidemiology (ep i dee mee OL uh jee) The branch of medicine dealing with the incidence, distribution, and control of disease in a population. It also involves the prevalence of disease in large populations, in addition to detection of the source and cause of epidemics of infectious disease.

etiology (ee tee OL uh jee) The study of the causes or origin of diseases.

histologic Pertaining to the study of body tissues.

impending A term used in the diagnosis of a condition that can be imminently threatening. For example, a patient showing signs of prediabetes may in the near future develop diabetes; therefore, in this case, diabetes is an impending condition.

medically necessary Accepted healthcare services that are appropriate for the evaluation and treatment of a disease, condition, illness or injury and are consistent with the applicable standard of care.

mortality The relative frequency of deaths in a specific population.

myxedema (mick suh DEE mah) Advanced hypothyroidism in adulthood.

reimbursement (ree im BURS ment) To make repayment for an expense or a loss incurred.

sequela (si KWEL uh) **(singular)**, **sequelae (plural)** An abnormal condition resulting from a previous disease.

specificity (spes uh FIS i tee) The quality or state of being specific.

A **diagnosis** has many purposes in healthcare. Patient treatment plans are based on the diagnosis. **Reimbursement** from insurance companies is based, in part, on the diagnosis. Researchers use diagnoses for their studies. Diagnostic coding has been used to standardize diagnoses. It was initially developed to study causes of **mortality**. Over time, diagnostic coding has been expanded to include all diseases and conditions. The World Health Organization (WHO) has established the International Classification of Diseases (ICD). This classification system is in its tenth revision and is known as the *International Classification of Diseases, 10th Revision, Clinical Modification* (ICD-10-CM). These codes are used for:

- mortality data
- **epidemiological** data
- billing purposes

The ICD-10-CM allows providers to be much more specific in diagnostic coding than was possible with previous revisions. This will, in turn, result in more accurate data collection and billing practices. Every year the Centers for Medicare and Medicaid Services (CMS) reviews the ICD-10-CM coding manual. The update is published on October 1. Additions, revisions, and deletions are made to many of the diagnostic codes, code descriptions, and guidelines. *You must always use the current year's coding manual to ensure accurate coding and to comply with regulatory guidelines.*

The Health Insurance Portability and Accountability Act (HIPAA) has mandated that specific code sets be used to help standardize the process of claims submission. The ICD-10-CM is the mandated diagnostic code set.

In this chapter we will look at the structure of the ICD-10-CM codes and how to accurately determine the correct code.

THE HISTORY OF MEDICAL CODING

Medical coding began as medical classification in 17th century England. John Graunt, a statistician, wanted to study causes of mortality in children under age 6, so he developed a medical classification system. In the mid-1800s, William Farr, a medical statistician, established a more organized disease classification to widen the system to patients of all ages. The principles of Farr's classification method, and those

of Jacques Bertillon, chief of statistics for the city of Paris, developed into the *International List of Causes of Death,* which was published in Chicago in 1893 by the International Statistics Institute. This list was revised every 10 years. After the League of Nations was established in 1920, its members saw the need for use of the classification system by a variety of stakeholders, including insurers, health administrators, hospitals, and military medical providers. The name of the list was changed to the *International List of Diseases.*

In 1946 the International Commission of the World Health Organization (WHO) established codes to define specific infectious diseases, parasites, symptoms, and causes of death. This code set was called the *Manual of the International Statistical Classification of Diseases, Injuries, and Causes of Death* (ICD).

(*Note:* It is important to understand the difference between the ICD and the *Clinical Modification* versions [i.e., ICD-10-CM]. The ICD is the international version, copyrighted and published by WHO. WHO authorized an adaptation for use in the United States, although all modifications had to conform to WHO conventions. The adaptation currently used in the United States is the ICD-10-CM. [Other countries also may apply for adaptations.] The *Clinical Modification* version provides much more detail and sometimes has separate sections for procedures.)

In 1995 WHO approved the development of the *International Classification of Diseases, Tenth Revision, Clinical Modification* (ICD-10-CM) code set. This code set has a different format from that of the ICD-9-CM. As of October 1, 2015, the ICD-10-CM has been used in the United States. The ICD-11 is currently being developed; according to WHO, the ICD-11 timeline will be adopted by member states no sooner than January, 2022.

Medical Coding in the United States

As history dictates, the original purpose of medical coding was to collect statistical data. The United States is the only country in the world that uses coding for health insurance reimbursement purposes. Providers are responsible for billing the insurance company for any services rendered during the *encounter* (i.e., any meeting between a patient and a healthcare provider), and the provider must use approved medical codes for these procedures and services to obtain reimbursement. This means that the provider must supply diagnostic information that demonstrates the need for the rendered procedures and/or services. The provider assigns a diagnosis through assessment of the patient.

All components of the encounter (i.e., diagnostic findings, procedures, and services) are used to determine the charges and to generate an insurance claim. This chapter focuses on the ways the medical assistant should gather diagnostic information and translate it into a diagnostic code. The ICD-10-CM coding manual is used for this purpose.

WHAT IS DIAGNOSTIC CODING?

Diagnostic coding changes written descriptions of diseases, illnesses, or injuries into alphanumeric codes. The ICD-10-CM code set uses up to seven characters to identify the disease or injury. Using the ICD-10-CM can help ensure both accurate health record documentation and efficient claims processing.

The ICD-10-CM code set is available through online resources, within the electronic health record (EHR) as an **encoder**, or as a print manual. The print manual is produced by several publishers and may use different layouts, symbols, color coding, and some other features. For the coding manual, however, the format, conventions, tables, appendices, content, and basic structure are the same.

When you use the ICD-10-CM, you will be choosing a standardized alphanumeric code for the **diagnostic statement** assigned by the provider. Diagnostic statements are found in:

- operative reports
- discharge summaries
- history and physical exam (H&P) reports
- reports on *ancillary diagnostic services* (e.g., radiology, pathology, and laboratory reports)

All of these should provide the patient's diagnosis or diagnoses. These reports are used by healthcare providers to code and report clinical information. Diagnostic coding is required for participation in Medicare and Medicaid programs and by most insurance companies. The diagnostic codes are used on insurance claims. The ICD-10-CM codes tell the insurance company why the procedures were done. These codes are linked to the procedures that are performed. If the diagnosis code does not match the procedure being provided, it may not be paid for. This linking can determine if a procedure or service is paid for. The diagnostic code can show that a procedure or service was **medically necessary**. If it was not medically necessary, the insurance company will not pay for it. For example, if diabetes mellitus is the diagnosis and the procedure is a throat culture, the insurance company would not pay it as it is not medically necessary for the treatment of diabetes mellitus. The ICD-10-CM is also used to keep track of various healthcare statistics related to disease and injury. Practice management software, clearinghouses, and insurance companies recognize these codes, which simplifies the coding process and speeds reimbursement to healthcare providers.

GETTING TO KNOW THE ICD-10-CM
Structure and Format of the ICD-10-CM

The ICD-10-CM has two sections:
- Alphabetic Index (the ICD-10-CM Index to Diseases and Injuries)
- Tabular List (officially, the ICD-10-CM Tabular List of Diseases and Injuries)

Determining an ICD-10-CM code starts in the Alphabetic Index and is confirmed in the Tabular List. These codes have three to seven characters (Fig. 16.1). Every ICD-10-CM code begins with an alphabetic letter that indicates the chapter in the Tabular List from which the code originates (Table 16.1). All the letters of the English alphabet are used except U, which WHO has reserved to assign to new diseases of uncertain **etiology**. Some conditions use more than one alphabetic letter in their code ranges. For example, the codes in Chapter 1, Certain Infectious and Parasitic Diseases (A00–B99), begin with the letter A or B. The second character is always numeric. The remaining characters can be a combination of letters and numbers. A decimal is required after the third character. There are only certain codes that require the 7th character. The following box describes the 7th character requirements in more detail.

ICD-10-CM 7th Character Requirements

Seventh characters are used for many ICD-10-CM codes. The following list shows the chapters that require a seventh character and what the character identifies:

- Chapter 13: Diseases of the Musculoskeletal System — Encounter
- Chapter 15: Pregnancy, Childbirth and the Puerperium — Fetus identification
- Chapter 18: Symptoms, Signs, and Abnormal Clinical and Laboratory Findings, Not Elsewhere Classified — Coma Scale
- Chapter 19: Injury, Poisoning, and Certain Other Consequences of External Causes — Encounter

---

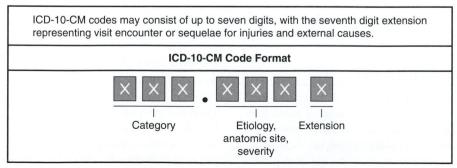

ICD-10-CM codes may consist of up to seven digits, with the seventh digit extension representing visit encounter or sequelae for injuries and external causes.

ICD-10-CM Code Format

Category — Etiology, anatomic site, severity — Extension

FIGURE 16.1 Code structure and format of ICD-10-CM codes.

TABLE 16.1   ICD-10-CM Tabular List of Diseases and Injuries

CHAPTER	TITLE	CODE RANGE	POSSIBLE DIAGNOSIS[a]	ICD-10-CM CODE
1	Certain Infectious and Parasitic Diseases	A00–B99	Measles	B05.9
2	Neoplasms	C00–D49	Colon cancer	C18.9
3	Diseases of the Blood and Blood-Forming Organs and Certain Disorders Involving the Immune Mechanism	D50–D89	Iron-deficiency anemia	D50.9
4	Endocrine, Nutritional, and Metabolic Diseases	E00–E89	Type I diabetes	E10
5	Mental, Behavioral, and Neurodevelopmental Disorders	F01–F99	Dementia	F03
6	Diseases of the Nervous System	G00–G99	Parkinson's disease	G20
7	Diseases of the Eye and Adnexa	H00–H59	Glaucoma	H40.9
8	Diseases of the Ear and Mastoid Process	H60–H95	Otitis media, left ear	H60.92
9	Diseases of the Circulatory System	I00–I99	Hypertensive heart disease	I11.9
10	Diseases of the Respiratory System	J00–J99	Acute sinusitis	J01.91
11	Diseases of the Digestive System	K00–K95	Inguinal hernia	K40
12	Diseases of the Skin and Subcutaneous Tissue	L00–L99	Pressure ulcer of right heel	L89.619
13	Diseases of the Musculoskeletal System and Connective Tissue	M00–M99	Rheumatoid arthritis	M05
14	Diseases of the Genitourinary System	N00–N99	Endometriosis	N80.9
15	Pregnancy, Childbirth, and the Puerperium	O00–O94	Ectopic pregnancy	O00.9
16	Certain Conditions Originating in the Perinatal Period	P00–P96	Neonatal jaundice	P59.9
17	Congenital Malformations, Deformations and Chromosomal Abnormalities	Q00–Q99	Cleft lip	Q37.9
18	Symptoms, Signs and Abnormal Clinical and Laboratory Findings, Not Elsewhere Classified	R00–R99	Abdominal pain	R10.9
19	Injury, Poisoning and Certain Other Consequences of External Causes	S00–T88	Left ankle fracture	S82.92xA
20	External Causes of Morbidity	V00–Y99	Snowboard accident Fall from cliff Exposure to excessive natural cold	V00.318A W15 X31
21	Factors Influencing Health Status and Contact With Health Services	Z00–Z99	Pregnancy state	Z33.1

[a]All diagnoses presented are not otherwise specified (NOS).

- Chapter 20: External Causes of Morbidity – Encounter
- Chapter 21: Factors Influencing Health Status and Contact With Health Services – Encounter

As you can see, the seventh character most often indicates the encounter type. The letters most often used for an encounter type are A, D, and S:

- A: initial encounter
- D: subsequent encounter
- S: sequela, complications or conditions that occur as a direct result of a condition

The CMS prepares the Official Guidelines for Coding and Reporting to be used with the ICD-10-CM codes, in addition to instructions on how to report the codes on insurance claim forms. The guidelines are a set of rules that have been developed to accompany and complement the official conventions and instructions provided in the ICD-10-CM proper.

The Alphabetic Index

The Alphabetic Index consists of an alphabetic list of diagnostic terms and related codes. This index includes main terms, nonessential modifiers, essential modifiers, and subterms:

- *Main terms:* These terms appear in bold type.
- *Nonessential modifiers:* These terms follow the main term and are enclosed in parentheses. They are supplementary words or explanatory information. They do not need to be in the actual diagnostic statement.
- *Essential modifiers:* These terms are indented under the main term. They can modify the main term by describing different sites or etiology. They must be included in the diagnostic statement.

Fig. 16.2 shows an example of an entry in the Alphabetic Index:
- the main term
- nonessential modifiers
- essential modifiers

Let's use the example of **chronic** ischemic colitis shown in Fig. 16.2. You would start with the main term: Colitis. You can see that the main term is followed by the nonessential modifiers (acute, catarrhal, chronic, noninfective, hemorrhagic) that do not affect the code assignment. Follow the list to the modifying term: Ischemic. Indented under ischemic, you will find "chronic" with the code K55.1. You will look up K55.1 in the Tabular List.

CRITICAL THINKING APPLICATION   **16.1**

Mike is working with the ICD-10-CM manual and is trying to refresh his memory about nonessential and essential modifiers. In your own words define essential modifier and nonessential modifier. Compare your definitions with those of a classmate.

Supplementary Sections of the Alphabetic Index

The Alphabetic Index section includes two important tables.
- *Table of Neoplasms:* This table lists neoplasms by anatomic location. For coding purposes, neoplasms are further classified into six categories:
  - Malignant Primary
  - Malignant Secondary
  - Ca (cancer) in situ
  - Benign
  - Uncertain Behavior
  - Unspecified Behavior
- *Table of Drugs and Chemicals:* This table presents a classification of drugs and other chemical substances; it is used to identify poisonings and external causes of adverse effects. The six coding classifications are:
  - Poisoning, Accidental (Unintentional)
  - Poisoning, Intentional Self-Harm
  - Poisoning, Assault
  - Poisoning, Undetermined
  - Adverse Effect
  - Underdosing

The Tabular List

The Tabular List is divided into 21 chapters. Most chapter titles specify a particular group of diseases and injuries, and all titles are followed by a code range in parentheses; for example, Chapter 1, Certain Infectious and Parasitic Diseases (A00–B99) (see Table 16.1).

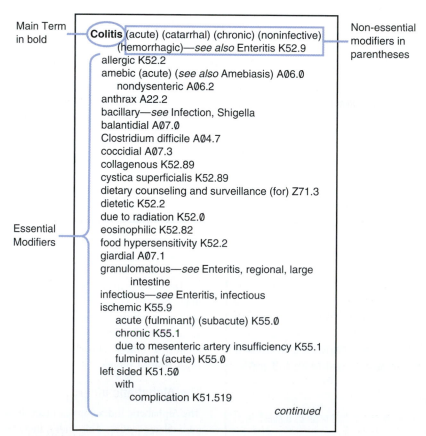

Main Term in bold → **Colitis** (acute) (catarrhal) (chronic) (noninfective) (hemorrhagic)—*see also* Enteritis K52.9 ← Non-essential modifiers in parentheses

Essential Modifiers →
allergic K52.2
amebic (acute) (*see also* Amebiasis) A06.0
    nondysenteric A06.2
anthrax A22.2
bacillary—*see* Infection, Shigella
balantidial A07.0
Clostridium difficile A04.7
coccidial A07.3
collagenous K52.89
cystica superficialis K52.89
dietary counseling and surveillance (for) Z71.3
dietetic K52.2
due to radiation K52.0
eosinophilic K52.82
food hypersensitivity K52.2
giardial A07.1
granulomatous—*see* Enteritis, regional, large intestine
infectious—*see* Enteritis, infectious
ischemic K55.9
    acute (fulminant) (subacute) K55.0
    chronic K55.1
    due to mesenteric artery insufficiency K55.1
    fulminant (acute) K55.0
left sided K51.50
    with
        complication K51.519

continued

FIGURE 16.2 ICD-10-CM Alphabetic Index with main term, nonessential modifiers, and essential modifiers.

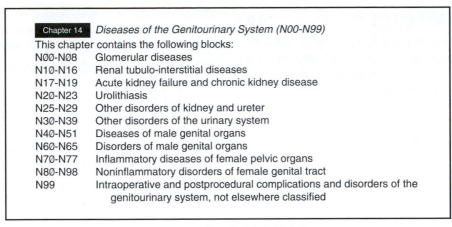

Diseases of the Genitourinary System (N00-N99)
This chapter contains the following blocks:
N00-N08   Glomerular diseases
N10-N16   Renal tubulo-interstitial diseases
N17-N19   Acute kidney failure and chronic kidney disease
N20-N23   Urolithiasis
N25-N29   Other disorders of kidney and ureter
N30-N39   Other disorders of the urinary system
N40-N51   Diseases of male genital organs
N60-N65   Disorders of male genital organs
N70-N77   Inflammatory diseases of female pelvic organs
N80-N98   Noninflammatory disorders of female genital tract
N99   Intraoperative and postprocedural complications and disorders of the genitourinary system, not elsewhere classified

FIGURE 16.3 Chapter blocks in the Tabular List.

Some chapters use a body part or an organ system to group the codes; for example:

- Chapter 7, Diseases of the Eye and Adnexa (H00–H59)
- Chapter 9, Diseases of the Circulatory System (I00–I99)

Other chapters group conditions by etiology or the nature of the disease process; for example:

- Chapter 2, Neoplasms (C00–D49)
- Chapter 15, Pregnancy, Childbirth, and the Puerperium (O00–O94) – groups codes related to the prenatal and postnatal periods
- Chapter 20, External Causes of Morbidity (V00–Y99) – also groups codes related to external causes of injury and poisoning
- Chapter 21, Factors Influencing Health Status and Contact with Health Services (Z00–Z99)

Each chapter is divided into subchapters, or blocks, and each subchapter has a designated 3-character code. These subchapter codes and code ranges form the foundation of the ICD-10-CM code set.

In each chapter, all the 3-character block codes begin with the alphabetic letter assigned to that chapter. For example, in Chapter 6, Diseases of the Nervous System (G00–G99), all the block codes (and their versions) begin with G. If a chapter's code range includes two letters [e.g., Chapter 1, Certain Infectious and Parasitic Diseases (A00–B99)], each 3-character block code begins with one of those two letters. The letter is followed by a 2-character number. A summary of the blocks (Fig. 16.3) at the beginning of each chapter provides an overview of the chapter.

As mentioned, the ICD-10-CM manual is produced by a variety of publishers, but many of the optional features are similar (remember, the important elements are always the same, regardless of the publisher). For instance, to enable the coder to better maneuver through the Alphabetic Index, each page has *guide words*, which are the first and last words on that page (this is the same arrangement used for the pages of a dictionary). Each chapter of the Tabular List has a different-colored border strip; in some manuals, this strip shows the chapter title and the range of codes found on that specific page. In the chapters in the Tabular List, the codes for each category/block are arranged alphabetically (by the initial alpha character) and then numerically. Familiarizing yourself with these tools can help you

improve your proficiency as you work through the manual to find the most accurate code.

It is important to note that some codes do not need to be extended beyond the 3-character code, and these are considered valid codes as is; for example, code **I10**

{Essential (primary) hypertension}

If a code has only three characters, do not add a decimal after the 3rd character. If a code has more than three characters, add a decimal point after the 3rd character; for example, **K11.7**

{Disturbances of salivary secretion}

Most ICD-10-CM codes have 4 to 7 characters.

Reporting NEC and NOS Codes

In some cases, because of limited documentation in the patient's health record, the medical assistant coder can find it difficult to assign an ICD-10-CM code with a higher **specificity**. The ICD-10-CM code set accommodates these coding circumstances by establishing "not elsewhere classified" (NEC) and "not otherwise specified" (NOS) guidelines.

- *NEC* means that the diagnostic statement contains specific wording, but no specific classification exists to match the wording. For example, an NEC code would be assigned if a patient seeks medical attention for **chronic** postoperative pain. The ICD-10-CM code would be **G89.28 {Other chronic postprocedural pain}**
  - For all NEC codes, the last character is always 8.
- *NOS* means that the diagnostic statement does not contain any more specific wording. For example, sinusitis with no documentation of the specific sinus site is assigned the NOS code **J32.9 {Chronic sinusitis, unspecified}**

The coder should keep in mind that the lack of documentation does not mean that all the patient's sinuses are inflamed. There must be no documentation of the exact site of the sinusitis for a non-NOS code to be assigned. As providers recognize that ICD-10-CM codes are more specific than ICD-9-CM codes, their documentation also is becoming more specific.

- For all NOS codes, the last character is always 9.

CRITICAL THINKING APPLICATION   16.2

Mike is reviewing the Tabular List of the ICD-10-CM coding manual. He notices that each chapter begins with a list of diagnostic categories with a corresponding range of codes. What is this called? How can this feature be used as a tool for accurate ICD-10-CM code assignment?

Conventions Used in the Tabular List

Conventions are abbreviations, punctuation, symbols, instructional notations, and related entities that help the coder select an accurate, specific code. Conventions are found in the Tabular List, but not in the Alphabetic Index. Understanding their meaning and using them as guides are crucial to accurate coding. Table 16.2 lists the most common conventions.

CRITICAL THINKING APPLICATION   16.3

Mike is looking for the ICD-10-CM code for morbid obesity. From the Alphabetic Index, Mike finds the code E66. When he goes to verify the code in the Tabular List, he finds that the main term, Overweight and obesity, has a symbol indicating that a 4th character is needed. What is Mike's next step to assign the most accurate code? Can Mike just use E66? Why or why not? Share your answer with the class.

Coding Guidelines

The coding manual begins with the ICD-10-CM Official Guidelines for Coding and Reporting. Every coding guideline for the entire ICD-10-CM code set is included in this section. The guidelines are a set of rules that have been developed to complement the official conventions and instructions provided in the ICD-10-CM proper. The guidelines are organized into four sections.

Section I. Conventions, General Coding Guidelines and Chapter Specific Guidelines: This section covers the structure and conventions of the ICD-10-CM classification system, in addition to the general guidelines that apply to the entire system. It also contains chapter-specific guidelines for each of the Tabular List's 21 chapters.

Section II. Selection of Principal Diagnosis: This section includes guidelines for selection of a principal diagnosis for non-outpatient settings.

Section III. Reporting Additional Diagnoses: This section includes guidelines for reporting additional diagnoses in non-outpatient settings.

Section IV. Diagnostic Coding and Reporting Guidelines for Outpatient Services: As the title indicates, this section includes diagnostic coding and reporting guidelines for outpatient services.

The coding guidelines start with a table of contents for each of the four sections, including the related chapters of disease and injury. After the table of contents, the coding guidelines are presented in section order (i.e., Sections I through IV). For the purposes of outpatient medical office billing, you are most likely to need Sections I and IV.

PREPARING FOR DIAGNOSTIC CODING

Now that you have a basic understanding of the ICD-10-CM system, let's take a look at how you find the information you need to determine diagnostic codes.

TABLE 16.2	**Commonly Used Conventions in the Tabular List**	
CONVENTION	**EXPLANATION**	**EXAMPLE**
Placeholder Character	ICD-10-CM uses the dummy placeholder X in two different ways. The dummy placeholder can be used as the 5th character in certain 6-character codes; this allows for future expansion of the code set without interruption of the 6-character structure. Specific categories have a 7th character, but may not use the 4th, 5th, or 6th characters. In these cases, the dummy placeholder X is used to fill the empty character spaces. Note that a dummy placeholder would not be needed for codes with fewer than 7 characters.	T43.4X1A Poisoning by butyrophenone and thiothixene neuroleptics, accidental, initial encounter (unintentional) S50.01XA Contusion of right elbow
Punctuation	Four basic forms of punctuation are used in the Tabular List: brackets, parentheses, colons, and braces. Each form serves a different purpose to help you read and understand the code descriptions.	[ ] Brackets enclose synonyms, alternative wording, or explanatory phrases ( ) Parentheses are used to enclose supplementary words, which may be present or absent in the statement of a disease or procedure : Colons are used in the Tabular Index after an incomplete term that needs one or more of the modifiers or adjectives that follow to make it assignable { } Braces enclose a series of terms, each of which is modified by the statement appearing to the right of the brace

TABLE 16.2 Commonly Used Conventions in the Tabular List—*continued*

CONVENTION	EXPLANATION	EXAMPLE

Instructional Notations	Instructional notations, which are found in both the Alphabetic Index and the Tabular List, are critical to correct coding practices. They are located directly under the main term.	**Includes**: Further defines or gives examples of the content of the category
		Excludes: The ICD-10-CM uses two types of exclusion notes:
		  Excludes1: This is a clear "NOT CODED HERE!" message. It means that the excluded code should never be used with the code above the Excludes1 note. For example, code **G14**
		  {Postpolio syndrome}
		  has this Excludes1 note:
		  sequelae of poliomyelitis (B91)
		  Excludes2: This means "not included here." The excluded condition is not part of the condition represented by the code; however, a patient may have both conditions. When an Excludes2 note is present, the coder may code both conditions if the patient presents with both. For example, code F02
		  {Dementia in other diseases classified elsewhere}
		  has the following Excludes2 note: **vascular dementia** (F01.5). This means that vascular **dementia** is not part of the condition coded as F02; therefore, you can code both dementia (F02) and vascular dementia (F01.5) if the patient has both.
		Code first/Use additional code: *Code first* notes appear under *manifestation* codes. Manifestation codes specify the way in which an underlying condition appears, or manifests, as a result of an underlying etiology; the main terms of most manifestation codes include the words "in diseases classified elsewhere." A *Code first* note indicates that the underlying condition must be coded first. For example, Code F02
		{Dementia in other diseases classified elsewhere}
		states, Code first the underlying physiological condition, such as: Alzheimer's (G30.-)

Relational Terms	These terms are used in both the Alphabetic Index and the Tabular List to clarify the context of the disease or injury.	• *And*: In the Tabular List code titles, *and* should be interpreted as meaning "and/or." • *With*: The term *with* should be interpreted as meaning "associated with" or "due to" when it appears in the Alphabetic Index, or in an instructional note or code title in the Tabular List. In the Alphabetic Index, the word *with* follows immediately after the main term, not in alphabetical order. • *Due to*: In both the Tabular List and the Alphabetic Index, the term *due to* signifies relationship between two conditions. This assumption can be made when both conditions are present or when the diagnostic statement indicates this relationship.

Abstracting Diagnostic Statements

To prepare for diagnostic coding, you must analyze the patient's health record and **abstract** the diagnostic statement documented in the various reports. Sources of diagnostic statements include the encounter form, treatment notes, discharge summary, operative report, and radiology, pathology, and laboratory reports. Let's take a look at those documents.

Encounter Form

The **encounter form** (also known as a *superbill*) can be viewed in the EHR or as a paper document. The most commonly used diagnostic and procedure codes are listed. The provider then indicates what services and/or procedures were done and the diagnosis code for the visit. It is important to update the encounter form with the new diagnostic and procedure codes. If outdated codes are used, it can delay or reduce the amount paid by the insurance company.

History and Physical Exam

The history and physical exam (H&P) are the starting point of the patient's medical evaluation. The H&P begins with a statement in the patient's own words that describes the reason for the visit. This statement, called the *chief complaint* (CC), is often abbreviated in the history documentation in the health record. After the chief complaint, the provider documents any other pertinent history:

- Medical, current illness and past medical history
  - History of present illness (HPI)
  - Previous illnesses
  - Previous hospitalizations
  - Previous surgeries
- Family history
  - Family members
    - Current ages
    - If deceased, age of death
    - Any medical conditions
- Social history
  - Tobacco use
  - Alcohol use
  - Drug use

After recording the patient's history, the provider performs a physical examination. This includes both objective and subjective assessments of the patient's physical status. The final sections of an H&P include an assessment and a plan. The assessment is the provider's evaluation of the findings from the H&P, and it includes a diagnostic statement. The plan is the treatment plan for the conditions noted in the assessment; it may include x-ray studies, laboratory tests, surgery, administration of medications, or other treatments.

Progress Notes

Progress notes are the second most common medical document from which diagnostic statements can be extracted. The format healthcare providers most commonly use for their notes is *SOAP notes*, a system of charting in which information is divided into *s*ubjective findings, *o*bjective findings, *a*ssessment, and *p*lan for treatment. Just as in the H&P, the diagnostic statement can most often be found in the assessment section of the SOAP notes.

Discharge Summary

The discharge summary is used primarily for abstracting diagnostic information for patients who were hospitalized, rather than those seen in a provider's office. The main elements of a discharge summary are:

- admission date
- date of discharge
- H&P findings
- clinical course during hospitalization
- health condition on discharge
- discharge diagnosis
- aftercare plan

Diagnostic statements are abstracted from the discharge diagnosis section. This diagnosis would be used to bill for the provider's visits to the patient while the person was in the hospital. The medical office can use a discharge summary as an overview of the patient's condition, especially if the discharge was recent.

Operative Report

For patients who have surgery as an outpatient or inpatient, the operative report also is used to abstract diagnostic statements. An operative report includes:

- preliminary diagnosis
- final diagnosis

- detailed description of the operative procedure from start to finish

The medical assistant uses the final diagnosis when searching for and selecting a diagnostic code.

Radiology, Laboratory, and Pathology Reports

Radiology, laboratory, and pathology reports are used to support and/or establish the diagnostic statement. Any findings from these reports must be documented in the progress notes in the health record so that they can be used for diagnostic coding, charge entry, or insurance billing purposes.

CRITICAL THINKING APPLICATION 16.4

While reviewing an encounter form, Mike notices that the diagnostic statement indicated that the patient needed to be treated for a left inguinal hernia. However, Mike also notes that the surgical report indicates that the left inguinal hernia was obstructed. What should Mike use as the final diagnostic statement? Should he ask the provider which diagnostic statement to use?

STEPS IN ICD-10-CM CODING

Accurate ICD-10-CM coding requires eight basic steps (Table 16.3). The first step involves abstracting the diagnostic statement from the health record and figuring out the main and modifying terms. Use the Alphabetic Index to search for the code or code ranges that best fit the diagnostic statement. The remaining steps are performed using the Tabular List to verify and confirm that the code or codes located in the Alphabetic Index fully match the diagnostic statement and that they are the most specific and accurate diagnostic codes. Procedure 16.1 on p. 350 details the basic coding steps using the ICD-10-CM manual and also encoder software (i.e., TruCode).

Using the Alphabetic Index

After the diagnostic statement has been abstracted from the health record, identify the main term and start searching for the best code, or code range, in the Alphabetic Index. It is important to note that the Alphabetic Index should be used only as a tool to locate the appropriate code or code range. The Tabular List, with its conventions, punctuation, notes, and guidelines, must always be used to confirm that the code or codes selected are accurate and specific and that there are no contraindications to the use of the code found in the Alphabetic Index. For this reason, never assign a code directly from the Alphabetic Index. Even if only one code is found in the Alphabetic Index, it may be used only if a thorough review of the conventions and instructional notations in the Tabular List does not **contraindicate** it.

Fig. 16.4 shows an excerpt from the Alphabetic Index for the main term **Cyst.** The first essential modifier is "eyelid." Note the nonessential modifier – sebaceous – in parentheses after eyelid. (Remember, nonessential modifiers add detail, but they do not have to be present in the diagnostic statement for the code to be acceptable for use.) Directly below the essential modifier eyelid are the subterms. Note that there are separate subterms for the left eye and for the right eye. In addition, the diagnostic codes for each eye are further modified by the location of the cyst (upper or lower).

TABLE 16.3	Diagnostic Coding Step-by-Step: Parkinson's Disease
Step 1	Determine the correct diagnosis from the diagnostic statement. Parkinson's Disease
Step 2	Use the main term to look up the diagnosis in the Alphabetic Index. Parkinson's disease, syndrome or tremor—see Parkinsonism
Step 3	Look up the "see" term in the Alphabetic Index. Parkinsonism (idiopathic) (primary) G20

Step 4	• *Review the essential modifiers under the main term.*
	Parkinsonism (idiopathic) (primary) G20
	with neurogenic orthostatic hypotension (symptomatic) G90.3
	arteriosclerotic G21.4
	dementia G31.83 *[F02.80]*
	   with behavioral disturbance G31.83 *[F02.81]*
	due to
	   drugs NEC G21.19
	      neuroleptic G21.11
	neuroleptic induced G21.11
	postencephalitic G21.3
	secondary G21.9
	   due to
	      arteriosclerosis G21.4
	      drugs NEC G21.19
	         neuroleptic G21.11
	      encephalitis G21.3
	      external agents NEC G21.2
	      syphilis A52.19
	   specified NEC G21.8
	syphilitic A52.19
	treatment-induced NEC G21.19
	vascular G21.4

Step 5	• *Choose the correct essential modifier based on the diagnostic statement.* Because the diagnostic statement only indicates Parkinson's Disease, code G20 should be chosen.
Step 6	• *Look up code G20 in the Tabular List.* **G20 Parkinson's disease**

Step 7	• *Check for any coding guidelines, conventions, inclusion or exclusion notes, or an additional character symbol.*
	Includes Hemiparkinson's
	Excludes1 Idiopathic Parkinsonism or Parkinson's disease
	                         Paralysis agitans
	                         Parkinsonism or Parkinson's disease NOS
	                         Primary Parkinsonism or Parkinson's disease dementia with Parkinsonism (G31.83)

Step 8	• *Assign the final ICD-10-CM code.* **G20 Parkinson's disease**

```
Cyst—continued
    eyelid (sebaceous) H02.829
        infected—see Hordeolum
    left H02.826
        lower H02.825
        upper H02.824
    right H02.823
        lower H02.822
        upper H02.821
```

FIGURE 16.4 Excerpt from the Alphabetic Index: Cyst (main term), eyelid (essential modifier), sebaceous (nonessential modifier).

```
H02.82    Cysts of eyelid
            Sebaceous cyst of eyelid
    H02.821    Cysts of right upper eyelid
    H02.822    Cysts of right lower eyelid
    H02.823    Cysts of right eye, unspecified eyelid
    H02.824    Cysts of left upper eyelid
    H02.825    Cysts of left lower eyelid
    H02.826    Cysts of left eye, unspecified eyelid
    H02.829    Cysts of unspecified eye, unspecified
               eyelid
```

FIGURE 16.5 Excerpt from the Tabular List: H02.82 Cysts of eyelid.

Using the Tabular List

Once you have identified at least the first three characters of the code in the Alphabetic Index, turn to the Tabular List. The chapters in the Tabular List are arranged alphabetically according to the initial letter of the 3-character code or codes assigned to each chapter. For example, Chapter 1 has code range A00–B99; Chapter 2 has code range C00–D49; Chapter 3 has code range D50–D89, and so on.

From the above example, you've determined that the code you probably need is in the H02 code range. Turn to the chapter that includes that range (Chapter 7). Fig. 16.5, an excerpt from the Tabular List, shows **Cysts of eyelid** as a main term, with the code H02.82. (Note that the nonessential modifier, sebaceous, is not shown in parentheses; rather, it appears under the main term in the nonbold phrase "Sebaceous cyst of eyelid.")

In the coding manual you would see the "additional character" symbol, which indicates that code H02.82 requires one more character. All possible diagnoses with 6-character codes are indented below the main term. A closer look at the disorders and their codes shows that the 6th character specifies the right or left eye and the location of the cyst on the eyelid (upper or lower). For the not-specified code, 9 would be the 6th character position.

Encoder Software

Encoder software (e.g., TruCode) is a tool commonly used by coders to assist in medical coding. This software performs computer-aided coding to assign the most accurate code possible. (TruCode is especially helpful to students because it allows them to search the ICD-10-CM manual using a few key terms.) The coder types a few key words into a search box, and the software finds the most likely matches in the

Alphabetic Index. The coder then clicks on a specific code, and the software searches the Tabular List. From the Tabular List, the coder can scroll up and down to determine the most accurate code. Encoder software can increase the speed and efficiency of coding for a wide variety of medical cases.

CRITICAL THINKING APPLICATION   **16.5**

Mike has determined a diagnostic statement to be "Perforation of the tympanic membrane in the left ear." What keyword should be used for the TruCode software search box? What main term will the encoder go to in the Alphabetic Index? What should Mike click to get to the Tabular List? At what point can Mike be sure that he has assigned the most accurate and specific code?

UNDERSTANDING CODING GUIDELINES

All ICD-10-CM coding manuals, regardless of the publisher, have comprehensive instructional notations and conventions to help the coder select the most accurate diagnostic code or codes. When there is a difference between reference sources (including this text), the current year's ICD-10-CM coding manual is the final authority – this fact cannot be emphasized enough. When coding, you must always refer to and thoroughly review the conventions, instructional notations, code definitions, and other guidelines in the Alphabetic Index and Tabular List in the current year's version of the ICD-10-CM.

The following instructions are designed to provide some additional guidance in selecting diagnostic codes from various chapters in the ICD-10-CM. But they are not to be considered a replacement for the ICD-10-CM manual, nor do they provide all the coding information, definitions, or explanations found in the manual. The steps for diagnostic coding (see Procedure 16.1 on p. 350) are the same for all chapters of the ICD-10-CM; however, special rules and considerations apply to some chapters that affect the code selection process.

Coding of Signs and Symptoms

Signs and symptoms are coded only if the provider has not yet determined the final diagnosis. For example, if the provider's notes state "rule out," "suspected," "probable," or "suspected" the coder should use the patient's documented signs and symptoms, including subjective and objective findings. *Subjective findings* include the patient's chief complaint or statements about why the patient is seeking medical care. *Objective findings* are any measurable indicators found during the physical examination. If a patient comes in to see the provider because he or she has had a sore throat and fever for the past 3 days and the provider states "suspected strep throat" as the diagnosis, you would code sore throat and fever.

In the Tabular List, ill-defined conditions, signs, and symptoms are found in Chapter 18, Symptoms, Signs, and Abnormal Clinical and Laboratory Findings, Not Elsewhere Classified (R00–R99).

Conditions, signs, and symptoms found in Chapter 18 include the following:

- Not elsewhere classified (NEC) cases, even after all the facts of the medical case have been examined
- Signs or symptoms that existed on the first encounter but were temporary and for which causes could not be determined

- Conditional diagnosis for a patient who failed to return for further care and the cause of whose condition had not yet been determined
- Medical cases referred elsewhere for treatment before a diagnosis could be made
- Not otherwise specified (NOS) cases in which a more precise diagnosis was not available for any reason
- Certain symptoms, for which supplementary information is provided, that represent important problems in the medical care provided

Coding the Etiology and Manifestation

Etiology refers to the underlying cause or origin of a disease. *Manifestation* describes the signs and symptoms of the disease. In the Alphabetic Index, the etiology and manifestation codes are listed together. The etiology code is always listed first, and the manifestation code is listed beside it in italics and enclosed within brackets. If the diagnosis in the health record indicated **cataract** due to **myxedema**, you would find the following listed in the Alphabetic Index:

- **cataract** (cortical) (immature) (incipient) H26.9
- the essential modifier would be myxedema E03.9 *[H28]*

E03.9 takes you to the Other hypothyroidism section, which is the etiology for this cataract. H28 takes you to the cataract, which is the manifestation. You would need to verify both codes in the Tabular List and list both codes in the documentation.

Multiple Coding

In addition to the signs and symptoms that require two codes to fully describe a single condition affecting multiple body systems, other single conditions may require more than one code. In the Tabular List, *Use additional code* notes appear with codes that are not part of an etiology/manifestation pair, but in which a secondary code is useful to fully describe a condition. The sequencing rule is the same as for the etiology/manifestation pair: *use additional code* indicates that a secondary code should be added after the condition code.

For example, consider a bacterial infection that is not included in Chapter 1, Certain Infectious and Parasitic Diseases (A00–B99). A secondary code may be required to identify the organism causing the infection. This secondary code may come from category **B95**

{*Streptococcus, Staphylococcus,* and *Enterococcus* as the cause of diseases classified elsewhere}

or from category **B96**

{Other bacterial agents as the cause of diseases classified elsewhere}

A *use additional code* note normally is found at the infectious disease code, indicating that the organism code must be added as a secondary code.

As mentioned, *code first* notes are used for certain conditions that involve both an underlying etiology and multiple body system manifestations caused by that etiology. In such cases, the underlying condition should be sequenced first, before the manifestations.

A *code, if applicable, any causal condition first* note indicates that this code may be assigned as a principal diagnosis when the causal condition is unknown or not applicable. If the causal condition is known, the code for that condition should be sequenced as the principal, or first-listed, diagnosis.

Multiple codes may be needed for sequelae, and complication codes and obstetric codes may be needed to more fully describe a condition. See the specific guidelines for these conditions.

Sequela (Late Effects) Codes

Sequelae are the lingering effects produced by a health condition after the acute phase of an illness or injury has ended. The acute phase is considered the first 30 days of a condition with no improvement. There is no time limit on when a **sequela** code can be used. The residual effect may be apparent early (e.g., another stroke), or it may occur months or years later (e.g., the consequences of a previous injury). Coding of sequelae generally requires two codes sequenced in the following order: the original condition or nature of the sequela is sequenced first; the sequela code is sequenced second.

An exception to the above guidelines are instances in which the code for the sequela is followed by a manifestation code identified in the Tabular List; or, the sequela code has been expanded (at the 4th, 5th, or 6th character) to include the manifestation or manifestations. The code for the acute phase of an illness or injury that led to the sequela is never used with a code for the late effect. The following box presents the rules for coding **impending**, or threatened, conditions.

Rules for Coding Impending or Threatened Conditions

Code any condition described at the time of discharge as "impending" or "threatened."

1. If it did occur, code as a confirmed diagnosis.
2. If it did not occur, consult the Alphabetic Index to determine whether the condition has a subterm for impending or threatened; also check main term entries for Impending and threatened.
3. If the subterms are listed, assign the given code.
4. If the subterms are not found, code the existing underlying condition or conditions, signs, or symptoms, and not the condition described as "threatened" or "impending."

Coding Complications of Care

A complication from medical care generally requires additional procedures or services for a patient, but often the complication is not mentioned as part of the diagnostic statement; this can result in reduced reimbursement. It is important to review the medical documentation to determine whether a complication exists and to code the complication in addition to the diagnostic statement. Keep in mind, not all conditions that occur during or after medical care or surgery are classified as complications. Two criteria must be met: a cause-and-effect relationship must be established between the care provided and the condition; and the documentation must indicate that the condition is a complication.

Coding Infectious and Parasitic Diseases

Multiple diagnostic codes are needed to code infectious or parasitic diseases. The first code identifies the disease or condition (e.g., throat infection), and the second code identifies the organism causing the disease (e.g., enterovirus). The second code can be found in the Tabular List in Chapter 1. The basic coding principles for the use of either combination or multiple codes apply throughout this section of the ICD-10-CM.

Coding Organism-Caused Diseases

The two-step process of coding organism-caused diseases begins with the affected anatomic site. In the case of a throat infection caused by enterovirus, you should first assign the diagnostic code for throat infection, or pharyngitis. In the Tabular List, code **J02.8**

> {**Acute pharyngitis due to other specified organism**}

is accompanied by the following *Use additional code* note: "Use additional code (B95–B97) to identify infectious agent" (Fig. 16.6). In the Tabular List, the B95–B97 category/block (found in Chapter 1) is titled Bacterial and Viral Infectious Agents. Starting with code B95, search for the code that specifies enterovirus; this happens to be code **B97.1**

> {**Enterovirus as the cause of diseases classified elsewhere**}

Note that code B97.1 requires a 5th character; however, no other information is provided by the medical record. Therefore, you can assign code **B97.19**

> {**Other enterovirus as the cause of diseases classified elsewhere**}

as the final organism code.

Coding Human Immunodeficiency Virus (HIV) Infection and Acquired Immunodeficiency Syndrome (AIDS)

To correctly code HIV infection and AIDS, it is essential to first understand the descriptions of the codes available. The key is whether the patient has symptoms.

- HIV: This indicates only that the virus is present.
- AIDS: AIDS is a syndrome; a *syndrome* is defined as a "group of symptoms occurring together." AIDS is the manifestation of signs and/or symptoms that can occur as a result of HIV infection.

Never code a patient as having HIV infection unless it is clearly documented as confirmed. Probable and suspected cases are never coded; instead, the signs and symptoms present should be coded. If a patient is seen for an HIV-related condition, the principal diagnosis should be **B20**

> {**Human immunodeficiency virus [HIV] disease**}

followed by additional diagnostic codes for all reported HIV-related conditions.

Remember that strict restrictions are placed on the disclosure of medical information about patients with HIV infection and/or AIDS. Make sure the patient has signed the appropriate release of medical information form before any disclosures are made to third parties.

Coding Neoplasms

A *neoplasm*, or new growth, is coded by the site or location of the neoplasm and its behavior. The Table of Neoplasms (Fig. 16.7) is located just after the Alphabetic Index in the coding manual. This table lists the ICD-10-CM codes for neoplasms by anatomic site in alphabetic order. Six possible code numbers exist for each anatomic site, depending on whether the neoplasm is malignant or benign, exhibits uncertain behavior, or is of an unspecified nature. In the Table of Neoplasms, malignant neoplasms are categorized into three separate subclassifications: Malignant Primary, Malignant Secondary, and Ca in situ (carcinoma in situ).

Terms Defining Malignant Neoplasm Sites

- *Primary:* Identifies the originating anatomic site of the neoplasm. A primary malignancy is defined as the original site or sites of the cancer.
- *Secondary:* Identifies sites to which the primary neoplasm has metastasized (spread). A secondary malignancy is defined as a second location to which the cancer has spread from the primary location.
- *Ca in situ:* Carcinoma in situ is defined as the absence of invasion of surrounding tissues. Tumor cells are undergoing malignant changes but are still confined to the point of origin, without invasion of surrounding normal tissue. The *Ca in situ* column is used only if the provider documents that precise terminology.

Definitions of Benign, Uncertain Behavior, and Unspecified Nature Neoplasms

- *Benign:* The growth is noncancerous, nonmalignant, and has not invaded adjacent structures or spread to distant sites.
- *Uncertain Behavior:* The pathologist is unable to determine whether the neoplasm is benign or malignant.
- *Unspecified Nature:* Neither the behavior nor the **histologic** type of neoplasm is specified in the diagnostic statement.

Most coding decisions on malignant neoplasms are between the primary and secondary classifications. Other terms are used in the following cases:

- *In situ* is used only when the diagnostic statement contains that exact phrase.
- *Unspecified* is used only when no pathologic study has been done, and the neoplasm is still described with a term such as "tumor" or "growth."
- *Uncertain* is used by the provider when it has not been determined whether the neoplasm is malignant or benign.

Six Steps for Coding Neoplasms

The following steps can help determine the most specific and accurate diagnostic code for a neoplasm. These steps can be used in addition to the basic diagnostic steps:

1. In the Table of Neoplasms, find the site (anatomic location) of the neoplasm.

- J02.8 Acute pharyngitis due to other specified organisms

      Use additional code (B95-B97) it identify infectious agent
      Excludes1   pharyngitis due to coxsackie virus (B08.5)
                  pharyngitis due to gonococcus (A54.5)
                  acute pharyngitis due to herpes [simplex] virus (B00.2)
                  acute pharyngitis due to infectious mononucleosis (B27.-)
                  enteroviral vesicular pharyngitis (B08.5)

FIGURE 16.6 Excerpt from the Tabular List: J02.8 Acute pharyngitis due to other specified organisms.

	Malignant Primary	Malignant Secondary	Ca in situ	Benign	Uncertain Behavior	Unspecified Nature		Malignant Primary
bladder (urinary)	C67.9	C79.11	D09Ø	D30.3	D41.4	D49.4	marrow NEC	C96.9
dome	C67.1	C79.11	D09Ø	D30.3	D41.4	D49.4	unspecified side	C40.10
neck	C67.5	C79.11	D09Ø	D30.3	D41.4	D49.4	marrow NEC	C96.9
orifice	C67.9	C79.11	D09Ø	D30.3	D41.4	D49.4	cartilage NEC	C41.9
ureteric	C67.6	C79.11	D09Ø	D30.3	D41.4	D49.4	clavicle	C41.3
urethral	C67.5	C79.11	D09Ø	D30.3	D41.4	D49.4	marrow NEC	C96.9
overlapping lesion	C67.8	—	—	—	—	—	clivus	C41.Ø
sphincter	C67.8	C79.11	D09Ø	D30.3	D41.4	D49.4	marrow NEC	C96.9
trigone	C67.Ø	C79.11	D09Ø	D30.3	D41.4	D49.4	coccygeal vertebra	C41.4
urachus	C67.7	—	D09Ø	D30.3	D41.4	D49.4	marrow NEC	C96.9
wall	C67.9	C79.11	D09Ø	D30.3	D41.4	D49.4	coccyx	C41.4
anterior	C67.3	C79.11	D09Ø	D30.3	D41.4	D49.4	marrow NEC	C96.9
lateral	C67.2	C79.11	D09Ø	D30.3	D41.4	D49.4	costal cartilage	C41.3
posterior	C67.4	C79.11	D09Ø	D30.3	D41.4	D49.4	costovertebral joint	C41.3
blood vessel—*see* Neoplasm, connective tissue							marrow NEC	C96.9
							cranial	C41.Ø

FIGURE 16.7 Excerpt from the Table of Neoplasms.

2. Determine, from the documentation, whether the neoplasm is malignant or benign.
3. If the neoplasm is benign, select the correct column in the table by reviewing the diagnostic statement.
4. If the neoplasm is malignant, select the column in the table that best fits its behavior: Malignant Primary, Malignant Secondary, or Ca in situ.
5. Link the appropriate column to the appropriate row.
6. Check the code shown in the table with the code in the Tabular List, to make sure it complies with the guidelines, conventions, and instructional notations of the latter.

The ICD-10-CM manual always provides additional information, definitions, and guidelines for coding neoplasms in the Tabular List, just as it does for all other diseases, illnesses, and injuries.

Coding for Diabetes Mellitus

Diabetes mellitus (DM) is classified as type 1 or type 2. Patients with DM type 1 develop the disease because the pancreas is unable to produce insulin. In individuals with DM type 2, the pancreas has become unable to maintain the level of insulin the body needs to function, or the person has developed target cell resistance to insulin.

The diabetes mellitus codes are combination codes. This means that they include the type of diabetes mellitus, the body system affected, and the complications affecting that body system. Use as many codes within a particular category/block as necessary to describe all the complications of the disease. These codes should be sequenced according to the reason for a particular encounter. Assign as many codes from category/block E08–E13 (Diabetes Mellitus) as needed to identify all the patient's associated conditions.

Diabetes Mellitus and the Use of Insulin

In the ICD-10-CM, the primary codes for diabetes mellitus (E08–E13) do not include whether the individual is using insulin. Therefore, if insulin use is documented in the health record, a second code is required: **Z79.4**

> **{Long term (current) use of insulin}**

Code Z79.4 should not be assigned if insulin is given temporarily during an encounter to bring the blood glucose level under control in a patient with DM type 2.

Gestational Diabetes

Gestational, or pregnancy induced, diabetes can occur during the second and third trimesters of pregnancy in women who were not diabetic before pregnancy. Gestational diabetes can cause complications in the pregnancy similar to those of pre-existing diabetes mellitus. It also puts the woman at greater risk of developing diabetes after the pregnancy. Codes for gestational diabetes are in subcategory **O24.4**

> **{Gestational diabetes mellitus}**

No other code from category **O24**

> **{Diabetes mellitus in pregnancy, childbirth, and the puerperium}**

should be used with a code from subcategory O24.4. The codes under subcategory O24.4 include diet controlled (O24.410) and insulin controlled (024.414). If a patient with gestational diabetes is treated with both diet and insulin, only the code for insulin controlled is required.

Code **Z79.4**

> **{Long-term (current) use of insulin}**

should also be assigned with codes from subcategory O24.4 if the patient is being treated with insulin.

An abnormal glucose tolerance level in pregnancy is assigned a code from subcategory **O99.81**

> **{Abnormal glucose complicating pregnancy, childbirth, and the puerperium}**

Coding for the Circulatory System

Providers use a wide variety of terms and phrases to identify components of the circulatory system. To code disorders of the circulatory system accurately, the coder must carefully review all inclusions, exclusions, conventions, guidelines, and instructional notations associated with each potential code selected.

Myocardial Infarction

A myocardial infarction (MI) is coded as follows:

- As *acute* if it is documented as such in the diagnostic statement or has a stated duration of 8 weeks or less.
- As *chronic* if it is so stated in the diagnostic statement or if symptoms persist after 8 weeks.

Other MI coding considerations include the following:

1. If an MI is specified as "old" or "healed" without any current or presenting symptoms, it should be coded using category **I21** {**ST elevation (STEMI) and non-ST elevation (NSTEMI) myocardial infarction**}
2. A history of an MI uses code **I25.2** {**Old myocardial infarction**}

   This code is used only if the patient has no symptoms and only if the old MI was diagnosed by means of an electrocardiogram.
3. If the patient is symptomatic, code the underlying condition or symptoms only if the underlying condition is not known: **I21.3** {**ST elevation (STEMI) myocardial infarction of unspecified site**}

Hypertensive Disease

A distinction is made in the ICD-10-CM between "elevated" and "high" blood pressure. High blood pressure is defined as hypertension [**I10 Essential (primary) hypertension**]. If a diagnostic statement does not contain the word "hypertension" or the phrase "high blood pressure," the condition is coded as elevated blood pressure [**R03.0 Elevated blood-pressure reading, without diagnosis of hypertension**], not hypertension.

Hypertension frequently is the cause of various forms of heart and vascular disease; however, the mention of hypertension in the diagnostic statement does not mean that a combination code for hypertensive heart disease should be used. If a cause-and-effect relationship exists between the hypertension and the heart disease, it should be clearly documented in the clinical record or diagnostic statement.

The hypertension table in the ICD-9-CM was not included in the ICD-10-CM. Heart conditions classified to category **I50** {**Heart failure**} or subcategories I51.4–I51.9 are assigned to a code from category **I11** {**Hypertensive heart disease**} when a causal relationship is stated in the health record ("as a result of hypertension") or implied ("hypertensive"). Use an additional code from category I50 to identify the *type* of heart failure in patients with heart failure.

The same heart conditions (category I50 or subcategories I51.4–I51.9) with hypertension, but without a stated causal relationship, are coded separately. The codes should sequence according to the circumstances of the admission or encounter.

Coding for Chronic Kidney Disease

Assign codes from category **I12** {**Hypertensive chronic kidney disease**}

when both hypertension and a condition classifiable to category **N18** {**Chronic kidney disease (CKD)**} are present. Unlike for hypertension with heart disease, the ICD-10-CM presumes a cause-and-effect relationship and classifies chronic kidney disease with hypertension as hypertensive chronic kidney disease.

The appropriate code from category N18 should be used as a secondary code with a code from category I12 to identify the stage of chronic kidney disease.

If a patient has hypertensive chronic kidney disease and acute renal failure, an additional code for the acute renal failure is required.

Coding for Atherosclerotic Cardiovascular Disease

The ICD-10-CM has combination codes for atherosclerotic heart disease with angina pectoris. The subcategories for these codes are **I25.11** {**Atherosclerotic heart disease of native coronary artery with angina pectoris**} and **I25.7** {**Atherosclerosis of coronary artery bypass graft(s) and coronary artery of transplanted heart with angina pectoris**}

When you use one of these combination codes, you do not need to use an additional code for angina pectoris. A causal relationship can be assumed in a patient with both atherosclerosis and angina pectoris, unless the documentation indicates that the angina is due to something other than the atherosclerosis.

If a patient with coronary artery disease is admitted because of an acute myocardial infarction (AMI), the AMI should be sequenced before the coronary artery disease.

Coding for Skin Ulcers

Codes from category **L89** {**Pressure ulcer**}

are combination codes that identify the site of the pressure ulcer and the stage of the ulcer. The ICD-10-CM classifies pressure ulcer stages based on severity, which is designated by stages 1 to 4; unspecified stage; or unstageable. Unspecified and unstageable codes are used for pressure ulcers in which the stage cannot be clinically determined (e.g., the ulcer has been treated with a skin or muscle graft). These codes also are used for pressure ulcers documented as a deep tissue injury, but not documented as being due to trauma. The modifying term defines each stage, depending on the location of the ulcer (Fig. 16.8).

Coding for Complications of Pregnancy, Childbirth, and the Puerperium

Coding for the obstetric patient is like using a specialty codebook within the ICD-10-CM coding manual. This is challenging for coders who do not code obstetrics often. Some important clinical terms regarding pregnancy are:

- *antepartum*: Pregnancy (applies as soon as a pregnancy test result is positive)
- *childbirth*: Delivery
- *postpartum*: The *puerperium*, or first 6 weeks after delivery
- *peripartum*: The period from the last month of pregnancy to 5 months postpartum

L89.21   **Pressure ulcer of right hip**
     L89.210   Pressure ulcer of right hip, unstageable
     L89.211   Pressure ulcer of right hip, stage I
          Healing pressure ulcer of right hip back, stage I
          Pressure pre-ulcer skin changes limited to persistent focal edema, right hip
     L89.212   Pressure ulcer of right hip, stage II
          Healing pressure ulcer of right hip, stage II
          Pressure ulcer with abrasion, blister, partial thickness skin loss involving epidermis and/or dermis, right hip
     L89.213   Pressure ulcer of right hip, stage III
          Healing pressure ulcer of right hip, stage III
          Pressure ulcer with full thickness skin loss involving damage or necrosis of subcutaneous tissue, right hip
     L89.214   Pressure ulcer of right hip, stage IV
          Healing pressure ulcer of right hip, stage IV
          Pressure ulcer with necrosis of soft tissues through to underlying muscle, tendon, or bone, right hip
     L89.219   Pressure ulcer of right hip, unspecified stage
          Healing pressure ulcer of right hip NOS
          Healing pressure ulcer of right hip, unspecified stage

FIGURE 16.8 Coding Example: L89.21 Pressure ulcer of right hip.

Obstetrics cases use codes from Chapter 15, Pregnancy, Childbirth and the Puerperium (O00–O9A). Additional codes from other chapters may be used in conjunction with Chapter 15 codes to further specify conditions.

If the provider documents that the pregnancy is incidental to the encounter, code **Z33.1**

{Pregnant state, incidental}

should be used instead of any Chapter 15 codes. This would be the case if the patient were being seen for a sprained ankle. The sprained ankle is not related to the pregnancy but is an incidental diagnosis. It is the provider's responsibility to state that the condition being treated is not affecting the pregnancy. Codes from Chapter 15 are documented only in the maternal health record; they are never used in the health record of the newborn.

Most of the codes in Chapter 15 have a 6th character, which indicates the trimester of pregnancy. Assignment of the final character for trimester should be based on the provider's documentation of the trimester (or number of weeks) for the encounter. This applies to the assignment of trimester for preexisting conditions, in addition to those that develop during or are due to the pregnancy. The provider's documentation of the number of weeks may be used to assign the appropriate code identifying the trimester. The 7th character in this chapter is used to identify the fetus when there is more than one.

7th Character for Fetus Identification

Some codes in Chapter 15, Pregnancy, Childbirth and the Puerperium (O00–O9A), require a 7th character. In this chapter the 7th character is used when there are multiple fetuses to indicate which fetus is affected. The 7th character options are:
    0 not applicable or unspecified
    1 for the fetus identified as 1
    2 for the fetus identified as 2
    3 for the fetus identified as 3
    4 for the fetus identified as 4
    5 for the fetus identified as 5
    9 other fetus

Outcome of Delivery and Liveborn Infant Codes

When a delivery occurs, the principal diagnosis should correspond to the main circumstances or complication of the delivery. In cases of cesarean delivery, the selection of the principal diagnosis should be the condition assigned after the encounter that was responsible for the patient's admission. If the patient was admitted with a condition that resulted in the performance of a cesarean procedure, that condition should be selected as the principal diagnosis. If the reason for the admission was unrelated to the condition resulting in the cesarean delivery, the condition related to the reason for the admission/encounter should be selected as the principal diagnosis.

For example, a maternity patient was admitted to the hospital for pneumonia, but because of complications, a cesarean section was performed. In this case, the pneumonia would be the primary diagnosis. A code from category **Z37**

{Outcome of delivery}

should always be included in the maternal health record when a delivery has occurred. Codes from category Z37 are not to be used in subsequent records or in the newborn's health record.

Code **O80**

{Encounter for full-term uncomplicated delivery}

should be assigned when a woman is admitted for a full-term vaginal delivery and delivers a single, healthy infant without any complications antepartum, during the delivery, or postpartum during the delivery episode. Code O80 is always a principal diagnosis.

Newborn Coding

Chapter 16, Certain Conditions Originating in the Perinatal Period (P00–P96), also is used for coding and reporting purposes. The perinatal period extends from just before the birth through day 28 after the birth. When you code the birth episode in a newborn's health record, assign a code from category **Z38**

{Liveborn infants according to place of birth and type of delivery}

as the principal diagnosis. A code from category Z38 is assigned only once, to a newborn at the time of birth. If a newborn is transferred to another institution, a code from category Z38 should not be used at the receiving hospital. When a newborn is admitted to another hospital, the newborn's admitting diagnosis is the health condition that required the hospital transfer.

Coding for Injuries

When you code injuries, assign separate codes for each injury unless a combination code is provided, in which case the combination code is assigned. Code **T07**

> **{Unspecified multiple injuries}**

should not be assigned in the inpatient setting unless documentation for a more specific code is not available. Traumatic injury codes (S00–T14.9) are not to be used for normal, healing surgical wounds or to identify complications of surgical wounds.

The code for the most serious injury, as determined by the provider and the focus of treatment, is sequenced first.

Superficial Injuries

Superficial injuries, such as abrasions and contusions, are not coded when they are associated with more severe injuries at the same site.

Primary Injury With Damage to Nerves and/or Blood Vessels

When a primary injury results in minor damage to peripheral nerves or blood vessels, the primary injury is sequenced first. Any additional code or codes for injuries to nerves and the spinal cord and/or injury to vessels or nerves are coded as secondary.

Coding for Traumatic Fractures

The principles of multiple coding of injuries should be followed in the coding of fractures. Fractures of specified sites are coded individually by site in accordance with the level of detail furnished by the health record. The traumatic fracture categories include the following: A02, S12, S22, S32, S42, S49, S52, S59, S62, S72, S82, S89, and S92. A fracture not indicated as open or closed should be coded as closed. A fracture not indicated as displaced or not displaced should be coded as displaced.

Coding for Burns and Corrosions

The same principles for multiple coding apply to burns. Code each burn separately unless specific combination codes are given in the Tabular List. There are many combination codes. Most burn codes are found in Chapter 19 (Injury, Poisoning, and Certain Other Consequences of External Origin); the applicable codes are T20–T32. Because burns are coded by site and degree and by the extent of body surface involvement, all burn cases should have at least two codes, and a third if the wound is infected. Other types of wounds, lacerations, punctures, and so on use a different 5th character to show that they are infected and, therefore, complicated. However, burn codes use the 5th character for other information. Therefore, these diagnoses require an additional code to indicate infection.

The ICD-10-CM makes a distinction between burns and corrosions. The burn codes are used for the following: thermal burns (except sunburns) caused by a heat source, such as a fire or hot appliance; burns resulting from electricity; and burns resulting from radiation. Corrosions, on the other hand, are burns caused by chemicals. The guidelines are the same for burns and corrosions.

Current burns (T20–T25) are classified by depth, extent, and burn agent (X code). Depth is categorized as first degree (redness), second degree (blistering), and third degree (full-thickness involvement).

Burns of the eye and internal organs (T26–T28) are classified by site but not by degree.

Coding for Drug Toxicity

Chapter 19 also includes coding for the following drug toxicity classifications:

- *Poisoning* (T36–T50): A reaction to the improper use of a medication, which can be the result of an error made by the prescribing provider, intentional overdose, interaction with drugs or alcohol, or a reaction caused when a nonprescribed medication interacts with a prescribed and properly administered medication.
- *Adverse effect:* An unfavorable side effect that occurs even though a medication is correctly prescribed and properly administered.
- *Underdosing:* Patient takes less of a medication than is prescribed by the provider or by the manufacturer's instructions.
- *Toxic effect:* Patient ingests or comes in contact with a toxic substance.

Codes in categories T36–T65 are combination codes that include the substance taken and the intent. No additional external cause code is required for poisonings, toxic effects, adverse effects, and underdosing codes. When you are coding, do not code directly from the Table of Drugs and Chemicals. Always refer back to the Tabular List.

Coding for External Causes of Morbidity

External cause codes are intended to provide data for research on injuries and for evaluation of injury prevention strategies. These codes capture:

- how the injury or health condition happened (cause)
- the intent (unintentional or accidental; or intentional, such as suicide or assault)
- the place where the event occurred
- the activity of the patient at the time of the event, and the person's status (e.g., civilian, military)

These codes are often used for workers' compensation claims.

Place of Occurrence Guideline

Codes from category **Y92**

> **{Place of occurrence of the external cause}**

are secondary codes. They are used after other external cause codes to identify the location of the patient at the time of the injury or other condition.

A place of occurrence code is used only once, at the initial encounter for treatment. No 7th character is used in Y92 codes. Only one code from category Y92 should be recorded on the patient's health record. Do not use place of occurrence code **Y92.9**

> **{Unspecified place or not applicable}**

if the place is not stated or if it is not applicable.

Activity Codes

Category **Y93** codes

> **{Activity codes}**

are used to define the activity the patient was involved in at the time of injury or when the health condition developed. Only one code from category Y93 should be recorded in the patient's health record. An activity code should be used in conjunction with a place of occurrence code (Y92). The activity codes are not applicable to poisonings, adverse effects, misadventures, or sequelae.

Do not assign code **Y93.9**

{Unspecified activity}

if the activity is not stated.

A code from category Y93 can be used with external cause (Y99) and occurrence (Y92) codes if identifying the activity provides additional information about the event. For example, you are coding a closed ankle fracture that occurred while the patient was playing soccer in a public park. First, you must identify what should be coded first. In this case, the ankle fracture is coded first: **S92.111A**

{Displaced fracture of neck of right talus}

(Remember, "A" indicates initial encounter). The second code is the activity code; the patient was playing soccer, so the code for this activity is **Y93.66**

{Activity, soccer}

Remember, if the report did not state an activity, do not add **Y93.9**

{Unspecified activity}

Finally, when an activity code is used, a place of occurrence code should also be used. In this scenario, the patient was playing in a public park; therefore, the place of occurrence code is **Y92.830**

{Public park}

Coding for Health Status and Contact With Health Services

In the ICD-10-CM, Chapter 21, Factors Influencing Health Status and Contact with Health Services (Z00–Z99) are used to describe circumstances or encounters with a healthcare provider when no current illness or injury exists. The 16 categories of Z codes include contact/exposure, inoculations and vaccinations, health status, history of screening, observation, aftercare, follow-up, donor counseling, encounters for obstetric and reproductive services, newborns and infants, routine and administrative examinations, and other health encounters that do not fall into any one of the mentioned categories.

MAXIMIZING THIRD-PARTY REIMBURSEMENT

The most important thing to remember in using the ICD-10-CM is to code the diagnosis to the highest level of specificity. Obtaining the correct reimbursement is important to the practice's cash flow, and it depends on proper coding and billing techniques. Some other crucial points to remember when submitting diagnostic codes for claims include:

- Use the current year ICD-10-CM manual and stay informed of all changes, revisions, and additions published for that year to both the codes and the official coding guidelines.
- Code accurately from documented information, making sure the appropriate code or codes are assigned for all parts of the diagnostic statement, with no additions or omissions.
- Be sure the diagnosis corresponds to the symptoms and treatment. Many codes are specific to age and gender.
- Review data entry to make sure no digits have been transposed.
- Know the insurance carrier's rules and requirements for completion and submission of claims.
- Incomplete or inaccurate codes may result in delay or denial of reimbursement. An inaccurate diagnosis may have a lifelong negative effect on the patient.

PROVIDERS AND ACCURATE CODING

Detailed documentation in the patient's health record can help coders to code to the highest specificity. Therefore, providers should be trained in how to document patient health records appropriately. Respectfully discuss with providers that diagnostic codes cannot be assigned unless clear documentation is found in the patient's health record. Some providers may feel that because they care for the same type of cases, specialized diagnostic statements should be implied. However, the medical assistant should stress to providers the importance of detailed documentation and how developing this practice not only improves ICD-10-CM code assignment but may also result in higher health insurance reimbursements.

Staff meetings to review third-party requirements should be held regularly by the medical billing supervisor. Medical assistants should be respectful to the healthcare provider when discussing third-party requirements for more detailed documentation. An understanding and patient attitude toward the healthcare provider goes a long way in building a trusting relationship.

Ethical Standards of Medical Coding

At times coders can feel pressured by decreasing insurance reimbursements and their employers to use fraudulent coding practices. However, if a medical practice is convicted of fraudulent billing, the coders may lose their coding license and face federal fines. A number of ethical standards have been established for medical coding, and most of these can help coders identify unethical coding behaviors. The following tips explain how to proceed in scenarios that may pose ethical dilemmas.

1. **Understand what ethical coding standards mean.** Coders face stress from all sides: financial issues, providers, and other coders. However, stress cannot be a compelling reason coders intentionally report diagnoses and/or higher specificity codes without sufficient documentation.
2. **Stand your ground.** When coding, be true to yourself, even though it can be hard in a stressful environment. When you know a record needs additional documentation to justify reporting certain codes, don't be afraid to speak up to the provider. Conduct research ahead of time to strengthen your case. For example, search through and print out applicable issues of *Coding Clinic* from the American Hospital Association website: *ahacentraloffice.org*. The more backup documentation you have, the more likely it is that management will support your ethical coding decision.
3. **Say something.** Other coders may not follow the same ethical coding standards as you. If you observe unethical coding practices, bring it to the attention of the coder and allow him or her to make the needed adjustments. Broaching this issue with a colleague can be challenging but encourage the other coder to reflect on the ethics of his or her actions. If the unethical coding practices continue, be sure to inform the next person in command.
4. **Keep in communication with the office manager.** Some coding situations require more management involvement than others. For example, if your conversation with a colleague does nothing to dissuade unethical behavior, bring your manager into the loop. Or, if you know you need to query a provider about a health record that might yield a higher reimbursement, but that provider is on vacation for 7 days, enlist your office manager's

help in flagging the health record until the provider returns to clarify it.

5. **Review notes from other health providers.** In most scenarios, coders are not allowed to code from documentation by anyone other than a provider; however, notes from ancillary staff members may encourage a coder to ask the provider whether the diagnosis does exist. For example, if a consultation with a dietitian suggests that a patient is malnourished, but the provider does not document this anywhere, you may be able to use the dietitian's clinical information as the basis for querying the provider. The diagnosis cannot be coded based solely on the dietitian's clinical information; the code can be assigned only after the provider confirms the diagnosis.

CLOSING COMMENTS

Diagnostic coding using the ICD-10-CM, with its almost 70,000 codes, can seem overwhelming. Successful medical coders follow specific steps to assign the most accurate ICD-10-CM code. Encoder software (e.g., TruCode) can search ICD-10-CM electronically to aid in faster coding. Detailed documentation in the patient's health record and accurate coding work hand-in-hand to maximize reimbursement for services provided. When you work with providers on issues related to coding and documentation, show respect and patience. Medical assistants are expected to follow ethical standards by assigning and reporting only codes that are clearly supported by the documentation in the patient's record. When in doubt, a medical assistant should consult the provider for clarification. A coding professional is responsible for maintaining and continually enhancing his or her coding skills and for staying current with the changes in the codes, guidelines, and regulations.

Patient Coaching

Most patients know very little about medical coding, so they may not understand how the codes on their encounter forms relate to their diagnosis. If the patient has questions, explain that the codes represent his or her diagnosis to the most specific and accurate level. Because the coding system is much like a foreign language to patients, be patient when explaining this process and answering questions, so that the patient is able to understand the insurance billing process.

Legal and Ethical Issues

Using the medical coding system allows providers to express the simplicity or complexity of a medical treatment or procedure. This specificity leads to the maximum reimbursement to the provider. The medical assistant must perform coding procedures accurately so that they reflect exactly what happened during the treatment. Codes must not be exaggerated to increase reimbursement to the provider.

Professional Behaviors

Although providers may be overly concerned about the need to maximize insurance reimbursements, coders should never feel coerced into fraudulent coding practices. Successful coders rely solely on medical documentation as the source of diagnostic statements. Coders should never assume that additional complications or conditions exist if they are not documented. In these cases, strong communication between the coder and the provider is necessary to clarify the appropriate diagnoses.

SUMMARY OF SCENARIO

Mike's experience using the ICD-10-CM coding manual and encoder software on actual medical office cases has made him even more enthusiastic about his new responsibilities, and he enjoys the coding process more. He knows that as he gains experience in ICD-10-CM coding, he will be able to set a positive example for the staff. As Mike progresses with diagnostic coding, he will also be able to help the providers and medical assistant staff be attentive to details when documenting in a health record.

Although the electronic encounter form for entering billing codes is an easy tool, Mike has learned that knowing how to use the ICD-10-CM Alphabetic Index and Tabular List is a necessary skill to ensure accurate coding. He also knows

that it is important when coding a diagnosis to make sure the medical documentation matches the encounter form and that all elements of the diagnostic statement are included. Furthermore, he must ensure that the diagnosis listed on the encounter form is fully documented in the patient's health record. Mike is feeling more comfortable about referring to coding guidelines to ensure the most accurate code and to make certain that every character for the ICD-10-CM code is present. Every feature of the manual provides guidance in choosing and confirming a diagnostic code that matches the diagnostic statement on the encounter form and in the health record. Searching for codes in the encoder also has helped Mike develop his coding skills more quickly.

SUMMARY OF LEARNING OBJECTIVES

1. **Describe the historical use of the International Classification of Disease (ICD) in the United States and describe how diagnostic coding is related to medical necessity.**
   In 1946, the International Commission of the World Health Organization (WHO) established a code set called the *Manual of the International Statistical Classification of Diseases, Injuries, and Causes of Death* (ICD). Eventually, WHO approved an adaptation of this code set for use in the United States; the ninth edition, the *International Classification of Diseases, Ninth Revision, Clinical Modification* (ICD-9-CM), was approved and put into use in 1975. The United States adopted ICD-10-CM diagnostic coding on October 1, 2015.

The diagnostic code tells the insurance company why a procedure was done. If the diagnosis does not match the procedure, then the insurance company can say that it was not medically necessary and not pay for the procedure.

2. **Identify the structure and format of the *International Classification of Diseases, 10th Revision, Clinical Modification* (ICD-10-CM).**

Depending on the publisher, the ICD-10-CM coding manual will vary somewhat in layout, symbols, color coding, and some other features. However, the format, conventions, tables, appendixes, content, and basic structure are always the same.

Every ICD-10-CM code begins with an alphabetic letter that indicates the chapter of disease and injury in which the code is listed. (All the letters in the English alphabet are used except U, which WHO has reserved to assign to new diseases with uncertain etiologies.) Codes contain up to 7 alphanumeric characters; the first 3 characters are followed by a period. Codes that require a 7th character may use an X as a placeholder for the 4th, 5th, and 6th characters if no other code can be used for those characters.

3. **Describe how to use the Alphabetic Index to select main terms, essential modifiers, and the appropriate code (or codes) and code ranges.**

The ICD-10-CM Index to Diseases and Injuries (commonly called the *Alphabetic Index*) consists of an alphabetic list of diagnostic terms and related codes. This index includes main terms, nonessential modifiers, essential modifiers, and subterms. Fig. 16.3 provides an example of the *main term* **Colitis**; which is followed by the *nonessential modifiers* (acute), (catarrhal), (chronic), (noninfective), and (hemorrhagic). The second *essential modifier* listed under the main term is "amebic (acute)," and the *subterm* listed under amebic is "nondysenteric." The *main term* is bold face; the *nonessential modifiers* that follow it are enclosed in parentheses; the *essential modifier* is indented one space under the main term; and the *subterm* is indented one space under the essential modifier (two spaces under the main term). The nonessential modifiers (i.e., acute, catarrhal, chronic, noninfective, and hemorrhagic) do not affect the code assignment. The hyphen (-) at the end of the code indicates that additional characters are required to complete the code.

4. **Do the following related to the Tabular List:**
   - *Explain how to use the Tabular List to select main terms, essential modifiers, and the appropriate code (or codes) or code ranges.*

     The ICD-10-CM Tabular List of Diseases and Injuries (commonly called simply the *Tabular List*) is divided into 21 chapters. Each chapter is divided into categories, or *blocks,* that have been assigned 3-character codes. These codes form the foundation of the ICD-10-CM code set.

     In most of the chapters, the title is composed of a group of diseases and injuries, followed by a code range in parentheses. For example, Chapter 1 is: Certain Infectious and Parasitic Diseases (A00–B99). However, some chapter titles use a part of the body or an organ

system to group the codes; for example: Chapter 9, Diseases of the Circulatory System (I00–I99). Still other chapters group conditions together by etiology or the nature of the disease process, as in Chapter 2, Neoplasms (C00–D49). Chapter 15, Pregnancy, Childbirth, and the Puerperium (O00–O9A), groups codes related to the prenatal and postnatal periods. Chapter 20, External Causes of Morbidity (V00–Y99), replaces the V and E codes used in the ICD-9-CM. Chapter 20 also groups codes related to external causes of injury and poisoning. Chapter 21 is Factors Influencing Health Status and Contact with Health Services (Z00–Z99).

   - *Summarize coding conventions as defined in the ICD-10-CM coding manual.*

     Conventions are abbreviations, punctuation, symbols, instructional notations, and related elements that help the coder select an accurate, specific code. Conventions are found in the Tabular List, but not in the Alphabetic Index. Understanding their meaning and using them as guides are crucial to accurate coding.

5. **Review the Official Coding Guidelines to assign the most accurate ICD-10-CM diagnostic code.**

An important section of the coding manual is the ICD-10-CM Official Guidelines for Coding and Reporting. Every coding guideline for the entire ICD-10-CM code set is included in this Coding Guidelines section at the beginning of the manual. These guidelines are a set of rules developed to accompany and complement the official conventions and instructions provided in the ICD-10-CM proper.

6. **Explain how to abstract the diagnostic statement from a patient's health record.**

To prepare for medical coding, the medical assistant must analyze and abstract the diagnostic statements documented in the various reports in the patient's health record. Sources of diagnostic statements include the encounter form; treatment notes; discharge summary; operative report; and radiology, pathology, and laboratory reports.

7. **Describe how to use the most current diagnostic codes and perform diagnostic coding.**

Eight basic steps are required for accurate ICD-10-CM coding (see Table 16.3). The first step involves abstracting the diagnostic statement from the health record and determining the main and essential modifiers from the various medical reports. The next steps are performed using the Alphabetic Index to search for the code, codes, or code ranges that best fit the diagnostic statement. The remaining steps are performed using the Tabular List to verify and confirm that the code or codes located in the Alphabetic Index fully match the diagnostic statement and are the most specific and accurate diagnostic codes. The medical assistant's knowledge of accurate diagnostic coding contributes to the legal and financial health of the practice. In most cases, ICD-10-CM codes are found on the encounter form. However, with literally thousands of current diagnostic codes, it may be necessary to code from the ICD-10-CM manual. The process for diagnostic coding is outlined in Procedure 16.1 on p 278.

Continued

SUMMARY OF LEARNING OBJECTIVES—*continued*

8. **Identify how encoder software can help the coder assign the most accurate diagnostic code.**

   Encoder software is computer-aided coding, which helps determine the most accurate code possible. The coder types a few key words into a Search box, and the software matches the entry with main terms in the Alphabetic Index. The coder then clicks on a specific code to hyperlink to the Tabular List.

9. **Explain the importance of coding guidelines for accuracy, discuss special rules and considerations that apply to the code selection process, and describe how to maximize third-party reimbursement.**

   All ICD-10-CM coding manuals, regardless of the publisher, have comprehensive instructional notes and conventions to help the coder select the most accurate diagnostic code or codes. When a discrepancy occurs between reference sources, including this text, the current year's ICD-10-CM coding manual is the final authority. When coding,

   the medical assistant must always refer to and thoroughly review the conventions, instructional notations, code definitions, and other guidelines in the Alphabetic Index and Tabular List.

   The most important thing to remember in using the ICD-10-CM is to code the diagnosis to the highest level of specificity in order to maximize third-party reimbursement.

10. **Review medical coding ethical standards.**

    At times medical coders can feel pressure from decreasing insurance reimbursements and their employers that they justify fraudulent coding practices. If a medical practice is convicted of fraudulent billing, it will lose its coding license, and it and the coder also may face federal fines. A number of standards have been established for ethical coding, and most of these can help coders recognize unethical coding behaviors.

PROCEDURE 16.1   Perform Coding Using the Current ICD-10-CM Manual or Encoder

Task: To perform accurate diagnosis coding using the ICD-10-CM manual.

Scenario: The encounter form and progress notes both show that the diagnosis for this patient encounter is acute colitis. Locate the most accurate ICD-10-CM code for this diagnostic statement.

EQUIPMENT and SUPPLIES

- ICD-10-CM manual (current year), or
- Encoder software, such as TruCode

PROCEDURAL STEPS

Alphabetic Index

1. Determine and locate the main terms from the diagnostic statement in the Alphabetic Index.
   PURPOSE: To provide a starting point for searching the Alphabetic Index.
2. Locate the essential modifiers listed under the main term in the Alphabetic Index.
   PURPOSE: To ensure further specificity of the codes found in the Alphabetic Index.
3. Review the conventions, punctuation, and notes in the Alphabetic Index.
   PURPOSE: To ensure that no additional searches, exclusions, or similar terms are needed to complete the search in the Alphabetic Index.
4. Choose a tentative code, codes, or code range from the Alphabetic Index that matches the diagnostic statement as closely as possible.
   PURPOSE: To prevent backtracking and repeated searches in the Alphabetic Index.

Tabular List

1. Look up the codes chosen from the Alphabetic Index in the Tabular List.
   PURPOSE: To begin the process of determining whether the codes selected from the Alphabetic Index are appropriate and accurate.
2. Review notes, conventions, and the Official Coding Guidelines associated with the code and code description in the Tabular List.
   a. Review conventions and punctuation.
   b. Review instructional notations:
      - *Includes* and *excludes* notes
      - *Code first, code also,* and *code additional* notes
      - *and, or,* and *with* statements
   PURPOSE: To ensure that the code or codes selected are appropriate for use and to determine whether they require additional codes or further specificity or are excluded from use.
3. Verify the accuracy of the tentative code in the Tabular List.
   a. Make sure all elements of the diagnostic statement are included in the codes selected.
   b. Make sure the code description does not include anything not documented in the diagnostic statement.
   PURPOSE: To ensure that the most accurate and specific code is selected and that no contraindication exists to use of the code or codes selected.

PROCEDURE 16.1   Perform Coding Using the Current ICD-10-CM Manual or Encoder—*continued*

4. Extend the codes to their highest level of specificity (up to the 7th character, if required). If a 7th character is required, and no codes are present for the 4th, 5th, or 6th characters, it is appropriate to use the dummy placeholder X for these positions.

5. Assign the code (or codes) selected from the Tabular List as the appropriate code for the patient's condition by documenting it in the patient's health record.

<u>PURPOSE</u>: To ensure that the health record and/or electronic encounter form contain documentation of the code or codes assigned.

Using the TruCode Encoder Software

1. Type in the main term from the diagnostic statement in the search box, as in the following figure.

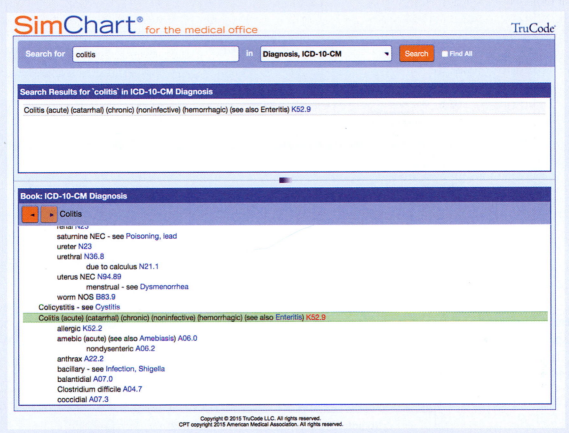

1

2. The software will provide a list of main terms that could be related to the diagnosis typed in the search box. The coder chooses the main term that best represents the diagnostic statement.

3. Based on the main term chosen, a list of essential modifiers is presented (see the following figure). The coder must review the diagnostic statement to ensure that all documented modifying terms are identified. If the provider does not document a modifying term, the coder should not assume that a modifying term was implied.

Continued

PROCEDURE 16.1   Perform Coding Using the Current ICD-10-CM Manual or Encoder—*continued*

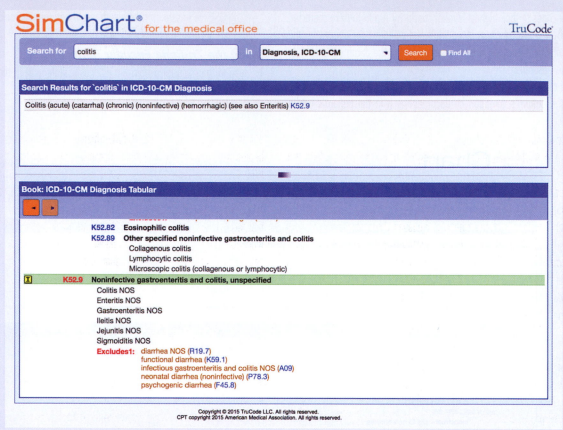

2

4. In the preceding figure, note the yellow on the left of the chosen diagnosis. In the TruCode program, click on the yellow area, and an instructional notes textbox, which includes coding guidelines, will appear, as in the following figure. To determine the most accurate code, follow these coding guidelines.

5. Once all the menus of essential modifiers have been presented, choose the most accurate and specific code based on the diagnostic statement.

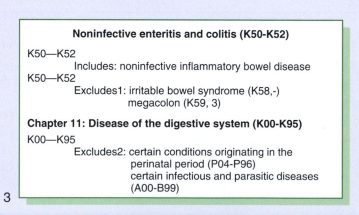

Noninfective enteritis and colitis (K50-K52)

K50—K52
       Includes: noninfective inflammatory bowel disease
K50—K52
       Excludes1: irritable bowel syndrome (K58,-)
           megacolon (K59, 3)

Chapter 11: Disease of the digestive system (K00-K95)

K00—K95
       Excludes2: certain conditions originating in the
           perinatal period (P04-P96)
           certain infectious and parasitic diseases
           (A00-B99)

3

SCENARIO

Sherald Vogt, a medical assisting student, works at Walden-Martin Family Medical Clinic (WMFM). Sherald really enjoyed learning about diagnostic coding in the *International Classification of Diseases, 10th Revision, Clinical Modification* (ICD-10-CM), and now she looks forward to learning about procedural coding. Sherald recognizes that a strong understanding of anatomy and physiology are vital to correct diagnostic coding. She also believes the knowledge she has gained will help her in procedural coding. Sherald will be using the *Current Procedural Terminology* (CPT) coding system for most procedures and services provided in the medical office. In addition, she will use the *Healthcare Common Procedure Coding System* (HCPCS; pronounced "hic-pix") for medical products and services not found in the CPT.

As she did with the ICD-10-CM, Sherald is learning that accurate coding begins with the proper analysis of documentation found in the health record. With that information, she will abstract the correct data to assign an accurate procedure code. As does the ICD-10-CM, the CPT has coding guidelines, symbols, and formal steps specific to procedural coding. However, unlike in ICD-10-CM diagnostic coding, in CPT and HCPCS coding Sherald must determine how and when to use modifiers. The office manager wants to give Sherald some experience, so he allows her to review some healthcare records, so she can practice coding.

While studying this chapter, think about the following questions:
- What code set will be used for outpatient procedural coding?
- What will Sherald find similar to what she learned with the ICD-10-CM as she performs procedural coding?
- What will help Sherald select the most specific and accurate CPT code?
- What are the differences between CPT coding and HCPCS coding?
- How will Sherald use and apply modifiers in CPT and HCPCS coding?
- What will Sherald learn about the legal implications of inaccurate coding?

LEARNING OBJECTIVES

1. List and describe the three code categories in the *Current Procedural Terminology* (CPT) manual.
2. Distinguish between the Alphabetic Index and the Tabular List in the CPT code set. Also, list the six different sections of the Tabular List.
3. Discuss special reports and explain the importance of modifiers in assigning CPT codes.
4. Review various conventions in the CPT code set.
5. Identify the required medical documentation for accurate procedural coding.
6. Describe the steps that should be taken in order to be efficient with CPT procedural coding. Also discuss how to use the alphabetic index and the tabular list.
7. Identify CPT coding guidelines for evaluation and management (E/M) procedures. In addition, perform procedural coding of an office visit and an immunization.
8. Identify CPT coding guidelines for anesthesia procedures.
9. Identify CPT coding guidelines for surgical procedures.
10. Discuss coding factors for the integumentary system and muscular system, and for maternity care and delivery.
11. Identify CPT coding guidelines for the Radiology, Pathology and Laboratory, and Medicine sections.
12. Do the following related to the HCPCS code set and manual:
    - Identify procedures and services that require HCPCS codes.
    - Describe how to use the most current HCPCS level II coding system.
13. Summarize common HCPCS coding guidelines.

VOCABULARY

bilaterally (bie LAT er uhl ee) Pertaining to, involving, or affecting two or both sides.

Certified Registered Nurse Anesthetist (CRNA) A nursing healthcare professional who is certified to administer anesthesia.

chief complaint A statement in the patient's own words that describes the reason for the visit.

CPT Assistant An online CPT coding journal, supported by the AMA, that addresses subjects such as appealing insurance denials, validating coding to auditors, training staff members, and answering day-to-day coding questions.

debridement The surgical removal of dead, damaged, or infected tissue to improve the function of healthy tissue.

eponym (EP uh nim) In medical terms, a medical diagnosis or procedure named for the person who discovered it.

global services For purposes of CPT coding, medical services and procedures performed for the patient before, during, and after a surgical procedure, that are included with the assigned CPT code.

performance measurement The regular collection of data to assess whether the correct processes are being performed and desired results are being achieved.

review of systems (ROS) A list of questions related to each organ system, designed to uncover potential disease processes.

special report Additional medical documentation required to confirm the need for the use of unlisted, unusual, or newly adopted medical procedures code.

specificity (spes i FIS i tee) The quality or state of being specific.

Procedural coding changes the written descriptions of procedures and services delivered in a healthcare facility into numeric or alphanumeric codes. These codes are used for a variety of different purposes. They can be used to track the services that are being provided to patients and on claims sent for payment from insurance companies. There are three procedure code sets used for these purposes:

- *International Classification of Diseases, 10th Revision, Procedural Coding System* (ICD-10-PCS)
- *Current Procedural Terminology* (CPT)
- *Healthcare Common Procedure Coding System* (HCPCS)

Table 17.1 compares the three different code sets. Medical assistants most often work in an outpatient setting. This chapter will focus on the CPT and HCPCS code sets. The medical biller is responsible for maintaining accurate medical records and for processing insurance claims. This can be done efficiently by using the CPT and HCPCS codes. These codes identify procedures and services commonly used in an outpatient healthcare facility.

INTRODUCTION TO THE CPT MANUAL

The Current Procedural Terminology (CPT) system was developed and is maintained by the American Medical Association (AMA). It

is updated each year and released on October 1. The CPT coding manual consists of descriptive terms and identifying codes for reporting professional and technical services. CPT codes convert written descriptions of procedures and services into numeric codes. They establish a standard system that accurately describes medical and surgical services.

CODE CATEGORIES IN THE CPT MANUAL

There are three different categories of codes in the CPT. Category I codes are used most frequently and are required for insurance claim submission. Category II and Category III codes are used for data collection.

Category I Codes

Category I codes are located in the Tabular List of the CPT manual and arranged by sections. For example, codes beginning with 7 (e.g., 70100—radiologic examination of the mandible, partial, with less than four views) are located in the Radiology section of the manual. Each code has a description of the service or procedure performed. These codes are 5-digit numeric codes.

TABLE 17.1 Comparison of Procedural Code Sets

CODE SET	USED FOR	CODE FEATURES	EXAMPLE	DESCRIPTION	DEVELOPER	UPDATED
ICD-10-PCS	Inpatient hospital procedures	7-digit alphanumeric code	0TTJ0ZZ	Appendectomy	National Center for Health Statistics	Annually, October 1
CPT	Outpatient procedures; professional and technical services	5-digit numeric code; a 2-digit modifier can be added	44970	Laparoscopic appendectomy	American Medical Association (AMA)	Annually, January 1
HCPCS	Auxiliary medical treatment, including vaccines, medical transport, drugs, durable medical equipment	5-digit alphanumeric code; a 2-digit modifier can be added	A0428	Ambulance service, basic life support, nonemergency transport	Centers for Medicare and Medicaid Services (CMS)	Annually, October 1

Format of the CPT Coding Manual

- Comprehensive instructions for using the manual, including the steps for coding
- Tabular List, which includes the following six sections:
  - Evaluation and Management
  - Anesthesia
  - Surgery
  - Radiology
  - Pathology and Laboratory
  - Medicine
- Coding Guidelines, Conventions, and Notes
- Appendices (16; A–P)
- The Alphabetic Index

Fracture

Acetabulum	
Closed Treatment	27220-27222
Open Treatment	27226-27228
with Manipulation	27222
without Manipulation	27220
Alveolar Ridge	
Closed Treatment	21440
Open Treatment	21445
Ankle	
Bimalleolar	27808, 27810, 27814
Lateral	27786, 27788, 27792, 27808, 27810, 27814
Medial	27760, 27762, 27766, 27808, 27810, 27814
Posterior	27767-27769, 27808, 27810, 27814
Trimalleolar	27816, 27818, 27822-27823
Ankle Bone	
Medial	27760-27762
Bennett's	
See Thumb, Fracture	
Blow-Out Fracture	
Orbital Floor	21385-21387, 21390, 21395
Bronchi	
Reduction	31630
Calcaneus	
Closed Treatment	28400-28405
Open Treatment	28415-28420
Percutaneous Fixation	28406
with Manipulation	28405-28406
without Manipulation	28400

FIGURE 17.1 Alphabetic Index: Fractures.

Category II Codes

Category II codes are a set of supplemental tracking codes that healthcare facilities use for **performance measurement**. Category II codes are optional. They cannot be used as a substitute for Category I codes, and they are not used as part of the insurance billing process. When these codes are used, it can reduce the need for abstracting information from the health record. These codes describe clinical components that may be typically included in Evaluation and Management services, or clinical services. In a Category II code, the 5th digit is the letter F. If a patient was seen by the provider for asthma, a Category I code of 99213 could be used for the visit. In addition, a Category II code of 2015F Asthma impairment assessed (Asthma) could be used.

Category II codes are described and listed in their own section, which is located after the Medicine section and before the appendices. Category II codes are reviewed by the Performance Measures Advisory Group. This group is composed of members from various medical organizations and government agencies.

Category III Codes

Category III codes are temporary codes used for emerging and new technology, services, and procedures that have not been officially added to the Tabular List. The 5th digit in a Category III code is the letter T. Category III codes may be used in billing and reporting if:

- no code in the Tabular List correctly describes the technology, service, or procedure performed.
- no Category I code matches the documentation.

In most publishers' editions of the CPT manual, Category III codes are also listed in their own section, after the Medicine section and before the appendices.

ORGANIZATION OF THE CPT MANUAL

The CPT coding manual is separated into the Alphabetic Index and the Tabular List.

The Alphabetic Index

CPT coding starts with the Alphabetic Index. It is found in the back of the CPT manual and is an alphabetic listing of main terms. These terms represent the type of surgery, the anatomic site, or **eponym** (Fig. 17.1). Much like the Alphabetic Index in the ICD-10-CM manual, the Alphabetic Index in the CPT gives a code, codes, or a code range that must be verified in the Tabular List of the CPT manual.

CRITICAL THINKING APPLICATION 17.1

To practice her coding skills, Sherald is reviewing a surgical report for a gallbladder removal. Will she be able to find the main term "gallbladder" in the Alphabetic Index? Why or why not? What other main term could she be looking for? Once she finds the range of codes in the Alphabetic Index, what is her next step?

The Tabular List

The Tabular List is divided into six sections, with codes listed in numeric order in each section. As in the ICD-10-CM, the codes in the Tabular List include definitions, guidelines, and notes. These enable the coder to select the most specific code based on the procedural statement and service descriptions documented in the health record. The six sections of the Tabular List and their CPT code ranges are:

- Evaluation and Management (99201–99499)
- Anesthesia (00100–01999, 99100–99140)
- Surgery (10021–69990)
- Radiology, including nuclear medicine and diagnostic ultrasound (70010–79999)
- Pathology and Laboratory (80047–89398)
- Medicine (90281–99199, 99500–99607)

Sections are subdivided into *subsections*; *subsections* are subdivided into *subheadings*; and *subheadings* can be subdivided into *categories*. Each level of a section provides more **specificity** about the procedure or service performed and the anatomic site or organ system involved. Each section and subsection provides coding guidelines and, if needed, a reference to the **CPT Assistant**. In most instances, all four levels are found, although this is not a hard-and-fast rule.

Format of Tabular List

Section: Surgery (10021–69990)
Subsection: Integumentary System
Subheading: Skin Subcutaneous and Accessory Structures
Category: Debridement

In the CPT manual, the subsection is listed below the section and indented. The subsection usually describes an anatomic site or an organ system, as in the following examples:

- Anatomic site: heart, femur, or skull
- Organ system: digestive, integumentary, or cardiovascular

A subheading is listed below the subsection. It generally refers to a specific procedure or service, but it can also indicate a more specific anatomic site:

- Procedures: esophagoscopy, incision and drainage, or cardiac catheterization
- Specific anatomic site: mitral valve, distal femur, or occipital bone

Category is the lowest level of code description.

UNLISTED PROCEDURE OR SERVICE CODE

Occasionally, even with the most detailed documentation, an accurate code to match the procedure or service performed cannot be found in the CPT manual. For this reason, in each section, nonspecific codes have been provided. These codes are known as Unlisted Procedures and Services. For example, code 29999 is found in the Surgery section, Musculoskeletal subsection. It describes an "unlisted procedure, arthroscopy." Unlisted codes can be used only when no other Category I or Category III code exactly matches the documentation. When an unlisted code is used, a **special report** must be sent with the insurance claim that describes the procedure or service in detail.

GENERAL CPT CODING GUIDELINES

At the beginning of each section and some subsections are coding guidelines. These guidelines add definitions and descriptions needed to interpret and report the procedures and services in that section or subsection. Coding guidelines enhance the coder's understanding of when and under what circumstances specific codes may be used. It is important to thoroughly read and apply the coding guidelines provided. Because coding guidelines are updated every year on October 1, it is also important to reread the guidelines after every new edition is released. Selecting a code without reading the guidelines usually leads to selection of the wrong code. Not only will this result in possibly delayed or denied reimbursement, but also, continued

inappropriate code selection can be considered fraud or abuse and can result in serious civil or criminal penalties.

Terms related to inaccurate coding are upcoding and downcoding. *Upcoding* is the use of a higher level procedure code than is supported in the documentation or medical necessity. A documentation example would be using Evaluation and Management (E/M) code 99213 (detailed history, detailed examination, and low complexity medical decision making) when the documentation supports 99202 (Expanded problem focused history and examination, and straightforward medical decision making). As mentioned in the diagnostic coding chapter, diagnosis and procedure codes are linked on the claim. For example, a patient undergoes a rhinoplasty for cosmetic reasons, but the diagnosis code for a deviated septum is submitted. A deviated septum would be considered medically necessary and could be paid by the insurance company. It is likely that the insurance company would request the records for this procedure and see in the documentation that the patient requested a cosmetic rhinoplasty. These examples would be considered fraud.

Downcoding is the use of a lower level procedure code than is justified. This also can be damaging to the healthcare facility, because it would result in lower reimbursement.

In procedural coding, the coder must always choose the code that most accurately describes the services provided.

Modifiers

Category I code *modifiers* are two-digit, numeric codes that report or indicate specific criteria, a specific condition, or a special circumstance.

Category II code modifiers are alphanumeric. Category I or Category II modifiers are used with CPT codes to indicate that a service or procedure performed was altered by specific circumstances (Table 17.2). Modifiers are included with the 5-digit CPT code to supply additional information or to describe extenuating circumstances that affected the procedure or service. For instance, modifier –50

TABLE 17.2	Commonly Used CPT Code Modifiers
MODIFIER	**DESCRIPTION**
–50	Bilateral procedure. If the procedure was performed on both sides of the body (e.g., both knees, both eyes) and the code description does not indicate that the procedure or service was performed bilaterally, modifier –50 is used.
–62	Two surgeons. When two surgeons work together as primary surgeons performing distinct parts of a procedure, each surgeon should report the procedure he or she performed to the insurance carrier using modifier –62. This prevents the insurance carrier from possibly rejecting a surgical charge as a duplicate.
–26	Professional component. This modifier is used when a technician performs the service to provide his or her professional opinion.
–RT, –LT	Indicates the side of the body on which the procedure took place. (e.g., 19100–LT – Breast biopsy, left side)

Symbols

▲	Revised code
●	New code
►◄	New or revised text
➜	Reference to *CPT Assistant, Clinical Examples in Radiology,* and *CPT Changes*
✚	Add-on code
⊘	Exemptions to modifier 51
⊙	Moderate sedation
✗	Product pending FDA approval
○	Reinstated or recycled code
#	Out-of-numerical sequence code

FIGURE 17.2 CPT conventions.

adds the detail that a procedure was performed **bilaterally**, or on both sides of the body. When an assistant surgeon is needed for a surgical procedure, modifier –80 is used. This allows the assistant surgeon to submit charges for his or her time. Modifiers can also show which side of the body a medical procedure was performed on. For example, the code 19100–RT indicates that the right breast was biopsied. A list of modifiers can be found in the CPT coding manual in Appendix A.

CPT CONVENTIONS

Conventions, or special symbols (Fig. 17.2), are used to provide additional information about specific codes. Let's look at a skin graft procedure for a wound that is 50 sq cm:

- Code 15271, Application of skin substitute graft to trunk, arms, legs, total wound surface area up to 100 sq cm; first 25 sq cm or less wound surface area
- Code +15272, each additional 25 sq cm wound surface area, or part thereof

To accurately code for this skin graft, two codes would be used: 15271 and 15272.

In the Tabular List in most CPT manuals, the legend explaining the meanings of the convention symbols is found at the bottom of each page.

CRITICAL THINKING APPLICATION   **17.2**

Sherald is trying to look up the CPT code for a left arm cyst biopsy. She has found the code, but how can she show that the procedure took place on the left side?

Sherald also came across CPT code 32440 (removal of lung, pneumonectomy), but she needs to also code for the repair of a portion of the bronchus. The code has a (+) in front of it; what does this mean?

APPENDICES

The CPT coding manual uses appendices to organize changes to the original code set. There are 16 appendices. A list of appendices and the codes they contain can be found in Table 17.3.

DOCUMENTATION FOR CPT CODING

Medical records used for procedural coding can include any or all of the following:

- Encounter form (Fig. 17.3)
- History and physical report (H&P)
- Progress notes
- Discharge summary
- Operative report
- Pathology report
- Anesthesia record
- Radiology report

When you compare the documentation to the codes, make sure all the elements of the description match substantially, with nothing added or missing. For example, review CPT codes 21315 and 21320. Both codes describe the closed treatment of a nasal bone fracture. However, 21315 indicates that there is no stabilization, and 21320 indicates that there is stabilization. The coder reviews the procedures and then assigns the CPT code with the description that most closely resembles the documentation.

Some providers have CPT and ICD-10-CM codes printed on their encounter forms; however, these codes should be treated only as a reference. Medical coders must also review the health record carefully, abstracting all the procedures and services rendered during an encounter. For example, a provider may circle the procedure for a preventive health visit for a 4-year-old on the encounter form but forget to record the injections provided during the encounter. When the medical assistant reviews the patient's electronic health record (EHR), he or she discovers that the provider's notes state routine injections were administered. If the medical assistant had not reviewed the EHR, the clinic would have lost reimbursement because the claim would not have included all the CPT codes for the visit. Encounter forms should be updated annually to ensure that code additions, changes, and revisions are current.

STEPS FOR EFFICIENT CPT PROCEDURAL CODING

The CPT coding process, which includes use of the Alphabetic Index and the Tabular List, applies to all sections of the CPT manual, except for the E/M and Anesthesia sections.

To start the procedural coding process, you must first determine the procedures or services that were provided. This is accomplished with two basic steps:

1. Analyze and abstract the procedural statement documented in the health record.
2. Compare it with the encounter form, operative report, or other documentation to ensure that all services and procedures have been recorded.

For practice on CPT surgery coding, refer to Procedure 17.1 on p. 371.

Abstracting

The term *abstract*, used as a verb in this context, is the process of collecting pertinent medical information needed to assign the correct code.

Abstracting ensures that all medical procedures and services are identified, and none are omitted. The abstracted data are then broken

TABLE 17.3   Appendices of the CPT Manual

APPENDIX	TITLE	DESCRIPTION
A	Modifiers	All modifiers applicable to CPT codes
B	Summary of Additions, Deletions, and Revisions	Shows the actual changes made to the annual CPT manual
C	Clinical Examples	Provides helpful narrative examples to aid selection of the correct and most specific level of E/M codes
D	Summary of CPT Add-on Codes	A list of CPT add-on codes
E	Summary of CPT Codes Exempt from Modifier 51	CPT codes that cannot use modifier 51, which indicates multiple procedures
F	Summary of CPT Codes Exempt from Modifier 63	CPT codes that cannot use modifier 51, which indicates procedures done on infants weighing < 4 kg
G	Summary of CPT Codes That Include Moderate (Conscious) Sedation	A list of CPT codes that do not use an additional code for conscious sedation
H	Alphabetic Listing of Performance Measures	Contains an alphabetic index of performance measures by clinical condition or topic
I	Genetic Testing Modifiers	Contains genetic testing modifiers
J	Electrodiagnostic Medicine Listing of Sensory, Motor, and Mixed Nerves	A list in which each sensory, motor, and mixed nerve is assigned its appropriate nerve conduction study code, to enhance accurate reporting of codes 95907 to 95913
K	Product Pending FDA Approval	Vaccine products that have been assigned a CPT code in anticipation of approval from the Food and Drug Administration (FDA)
L	Vascular Families	A diagram of veins to the first, second, and third order. assuming that the starting point is catheterization of the aorta
M	Renumbered CPT Codes– Citations Crosswalk	A summary of crosswalked, deleted, and renumbered codes, in addition to descriptors with the associated *CPT Assistant* references for the deleted codes
N	Summary of Resequenced CPT Codes	A list of CPT codes that do not appear in numeric sequence, which allows existing codes to be relocated to an appropriate location
O	Multianalyte Assays with Algorithmic Analysis	A list of CPT codes that includes a set of administrative codes for Multianalyte Assays with Algorithmic Analyses procedures; these typically are unique to a single clinical laboratory or manufacturer
P	CPT Codes That May Be Used for Synchronous Telemedicine Services	A list of CPT codes that may be used for reporting real-time telemedicine services when appended by modifier 95

down into main terms and modifying terms. A main term is usually the primary procedure or service performed, and a modifying term further defines or adds information to the main term. Next, the main and modifying terms are used to find the code or code ranges in the Alphabetic Index. Last, the code selected is confirmed by reviewing the guidelines, notes, and conventions in the Tabular List to verify that the most accurate code has been chosen.

USING THE ALPHABETIC INDEX

Procedural coding starts with identifying the main term and then locating it in the Alphabetic Index. Although the Alphabetic Index is a comprehensive, alphabetic listing of all main terms, there are

no code descriptions. It is not effective to assign a CPT code simply by finding it through the Alphabetic Index. The Alphabetic Index is not a substitute for the Tabular List. Even if an individual is only looking for one code, the Tabular List must be used to ensure the code is accurate.

The Alphabetic Index is used as a guide to search for one or more codes or code ranges. The index is similar to that found in the back of any textbook; it is an alphabetic list of main and modifying terms found in the Tabular List of the coding manual. In a typical index, the term or concept listed in the index is followed by the page numbers on which detailed information is presented in the body of the book. The Alphabetic Index in the CPT coding manual is used in the same way, except that it provides codes or code ranges rather

Julie Walden, M.D.   David Kahn, M.D.
James Marin, M.D.   Jean Burke, N.P.
Angela Perez, M.D.

YOUR NAME CLINIC
Walden-Martin Family Medical Clinic,
1234 Anystreet, Anytown AK 12345
Phone: 123-123-1234   Fax: 123-123-5678

TELEPHONE:
FAX:

PATIENT'S NAME			CHART #			DATE			☐ MEDI-MEDI ☐ MEDICAL
									☐ MEDICARE ☐ PRIVATE
									☐ SELF PAY ☐ HMO _____

✔	CPT/Md	DESCRIPTION	FEE	✔	CPT/Md	DESCRIPTION	FEE	✔	CPT/Md	DESCRIPTION	FEE	✔	CPT/Md	DESCRIPTION	FEE
	OFFICE VISIT—NEW PATIENT				**LAB STUDIES**				**PROCEDURES (continued)**				**INJECTIONS**		
	99202	Focused Ex.			36415	Venipucture			93235	Holter, 24 Hour			90724	Influenza	
	99203	Detailed Ex.			81000	Urinalysis			10061	I & D Abscess Comp.			90732	Pneumococcal	
	99204	Comprehensive Ex.			81003	—w/o Micro			10060	I & D Abscess Simple			J0295	Ampicillin, 1 gr	
	99205	Complex Ex.			84703	HCG (Urine, Pregnancy)			94761	Oximetry w/Exercise			J0696	Rocephine	
	OFFICE VISIT—ESTABLISHED PATIENT				82948	Glucose			93720	Plethysmography			J1030	Depomedrol 40 mg	
	99212	Focused Ex.			82270	Hemoccult			94760	Pulse Oximetry			J2000	Lidocaine 50 cc	
	99213	Expanded Ex.			85023	CBC-diff.			10003	Rem. Sebaceous Cyst			J2175	Demerol	
	99214	Detailed Ex.			85024	CBC w/part diff			11100	Skin Bx			J3360	Valium 5 mg	
	99215	Complex Ex.			85018	Hemoglobin			94010	Spirometry			J1885	Toradol 30 mg IV	
	PREVENTATIVE MEDICINE—NEW PATIENT				88155	Pap Smear			92801	Visual Acuity			J1885	Toradol 60 mg IM	
	99381	< 1 year old			87210	KOH/Saline Wet Mount			17100	Wart Removal			90720	DTP–HIB	
	99382	1–4 year old			87430	Strep Antigen			17101	Wart Removal, 2nd			90746	HEP B—HIB	
	99383	5–11 year old			87060	Throat Culture			17102	Wart Removal, 3–15			90707	MMR	
	99384	12–17 year old			80009	Chem profile			11042	Wound Debrid.			86580	PPD	
	99385	18–39 year old			80061	Lipid profile			**X-RAY**				86580	PPD w/control	
	99386	40–64 year old			82465	Cholesterol			70210	Sinuses			90732	Pneumovax	
	99387	65+ year old			99000	Handling fee			70360	Neck Soft Tissue			90716	Varicella	
	PREVENTATIVE MEDICINE—ESTABLISHED PATIENT				**PROCEDURES**				71010	CXR (PA only)			82607	Vitamin B12 Inj.	
	99391	< 1 year old			92551	Audiometry			71020	Chest 2V			90712	Polio	
	99392	1–4 year old			29705	Cast Removal			72040	C-Spine 2V			90788	TD Adult	
	99393	5–11 year old			2900_	Casting (by location)			72100	Lumbrosacral			95115	Allergy inj., single	
	99394	12–17 year old			92567	Ear Check			73030	Shoulder 2V			95117	Allergry inj., multiple	
	99395	18–39 year old			69210	Ear Wax Rem. 1 2			73070	Elbow 2V					
	99396	40–64 year old			93000	EKG			73120	Hand 2V					
	99397	65+ year old			93005	EKG tracing only			73560	Knee 2V					
					93010	EKG. Int. and Rep			73620	Foot 2V					
					11750	Excision Nail			74000	KUB					
					94375	Flow Volume									

DESCRIPTION   ICD-10-CM

____ Abdominal pain/unspec...... R10.9
____ Abscess...................... L02._
____ Allergic reaction............... T78.40_
____ Alzheimer's disease.......... G30
____ Anemia/unspec............... D64.9
____ Angina/unspec................. I20.9
____ Anorexia...................... R63.0
____ Anxiety/unspec............... F41.9
____ Apnea, sleep.................. G47.30
____ Arrhythmia, cardiac.......... I49.9
____ Arthritis, rheumatoid.......... M06.9
____ Asthma/unspec............... J45.909
____ Atrial fibrillation.............. I48.0
____ B-12 deficiency............... E53.8
____ Back pain, low............... M54.5
____ BPH.......................... N40
____ Bradycardia/unspec.......... R00.1
____ Broncitis, acute.............. J20._
____ Bronchitis, chronic.......... J42
____ Bursitis/unspec.............. M71.9
____ CA, breast.................... C50._
____ CA, lung...................... C34._
____ CA, prostate.................. C61
____ Cellulitis...................... L03._
____ Chest pain/unspec........... R07.9
____ Cirrhosis, liver/unspec...... K74.60
____ Cold, common................ J00
____ Colitis/unspec................ K51.90
____ Confusion.................... R41.0
____ CHF.......................... I50.9
____ Constipation................. K59.00
____ COPD......................... J44.9
____ Cough........................ R05
____ Crohn's disease/unspec.... K50.90
____ CVA.......................... I63.9
____ Decubitus ulcer............. L89._
____ Dehydration................. E86.0

____ Dementia/unspec............... F03
____ Depression, major/unsp...... F32.9
____ Diab I, no complications...... E10.0
____ Diab II, no complications..... E11.9
____   w/kidney complic........... E11.2_
____   w/ophthalmic compl...... E11.3_
____   w/neurolog compl.......... E11.4_
____   w/circulartory compl...... E11.5_
____ Insulin use.................... Z79.4
____ Diarrhea/unspec.............. R19.7
____ Diverticulitix................. K57.92
____ Diverticulosis................ K57.90
____ Dizziness..................... R42
____ Dysuria....................... R30.0
____ Edema/unspec................ R60.9
____ Endocarditis................. I38
____ Esophageal reflux........... K21.0
____ Fatigue (lethargy).......... R53.83
____ FUO.......................... R50.9
____ Gastritis..................... K29.70
____ Gastroenteritis (colitis)...... K52.9
____ G.I. bleed................... K92.2
____ Gout/unspec................. M10.9
____ Headache.................... R51
____ Health exam................. 200._
____ Hematuria/unspec........... R31.9
____ Herpes simplex............. B00.9
____ Herpes zoster.............. B02.9
____ Hiatal hernia............... K44.9
____ HTN (HBP)................... I10
____ Hyperlipidemia/unspec...... E78.5
____ Hypothyroidism/unspec...... E03.9
____ Impotence................... N52._
____ Influenza, respiratory...... J10.1
____ Insomnia.................... G47.0
____ IBS, diarrhea............... K58.
____ Lupus, systemic erythim...... M32.9

____ MI, acute..................... I21._
____ MI, old....................... I25.2
____ Migraine..................... G43.9
____ Myalgia...................... M79.1
____ Neck pain................... M54.2
____ Neuropathy................. G62.9
____ Nausea...................... R11.1
____ Nausea/vomitting........... R11.0
____ Obesity/unspec............. E66.9
____ Osteoarthritis (site)........ M19._
____ Otitis media............... H66.9
____ Parkinson's disease........ G20
____ Pharyngitis, acute......... J02.9
____ Pleurisy..................... R09.1
____ Pneumonia.................. J18.9
____ Pneumonia, viral........... J12.9
____ Prostatitis/unspec.......... N41.9
____ PVD.......................... I73.9
____ Radiculopathyp............. M54.1_
____ Rectal bleeding............ K62.5
____ Renal failure............... N19
____ Sciatica..................... M54.3_
____ Shortness of breath........ R03.02
____ Sinusitis, chr./unspec...... J32.9
____ Syncope..................... R55
____ Tachycardia/unspec........ R00.0
____ Tachy., supraventric....... I47.1
____ Tedinitix/unspec........... M77.9
____ TIA.......................... G45.9
____ Ulcer, duodenal/unspec.... K26.9
____ Ulcer, gastric/unspec...... K25.9
____ Ulcer, peptic/unspec....... K27.9
____ URI/unspec.................. J06.9
____ UTI.......................... N39.0
____ Vertigo...................... R42
____ Weight gain................ R63.5
____ Weight loss................ R63.4

DIAGNOSIS: (IF NOT CHECKED ABOVE)		**TODAY'S FEE**
		AMT. REC'D.
PROCEDURES: (IF NOT CHECKED ABOVE)	RETURN APPOINTMENT INFORMATION:	REC'D BY:
		☐ CASH
		☐ CR. CARD
	(DAYS)(WKS.)(MOS.)(PRN)	☐ CHECK # _____ BALANCE

FIGURE 17.3 Encounter form.

than page numbers. As discussed earlier, the Tabular List is divided into sections, and the procedures and services are listed in numeric order by the Category I code.

The Alphabetic Index is organized by main terms and modifying terms that are indented below the main term. Modifying terms further describe and add information needed to narrow the search for an appropriate procedure or service code. A main term can be a procedure, such as an excision. Each modifying term could provide further information such as:

- anatomic location
- organ excised
- type of instrument used
- special technique
- other procedures performed at the same time (e.g., obtaining biopsy tissue for examination)

Modifying terms affect the selection of appropriate codes; therefore, it is important to review the list of modifying terms when selecting a code or code range.

Searching the Alphabetic Index

Begin the search of the Alphabetic Index by using one of the four primary classifications (or types) of main and modifying terms:

- Procedure or service (e.g., examination, excision, scope, revision, repair, drainage)
- Organ or anatomic site (e.g., clavicle, mandible, humerus, liver, colon, uterus)
- Condition, illness, or injury (e.g., cholelithiasis, ulcer, fracture, pregnancy, fever)
- Eponym, synonym, abbreviation, or acronym (e.g., Naffziger operation, MRI [magnetic resonance imaging], TURP [transurethral resection of the prostate])

When searching the Alphabetic Index, use:

- the name of the performed procedure or service (anastomosis, splint, repair, stress test, therapy, vaccination)
- the organ or other anatomic site of the procedure (tibia, colon, salivary gland, aorta)
- the condition, illness, or injury (abscess, fracture, cholelithiasis, strabismus)
- synonyms, eponyms, or abbreviations (ECG [electrocardiography], Stookey-Scarff procedure, Mohs' micrographic surgery)

Sometimes searching for a main term may not yield any results. When a main term cannot be found, search by another primary classification in the Alphabetic Index. Let's search the following procedural statement: Removal of Skin Tags on Neck. Begin by identifying the main terms that closely match the four primary classifications in the Alphabetic Index:

1. Procedure or Service: Removal
2. Organ or Anatomic Site: Neck Skin
3. Condition, Illness, or Injury: Skin Tag
4. Eponym: None in this case

Once all possible main terms have been abstracted, the coder can quickly search through the Alphabetic Index for the code or code range that matches the procedural statement.

Using *See* and *See Also* in the Alphabetic Index

The *see* statement in the Alphabetic Index points to another location in the Alphabetic Index to find the code or code range. The *see also* statement points to additional codes or code ranges in the Alphabetic Index that may be useful to the code found in the original search.

Single Codes and Code Ranges

In the Alphabetic Index, a procedure or service may list a single code or a range of possible codes that may match the documentation. Remember that the Alphabetic Index is an index; it is designed as a guide to the most suitable codes that match the documentation. At this point, the search is only for the closest match or matches to the procedural statement.

Some medical procedures and diagnostic tests can be quite complex. There may be a single code or a code range that may include one main term but has several modifying terms for the main term. For example, the code for Acromioplasty has a range of codes: 23415–23420. The same main term, Acromioplasty, with a modifying term, partial, has a single code: 23130. The code range is shown with a hyphen to indicate that all codes within that range could be appropriate.

In some cases, a single code and a range of codes are listed for the same service or procedure. For example, Craterization, femur, lists both the single code 27360 and the code range 27070–27071. Once a single code or code range has been found in the Alphabetic Index, the next step is to look up each of those in the Tabular List. Select the code or codes that most closely match the documentation.

Steps for Using the CPT Alphabetic Index

1. Abstract the procedural statement from the medical documentation and determine the main and/or modifying terms.
2. Select the most appropriate main term to begin searching in the Alphabetic Index.
3. Once the main term has been located, select one or more modifying terms, if needed, to narrow the search.
4. If no main or modifying term produces an appropriate code or code range, repeat steps 2 and 3 using a different main term.
5. Find the code or code ranges that include all or most of the description of the procedure or service found in the medical record.

CRITICAL THINKING APPLICATION   **17.3**

Sherald is having trouble finding a procedural code in the Alphabetic Index for removal of a cataract. What are some options and/or alternative ways she can perform an Alphabetic Index search?

USING THE TABULAR LIST

Once the code or code ranges have been selected from the Alphabetic Index, the next stop is the Tabular List. This is where the procedural coding decision takes place. In the Tabular List, the conventions, symbols, guidelines, notes, and even the punctuation all play a part in choosing the most accurate code possible.

In the Tabular List, look up each code or code range found numerically in the Alphabetic Index. Read the description of each code thoroughly to ensure that the main terms abstracted from the procedural statement in the medical documentation are all included in the code description, with nothing substantial omitted or added. Read the section guidelines and notes to determine whether additional codes should be used, add-on codes or modifiers are required, or use of the code is contraindicated.

Use of the Semicolon

A semicolon (;) at the end of a main description indicates that modifying terms and descriptions follow. Every indented description below a stand-alone code is related to that stand-alone code. To get the full description for an indented code, you use the description of the stand-alone code up to the semicolon and then include the description of the indented code. Let's look at excision of the spleen as an example. In the CPT manual you will see the following entry:

Hemic and Lymphatic Systems
Spleen
Excision
38100 Splenectomy; total (separate procedure)
38101 partial (separate procedure)
38102 total, en bloc for extensive disease, in conjunction with other procedure (List in addition to code for primary procedure)

The description for code 38100 is a splenectomy, total. The description for code 38101 is splenectomy, partial. The description for code 38102 is splenectomy, total, en bloc for extensive disease, in conjunction with other procedure. If you were to use 38102, you would also have to have the code for the other procedure. You could not use just 38102.

For practice on CPT surgery coding, refer to Procedure 17.1 on p. 371.

Steps for Using the CPT Tabular List

Except for the special considerations required for coding from the E/M and Anesthesia sections, the following steps apply to all sections of the CPT manual.

1. Look up the code or code range from the Alphabetic Index. Search in the Tabular List numerically.
2. Compare the description of the code with the procedural statement from the documentation. Verify that all or most of the health record documentation matches the code description and that there is no additional element or information in the code description that is not found in the documentation.
3. Read the guidelines and notes for the section, subsection, and code to ensure that there are no contraindications to the use of the code.
4. Evaluate the conventions, especially add-on codes (+) and exemption from modifier −51.
5. Determine whether any special circumstances require the use of a modifier or whether a Special Report is required.
6. Record the CPT code selected in the health record documentation next to the procedure or service performed and in the appropriate block of the insurance claim form.

CPT CODING GUIDELINES: EVALUATION AND MANAGEMENT SECTION

Evaluation and Management codes are commonly referred to as E/M codes. These codes are used to reflect what the provider does during the time spent with the patient. To properly code for that, the medical assistant must apply different techniques from the basic steps outlined earlier. Assigning the correct E/M code includes:
- identifying the following for the procedure or service:
  - section
  - subsection
  - category
  - subcategory
- reviewing the reporting instructions and guidelines for the code chosen
- reviewing the level of E/M service
  - determining the extent of the history obtained and the examination performed
  - determining the complexity of medical decision making

The E/M section is divided into broad subsections, such as office visit, emergency room visit, hospital visit, and consultation. These subsections are further divided into subcategories, which include the place where the services were rendered, such as:
- provider's office
- hospital emergency department
- skilled nursing facility
- patient's home
- patient status
  - new
  - established

Procedure 17.2, Part A, on p. 373 explains how to perform CPT coding for an office visit. The first two steps in choosing an E/M code are:
1. Identify the place of service (POS)
2. Identify the patient status (new or established)

Identifying the Place of Service

The POS is the healthcare facility where the provider delivered care to the patient. The two most common places of service are "office" and "hospital." Table 17.4 presents a list of common POS locations and their 2-digit identifying numbers, or POS codes.

Identifying the Patient Status

The patient status choices are "new" or "established" patient. A new patient (NP) is one who has not received any professional services from the provider, or from another provider of the same specialty and subspecialty who belongs to the same group practice, within the past 3 years.

An established patient (EP) is one who has received professional services from the provider, or from another provider of the same specialty and subspecialty who belongs to the same group practice, within the past 3 years.

Once the POS and patient status have been established, the next step in selection of an E/M code is to determine the level of service provided.

TABLE 17.4   Commonly Used Place of Service (POS) Codes

CODE	NAME
01	Pharmacy
11	Office
12	Home
13	Assisted Living Facility
14	Group Home
15	Mobile Unit
17	Walk-In Retail Health Clinic
20	Urgent Care Facility
21	Inpatient Hospital
22	Outpatient Hospital
23	Emergency Room—Hospital
24	Ambulatory Surgery Center
31	Skilled Nursing Facility
34	Hospice
51	Inpatient Psychiatric Facility
60	Mass Immunization Center
65	End-Stage Renal Disease Treatment Facility
71	Public Health Clinic
72	Rural Health Clinic
81	Independent Laboratory

Select the Appropriate Level of E/M Services Based on the Following

1. For the following categories/subcategories, **all of the key components**, ie, history, examination, and medical decision making, must meet or exceed the stated requirements to qualify for a particular level of E/M service: office, new patient; hospital observation services; initial hospital care; office consultations, initial inpatient consultations; emergency department services; initial nursing facility care; domiciliary care, new patient; and home, new patient.

2. For the following categories/subcategories, **two of the three key components** (ie, history, examination, and medical decision making) must meet or exceed the stated requirements to qualify for a particular level of E/M services: office, established patient; subsequent hospital care; subsequent nursing facility care; domiciliary care, established patient; and home, established patient.

3. When counseling and/or coordination of care dominates (more than 50%) the encounter with the patient and/or family (face-to-face time in the office or other outpatient setting or floor/unit time in the hospital or nursing facility), then **time** shall be considered the key or controlling factor to qualify for a particular level of E/M services. This includes time spent with parties who have assumed responsibility for the care of the patient or decision making whether or not they are family members (eg, foster parents, person acting in loco parentis, legal guardian). The extent of counseling and/or coordination of care must be documented in the medical record.

FIGURE 17.4 Appropriate assignment of E/M codes.

- *Expanded problem-focused history:* The expanded problem-focused history includes:
  - symptoms, severity, and duration of the chief complaint
  - review of systems that relate to the chief complaint
  Usually the past, family, and social histories are not included.
- *Detailed history:* The detailed history includes:
  - chief complaint
  - extended history of present illness
  - problem-pertinent system review, including a review of a limited number of additional systems
  - pertinent past, family, and/or social histories directly related to the patient's problems.
- *Comprehensive history:* A comprehensive history includes:
  - chief complaint
  - extended history of present illness
  - ROS that is directly related to the problem or problems identified in the history of the present illness
  - review of all additional body systems, in addition to complete past, family, and social histories

Examination. The examination is the objective part of the patient's visit. The provider examines the patient, obtains measurable findings, and makes notes referring to body areas and/or organ systems as follows:

- *Body areas:* Head, including face and neck; chest, including breasts and axillae; abdomen; genitalia, groin, and buttocks; and back, including spine and extremities
- *Organs and organ systems:* General (e.g., vital signs, general appearance); eyes; ears, nose, throat, and mouth; cardiovascular;

Determining the Level of Service Provided

Key Components and Contributing Factors

The three key components for determining the level of service for E/M coding are history, examination, and medical decision making. The four contributing factors are counseling, nature of the presenting problem, coordination of care, time.

Counseling, the nature of the presenting problem, coordination of care, and time are secondary considerations. Fig. 17.4 presents criteria for choosing the appropriate E/M code.

History. To understand the history levels, it is important to know the definition and components of the patient's history. The history relates to the patient's clinical picture and depends on the patient for answers to specific questions.

The following are the four levels of history taking.

- *Problem-focused history:* A problem-focused history concentrates on the **chief complaint**; it looks at the symptoms, severity, and duration of the problem. It usually does not include a **review of systems (ROS)** or the family and social histories.

TABLE 17.5 Complexity of Medical Decision Making

NUMBER OF DIAGNOSES OR MANAGEMENT OPTIONS	AMOUNT AND/OR COMPLEXITY OF DATA TO BE REVIEWED	RISK OF COMPLICATIONS AND/OR MORBIDITY OR MORTALITY	TYPE OF MEDICAL DECISION MAKING
Minimal	Minimal or none	Minimal	Straightforward
Limited	Limited	Low	Low complexity
Multiple	Moderate	Moderate	Moderate complexity
Extensive	Extensive	High	High complexity

respiratory; gastrointestinal (GI); genitourinary; musculoskeletal; skin; neurologic; psychiatric; and hematologic, lymphatic, and immunologic

The examination is divided into the following levels:

- *Problem-focused examination:* The examination is limited to the affected body area or single system mentioned in the **chief complaint**.
- *Expanded problem-focused examination:* In addition to the limited body area or system, related body areas or organ systems are examined.
- *Detailed examination:* An extended examination is performed on the affected body area and related body areas or organ systems.
- *Comprehensive examination:* A complete multisystem examination is performed or a complete examination of a single organ system.

Medical Decision Making. When a provider makes medical decisions, the decisions are based on many years of education and experience. Three elements comprise the medical decision making process:

1. The number of diagnoses and/or management options
2. The amount and/or complexity of data obtained, reviewed, and analyzed
3. The risk of significant complications and/or morbidity and/or mortality

Number of Diagnoses and Management Options. The provider's notes during the history and examination should help identify whether the patient's problem is minor, acute, stable, or worsening. The documentation should also identify whether a new problem exists or whether the provider plans to order any diagnostic tests to further investigate the patient's illness or injury.

Amount and Complexity of Data Reviewed. The documentation should also identify what laboratory tests, x-ray diagnostic procedures, and other tests have been ordered or reviewed.

Risk of Complications and Morbidity or Mortality. Risk is often involved in medical care, either from the treatment given to the patient or from the lack of treatment and professional care. *Morbidity,* the relative incidence of disease, and *mortality,* which relates to the number of deaths from a given disease, are integral parts of the provider's assessment of risks.

Complexity Levels in Medical Decision Making. The complexity of medical decision making is categorized into four levels: straightforward, low complexity, moderate complexity, and high complexity.

Table 17.5 presents descriptions of the different levels of complexity of medical decision making.

Factors That Contribute to E/M Complexity

Counseling

Counseling is a discussion with a patient and/or family members about diagnostic results, impressions, recommended diagnostic studies, prognosis, risks and benefits of management or treatment options, instructions for management, treatment, and/or follow-up.

Almost all E/M services involve a degree of counseling with the patient and/or family. This is factored into the E/M code. As long as the counseling does not exceed 50% of the time spent with the patient, it is included in the E/M code. It can be considered a contributing factor when the counseling exceeds 50% of the encounter.

Nature of the Presenting Problem

The presenting problem is usually explained in the chief complaint. It can range from something as simple as a cold in an otherwise healthy patient to a life-threatening problem. Unless dealing with the nature of the presenting problem exceeds half of the patient encounter, it is included in the E/M code description and is not a factor in selecting the level of service.

Coordination of Care

Some patients need help in arranging for care beyond the visit or hospitalization. Some will need care in a skilled nursing facility or home health care. Others will need hospice care. The primary provider usually coordinates this care. Coordination of care is also factored into the E/M code and is a consideration for determining the level of service only when it exceeds 50% of the patient encounter.

Time

Time is included in the E/M code descriptions only to assist providers in selecting the most appropriate level of E/M service. The times stated in the code descriptions are averages. Time is not a determining factor in code selection unless counseling exceeds more than 50% of the encounter. Only then can time be used as a determining component to code level selection.

At first, E/M coding can be difficult to understand and put into practice. The E/M coding process provided here can serve as a guide to help medical assistants in determining place of service, patient status, and level of care provided.

You can then select the most accurate E/M code. Using the clinical examples in Appendix C of the CPT manual and comparing them to the medical documentation also can help medical assistants acquire a better understanding of E/M coding.

CPT CODING GUIDELINES: ANESTHESIA

Anesthesiologists and **Certified Registered Nurse Anesthetists (CRNAs)** use codes in the Anesthesia section. These codes always start with a zero (0) (except for Qualifying Circumstances for Anesthesia [99100–99140]) and identify the anatomic location of the surgery performed. CPT codes are used for unconscious sedation or for putting patients to sleep during the medical procedure; codes for conscious sedation are found in the Medicine section.

Anesthesia coding differs from any other form of coding in the way anesthesia services are billed. These professionals are paid a standard amount per unit compared to surgeons, who are paid by the procedure. A standard formula has been established to determine the number of units they can bill for each procedure for which they provide anesthesia.

Basic unit value + Time units + Modifying units (B + T + M)

Basic Unit Value (B)

The Anesthesia Society of America (ASA) publishes a Relative Value Guide (RVG) that lists the codes for anesthesia services. The RVG compares anesthesia services and assigns a numeric value to each service based on the level of complexity; this numeric value is called the *basic unit value.*

Time Units (T)

Anesthesia services are provided based on the time during which the anesthesia was administered, in hours and minutes. Typically, 15 minutes equals 1 time unit, although this can vary because insurance carriers make that determination independently. The time starts when the anesthesiology provider begins preparing the patient to receive anesthesia, continues through the procedure, and ends when the patient is no longer under the professional care of the anesthesiology provider. The hours and minutes during which anesthesia was administered are recorded in the patient's anesthesia record.

Modifying Units (M)

Modifying units reflect circumstances or conditions that change or modify the environment in which the anesthesia service was provided. The two modifying characteristics for anesthesia services are qualifying circumstances and physical status modifiers.

Qualifying Circumstances (QC)

Sometimes anesthesia is provided in situations that make administration more difficult. These types of cases include provision of anesthesia in emergency situations, to patients of extreme age, during the use of controlled hypotension, and with hypothermia. There are four qualifying circumstances (QC) codes. Each of the 5-digit codes is preceded by a plus sign symbol (+), indicating that it is an add-on code; these codes are used in addition to the Category I anesthesia code. Table 17.6 presents a list of the Qualifying Circumstances CPT codes.

TABLE 17.6 Anesthesia Qualifying Circumstances and Physical Status Modifiers

MODIFIER	DESCRIPTION
Qualifying Circumstances CPT Codes[a]	
99100	Anesthesia for a patient of extreme age (i.e., <1 yr or >70 yr)
99116	Anesthesia complicated by utilization of total body hypothermia
99135	Anesthesia complicated by utilization of controlled hypothermia
Physical Status Modifiers[b]	
P1	A normal healthy patient
P2	A patient with mild systemic disease
P3	A patient with severe systemic disease
P4	A person with severe systemic disease that is a constant threat to life
P5	A moribund patient who is not expected to survive without the procedure
P6	A declared brain-dead patient whose organs are being removed for donor purposes

[a]Use a qualifying circumstances modifier code, if appropriate, in addition to the primary CPT Category I Anesthesia code.
[b]A physical status modifier is required for performing anesthesia calculations.

Physical Status Modifiers

Physical status modifiers are used to indicate the patient's physical condition at the time anesthesia was provided. There are five physical status modifiers, each composed of two characters: first the letter P, followed by a ranking of 1 to 6 (e.g., P1, P2, P3, and so on). P1 represents a normal, healthy patient, and P6 represents a brain-dead patient whose organs are being harvested. Table 17.6 also presents a list of physical status modifiers and their descriptions; a list also can be found in the Anesthesia section of the CPT manual.

Conversion Factors

A *conversion factor* is the dollar value of each basic unit value. Each third-party payer issues a list of conversion factors. The conversion factor for any given geographic location is multiplied by the number of basic unit values assigned to each procedure (Fig. 17.5).

Calculating Anesthesia Services

Using the basic unit value (B), modifying unit (M), time unit (T), physical status (PS) modifier, if applicable, and the conversion factor (Fig. 17.6), the fee for anesthesia services is calculated according to the anesthesia billing formula:

(B + M + T + PS) × Conversion factor

Locality Name	Anesthesia Conversion Factor
Manhattan, NY	22.65
NYC suburbs/Long I., NY	22.74
Queens, NY	22.28
Rest of New York	19.91
North Carolina	20.23
North Dakota	19.70

FIGURE 17.5 Anesthesia conversion factors.

Medical Narrative

A 25-year-old female patient in good physical condition has anesthesia services while undergoing laparoscopy (CPT-4 Code 00840). The time for the anesthesia administration was 2 hours. For the purposes of this example the RBV basic unit value will be 4.

Basic Unit Value = 4
+ Modifying Units: PS = 0
+ QC = 0
+ Time Units = 8
= 12 Total Units

The total units value of 12 is then multiplied by the conversion factor for the geographic location of the anesthesiologist's office. For the purposes of this exercise, the conversion factor for Manhattan, NY, will be $20.48, and for North Carolina, $15.77. For the office located in Manhattan, NY, multiply $20.48 by 12. The fee for the anesthesia services would be $245.76. For the office located in North Carolina, multiply 12 times $15.77, for a fee of $189.24.

FIGURE 17.6 Anesthesia formula and calculation.

CPT CODING GUIDELINES: SURGICAL SECTION

Specific guidelines and notes related to surgery coding must be considered when assigning a CPT code. Always review the current year's guidelines for the Surgery section for the most up-to-date information. The following sections discuss a few of the more common guidelines. When coding procedures and services, be sure to read the guidelines and notes thoroughly for accurate coding assignment.

Surgical Package Definition

The CPT code set is designed to include patient prep, surgical care, and postsurgical care in a single code. These are considered **global services** because they are already built into the surgical package cost of the assigned CPT code. Medical coders who include any of these global services as a separate CPT code are committing fraud. The CPT code descriptions of global surgical services typically include the following:

- Local infiltration, digital block, and/or topical anesthesia
- After the decision for surgery, one related E/M encounter on the day of, or the day before, the date of the procedure

- Immediate postoperative care, including documentation in the patient's health record and talking with family and/or other physicians
- Writing orders for postsurgical care
- Evaluating the patient in the postanesthesia recovery area
- Typical postoperative follow-up care (includes care for approximately 6 to 8 weeks after surgery and is usually done at the provider's office)

NCCI Edits and Unbundled Codes

In 1996, in an effort to prevent fraudulent medical coding, the Centers for Medicare and Medicaid Services (CMS) established the National Corrective Coding Initiative (NCCI) edit list. This list contains two columns of codes, and the codes in the two columns are mutually exclusive. Submitted claims that contain mutually exclusive codes are automatically rejected.

When a CPT procedure is billed, this code includes services related to prepping the patient for the procedure, performing the procedure, and suturing to complete the procedure; the single code for the procedure is called a *bundled code* because it represents all of the stages of surgery. When each step of the procedure is listed separately, these are called *unbundled codes*. Unbundled codes are used when the components of a major procedure are separated and reported separately. When these codes are separated and used individually, a special report should be used to describe the circumstances that made the unbundling necessary; the reason for this is that unbundled CPT codes have higher reimbursements because each code is paid separately. Medical billers who regularly unbundle CPT codes may be cited for fraud and/or abuse.

Integumentary System – Excision of Lesions—Benign or Malignant

Excision of benign lesions includes a simple closure and anesthesia. If a wound (incision, excision, or traumatic lesion) requires intermediate or complex closure, the repair by intermediate or complex closure is coded and reported separately from the incision or excision. For example, if the provider excised a benign lesion measuring 1 cm from the patient's arm that required intermediate repair (closure), two codes would be used:

- 11401 – Excision, benign lesion including margins; excised diameter 0.6 to 1 cm
- 12031 – Repair, intermediate, wounds of scalp, axillae, trunk and/or extremities (excluding hands and feet); 2.5 cm or less

Levels of Closure (Repair)

- *Simple repair:* Performed when the wound is superficial (epidermis, dermis, or subcutaneous) without significant involvement of deeper structures. This includes local anesthesia and chemical or electrocauterization of wounds not closed.
- *Intermediate repair:* Includes simple repair with a need for a layered closure of one or more of the deeper layers of subcutaneous tissue and superficial fascia in addition to the skin closure. Single-layer closure of heavily contaminated wounds that required extensive cleaning or removal of particulate matter also constitutes an intermediate repair.
- *Complex repair:* Includes wounds that require more than layered closure (e.g., scar revision, extensive undermining, or stents or

retention sutures). Necessary preparation includes creation of a limited defect for repairs or **debridement** of complicated lacerations. Complex repair does not include excision of benign or malignant lesions, excisional preparation of a wound bed, or debridement, or the removal of damaged tissue or foreign objects from a wound, an open fracture, or an open dislocation.

Listing Services for Wound Repair

- The repaired wound or wounds should be measured and recorded in centimeters; it also should be indicated whether the wound was curved, angular, or in a star-like pattern.
- When multiple wounds are repaired, add together the lengths of those in the same classification (simple, intermediate, or complex) and from all anatomic sites that are grouped together into the same code descriptor.
- When wounds of more than one classification are repaired, list the more complicated repair as the primary procedure and the less complicated repair as the secondary procedure, using modifier –59.
- Debridement is considered a separate procedure only when gross contamination requires prolonged cleansing; when a large amount of dead or contaminated tissue must be removed; or when debridement is carried out separately without immediate primary closure.
- Wound repair that involves nerves, blood vessels, and/or tendons should be reported under the appropriate system for repair of those structures. The repair of these associated wounds is included in the primary procedure unless it qualifies as a complex repair, in which case modifier –59 applies.

Musculoskeletal System

Fractures

- *Closed fracture:* The fractured bone does not protrude through the dermis or epidermis.
- *Open fracture:* The fractured bone cuts through the skin layers and can be directly visualized.
- *Closed treatment:* The fracture site is not surgically opened. The three methods of closed treatment of fractures are:
  - without manipulation
  - with manipulation
  - with or without traction
- *Manipulation:* Attempted reduction or restoration of a fracture or dislocated joint into its normal anatomic alignment by manually applied forces.
- *Open treatment:* Used when (1) the fractured bone is surgically opened or (2) an opening is made remote from the fracture site to insert an intramedullary nail across the fracture site.
- *Percutaneous skeletal fixation:* Fracture treatment that is neither open nor closed. The fracture fragments are not visualized, but a fixation device (e.g., pins) is placed across the fracture site, usually under x-ray imaging.

Maternity Care and Delivery

The services normally provided in uncomplicated maternity cases include antepartum care, delivery, and postpartum care.

- *Antepartum* care includes:
  - initial and subsequent history
  - physical examinations
  - recording of weight, blood pressure, and fetal heart tones
  - routine chemical urinalysis
  - monthly visits up to 28 weeks' gestation
  - biweekly visits to 36 weeks' gestation
  - weekly visits until delivery.

Any other visits or services provided within this period should be coded separately, including any routine tests (e.g., sonography, routine laboratory tests).

- *Delivery* includes:
  - admission to the hospital, the admission history, and the physical examination
  - management of uncomplicated labor
  - vaginal delivery (with or without forceps or episiotomy), or cesarean delivery.

Medical problems complicating labor and delivery should be identified by using the codes in the Medicine and E/M sections in addition to codes for maternity care.

- *Postpartum* care includes:
  - hospital and office visits after vaginal or cesarean section delivery

CPT CODING GUIDELINES: RADIOLOGY SECTION

Assigning CPT codes for the Radiology section follows the same procedure as for the Surgery section. The Radiology section contains all diagnostic imaging codes, including x-ray studies, ultrasound, MRI, and nuclear medicine procedures, in addition to radiation oncology and several other types of diagnostic imaging procedures, services, and therapies. The Radiology section is divided into subsections: head and neck; chest, spine, and pelvis; upper and lower extremities; abdomen, gastrointestinal and urinary tracts; and gynecologic, obstetric, heart, and vascular procedures. The next subdivision, categories, defines the types or functions of various procedures (e.g., diagnostic ultrasound, radiation oncology, and so on) unique to the anatomic site subsection. In addition to the radiology procedure codes, codes are included for physician supervision and interpretation of diagnostic imaging data and for clinical and radiation treatment planning and administration of contrast materials during radiologic procedures.

CPT CODING GUIDELINES: PATHOLOGY AND LABORATORY SECTION

Assigning CPT codes for the Pathology section also follows the same procedure as for the Surgery section. For purposes of coding from the Laboratory section, organ or disease panels are groupings of numerous tests performed to diagnose the health or disease status of specific organ systems. A panel code can be used only if all the tests listed under the code selected were performed. These are considered *bundled codes* and must be billed under the single CPT code. If they are not all present, the individual tests should be billed using a separate code for each. There are two types of drug testing, qualitative and quantitative. The codes for drug testing are *qualitative;* that is, they are based on the type of drug found. *Quantitative* assays, on the other hand, are performed to determine the amount of drug present.

CPT Tabular List Basic Metabolic Panel

80047 Basic metabolic panel (Calcium, ionized)
  This panel must include the following:
  Calcium, ionized (82330)
  Carbon dioxide (bicarbonate) (82374)
  Chloride (82435)
  Creatinine (82565)
  Glucose (82947)
  Potassium (84132)
  The codes in parentheses after the individual tests are CPT codes. Those CPT codes would be used if not all of these tests were ordered at the same time.
Other Basic Metabolic Panel Components
  Sodium (84295)
  Urea Nitrogen (BUN) (84520)

CRITICAL THINKING APPLICATION   17.4
Sherald reviewed a coded medical record for a Basic Metabolic Panel with total Calcium that had listed specific CPT codes for each panel test. Is this the correct way to code for the organ panel? According to the box above, how should this organ panel be coded?

CPT CODING GUIDELINES: MEDICINE SECTION

The Medicine section of the CPT contains codes for a variety of therapeutic procedures and diagnostic testing. This section also contains codes for dialysis, ophthalmology, acupuncture, chiropractic manipulation, and conscious sedation. The steps for determining Medicine codes are similar to those for choosing Surgery codes.

Immune Globulins

When you code administration of immune globulins, identify the immune globulin product administered (CPT codes 90281–90399) and the method of administration using the codes in the hydration, therapeutic, prophylactic, and diagnostic injections and infusions subsection.

Hydration codes are intended to report a hydration intravenous (IV) infusion consisting of prepackaged fluid and electrolytes; they are not used to report the infusion of drugs or other substances. When multiple drugs are administered, report the service or services and the specific materials or drugs for each.

Immunization for Vaccines or Toxoids

The immunization for vaccines or toxoids codes (CPT codes 90460, 90461, 90471–90474) are for the administration of vaccines and toxoids only and should be reported in conjunction with the appropriate codes in the immunization administration for vaccine/toxoids subsection.

Vaccines/Toxoids Codes

These codes identify the vaccine product only (CPT codes 90476–90749). Codes in the immunization administration for

vaccines/toxoids subsection must be used in addition to the vaccine or toxoid product codes. To meet the reporting requirements of immunization registries, vaccine distribution programs, and reporting systems, the exact vaccine product administered must be reported on the insurance claim.

Home Health Procedures and Services

The home health procedures and services codes (CPT codes 99500–99602) are used by non-physician healthcare professionals only. They are used to report services provided in a patient's residence, including assisted-living apartments, group homes, nontraditional private homes, custodial care facilities, and schools.

HCPCS CODE SET AND MANUAL

HCPCS codes have 5 alphanumeric characters, beginning with one letter followed by 4 numbers. HCPCS uses coding conventions for special instructions relating to specific codes (Fig. 17.7). The modifiers for HCPCS are codes composed of 2 alphanumeric characters. The HCPCS modifiers do not change the description of the code, but rather provide additional information or describe extenuating circumstances. Like the CPT manual, the HCPCS manual is divided into an Alphabetic Index and a Tabular List. As with the CPT, procedures and services are looked up in the Alphabetic Index, and the code (or codes) is then confirmed as the most accurate and appropriate using the Tabular List. The HCPCS manual has no subsections, categories, or subcategories; it has only sections. An appendix contains all the HCPCS modifiers and their descriptions. The HCPCS codes are updated annually by the Centers for Medicare and Medicaid Services (CMS).

The coding steps for HCPCS are almost identical to those for CPT codes. Clinical documentation is the starting point for HCPCS

Humidifiers/Compressors/Nebulizers for Use with Oxygen IPPB Equipment

Code	Description
E0550	Humidifier, durable for extensive supplemental humidification during IPPB treatments or oxygen delivery
E0555	Humidifier, durable, glass or autoclavable plastic bottle type, for use with regulator or flowmeter
E0560	Humidifier, durable for supplemental humidification during IPPB treatment or oxygen delivery
E0561	Humidifier, nonheated, used with positive airway pressure device
E0562	Humidifier, heated, used with positive airway pressure device
E0565	Compressor, air power source for equipment which is not self-contained or cylinder driven
E0570	Nebulizer, with compressor
E0572	Aerosol compressor, adjustable pressure, light duty for intermittent use
E0574	Ultrasonic/electronic aerosol generator with small volume nebulizer
E0575	Nebulizer, ultrasonic, large volume
E0580	Nebulizer, durable, glass or autoclavable plastic, bottle type, for use with regulator or flowmeter
E0585	Nebulizer, with compressor and heater

FIGURE 17.7 Healthcare Common Procedure Coding System (HCPCS) Tabular List.

coding. The final code selected should add nothing to or omit anything from the description in the medical documentation. The final step is determining whether the code selected can stand alone or requires a modifier to further define or add needed information.

Sometimes HCPCS codes are used along with CPT codes, especially in the medical office setting. For example, a well-baby visit would include the E/M code for the patient visit and also HCPCS codes for the administration of immunizations. Procedure 17.2, Part B, on p. 374 explains how to code an office visit involving immunizations.

COMMON HCPCS CODING GUIDELINES

Ambulance Transport

HCPCS codes for ambulance transport range from A0021 to A0999. These codes require specific modifiers (Table 17.7) to be added to ensure code specificity. This section provides codes for a variety of medical transport, including ambulance services, nonemergency transportation, and medical supplies used during the transport. A waiting time calculation table also is available, if needed.

Medical and Surgical Supplies

HCPCS codes for medical and surgical supplies range from A4000 to A6513. The HCPCS manual provides some figures that offer guidance as to what the medical and surgical supplies look like, so

that they can be billed properly. Medical assistants can code only for surgical supplies purchased by the medical office. For example, pharmaceutical and medical equipment representatives can provide the medical office with some supplies that can be used for patient care. However, it is unethical to bill the patient's insurance company for supplies that were given to the provider for free. All medical and surgical supplies used during patient care should be documented on the encounter form in the patient's health record.

Durable Medical Equipment

HCPCS codes for durable medical equipment range from E0100 to E1841. Examples of durable medical equipment include crutches, wheelchairs, walkers, and other products that assist patients with mobility. Some equipment is kept in the medical office inventory. If the practice purchases the medical equipment wholesale, it is allowed to bill patients and/or their insurance company for the retail value of the equipment. Just as with medical and surgical supplies, it is important for the provider to document the dispensing of durable medical equipment on the encounter form or health record (see Procedure 17.3 on p. 375).

CLOSING COMMENTS

The CPT and HCPCS coding manuals are updated and published every year. The updated manuals should be ordered in the early fall so that they arrive in time for the medical assistant to review them. Always use the current year's manuals so that the codes are accurate. The Introduction in each manual discusses and highlights changes and/or new coding guidelines. Annual updates should be uploaded to reflect any coding changes in the encoder to ensure that all codes are up to date for the current year.

Legal and Ethical Issues

Medical assistants are responsible for keeping up to date on CPT coding to ensure that no fraud takes place in the coding and claims submission process. Medical assistants should also ensure that proper precautions are taken to avoid incorrect coding, data entry errors, and false claims submissions because these activities can be considered fraud.

Medical coders should be familiar with the NCCI edits, which are published every year by CMS. Medicare can cite a healthcare facility for fraud or abuse (or both) if claims submitted by the facility regularly show unbundled codes. Not only is unbundling an unethical practice, it incurs very stiff monetary penalties. According to the Civil Monetary Penalties Law, medical practices can be cited for penalties of up to $50,000 per violation, and assessments of up to three times the amount claimed for each item or service, or up to three times the amount of remuneration offered, paid, solicited, or received.

Patient-Centered Care

It is important for anyone who does coding to be able to explain to patients what those codes mean. When statements are sent to patients, many call the healthcare facility and ask for an explanation of the charges. A common question is "Why is the charge for my office visit so high?" By looking at the CPT E/M code, you can see the level of history taking, physical examination, and medical decision

TABLE 17.7	Modifiers Used for HCPCS Ambulance Transport Codes
TRANSPORTATION SERVICES MODIFIERS[a]	DESCRIPTION
D	Diagnostic or therapeutic site other than P or H when those are used as origin codes
E	Residential, domiciliary, custodial facility
G	Hospital-based dialysis facility (hospital or hospital related)
H	Hospital
I	Site of transfer (e.g., airport or helicopter pad) between modes of ambulance transport
J	Non-hospital-based dialysis facility
N	Skilled nursing facility
P	Physician's office
R	Residence
S	Scene of accident or acute event
X	Destination code only. Intermediate stop at physician's office on the way to hospital.

[a]Includes ambulance HCPCS origin modifiers.

making for that visit. You can help patients understand that it is not just the face-to-face time that determines the level of an office visit. If an extensive history and examination are done and a lot of tests must be reviewed, the E/M code will be at a higher level. That higher level warrants a higher charge. Most patients understand once all of the criteria have been explained to them. When you make these explanations with a pleasant attitude, patient satisfaction also improves.

Professional Behaviors

Two rules should be followed when you code any procedure or service:
1. Be as specific as possible in code selection and use all pertinent words in the description given in your documentation.
2. Never add or delete any words, modifying terms, or descriptors to the procedure or service code description that change the definition of the procedure or service or that are not documented.

SUMMARY OF SCENARIO

Sherald has learned that procedural coding using the CPT is similar in many ways to ICD-10-CM diagnostic coding. The two coding manuals have unique but also similar steps, conventions, and guidelines. She has learned that proper abstraction of procedural data from the health record is equally important for ICD-10-CM and CPT coding. Sherald also has learned that HCPCS codes are used to describe procedures and services not found in the CPT, such as vaccinations, ambulance services, and durable medical equipment.

Sherald uses documentation by the provider in the encounter form to identify the procedures performed. However, she realizes that she also must know how to use the CPT manual because some procedures or services must be coded from the documentation. As with diagnostic coding, Sherald reviews the patient's health record documentation if any questions come up about a claim. She knows that coding to the highest level of specificity helps to ensure accuracy and also enables the practice to obtain the maximum reimbursement allowed. She realizes the importance of keeping up to date with the CPT and HCPCS codes, so she plans to order the updated manuals every year. As Sherald continues to learn procedural coding, she envisions herself becoming well rounded in her knowledge of the practice's administrative operations.

SUMMARY OF LEARNING OBJECTIVES

1. **List and describe the three code categories in the *Current Procedural Terminology* (CPT) manual.**
   The CPT manual comprises three category codes: Category I, Category II, and Category III codes. Category I codes are 5-digit codes that are listed in the Tabular List. Category II codes are used for performance measurement, and their use is optional. Category III codes are temporary codes for emerging medical technologies.

2. **Distinguish between the Alphabetic Index and the Tabular List in the CPT code set. Also, list the six different sections of the Tabular List.**
   The CPT has two primary divisions, the Alphabetic Index and the Tabular List. The Alphabetic Index is like any other index in a textbook; it is simply a guide to finding data in the body of the textbook. The Tabular List is divided into six sections, and codes are listed in numeric order in each section.
   The six sections of the Tabular List are Evaluation and Management, Anesthesia, Surgery, Radiology, Pathology and Laboratory, and Medicine. Sections are divided into subsections; subsections are further divided into categories; and categories can be subdivided into subcategories.

3. **Discuss special reports and explain the importance of modifiers in assigning CPT codes.**
   When a bill is submitted for a service that is unlisted, unusual, or newly adopted, the third-party carrier requires a special consultation report. Modifiers are used in CPT codes to indicate that a service or procedure performed was altered by specific circumstances. Two-digit alphanumeric modifiers, included with the 5-digit CPT code, can be used to supply additional information or to describe extenuating circumstances that affected the rendered procedure or service.

4. **Review various conventions in the CPT code set.**
   Conventions are used to provide additional information about certain codes. Examples of conventions include triangular and round symbols, which indicate that a code or description was revised, removed, or added.

5. **Identify the required medical documentation for accurate procedural coding.**
   Medical records used for procedural coding can include any or all of the following: encounter form, history and physical report (H&P), progress notes, discharge summary, operative report, pathology report, anesthesia record, and/or radiology report. When the medical documentation is compared against any code description, all the elements of that code must substantially match, with nothing added or missing.

6. **Describe the steps that should be taken in order to be efficient with CPT procedural coding. Also discuss how to use the alphabetic index and the tabular list.**
   The basic steps in procedural coding are: (1) read, analyze, and abstract the procedure or service documented in the health record and (2) compare it with the encounter form, operative report, or other documentation to ensure that all services and procedures have been recorded. After searching the Alphabetic Index, the medical assistant should turn to the appropriate codes in the Tabular List to perform the final coding steps. Read the section thoroughly to determine the most accurate code to assign to the procedure or service, and then code the procedure or service. The process for procedural coding for surgery with the CPT code set is detailed in Procedure 17.1 on p. 371.

Continued

The Alphabetic Index is a comprehensive, alphabetic listing of all main terms used in procedural coding. However, it is not a substitute for the Tabular List. It is organized by main terms, and modifying terms are indented two spaces below that term. Begin the search of the Alphabetic Index by using one of the four primary classifications of main and modifying term entries. In the Tabular List, look up each code or code range found in the Alphabetic Index.

7. **Identify CPT coding guidelines for evaluation and management (E/M) procedures. In addition, perform procedural coding of an office visit and an immunization.**

   To properly code E/M services, the medical assistant must understand important differences, or variations, from the basic steps. Assigning the correct E/M code includes identifying the section, subsection, category, and subcategory of the procedure or service; reviewing the reporting instructions and guidelines for the code chosen; reviewing the level of E/M service; determining the extent of the history obtained and examination performed; and determining the complexity of medical decision making.

   To code an office visit, the coder first must determine the level of all key components, which include the history, examination, and medical decision making. (See Procedure 17.2, Part A on p. 373.)

   An immunization procedure is coded using the HCPCS code set. Coding for HCPCS is almost identical to coding for CPT because both manuals have an Alphabetic Index and a Tabular List. After searching the Alphabetic Index, the coder turns to the appropriate codes in the Tabular List to perform the final coding steps. The coder reads the section thoroughly to determine the most accurate code to assign to the procedure or service, and then codes the procedure or service. (See Procedure 17.2, Part B on p. 374.)

8. **Identify CPT coding guidelines for anesthesia procedures.**

   Anesthesia coding differs from any other form of coding in the way anesthesia services are billed. A standard formula has been established for payment of anesthesia services: Basic unit value (B) + Time units (T) + Modifying units (M) + Physical Status (PS): $B + T + M + PS$. The total number of units is then multiplied by the conversion factor.

9. **Identify CPT coding guidelines for surgical procedures.**

   Specific guidelines and notes related to surgery coding must be considered when assigning a CPT code. Always review the current year's guidelines in the Surgery section for the most up-to-date information.

10. **Discuss coding factors for the integumentary system and muscular system, and for maternity care and delivery.**

    Excision of benign lesions includes a simple closure and anesthesia. Different instructions are provided for each type of wound repair. Fractures are handled according to the type. The services normally provided in uncomplicated maternity cases include antepartum care, delivery, and postpartum care.

11. **Identify CPT coding guidelines for the Radiology, Pathology and Laboratory, and Medicine sections.**

    a. Assigning accurate CPT codes for the Radiology section is similar to the process for the Surgery section. The Radiology section contains all diagnostic imaging codes, including x-ray studies, ultrasound, magnetic resonance imaging (MRI), and nuclear medicine procedures, in addition to radiation oncology and several other types of diagnostic imaging procedures, services, and therapies.

    b. Assigning accurate CPT codes for the Pathology and Laboratory section also is similar to the process for the Surgery section. The subcategories for the Pathology section include organ panels and disease panels, drug testing, therapeutic drug assays, evocative or suppression testing, consultations, urinalysis, chemistry, molecular diagnostics, infectious agents, microbiology, anatomic pathology, cytopathology, cytogenetic studies, and surgical pathology. In the Laboratory section, organ or disease panels are groupings of numerous tests performed to diagnose the health or disease status of specific organ systems.

    c. The Medicine section contains codes for a variety of therapeutic procedures and diagnostic testing. This section also contains codes for Dialysis, Ophthalmology, Acupuncture, Chiropractic Manipulation, and Conscious Sedation. The steps for determining codes in the Medicine section are similar to those for determining codes in the Surgery section.

12. **Do the following related to the HCPCS code set and manual:**

    - *Identify procedures and services that require HCPCS codes.*
      HCPCS is a collection of codes and descriptions that represent procedures, supplies, products, and services not covered by or included in the CPT coding system. HCPCS codes, like CPT codes, are updated annually by the CMS. These codes are designed to promote standardized reporting and collection of statistical data on medical supplies, products, services, and procedures.

    - *Describe how to use the most current HCPCS coding system.*
      Like the CPT manual, the HCPCS manual is divided into two parts: the Alphabetic Index and the Tabular List. As with the CPT, procedures and services are looked up in the Alphabetic Index, and the Tabular List then is used to confirm that the code is the most accurate and appropriate one. The HCPCS manual has no subsections, categories, or subcategories; it has only sections. An appendix contains all the HCPCS modifiers and their descriptions. The coding steps for HCPCS are almost identical to those for CPT Category I codes.

13. **Summarize common HCPCS coding guidelines.**

    Ambulance Transport codes require specific modifiers to ensure code specificity. The HCPCS manual provides some figures that offer guidance as to what the medical and surgical supplies look like, so they can be billed properly. Medical assistants can only bill for surgical supplies that were purchased by the medical office. The medical office can purchase the medical equipment wholesale but still bill patients and/or their insurance companies for the retail value of the equipment. When the insurance company is billed, it is vital that the medical assistant fill in the "Number of Units" box on the health insurance claim form for equipment provided to the patient.

PROCEDURE 17.1   Perform Procedural Coding: Surgery

Task: To use the steps for CPT procedural coding to find the most accurate and specific CPT surgery code.

EQUIPMENT and SUPPLIES

- CPT coding manual (current year) or
- TruCode encoder software
- Operative report (see the following figure)

Operative Report

PATIENT NAME: Sonia Sample
ROOM NUMBER: 222 West
MR NUMBER: 12-34-56

DATE OF PROCEDURE: 04/22/20XX
PREOPERATIVE DIAGNOSIS: Acute cholecystitis
POSTOPERATIVE DIAGNOSIS: Acute cholecystitis
NAME OF PROCEDURE: 1. Laparoscopic cholecystectomy
                           2. Intraoperative cystic duct cholangiogram
SURGEON: Claude St. John, M.D.
ASSISTANT: Mark Weiss, D.O.
ANESTHESIOLOGIST: Angela Adams, M.D.
ANESTHESIA: General

DESCRIPTION OF THE OPERATION:

The patient was placed in the supine position under general anesthesia. The oral gastric tube was placed. The Foley catheter was placed. The patient received appropriate antibiotics. The abdomen was prepped with iodine and draped in the usual fashion. Using a midline subumbilical incision, we entered the subcutaneous fat to find the aponeurosis of the rectus abdominis. Two stay sutures were placed 0.5 cm from the midline bilaterally and we left on these sutures, creating an opening in the linea alba.

Under direct vision, the catheter was placed. The Hasson cannula was placed in the abdominal cavity and all was normal except an acute necrotizing and probably gangrenous gallbladder. There were multiple omental adhesions. Three other trocars were placed in the right subcostal plane in the midline, midclavicular line, and midaxillary line using a #10, #5, and #5 mm trocar, respectively. The gallbladder was punctured and emptied of clear white bile indicating a hydrops of the gallbladder. It was grasped at its fundus and at Hartmann's pouch retracted cephalad and to the right, respectively. We found the cystic duct and the cystic artery after circumferential dissection and isolated the cystic duct completely.

When we were sure that this structure was a deep cystic duct, the clip was placed at the most distal aspect to make an opening immediately proximally and we placed a Reddick cholangiocatheter into it via #14 gauge percutaneous catheter. The cholangiogram showed normal arborization of the liver radicals. Normal bifurcation of the common hepatic duct. Normal common hepatic duct. Long large cystic duct. The common bile duct had numerous stones within it. They could not be emptied from the common bile duct. There was good flow into the duodenum.

The impression was choledocholithiasis. This was corroborated by the radiologist. The decision was made to prepare the patient most probably for endoscopic retrograde cholangiopancreatography postoperatively, and no further intervention of the common bile duct was done in this setting.

The cholangiocatheter was removed. An attempt was made to milk the bile out, but no stones came out. Three clips were placed on the proximal aspect of the cystic duct and the duct was then cut distally. The artery was isolated and double clipped proximally and single clipped distally and cut in the intervening section. We then peeled the gallbladder off the gallbladder bed with some difficulty because of the intense edema and inflammation. It was then removed from the liver bed completely. Cautery, suctioning and irrigation were used copiously to create a bloodless field. A last check was made and there was no bleeding and no bile leaking. A #15 Jackson-Pratt type drain was placed into Morrison's pouch and brought out through the lateral most port. We then removed, with great difficulty, the gallbladder from the umbilicus. Because of its enormous size and a 3 cm stone within it that was very difficult to macerate, the opening of the umbilicus had to be enlarged.

As this was done, we removed the gallbladder completely and sent it for pathologic section. Two separate figure-of-eight 0 PDS were used to close the abdominal fascia. The Jackson-Pratt drain was then sutured in place with 2.0 nylon. The skin was closed throughout with subcuticular 3-0 PDS after copious irrigation of the subcutaneous plane. Mastisol and Steri-Strips were placed on the wound. The patient remained stable although she did have bigeminy during surgery and was on a Lidocaine drip. She will be going to the intensive care unit but as she left, she was extubated in the recovery room and was fully alert. She is moving all limbs.

I will discuss with the gastroenterologist postoperative endoscopic retrograde cholangiopancreatography.

SPECIMEN: Gallbladder.

Claude St. John, M.D.
CSJ/ld:
D: 04/22/20XX
T: 04/22/20XX 9:21 a.m.
CC: Maria Acosta, M.D.

Continued

PROCEDURE 17.1 | Perform Procedural Coding: Surgery—*continued*

PROCEDURAL STEPS

Using the CPT Coding Manual

1. Abstract the procedures and/or services from the procedural statement in the surgical report.
2. Select the most appropriate main term to begin the search in the Alphabetic Index.
3. Once the main term has been located in the Alphabetic Index, review and select the modifying term or terms if required.
   PURPOSE: For additional specificity and to narrow the search for the most accurate CPT code or code range in the Alphabetic Index.
4. If the main term cannot be found in the Alphabetic Index, repeat steps 2 and 3 using a different main term possibly based on the procedural statement.
5. Once the CPT code or code range is identified in the Alphabetic Index, disregard any code or code range containing additional descriptions or modifying terms not found in the health record.
6. Record the code or code ranges that best match the procedural statements in the surgical report.
   PURPOSE: To prevent repeated reference to the Alphabetic Index by recording all possible matches to the code or code range sought. This saves time and prevents redundant effort.
7. Turn to the Tabular List and find the first code or code range from your search of the Alphabetic Index.
   PURPOSE: To begin the process of finding the most specific and accurate code.
8. Compare the description of the code with the procedural statement in the surgical report. Verify that all or most of the health record documentation matches the code description and that there is no additional information in the code description that is not found in the documentation.
9. Review the coding guidelines and notes for the section, subsection, and code to ensure that there are no contraindications to use of the code. Review the coding conventions and add-on codes, if any.
   PURPOSE: To ensure there are no instructions that would prevent the use of the code selected.

10. Determine whether a modifier is needed.
    PURPOSE: To select any appropriate modifiers that provide additional information for the chosen code to explain certain circumstances or provide additional detail.
11. Determine whether a Special Report is required.
    PURPOSE: To clarify and add additional detail when an unusual or extenuating circumstance exists or if a Category III or unlisted procedure Category I code is used.
12. Record the CPT code selected in the health record documentation next to the procedure or service performed and in the appropriate block of the insurance claim form.
    PURPOSE: To complete the documentation and recording requirements.

Using the TruCode Software

1. Abstract the procedures and/or services from the procedural statement in the surgical report.
2. Type the main term into the encoder Search box and select the CPT. Then click on Show All Results.
3. If the main term cannot be found through the search, repeat steps 2 and 3 using a different main term based on the procedural statement.
4. Choose the procedure description that is closest to the procedural statement in the surgical report (see the following figure).
   PURPOSE: To prevent upcoding or downcoding errors or other possible fraud and/or abuse circumstances.
5. Record the CPT code that best matches the procedural statements in the surgical report in the patient's health record.
   PURPOSE: To prevent repeated reference to the Alphabetic Index by recording all possible matches to the code or code range being sought. This saves time and prevents redundant effort.

PROCEDURE 17.1   Perform Procedural Coding: Surgery—*continued*

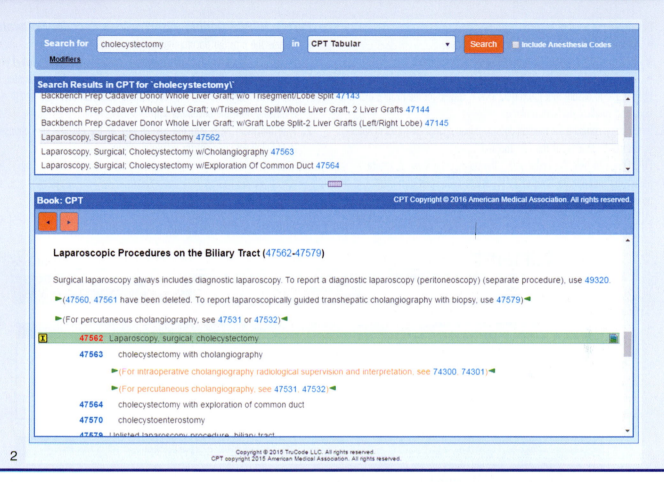

Search for [cholecystectomy] in [CPT Tabular ▾] [Search] ☐ Include Anesthesia Codes
Modifiers

Search Results in CPT for `cholecystectomy\`

Backbench Prep Cadaver Donor Whole Liver Graft; w/o Trisegment/Lobe Split 47143
Backbench Prep Cadaver Whole Liver Graft; w/Trisegment Split/Whole Liver Graft, 2 Liver Grafts 47144
Backbench Prep Cadaver Donor Whole Liver Graft; w/Graft Lobe Split-2 Liver Grafts (Left/Right Lobe) 47145
Laparoscopy, Surgical; Cholecystectomy 47562
Laparoscopy, Surgical; Cholecystectomy w/Cholangiography 47563
Laparoscopy, Surgical; Cholecystectomy w/Exploration Of Common Duct 47564

Book: CPT   CPT Copyright © 2016 American Medical Association. All rights reserved.

◀ ▶

Laparoscopic Procedures on the Biliary Tract (47562-47579)

Surgical laparoscopy always includes diagnostic laparoscopy. To report a diagnostic laparoscopy (peritoneoscopy) (separate procedure), use 49320.

►(47560, 47561 have been deleted. To report laparoscopically guided transhepatic cholangiography with biopsy, use 47579)◀

►(For percutaneous cholangiography, see 47531 or 47532)◀

47562   Laparoscopy, surgical; cholecystectomy
47563   cholecystectomy with cholangiography
►(For intraoperative cholangiography radiological supervision and interpretation, see 74300, 74301)◀
►(For percutaneous cholangiography, see 47531, 47532)◀
47564   cholecystectomy with exploration of common duct
47570   cholecystoenterostomy
47579   Unlisted laparoscopy procedure, biliary tract

PROCEDURE 17.2   Perform Procedural Coding: Office Visit and Immunizations

Task: To use the steps for CPT Evaluation and Management coding and HCPCS coding to find the most accurate and specific CPT E/M and HCPCS codes using the coding manuals or the TruCode encoder.

EQUIPMENT and SUPPLIES

- CPT coding manual (current year)
- HCPCS coding manual (current year) or
- TruCode encoder software
- Progress note

Progress Note for Daniel Miller (DOB 03/12/2012): 04/08/20XX Daniel was seen today for a follow-up visit for his recent case of otitis media in the left ear. The ear infection has completely cleared, and he is now able to receive his hepatitis B vaccine. The office visit involved a problem-focused history, problem-focused examination, and medical decision making of low complexity.

PROCEDURAL STEPS

Part A: CPT E/M Coding

1. Determine the place of service from the encounter form.
   PURPOSE: To determine the most accurate CPT E/M code, the place of service needs to be identified.
2. Determine the patient's status.
   PURPOSE: To determine the most accurate CPT E/M code, the patient should be identified as new or established.
3. Identify the subsection, category, or subcategory of service in the E/M section.
   PURPOSE: To ensure that the correct place of service and patient status are used and the appropriate level of service is selected.

Continued

PROCEDURE 17.2 | **Perform Procedural Coding: Office Visit and Immunizations**—*continued*

4. Determine the level of service:
- Determine the extent of the history obtained.
- Determine the extent of the examination performed.
- Determine the complexity of medical decision making.

<u>PURPOSE:</u> To ensure that the correct level is chosen for the history, examination, and medical decision making.

5. If necessary, compare the medical documentation against examples in Appendix C, Clinical Examples, of the CPT manual.

<u>PURPOSE:</u> To help the coder select the appropriate level of service.

6. Select the appropriate level of E/M service code, and document it in the patient's health record.

<u>PURPOSE:</u> To complete the documentation and reporting requirements.

Part B: HCPCS Coding with TruCode Encoder Software

1. Review the provider documentation.

<u>PURPOSE:</u> To ensure that all procedures and/or services are listed on the encounter form; that all procedures and services on the encounter form match the health record; and that nothing documented in the health record is missing from the encounter form.

2. Type the main term into the Search box of the encoder and choose the HCPCS Tabular code set for accurate coding.

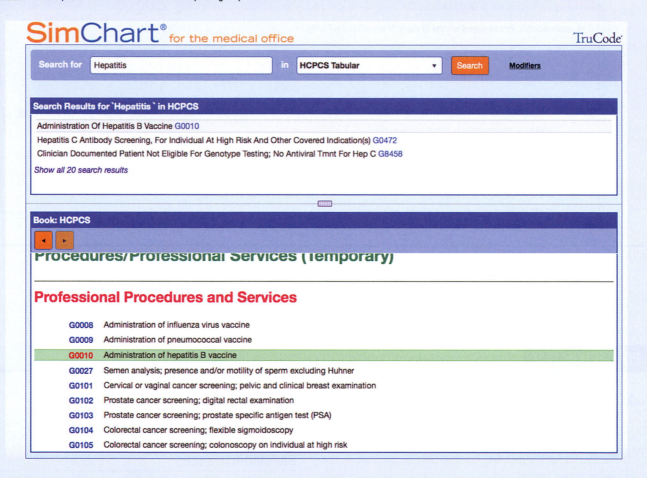

3. If no modifying term produces an appropriate code or code range, repeat steps 2 and 3 using a different main term.

<u>PURPOSE:</u> To help find the most appropriate code or code range by using alternative methods of searching the Alphabetic Index.

4. Compare the description of the code with the medical documentation.

<u>PURPOSE:</u> To avoid upcoding and downcoding errors and to ensure there are no contraindications to use of the code selected.

5. Select the appropriate HCPCS immunization code and document it in the patient's health record.

<u>PURPOSE:</u> To complete the documentation and reporting requirements.

PROCEDURE 17.3   Working with Providers to Ensure Accurate Code Selection

Using tactful communication skills means using good manners as you provide truthful, sensitive information to another person while considering the person's feelings. Tactful communication skills include verbal and nonverbal communication that shows respect, discretion, compassion, honesty, diplomacy, and courtesy. When you use tactful behaviors, you demonstrate professionalism and you preserve relationships by avoiding conflicts and finding common ground.

Many times, the medical coder is the expert on the accurate CPT and ICD code selections. The highest level of specificity must be used when coding so that appropriate reimbursement can occur. It is not uncommon for the medical coder to interact with providers and assist them in understanding the coding process. During these interactions, it is crucial that the medical coder provide the information in a professional, organized, and logical manner. Using tactful communication skills is critical to maintaining a healthy working relationship with the providers.

Using the following case study, role-play with two peers how you would use tactful communication skills with medical providers to ensure accurate code selection.

You are a new medical coder for the medical practice. You have been on the job for 6 weeks and have been seeing a trend of downcoding of charges. The required documentation is present in the health records, but the providers have been selecting less specific codes for the appointment types. Your goal is to explain to the providers accurate code selection for the appointment types.

18

MEDICAL BILLING AND REIMBURSEMENT ESSENTIALS

SCENARIO

Ann Snyder, a recent medical assisting graduate, has been hired to work in the billing office for Walden-Martin Family Medical (WMFM) Clinic. During her medical assistant program, her instructor, Grant Wilson, helped her realize that working with health insurance can be quite rewarding. Mr. Wilson worked with Ann and her classmates, answering their questions and helping them to see that medical insurance is not as complicated as it may seem.

Ann is detail oriented, and she enjoys billing and coding activities. She understands that performing these duties in the provider's office is crucial because tasks related to billing have a significant effect on the healthcare facility. She also understands that income generated is used to pay the clinic's expenses, including payroll, so the facility's staff indirectly counts on accurate and timely

billing. Medical assistants who continually develop their coding skills are assets to the practice and can look forward to a long and rewarding career.

Ann gained an understanding of the insurance process while in school. Mr. Wilson showed the students several different explanation of benefits (EOBs) forms from a variety of insurance companies so that the students could learn how the reimbursement process works for a variety of health insurance plans. Ann also learned about the importance of verifying patient billing information, in addition to the steps for obtaining precertification for medical procedures. She also learned how to discuss the patient's billing record professionally. Ann is looking forward to using all of the skills she gained in school.

While studying this chapter, think about the following questions:
- Why is it important to obtain accurate patient billing information?
- Why is it important to verify insurance eligibility and process precertification before the patient receives medical services?
- What steps are needed to complete a CMS-1500 Health Insurance Claim Form?
- What information is found on an EOB that is used to determine the patient's financial responsibility?
- How can you use sensitivity when informing patients of the financial responsibilities they face as a result of third-party requirements?

LEARNING OBJECTIVES

1. Describe the medical billing process, identify the types of information contained in the patient's billing record, and interpret information on an insurance card.
2. Discuss managed care policies and procedures, including precertification/preauthorization and referrals, and show sensitivity when communicating with patients regarding third-party requirements.
3. Identify steps for filing a third-party claim.
4. Explain how to submit health insurance claims, including electronic claims, to various third-party payers.
5. Review the guidelines for completing the CMS-1500 Health Insurance Claim Form and complete an insurance claim form.
6. Differentiate between fraud and abuse.
7. Discuss methods of preventing the rejection of claims.
8. Display tactful behavior when speaking with medical providers about third-party requirements.
9. Describe ways of checking a claim's status.
10. Review and read an Explanation of Benefits.
11. Discuss reasons for denied claims.
12. Define "medical necessity" as it applies to diagnostic and procedural coding and follow medical necessity guidelines.
13. Explain a patient's financial obligations for services rendered; also, inform a patient of these obligations, and show sensitivity when speaking with patients about third-party requirements.

VOCABULARY

adjudicate (uh JOO di kayt) To settle or determine judicially.
audit A process completed before claims submission in which claims are examined for accuracy and completeness.
capitation (ka pi TAY shun) A payment arrangement for healthcare providers. The provider is paid a set amount for each

enrolled person assigned to him or her, per period of time, whether or not that person has received services.
claims clearinghouse An organization that accepts the claim data from the provider, reformats the data to meet the specifications outlined by the insurance plan, and submits the claim.

VOCABULARY—continued

claim scrubbers Software that finds common billing errors before the claim is sent to the insurance company.

CMS-1500 Health Insurance Claim Form (CMS-1500) The standard insurance claim form used for all government and most commercial insurance companies.

copayment (copay) A set dollar amount that the patient must pay for each office visit. There can be one copayment amount for a primary care provider, a different copayment amount (usually higher) to see a specialist or be seen in the emergency department.

eligibility (el i ji BILL i tee) Meeting the stipulated requirements to participate in the healthcare plan.

endoscopy (en DOS kuh pee) Nonsurgical procedure that uses an endoscope to view inside the body.

explanation of benefits (EOB) A document sent by the insurance company to the provider and the patient explaining the allowed charge amount, the amount reimbursed for services, and the patient's financial responsibilities.

medical necessity Services or supplies (CPT and HCPCS codes) used to treat the patient's diagnosis (ICD codes) that meet the accepted standard of medical practice.

National Provider Identifier (NPI) An identifier assigned by the Centers for Medicare and Medicaid Services (CMS) that classifies the healthcare provider by license and medical specialties.

precertification The process of determining if a procedure or service is covered by the insurance plan and what the reimbursement is for that procedure or service.

provider Web portal A secure online website that gives contracted providers a single point of access to insurance companies. This allows the provider to determine patient eligibility and deductible status, submit preauthorizations/precertifications, and check the status of claims.

release of information A form completed by the patient that authorizes the medical office to release medical records to the insurance company for health insurance reimbursement.

Medical billing and reimbursement represent the financial lifeline of the healthcare facility. Collecting accurate patient health insurance information is essential to submitting accurate health insurance claims. Each health insurance company has its own claims submission policies and procedures for timely reimbursement. A successful medical assistant in insurance billing learns the insurance company requirements and submits accurate claims. Many health insurance companies have online **provider Web portals**. This has made the process of checking the status of a claim quick and easy. The medical assistant also needs to be able to look at a patient's insurance card and interpret the information found there, including **copayment (copay)** amounts. An **explanation of benefits (EOB)** from the insurance carrier will indicate the patient's deductible and/or co-insurance. Clear communication with the patient about his or her financial responsibilities takes patience and sensitivity.

MEDICAL BILLING PROCESS

The medical billing process starts when a patient makes an appointment and is complete when payment has been received. The following steps are typically taken for medical billing.

- Collect patient information when the patient calls to schedule an appointment. This includes information about the insured, his or her employer, demographic information, and health insurance data.
- When the patient arrives for the appointment, you should:
  - make a copy or scan both sides of the patient's insurance card and government-issued ID card.
  - if the patient has a copayment (copay) responsibility, collect it before services are provided (see Procedure 18.1 on p. 396).
- Verify the patient's **eligibility**, confirming that the patient's contract with the insurance company is valid for the date of service. Patient eligibility can be confirmed by:
  - calling the provider services phone number on the back of the health insurance ID card

- using the provider web portal sponsored by the patient's health insurance company
- Review patient benefits and exclusions for certain medical procedures and services.
  - If **precertification** is needed, contact the health insurance company to request it.
- After services have been provided to the patient, code the diagnosis and procedures and review the encounter form/superbill for completeness. The charges for the procedure or procedures should be provided automatically by the medical billing software.
- Complete the **CMS-1500 Health Insurance Claim Form (CMS-1500)** or an electronic claim form. Submit the form to the insurance company. Electronic claim information may be submitted to a **claims clearinghouse**.
- Review the electronic claims submission report to ensure that the claim was submitted accurately. Correct any discrepancies through the claims clearinghouse and resubmit denied claims.
- Meet the timely filing requirements of each of the different health insurance carriers. Health insurance companies do not pay claims submitted after the established filing period, and this balance cannot be billed to the patient.
- Post payments in the patient's account using the EOB to identify the line items that were paid, reduced, or denied. Patient account statements for the person's financial responsibility should be mailed out. Health insurance claims for patient accounts with secondary insurance should be submitted to the secondary carrier.

CRITICAL THINKING APPLICATION   18.1

The medical billing manager informs Ann that she has noticed an increase in the number of insurance claim rejections that state the patient cannot be identified. Which step of the medical billing process might be addressed to resolve this problem?

TYPES OF INFORMATION FOUND IN THE PATIENT'S BILLING RECORD

The claim submission process begins after the patient receives services from the provider. When a patient makes a first appointment, it is routine to ask the patient for insurance billing information. Much of this information is collected on the patient information form (Fig. 18.1). This form can be sent to the patient ahead of time or completed when the patient comes to the medical office for the first visit. This form should always be completed for every new patient. For established patients, demographic and insurance information should be verified.

Accurate patient information for submitting a health insurance claim is important, but a medical **release of information** form, signed by the patient, should also be kept in the person's health record. The release form allows the release of medical information to the insurance company. The Health Insurance Portability and Accountability Act (HIPAA) does not require this, but some state laws do. Many healthcare facilities will have a patient complete the form and keep it in the health record.

MANAGED CARE POLICIES AND PROCEDURES

Medical billers should be familiar with procedures commonly used by managed care organizations (MCOs), such as precertification. If the procedures are not followed, the MCO might not pay for the services. For example, pain management services typically require a preauthorization. If a pain management facility were to provide these services to the patient without preauthorization, the MCO could deny all insurance claims. To submit accurate health insurance claims, medical assistants should follow office procedures for applying MCO policies and procedures (see Procedure 18.2 on p. 396).

Precertification/Preauthorization

In an effort to control costs, many MCOs require precertification for certain procedures and services. *Precertification* is the process of proving to the insurance company that the service is medically necessary. The insurance company, in turn, will determine if it is a covered service and what the reimbursement will be. Precertification must be done before the procedure or service is performed.

To obtain precertification, the medical assistant:
- calls the provider services phone number on the back of the patient's health insurance ID card.
- provides the insurance company with procedures and/or services requested and the diagnoses.
- documents the outcome of the call in the patient's health record, including the precertification number.

Precertification does not guarantee payment of services. The process ensures that both the healthcare provider and the patient are informed both of the amount that the insurance company will pay and also the amount that the patient will have to pay.

Each insurance company has its own precertification requirements. Almost every MCO requires precertification, but medical assistants must confirm this by contacting the insurance company. Successful medical billers are diligent in obtaining precertification.

The precertification and preauthorization processes (see Procedure 18.3 on p. 398) are very similar. The insurance company is contacted after the primary care provider (PCP) recommends the procedure or service. In fact, many health insurance companies use the terms precertification and preauthorization interchangeably. However, precertification specifically determines whether the procedure is medically necessary, and *preauthorization* gives the provider approval to render the medical service. Precertification and preauthorization can be requested through an insurance company's online Web portal (see Procedure 18.3 on p. 398).

Preauthorization/Precertification Examples

1. Dr. David Kahn is the primary care provider (PCP) for Janine Butler, who has heartburn that has not improved with medication.
2. Because Ms. Butler's condition is not improving, Dr. Kahn requests preauthorization for her to see Dr. Eduard Hamilton, a gastrointestinal (GI) specialist. Ms. Butler is insured by a managed care organization (MCO).
3. The MCO authorizes Ms. Butler to see Dr. Hamilton; this authorization is sent to Ms. Butler, Dr. Kahn, and Dr. Hamilton. When Ms. Butler receives the authorization, she schedules an appointment with Dr. Hamilton.
4. After evaluating Ms. Butler, Dr. Hamilton orders an esophageal **endoscopy**. However, Ms. Butler is concerned about her financial responsibility. Therefore, Dr. Hamilton's office requests precertification for the endoscopy on Ms. Butler's behalf.
5. The MCO notifies Dr. Hamilton that the plan would reimburse a total of $1,500, and Ms. Butler would be financially responsible for $400. The precertification is sent both to Dr. Hamilton and Ms. Butler, who agree to its financial terms and schedule the procedure.

Referrals

Patients seeking specialized care must first visit their assigned PCP to obtain a referral to a specialist or for more specialized therapy or care. Patients with HMO plans can only obtain a referral to the specialist by visiting their assigned PCP. HMOs will measure how many patients are referred to specialists by individual PCPs. Approval or denial of a referral can take anywhere from a few minutes to a few days. The three types of referrals are as follows:

- A *regular referral* usually takes 3 to 10 working days for review and approval. This type of referral is used when the provider believes that the patient must see a specialist to continue treatment.
- An *urgent referral* usually takes about 24 hours for approval. This type of referral is used when an urgent but not life-threatening situation occurs.
- A *STAT referral* can be approved online when it is submitted to the utilization review department through the provider's Web portal. A STAT referral is used in an emergency situation as indicated by the provider.

A *regular referral* is the most common type and can be inconvenient for the patient. With most managed care plans, preauthorization needs to be obtained for a referral. Remember this cardinal rule: never tell the patient the referral has been approved unless you have a hard copy of the authorization. A referral is authorized after the approval has been received. When a referral is approved, the PCP's office and the patient should receive a copy of the authorization.

WALDEN-MARTIN
FAMILY MEDICAL CLINIC
1234 ANYSTREET | ANYTOWN, ANYSTATE 12345
PHONE 123-123-1234 | FAX 123-123-5678

Patient Information

Patient Information (Please use full legal name.)

Last Name: Tapia
First Name: Celia
Middle Initial: B
Medical Record Number: 11012373
Date of Birth: 05/18/1970
Age: 42
Sex: Female
SSN: 857-62-1594
Emergency Contact Name: Arnold Tapia

Address 1: 12 Highland Court
Address 2: Apt 101
City: Anytown
Country: United States   State/Province: AL
Zip: 12345-1234
Email: —
Home Phone: 123-858-1545
Driver's License: —
Emergency Contact Phone: 123-200-5006

Guarantor Information (Please use full legal name.)

Relationship of Guarantor to Patient: Spouse
Guarantor/Account #: Tapia, Arnold / 12088787
Account Number: 12088787
Last Name: Tapia
First Name: Arnold
Middle Initial: —
Date of Birth: 05/18/1970
Age: 42
Sex: Male
SSN: 812-93-1341
Employer Name: Anytown String Shop
School Name: —

Address 1: 12 Highland Court
Address 2: Apt 101
City: Anytown
Country: United States   State/Province: AL
Zip: 12345-1234
Email: —
Home Phone: 123-858-1545
Cell Phone: —
Work Phone: —

Provider Information

Primary Provider: James A. Martin, MD
Referring Provider: —
Date of Last Visit: August 28, 2013
Phone: 123-123-1234

Provider's Address 1: 1234 Anystreet
Provider's Address 2: —
City: Anytown
Country: United States   State/Province: AL
Zip: 12345-1234

Insurance Information (If the patient is not the Insured party, please include date of birth for claims.)

Insurance: Aetna
Name of Policy Holder: Arnold Tapia
SSN: 812-93-1341
Policy/ID Number: CT5487854
Group Number: 41554T

Claims Address 1: 1234 Insurance Way
Claims Address 2: —
City: Anytown
Country: United States   State/Province: AL
Zip: 12345-1234
Claims Phone: 180-012-3222

Secondary Insurance

Insurance: —
Name of Policy Holder: —
SSN: —
Policy/ID Number: —
Group Number: —

Claims Address 1: —
Claims Address 2: —
City: —
Country: —   State/Province: —
Zip: —
Claims Phone: —

"I hereby authorize direct payment of all insurance benfits otherwise payable to me for services rendered. I understand that I am financially responsible for all charges not covered by insurance for services rendered on my behalf to my dependents. I authorize the above prociders to release any information required to secure payment of benefits. I authorize the use of this signature on all insurace submissions."

Signature: Celia Japia   Date: 05/06/20XX

FIGURE 18.1 Complete patient registration form.

Always review the authorization thoroughly and confirm details, such as approved diagnosis and procedure codes and the exact period of time the authorization lasts. The patient will receive a letter with an authorization number and details regarding the approved services. The patient must bring the authorization to the specialist's office on the date of the appointment.

SUBMITTING CLAIMS TO THIRD-PARTY PAYERS

All health insurance companies accept:
- CMS-1500 as the standard claim form
- ICD-10-CM for diagnostic codes
- CPT and HCPCS procedural/supply codes

However, each health insurance company has its own policies and procedures for the submission of claims.

Guidelines for Medicare and Medicaid claims can be found on the administrator websites for each state. MCO plans associated with **capitation** agreements have specific guidelines on the types of medical services that are billable. Private health insurance plans have their own policies and procedures for submitting claims. The medical assistant should research the health plans commonly seen in the healthcare facility.

The medical assistant can successfully manage the requirements of the different insurance plans by keeping a medical billing manual. The manual should contain the billing policies and procedures for the most common third-party payers. The person in charge of the manual should make sure that every medical biller has a copy and that the policies and procedures are up to date. For example, Medicare's billing procedures and policies are updated on October 1. Whenever an update is released, the medical billing manual also should be updated.

Most providers are required to submit claims electronically for Medicare patients and are doing so for most other health insurance plans. If the majority of claims are submitted electronically, why is it important to learn the different fields of the CMS-1500 paper form? The data used to submit electronic claims are the same data used on the CMS-1500. A medical assistant who is familiar with a paper CMS-1500 will have no problem collecting the proper data for an electronic claim. Both methods will be discussed in the following sections.

GENERATING ELECTRONIC CLAIMS

Electronic claims are insurance claims that are transmitted over the internet from the provider to the health insurance company through *electronic data interchange*. Electronic data interchange is the electronic transfer of data between two or more entities. When submitting electronic claims, a healthcare facility transmits the data for the claim, and the health insurance company accepts it. Most medical billing software is designed to generate electronic claims.

As with paper claims, when electronic claims are submitted, accurate data are essential. When the medical assistant reviews the claim for accuracy, the claim is prepared for submission.

Electronic Claims Submission

Electronic claims are submitted in the 5010 format established by HIPAA and can be directly transmitted to the insurance carrier or to a claims clearinghouse.

Direct Billing

Direct billing is the process by which an insurance company allows a provider to electronically submit claims directly to the company. Most major insurance companies, including Medicare and Medicaid, provide software packages that are used to enter the following:
- Patient's information
- Insured's information
- Charges
- Provider details

Many carrier-direct systems are supplied free of charge to the provider, but the direct system can transmit only to specific carriers. If a majority of claims for the healthcare facility are submitted to just one insurance company, direct billing would be a good way to submit claims.

Clearinghouse Submissions

A claims clearinghouse is an organization that acts as a go-between for the healthcare facility and the insurance company. The clearinghouse:
- accepts electronically submitted claims information from healthcare agencies.
- **audits** the claims for completeness.
- reformats claims to meet insurance company specifications.

The claims are sorted by insurance plans and sent in batches electronically to the appropriate insurers. The insurance companies then send a report through the data clearinghouse to:
- confirm the receipt of claims.
- report the status of previously submitted claims.
- serve as claim payment notification.

A clearinghouse charges the healthcare facility a small fee for:
- sending and receiving claims transmissions.
- checking and preparing the claims for processing.
- consolidating claims so that one transmission can be sent to each carrier.
- submitting claims in correct data format to the appropriate insurance payer.

A typical fee is 25¢ per submitted claim. Other services that clearinghouses typically provide include:
- Reporting the number of claims submitted, and the number of errors and their specifics
- Forwarding claims to insurance carriers that accept electronic claims (e.g., Medicare, Medicaid, Blue Cross/Blue Shield, and others) or to another clearinghouse that may hold the contracts with specific payers
- Keeping provider offices updated as new carriers are added to the database
- Generating informative statistical reports

COMPLETING THE CMS-1500 HEALTH INSURANCE CLAIM FORM

The CMS-1500 Health Insurance Claim Form is the form required by HIPAA for paper claim submission. The form has 33 blocks. These blocks are divided into three sections:
- *Section 1: Carrier.* The first section indicates the type of insurance plan to which the claim is being submitted; this section includes only Block 1.

- *Section 2: Patient and Insured Information.* The second section contains information about the patient and the insured; it includes Blocks 1a through 13.
- *Section 3: Physician or Supplier Information.* The third section contains information about the provider or supplier; it includes Blocks 14 through 33.

Section 1: Carrier – Block 1 (Fig. 18.2)

Block 1 shows the type of insurance the patient has. Indicate the type of health insurance coverage for this claim by putting an X in the appropriate box, marking only one box. This information directs the claim to the correct payer.

Section 2: Patient and Insured Information – Blocks 1a through 13 (Fig. 18.3)

The CMS-1500 distinguishes between the patient and the insured. The insured is the individual who is directly contracted with the insurance company. For example, if an insurance claim for Lisa Parker is submitted and Blue Cross covers her through her employer, she is both the patient and the insured. However, if the insurance claim is for Johnny Parker, her son, Lisa Parker is the insured, and Johnny Parker, her dependent, is the patient. Every CMS-1500 requires the name, gender, and birth date of both the insured and the patient, even if they are different individuals. The blocks in Fig. 18.3 highlighted in yellow are for the patient's information, and the blocks highlighted in blue are for the insured's information.

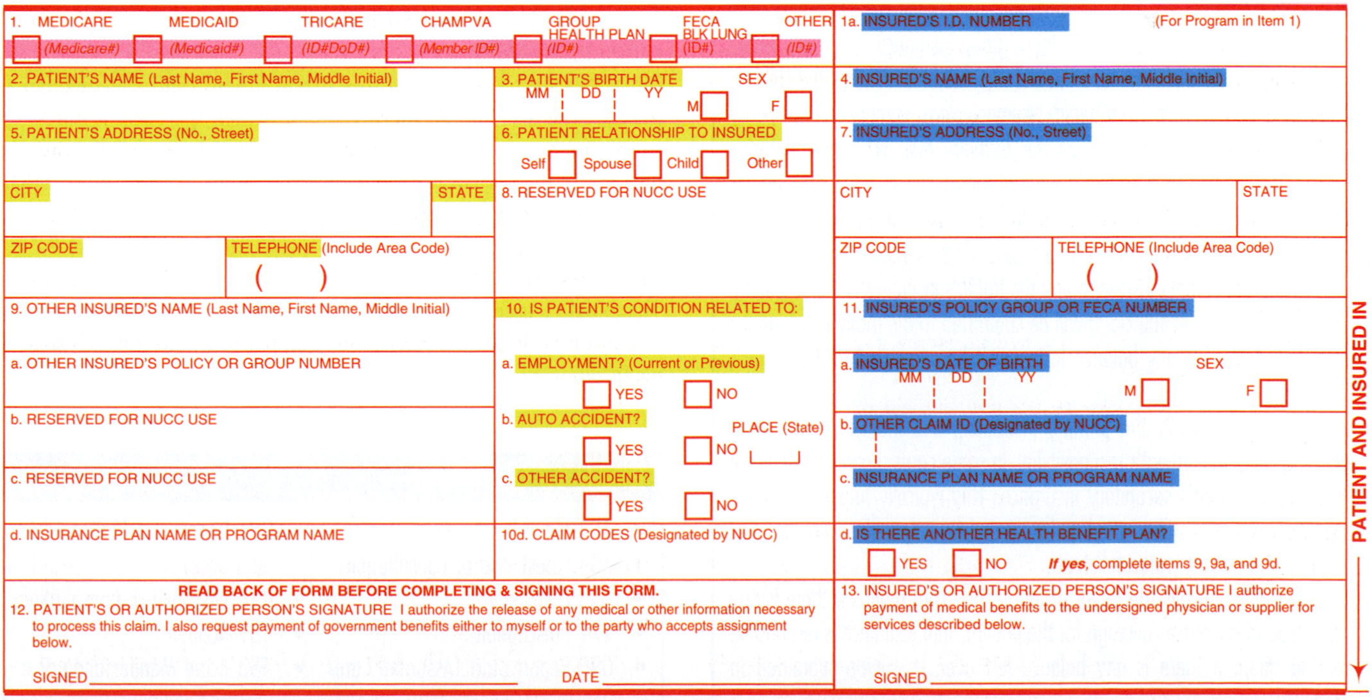

Blocks 1a, 4, 7, and 11 a–d

Information required for the insured includes:

- person's health plan ID number
- name
- address
- policy and group numbers
- birth date (MM/DD/YYYY) and gender
- employer's name (if applicable)
- name of the insurance plan
- whether the insured has another health benefit plan

HEALTH INSURANCE CLAIM FORM
APPROVED BY NATIONAL UNIFORM CLAIM COMMITTEE (NUCC) 02/12
PICA PICA
CARRIER
1. MEDICARE (Medicare #) | MEDICAID (Medicaid #) | TRICARE CHAMPUS (Sponsor's SSN) | CHAMPVA (Member ID#) | GROUP HEALTH PLAN (SSN or ID) | FECA BLK LUNG (SSN) | OTHER (ID)

FIGURE 18.2 Section 1 Carrier (Block 1).

1. MEDICARE (Medicare#) | MEDICAID (Medicaid#) | TRICARE (ID#DoD#) | CHAMPVA (Member ID#) | GROUP HEALTH PLAN (ID#) | FECA BLK LUNG (ID#) | OTHER (ID#)
1a. INSURED'S I.D. NUMBER (For Program in Item 1)
2. PATIENT'S NAME (Last Name, First Name, Middle Initial)
3. PATIENT'S BIRTH DATE MM DD YY SEX M F
4. INSURED'S NAME (Last Name, First Name, Middle Initial)
5. PATIENT'S ADDRESS (No., Street)
6. PATIENT RELATIONSHIP TO INSURED Self Spouse Child Other
7. INSURED'S ADDRESS (No., Street)
CITY STATE
8. RESERVED FOR NUCC USE
CITY STATE
ZIP CODE TELEPHONE (Include Area Code) ( )
ZIP CODE TELEPHONE (Include Area Code) ( )
9. OTHER INSURED'S NAME (Last Name, First Name, Middle Initial)
10. IS PATIENT'S CONDITION RELATED TO:
11. INSURED'S POLICY GROUP OR FECA NUMBER
a. OTHER INSURED'S POLICY OR GROUP NUMBER
a. EMPLOYMENT? (Current or Previous) YES NO
a. INSURED'S DATE OF BIRTH MM DD YY SEX M F
b. RESERVED FOR NUCC USE
b. AUTO ACCIDENT? YES NO PLACE (State)
b. OTHER CLAIM ID (Designated by NUCC)
c. RESERVED FOR NUCC USE
c. OTHER ACCIDENT? YES NO
c. INSURANCE PLAN NAME OR PROGRAM NAME
d. INSURANCE PLAN NAME OR PROGRAM NAME
10d. CLAIM CODES (Designated by NUCC)
d. IS THERE ANOTHER HEALTH BENEFIT PLAN? YES NO *If yes*, complete items 9, 9a, and 9d.
READ BACK OF FORM BEFORE COMPLETING & SIGNING THIS FORM.
12. PATIENT'S OR AUTHORIZED PERSON'S SIGNATURE I authorize the release of any medical or other information necessary to process this claim. I also request payment of government benefits either to myself or to the party who accepts assignment below.
SIGNED DATE
13. INSURED'S OR AUTHORIZED PERSON'S SIGNATURE I authorize payment of medical benefits to the undersigned physician or supplier for services described below.
SIGNED
PATIENT AND INSURED IN

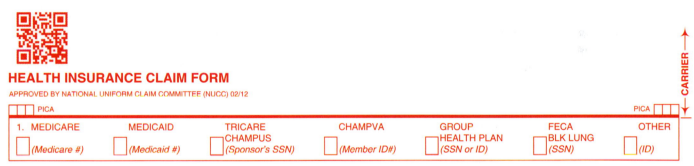

FIGURE 18.3 Section 2: Patient and Insured Information (Blocks 1a to 13).

Blocks 2, 3, 5, 6, and 10 a–c

Required information for the patient includes:

- person's name
- birth date (MM/DD/YYYY) and gender
- address
- relationship to the insured
- patient's status
- whether the patient's condition is related to his or her job, an automobile accident, or some other accident

---

CRITICAL THINKING APPLICATION   18.2

Ann is preparing an insurance claim to bill to Blue Cross. She notes that the patient is the dependent of the insured, so she reviews the patient registration intake form and finds that the date of birth for the insured is not present. Can Ann accurately complete the CMS-1500?

Block 9

Block 9 is for recording information about any secondary insurance plan that may be applicable. The data required includes:

- the other insured person's name
- policy or group number
- name of the other insurance plan.

Primary and Secondary Insurance Determination

When a patient is covered by more than one insurance policy, it is important to determine which policy is considered primary. The primary insurance pays the claim first, and if there is anything left over, it is submitted to the secondary insurance company. One of the most common situations is a patient with coverage under two policies, such as a dependent whose parents each have family coverage through employer group insurance.

In the case of a child whose mother and father both carry the child as a dependent on their employer health insurance plans, primary and secondary insurance status is determined by the *birthday rule*. Whichever parent's birth date falls first in a calendar year is considered to have the primary insurance. The year of the parent's birth is not used. If the mother's birth date is February 20 and the father's birth date is May 1, the mother's insurance is the primary insurance and the father's insurance is the secondary insurance. This means the claim will be submitted to the mother's insurance first, and if there is any balance left, it will be submitted to the father's insurance.

Medicare is usually the primary insurance, and there is a secondary policy to cover the patient's responsibility. In some cases, however, Medicare can be the patient's secondary insurance. This typically happens when a Medicare patient is still covered under an employer-sponsored group policy because the patient works full time.

Medicaid is always the payer of last resort. That means if there is any other type of insurance coverage for the patient, that insurance is responsible for the claim. If there is any balance left over, it will be submitted to Medicaid.

Blocks 12 and 13

Block 12 requires the signature of the *patient* or an authorized person, and Block 13 requires the signature of the *insured* or an authorized person. In Block 12, the signature authorizes the release of any medical or other information necessary to process or **adjudicate** the claim. In Block 13, the signature affirms that the insured has a signature on file authorizing payment of medical benefits directly to the provider (whose name appears in Block 31). The phrase "Signature on File" or "SOF" may be entered in these fields.

Assignment of Benefits

In the health insurance contract between the third-party payer and the patient, the patient receives the payment when a claim is submitted. For the healthcare facility to receive the reimbursement directly from the insurance company, the patient must sign an *assignment of benefits*. The assignment of benefits transfers the patient's legal right to collect benefits for medical expenses to the provider of those services, authorizing the payment to be sent directly to the provider. In other words, the assignment of benefits authorizes the provider to not only submit the insurance claim on behalf of the patient, but also to be reimbursed directly by the third-party payer. There is usually a statement about the assignment of benefits on the patient information form. When the patient has signed the assignment of benefits, the medical assistant completes Blocks 12 and 13 on the CMS-1500 form with the statement "Signature on File" or "SOF" and the claim filing date.

Section 3a: Physician or Supplier Information – Blocks 14 through 23 (Fig. 18.4)

Block 14: Date of current illness, injury, or pregnancy (LMP)

Block 14 requires the date of the current illness, injury, or pregnancy (LMP). The date should be the date on which the current illness or condition began; the date an injury occurred; or, in the case of pregnancy, the date of the last menstrual period (LMP), all in MM/DD/YYYY format.

Block 15: Other date

This block is used for another date related to the patient's condition or treatment. Enter the applicable qualifier to identify which date is being reported.

Block 15 Qualifiers

- 454 Initial Treatment
- 304 Latest Visit or Consultation
- 455 Last X-ray
- 471 Prescription
- 090 Report Start (Assumed Care Date)
- 091 Report End (Relinquished Care Date)
- 444 First Visit or Consultation
- 439 Accident
- 453 Acute Manifestation of a Chronic Condition

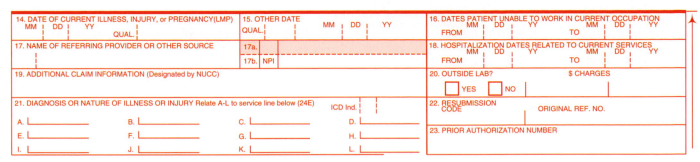

FIGURE 18.4 Section 3a: Physician or Supplier Information (Blocks 14 to 23).

Block 16: Dates patient unable to work in current occupation

These dates are used to help determine an employee's long- or short-term disability payments.

Blocks 17 and 17b: Name of referring provider or other source

Block 17 is for the name of the provider who referred or ordered the services or supplies. The following qualifier can be added:
- DN Referring Provider
- DK Ordering Provider
- DQ Supervising Provider

The provider's **National Provider Identifier (NPI)** is entered in Block 17b.

National Provider Identifier (NPI)

Government insurance claims require that National Provider Identifiers (NPIs) be used for the referring providers (Block 17b) and rendering providers (Block 24J). Every healthcare entity is required to have an NPI. The NPI is an identifier assigned by the CMS that classifies the healthcare provider by license and medical specialty. The Administrative Simplification provisions of the Health Insurance Portability and Accountability Act (HIPAA) required the adoption of standard unique identifiers for healthcare providers and health plans. The purpose is to improve the efficiency of electronic transmission of health information.

Some private insurance companies may require claims to be submitted with the NPI. However, each privately sponsored insurance plan in each state has its own policies and procedures. Medical assistants will find that some third-party payers require NPIs and others do not.

Block 18: Hospitalization dates related to current services

If inpatient services are provided, the admission and discharge dates are entered here.

Block 19: Additional claim information (designated by the National Uniform Claim Committee [NUCC])

Some insurance plans ask for specific identifiers in Block 19. The medical assistant should check the instructions from the applicable third-party payer.

Block 20: Outside lab charges

This block is used for diagnostic laboratory services purchased from an independent or a separate provider (who is listed in Block 32). Put an X in the YES box to indicate that the diagnostic test was performed by an entity other than the provider billing for the service (i.e., the provider listed in Block 33), and that the provider in Block 33 paid the laboratory directly. Include the amount the provider was charged by the diagnostic laboratory.

Block 21: Diagnosis or nature of illness or injury

The ICD-10-CM diagnosis code or codes are entered. Up to 12 diagnostic codes can be entered here. The primary diagnosis should be recorded in the first field. Do not include the decimal point in the diagnosis code. Relate lines A to L to lines of service in Block 24E by the letter of the line. This will link the diagnosis to the service provided.

Block 22: Resubmission code and/or original reference number

Both the resubmission code and the original reference number assigned by the insurance payer must be entered in this block. Resubmission codes:
- 7 Replacement of prior claim
- 8 Void/cancel of prior claim

Block 23: Prior authorization number

The preauthorization/precertification number obtained from the insurance company is entered.

Section 3b: Physician or Supplier Information – Blocks 24 through 33 (Fig. 18.5)

Procedure codes, such as the Current Procedural Terminology (CPT) codes and/or the Healthcare Common Procedure Coding System (HCPCS) codes, are listed in Block 24. Each procedure code is considered a line item; the line numbers are found to the left of Block 24. All data in one line belongs to the coordinated CPT/HCPCS code. For claims that require more than six line-items, a second CMS-1500 form should be generated. Check with the insurance company to confirm how to indicate that the claim has multiple pages; some insurance companies require the statement "Continued" or "Page 1 of 2" in Block 28, Total Charges.

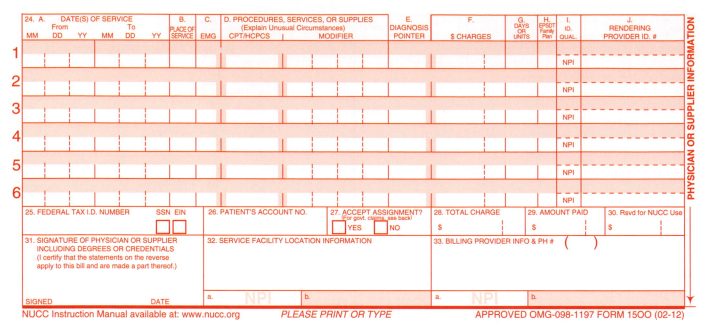

FIGURE 18.5 Section 3b: Physician or Supplier Information (Blocks 24 to 33).

Block 24: Procedures and charges

Block 24A – Date(s) of Service. Note that there is space for both "From" and "To" dates. If the service was provided on just one day, you would only enter a From date, in a MM/DD/YY format. If the service was provided on multiple days, such as an inpatient hospital stay, the first day the service was provided would be put in the From field and the last day the service was provided would be entered in the To field. The number of times that service was provided would be indicated in Block 24G.

Block 24B – Place of Service. The Place of Service (POS) codes indicate where the services were provided. As shown in Table 18.1, 11 would indicate that the procedure took place in a doctor's office.

Block 24C – EMG (emergency). A Y in this field indicates that the service was an emergency.

Block 24D – Procedures, Service or Supplies. There are two sections in this block, CPT/HCPCS and Modifier. There is space for a single 5-digit code and up to four separate 2-digit modifiers. No space is provided for a written description of the code; only the code is required.

Block 24E – Diagnosis Pointer. This block indicates which diagnosis is used for each line item. The letter from diagnosis listed in Block 21 should be used here to link the diagnosis to the service. Do not enter the ICD-10-CM codes in this block.

Block 24F – $ Charges. The dollar amount of the provider's fee for the service is entered here. This fee is calculated in the office based on work, expertise, and time. If a series of services was performed on any one line, multiply the number of days or units (Block 24G) by the charge for one procedure or service and enter the total amount for all days or units. This field is most commonly used for multiple visits, units of supplies, or anesthesia units.

Block 24G – Days or Units. The number of days or units is entered here. This block is used for multiple visits and units of supplies. If only one service is performed, 1 would be entered.

Block 24H – EPSDT/Family Plan. The acronym EPSDT stands for Early and Periodic Screening, Diagnosis, and Treatment, the child health program under Medicaid. This block identifies specific services covered under state health insurance plans. Refer to the appropriate insurance payer's guidelines (typically Medicaid or the Medicaid intermediary) for instructions on completing this block. Leave the block blank for Medicare, TRICARE, and the Civilian Health and Medical Program of the Department of Veterans Affairs (CHAMPVA) (military insurance plans), group health plans, Federal Employees Compensation Act (FECA)/Black Lung, and most other types of insurance.

Block 24I – ID Qual. This block is used if the number in Block 24J is not an NPI. The following are the qualifiers:

- 0B State License Number
- 1G Provider UPIN Number
- G2 Provider Commercial Number
- LU Location Number
- ZZ Provider Taxonomy

Block 24J – Rendering Provider ID #. Enter the NPI of the provider who rendered the service, as identification.

Blocks 25 to 33

Block 25 – Facility information. The Federal Tax ID Number of the provider filing the claim can be listed as a Social Security number (SSN) or an Employer Identification Number (EIN); mark the appropriate box with an X.

Block 26 – Patient's account no. Enter the account number or medical record number assigned to the patient by the provider of the service. This information will be included on the EOB from the insurance company to help with posting the payment.

Block 27 – Accept assignment? Put an X in the YES box if the provider will accept assignment; this means that he or she is a *participating provider* (PAR) and agrees to accept the terms of the agreement

TABLE 18.1 Common Place of Service Codes

CODE	DESCRIPTION	CODE	DESCRIPTION
11	Doctor's office	51	Inpatient psychiatry facility
12	Patient's home	52	Psychiatric facility—partial hospitalization
21	Inpatient hospital	53	Community mental health care (outpatient, 24-hour/day services, admission screening, consultation, and educational services)
22	Outpatient hospital		
23	Emergency department—hospital		
24	Ambulatory surgical center	54	Intermediate care facility/mentally retarded
25	Birthing center	55	Residential substance abuse treatment facility
26	Military treatment facility/uniformed service treatment facility	56	Psychiatric residential treatment center
31	Skilled nursing facility (swing bed visits)	60	Mass immunization center
32	Nursing facility (intermediate/long-term care facilities)	61	Comprehensive inpatient rehabilitation facility
33	Custodial care facility (domiciliary or rest home services)	62	Comprehensive outpatient rehabilitation facility
34	Hospice (domiciliary or rest home services)	65	End-stage renal disease treatment facility
35	Adult living care facilities (residential care facility)	71	State or local public health clinic
41	Ambulance—land	72	Rural health clinic
42	Ambulance—air or water	81	Independent laboratory
50	Federally qualified health center	99	Other unlisted facility

with the insurance company, and also to accept what the plan states as an allowed amount for the services provided.

Block 28 – Total Charge. This block shows the amount billed on the claim form for all services rendered. To arrive at this amount, add up the charges reported in Block 24F for all the lines of service on the claim form.

Block 29 – Amount Paid. The amount received from the patient or other payers.

Block 30 – Reserved for NUCC Use. Some secondary insurance claims use this box for the claim amount due after the primary insurance has paid.

Block 31 – Signature of Physician or Supplier. This block is for the signature of the authorized or accountable person for the services on the claim, verifying that he or she provided the services listed, and they have been checked for accuracy.

Block 32 – Service Facility Location Information. Enter the name, address, city, state, and ZIP code for the site where the services listed in the claim were provided. Enter the facility's NPI in Block 32a only if it is different from the Billing Provider NPI (Block 24J).

Block 33 – Billing Provider Info & PH #. Enter the address and phone number of the provider asking to be paid on this claim.

Block 33a – Enter the same NPI number listed in Block 24J. Procedure 18.4 on p. 398 demonstrates how to complete a health insurance claim form using the information from an insurance card and an encounter form (Fig. 18.6). Table 18.2 summarizes the

information required to complete the CMS-1500 Health Insurance Claim Form

---

CRITICAL THINKING APPLICATION   **18.3**

Ann is reviewing an encounter form that has one CPT code and two HCPCS codes with one diagnosis code for the same office visit. How many lines in Box 24 of the CMS-1500 will she need to use? Will all three CPT/HCPCS codes point to the same diagnosis? Why or why not?

ACCURATE CODING TO PREVENT FRAUD AND ABUSE

In any healthcare environment, accurate coding is essential to prevent fraud and abuse in reimbursement. According to HIPAA:

Fraud is defined as knowingly and willfully executing or attempting to execute a scheme to defraud any healthcare benefit program or to obtain by means of false or fraudulent pretenses, representations, or promises any of the money or property owned by any healthcare benefit program.

Abuse in medical billing would be actions that are contrary to ethical standards in the medical office. *Abuse* is an unintended action that directly or indirectly results in an overpayment to the healthcare provider. Abuse is similar to fraud, except that it is unclear if the unethical practice was committed on purpose. The term *intentional*

HEALTH INSURANCE CLAIM FORM

APPROVED BY NATIONAL UNIFORM CLAIM COMMITTEE (NUCC) 02/12

CARRIER

| PICA | | | | | | | PICA |

1. MEDICARE ☑ (Medicare#)   MEDICAID ☐ (Medicaid#)   TRICARE ☐ (ID#/DoD#)   CHAMPVA ☐ (Member ID#)   GROUP HEALTH PLAN ☐ (ID#)   FECA BLK LUNG ☐ (ID#)   OTHER ☐ (ID#)

1a. INSURED'S I.D. NUMBER (For Program in Item 1)
123-45-6789A

2. PATIENT'S NAME (Last Name, First Name, Middle Initial)
ROSE DAWSON

3. PATIENT'S BIRTH DATE MM 02 DD 17 YY XX   **SEX** M ☐ F ☑

4. INSURED'S NAME (Last Name, First Name, Middle Initial)
ROSE DAWSON

5. PATIENT'S ADDRESS (No., Street)
123 TITANIC PLACE

6. PATIENT RELATIONSHIP TO INSURED
Self ☑ Spouse ☐ Child ☐ Other ☐

7. INSURED'S ADDRESS (No., Street)
123 TITANIC PLACE

CITY NEW YORK   **STATE** NY

8. RESERVED FOR NUCC USE

CITY NEW YORK   **STATE** NY

ZIP CODE 10001   **TELEPHONE** (Include Area Code) ( )

ZIP CODE 10001   **TELEPHONE** (Include Area Code) ( )

9. OTHER INSURED'S NAME (Last Name, First Name, Middle Initial)
ROSE DAWSON

10. IS PATIENT'S CONDITION RELATED TO:

11. INSURED'S POLICY GROUP OR FECA NUMBER
123-45-6789A

a. OTHER INSURED'S POLICY OR GROUP NUMBER
123-45-6789

a. EMPLOYMENT? (Current or Previous) YES ☐ NO ☑

a. INSURED'S DATE OF BIRTH MM 02 DD 17 YY XX   **SEX** M ☐ F ☑

b. RESERVED FOR NUCC USE

b. AUTO ACCIDENT? YES ☐ NO ☑   PLACE (State)

b. OTHER CLAIM ID (Designated by NUCC)

c. RESERVED FOR NUCC USE

c. OTHER ACCIDENT? YES ☐ NO ☑

c. INSURANCE PLAN NAME OR PROGRAM NAME
MEDICARE

d. INSURANCE PLAN NAME OR PROGRAM NAME
AARP SECONDARY POLICY

10d. CLAIM CODES (Designated by NUCC)

d. IS THERE ANOTHER HEALTH BENEFIT PLAN?
YES ☑ NO ☐ If yes, complete items 9, 9a, and 9d.

READ BACK OF FORM BEFORE COMPLETING & SIGNING THIS FORM.

12. PATIENT'S OR AUTHORIZED PERSON'S SIGNATURE I authorize the release of any medical or other information necessary to process this claim. I also request payment of government benefits either to myself or to the party who accepts assignment below.

SIGNED SIGNATURE ON FILE   DATE 01/14/20XX

13. INSURED'S OR AUTHORIZED PERSON'S SIGNATURE I authorize payment of medical benefits to the undersigned physician or supplier for services described below.

SIGNED SIGNATURE ON FILE

PATIENT AND INSURED INFORMATION

14. DATE OF CURRENT ILLNESS, INJURY, or PREGNANCY (LMP) MM DD YY   QUAL.

15. OTHER DATE QUAL.   MM DD YY

16. DATES PATIENT UNABLE TO WORK IN CURRENT OCCUPATION FROM MM DD YY   TO MM DD YY

17. NAME OF REFERRING PROVIDER OR OTHER SOURCE
ROBERT WILSON, MD
17a.
17b. NPI 11122233344

18. HOSPITALIZATION DATES RELATED TO CURRENT SERVICES FROM MM DD YY   TO MM DD YY

19. ADDITIONAL CLAIM INFORMATION (Designated by NUCC)

20. OUTSIDE LAB? YES ☐ NO ☐ $ CHARGES

21. DIAGNOSIS OR NATURE OF ILLNESS OR INJURY Relate A-L to service line below (24E)   ICD Ind.
A. E11.22   B.   C.   D.
E.   F.   G.   H.
I.   J.   K.   L.

22. RESUBMISSION CODE   ORIGINAL REF. NO.

23. PRIOR AUTHORIZATION NUMBER

24. A. DATE(S) OF SERVICE						B. PLACE OF SERVICE	C. EMG	D. PROCEDURES, SERVICES, OR SUPPLIES (Explain Unusual Circumstances)		E. DIAGNOSIS POINTER	F. $ CHARGES		G. DAYS OR UNITS	H. EPSDT Family Plan	I. ID. QUAL.	J. RENDERING PROVIDER ID. #
From MM	DD	YY	To MM	DD	YY			CPT/HCPCS	MODIFIER							
01	14	XX	01	14	XX	11		99213		1	$125	00	1		NPI	11122233344
															NPI	
															NPI	
															NPI	
															NPI	
															NPI	

25. FEDERAL TAX I.D. NUMBER 098-76-5432   SSN ☐ EIN ☑

26. PATIENT'S ACCOUNT NO. RW125638

27. ACCEPT ASSIGNMENT? (For govt. claims, see back) YES ☑ NO ☐

28. TOTAL CHARGE $ 125 00

29. AMOUNT PAID $ 0

30. Rsvd for NUCC Use

31. SIGNATURE OF PHYSICIAN OR SUPPLIER INCLUDING DEGREES OR CREDENTIALS (I certify that the statements on the reverse apply to this bill and are made a part thereof.)
Robert Wilson, MD   01/14/XX
SIGNED   DATE

32. SERVICE FACILITY LOCATION INFORMATION
Feel Better Family Practice
101 Jack Place
New York, NY, 10001
(212) 555-1212
a. 22233344455   b.

33. BILLING PROVIDER INFO & PH # ( )
Robert Wilson, MD
101 Jack Place
New York, NY, 10001
(212) 555-1212
a. 11122233344   b.

PHYSICIAN OR SUPPLIER INFORMATION

NUCC Instruction Manual available at: www.nucc.org   **PLEASE PRINT OR TYPE**   APPROVED OMB-0938-1197 FORM 1500 (02-12)

FIGURE 18.6 Completed CMS-1500 Health Insurance Claim Form.

TABLE 18.2 Information Required for Completion of the CMS-1500 Health Insurance Claim Form

BLOCK	INFORMATION NEEDED	BLOCK	INFORMATION NEEDED
	Completed patient registration/intake form	12	Confirm that the patient's release of information form has been signed, dated, and is in the patient's record
	Photocopy of insurance card or cards (front and back)	13	Confirm that the insured's authorization of benefits form has been signed, dated, and is in the patient's record
	Encounter form		
	Preauthorization or precertification number (when applicable)	**Section 3: Physician or Supplier Information**	
Section 1: Carrier		14	Date current illness, injury, or pregnancy began
1	Type of insurance	15	Determine whether patient has had the same or similar symptoms
Section 2: Patient and Insured Information		16	From-To dates if patient was unable to work at current occupation
1a	Insured's identification (ID) number (primary insurance)	17	Name of ordering or referring provider
2	Patient's full name	17a	Not required
3	Patient's date of birth and gender	17b	Ordering or referring provider's NPI
4	Insured's name (primary insurance)	18	From-To dates if patient encounter included an inpatient hospital stay
5	Patient's address and telephone number • Permanent address (including apartment number if appropriate) • City, state, ZIP code • Telephone number	19	Determine whether insurance carrier in carrier block and Block 1 requires any information to be entered in this field
		20	Determine whether an outside laboratory was used; if so, enter charges billed to provider for outside lab services
6	Patient's relationship to insured	21	ICD-10-CM code or codes for patient's condition, illness, or injury (maximum of four per claim)
7	Insured's address and telephone number • Permanent address (including apartment number if appropriate) • City, state, ZIP code • Telephone number	22	Is Medicaid claim being resubmitted? If yes, provide reference number from original Medicaid claim submitted
		23	If prior authorization and/or referral is required, provide authorization (approval) number from insurance payer (preauthorization or precertification number)
9	Other insured's name (secondary insurance)[a]	24A	From-To dates of service for current encounter
9a	Policy or group number (secondary insurance)[a]	24B	Place of service (POS) code
9b	Secondary insured's date of birth and gender[a]	24C	If an emergency, put a Y in this box
9c	Secondary insured's employer or school name[a]	24D	CPT and/or HCPCS code CPT and/or HCPCS modifier(s) (maximum of four per charge line)
9d	Secondary insured's insurance plan or program name[a]		
10a-c	If patient's condition or illness is related to employment, auto accident, or some other type of accident, make sure information is obtained as outlined in Block 1	24E	Block 21 field or reference number (1, 2, 3 and/or 4)
10d	Claim codes as designated by NUCC	24F	Total charge for CPT- or HCPCS-coded services listed in Block 24D • If more than 1 day or unit is indicated in Block 24G, multiply the charge for the service(s) coded in Block 24D by the number of days/units in Block 24G; enter the result in Block 24F
11	Insured's policy, group, or FECA number (primary insurance)		
11a	Primary insured's date of birth and gender		
11b	Other claim ID designated by NUCC		
11c	Primary insured's insurance plan or program name		
11d	Determine whether the patient also is covered by a secondary health insurance plan		

Continued

TABLE 18.2   Information Required for Completion of the CMS-1500 Health Insurance Claim Form—*continued*

BLOCK	INFORMATION NEEDED	BLOCK	INFORMATION NEEDED
24G	Total number of days or units	30	Balance due (if any amount paid is shown in Block 29)
24H	EPSDT or Family Plan code (Medicaid or AFDC)	31	Signature of provider performing service or procedure
24I	Qualifier ID code (if no NPI available)	32	Address of facility where services were rendered
24J	Rendering (treating) provider's NPI—unshaded field PIN (if no NPI is available)—shaded field	32a	NPI number of service facility listed in Block 32
		32b	Qualifier ID number and PIN of facility listed in Block 32 (if no NPI available)
25	Rendering provider's federal tax ID number (EIN or SSN)		
26	Patient's account number with rendering provider	33	Name, address, and phone number of performing (rendering) provider
27	Determine whether contract or agreement between provider and insurance carrier allows provider to accept assignment	33a	NPI of provider listed in Block 33
28	Total charges from Block 24F, lines 1-6	33b	Qualifier ID number and PIN of provider listed in Block 33 (if no NPI available)
29	Amount paid by patient, insured, or other insurance		

ªOnly required if a secondary insurance exists and is to be submitted to the insurance carrier.
AFDC, Aid to Families with Dependent Children; *CPT,* Current Procedural Terminology coding system; *EIN,* Employer Identification Number; *EPSDT,* Early and Periodic Screening, Diagnosis, and Treatment; *FECA,* Federal Employees Compensation Act; *HCPCS,* Health Care Common Procedural Coding System coding method; *ICD-10-CM,* International Classification of Diseases, Tenth Revision, Clinical Modification coding method; *NPI,* National Provider Identifier; *PIN,* personal identification number; *POS,* place of service.

is important when determining whether fraudulent medical billing practices were done on purpose or were an accident.

Violations of the laws governing reimbursement may result in:
- nonpayment of claims.
- civil monetary penalties (CMPs).
- exclusion from the payer program.
- criminal and civil liability.
- in extreme cases, jail time.

These laws may be changed or updated. The person who is responsible for coding must pay close attention to detail and act as a sort of "medical detective" to prevent a case against a provider or clinic. The ICD-10-CM and CPT/HCPCS manuals are updated annually. New coding manuals have a few pages dedicated to the updates for that particular year. Accurate use of ICD-10-CM and CPT/HCPCS manuals is essential for correct translation of the claim information in the health record into the correct codes. However, as models of providing healthcare change, they can present some challenges for accurate coding and billing procedures.

Guidelines for Reviewing Claims Before Submission

The following guidelines can help ensure that clean insurance claims are submitted.
- Proofread the form carefully for accuracy and completeness.
- Make certain any necessary attachments are included with the completed form.
- Follow office policies and guidelines for claim review and signatures.

- Forward the original claim to the proper insurance carrier either by mail or electronically.
- Make sure the patient's and/or insured's name, address, and ID, group, and/or policy number are identical to the information printed on the insurance card.
- Make sure the patient's birth date and gender are the same as in the medical record.
- Section 2, Patient and Insured Information **(Blocks 1–13)**: Complete these blocks accurately, according to the insurance carrier's guidelines.
- **Block 11:** Enter the word NONE if Medicare is the primary payer.
- **Block 12:** Make sure the patient has authorized the release of information, and that Block 12 has a handwritten signature, the words "Signature on File," or the acronym SOF.
- **Blocks 17** and **17b:** If applicable, enter the referring provider's name and NPI number.
- Make sure the diagnosis is not missing or incomplete.
- Check that the diagnosis has been coded accurately, according to the ICD-10-CM coding manual, and is linked to the treatment.
- **Blocks 14–24J** (required fields for diagnosis and procedure): Make sure these blocks are completed accurately, according to the guidelines of the third-party payer or insurance company.
- List the fees for each charge individually; or, if more than 1 day or unit is entered in **Block 24G**, the fees must be computed correctly.
- **Block 25:** Double-check the provider's federal Social Security number (SSN) or Employer Identification Number (EIN) to ensure accuracy.

- **Block 27** (Accept Assignment?): Put an X in the YES box if the provider is a PAR provider or has an agreement with the insurance company to accept assignment.
- **Block 31:** Check for the provider's signature, which must be on the form.
- **Block 24J** and **Block 33a:** Make sure the provider's NPI, corresponding to the insurance carrier being billed, has been entered in Block 24J and again in Block 33a.

Patient-Centered Medical Home (PCMH)

Patient-centered medical home (PCMH) is a model of patient care. In this model, patient care is looked at from a holistic approach. The healthcare team wants to be able to assist the patient with any issues that come up about his or her care. This means having multiple team members available. The provider and the medical assistant would provide the primary care. There would also be a nurse who coordinates all of the care for the patient, including issues about home healthcare, financial issues, transportation issues, and so on. Many models include a clinical pharmacist who is available to discuss medication questions and concerns with the patient.

The goal of PCMH is to improve patient outcomes and reduce costs. There are accreditation processes that must be completed for a healthcare facility to be recognized as a PCMH.

Billing for the services provided can be a challenge for the medical biller. When do you bill for the pharmacist's visit or phone contact? It is important to have billing policies and procedures in place when your healthcare facility is a PCMH so that services are billed consistently and accurately.

PREVENTING REJECTION OF A CLAIM

It is important for the medical assistant to understand and comply with the specific guidelines for completing a CMS-1500 established by each insurance company. This prevents delays in reimbursement and denial of payment. The guidelines for Medicare, Medicaid, TRICARE, and workers' compensation can be found online at the websites for these healthcare insurers. Most practice management billing systems have built-in **claim scrubbers** that help in the process. If claims are sent electronically through a clearinghouse, claims auditing is done before the clearinghouse transmits the claim to the insurance company. Claims without errors of any type are called *clean claims*. Claims with incorrect, missing, or insufficient data are called *dirty claims*.

Communication With Providers About Third-Party Requirements

It can be challenging for a provider to keep up with the annual changes made by the government plans, private health insurance companies, and the coding updates. This is why healthcare providers trust their medical office staff to stay up to date on the various changes in the health insurance industry.

Some providers may be so focused on patient care that they feel uncomfortable with change. This may be the case with the encounter form/superbill used in patient care. A provider may feel comfortable using the same form, but over time, some codes may have changed or become obsolete, or new medical services offered may not be listed on the form.

A medical coder should tactfully discuss with the provider the benefits of using an updated encounter form. If the provider is still reluctant to change the form, even though it is outdated, the medical coder may suggest that the form will not be changed, just the codes on it. Adjust the encounter form to include an open text box for the provider to add medical procedures that he or she performs occasionally.

When communicating with the provider about coding issues, you must always have a respectful attitude. The many changes occurring in medical coding and billing can be overwhelming and confusing for some providers. The approach of coding professionals should be to guide them patiently through these changes.

CRITICAL THINKING APPLICATION 18.4

Being tactful means using good manners as you provide truthful, sensitive information or honest critical feedback to another person. Tactful behaviors include showing respect, discretion, compassion, honesty, diplomacy, and courtesy while you deliver a message. Tactful behaviors encompass both nonverbal and verbal communication, including what you say, how you say it, and your body language during the communication. A critical element of being tactful is considering the other person's feelings and reactions as you deliver the information. When you use tactful behaviors, you demonstrate professionalism and you preserve relationships by avoiding conflicts and finding common ground.

Many times the medical biller is the expert on the third-party requirements, and providers rely on the biller to help them understand the requirements. Being tactful with providers as you communicate third-party requirements is critical to your working relationship with the provider and also important in the overall financial scope of the agency. It is crucial to assist the provider in a tactful manner, understanding his or her role in meeting third-party requirements.

Using the following case study, role-play with two peers how you would display tactful behaviors when communicating with medical providers about third-party requirements.

You are the medical biller for your clinic. The two providers have not been communicating with you about procedures that need prior authorization from the insurance companies. As a result, multiple claims are being denied, and the clinic has had to write off much of the cost. Today you are talking with the providers, explaining common procedures that require prior authorizations and the process of getting preauthorizations.

CHECKING THE STATUS OF A CLAIM

The medical biller should keep track of every submitted claim to ensure timely reimbursement. Clearinghouses send a confirmation report after submission of a claim. The medical biller should always confirm that the claims submitted to the clearinghouse match the claims listed on the confirmation report. If direct billing is used, the medical biller must set up a system to track the claims that were submitted. Medical assistants should maintain this practice to ensure that every claim is submitted correctly.

The claim submission confirmation report also indicates claims that were rejected because they were incomplete. These claims should be corrected and resubmitted electronically immediately. Often these claims are rejected for data entry errors. The medical biller should compare the patient's information in the practice management software to the information on the patient's registration form and scanned insurance card, to ensure accuracy.

It typically takes 10 to 14 business days for insurance companies to process insurance claims electronically. If no response has been received from the insurance company after 30 days, the medical biller should inquire about the status of the claim. This can be done through the company's provider Web portal or by a call to the provider services number on the back of the patient's insurance ID card. To verify the claim status, you must provide the following:

- Insured subscriber's member number and birth date
- Patient's name and birth date
- Date of service

With this information, the insurance company should be able to tell if the claim has been paid, is still in process, was denied, or was never received. The medical biller will use this information for the proper follow-up. This could be:

- investigating the records at the clinic to see if the payment came in but was applied to the incorrect patient account.
- researching the denial and resubmitting the claim.
- determining why the claim was not received and resubmitting it.

The state insurance commission has standards that insurance companies must abide by, including claim processing times and payment guidelines. Medical assistants should keep the commission's contact information in the office medical billing manual as a reference, in case a claim should be reported.

EXPLANATION OF BENEFITS

An explanation of benefits is sent by the insurance company to the provider who submitted the insurance claim and to the patient. It comes with a check or a document indicating that funds were electronically transferred. Medicare sends a Remittance Advice (RA) with confirmation of electronic funds transfer. Although it has a different name, the document is the same as the EOB.

The healthcare facility cannot just deposit the check and disregard the EOB, which provides detailed accounting for the submitted insurance claim. The EOB breaks down each line item charge from Block 24 on the CMS-1500 into the charged amount, the amount allowable, and the amount paid. Most EOBs will also indicate how much was applied to the deductible, what the patient's co-insurance amount is, and if any services were denied.

Reading an Explanation of Benefits

The EOB contains essential information about the submitted health insurance claim. To properly apply payments to a patient's account, it is vital that the medical assistant understand all the elements of an EOB. When interpreting the EOB, review the following steps:

1. Verify that the EOB applies to the correct patient by comparing the account number and date of service on the EOB with the submitted claim.

2. Confirm that the EOB shows the same charged amount as the submitted claim. In other words, the line items and charges should match. Sometimes the EOB summarizes the entire claim in one charged amount. In this case, confirm that the total charged is the same as in the submitted claim.

3. Post the payment and adjusted amount per line item. In the practice management billing software, these are posted on the same line. The patient's responsibility, as determined by the primary insurance EOB, is calculated using the following equation:

$$\text{Charged amount} - \text{Payment amount} - \text{Adjustment amount} = \text{Patient's responsibility}$$

4. Once the patient's responsibility has been determined, check for a secondary insurance. If one is listed, submit a health insurance claim with the balance due determined by the primary insurance EOB. If no secondary insurance is listed, the patient is billed for the balance due.

5. Review the *remark codes* on the EOB for any additional messages or information about the claim. The remark codes area is where the insurance company indicates the conditions under which the claim was paid. For example, code 01 states that the claim amount allowed was established by the contract between the health insurance plan and the provider. Other remark codes give the reasons a claim was denied or rejected. Some remark codes indicate that the claim is pending, awaiting specific information.

6. All remark codes on pending or denied claims should be followed up immediately upon receipt of the EOB, to prevent further delay in payment for other claims.

Rejected Claims

The EOB provides detailed information on rejected claims. All rejected claims have a code, with a legend toward the bottom of the page. Some of the reasons claims are rejected:

- The time period for filing the claim had expired (check the insurance plan's billing policies manual for details).
- Incorrect ICD-10-CM, CPT, and/or HCPCS codes or combinations of codes were entered.
- The insurer claims that the ICD-10-CM code and the CPT/HCPCS codes do not match; that is, the claim lacks **medical necessity**.
- More than one CPT/HCPCS code was filed on the same date of service, and they are mutually exclusive when billed together.
- The claim was submitted to the wrong insurance company.

Rejected claims should be resubmitted as soon as possible to prevent further delay in reimbursement.

Denied Claims

The two main reasons for denial of payment are technical errors and insurance policy coverage issues. Technical errors include incorrect, incomplete information, data entry and/or mathematical errors. Common reasons for denial include:

- The patient was not covered by the insurance plan on the date of service.
- A listed procedure was not an insurance benefit.
- Preauthorization for the service was not obtained.
- Medical necessity

Medical Necessity

Insurance companies determine medical necessity based on the diagnostic and procedural codes submitted on the claim. The diagnostic code is the reason that the procedure was necessary. For example, if a claim submitted to the insurance company indicated that a bunionectomy was performed for tonsillitis, the insurer will deny the claim based on medical necessity. Procedure codes are linked to diagnostic codes in the claim. The health record must support the reason for each service provided.

If an insurance claim is denied for medical necessity, the medical assistant should review the claim information and the health record. If there is an error on the claim, such as the wrong diagnostic code on the encounter form, then a new claim should be submitted.

If an insurance claim is denied for medical necessity and the medical assistant believes that it was coded correctly, an appeal letter should be sent to the insurance company. The appeal letter should identify the denied claim and include a statement from the provider detailing the medical reasoning for performing the procedure. Additional medical reports (e.g., laboratory reports, operative reports, and history and physical examination findings [H&P]) should be sent if they support the provider's treatment decision (see Procedure 18.5 on p. 400).

THE PATIENT'S FINANCIAL RESPONSIBILITY

Most MCO health insurance contracts require patients to pay a copayment, which is collected at the time of service (Table 18.3). Copayments can range from $10 to $75 for office visits. They vary, depending on whether the patient is seen by a PCP or a specialist, in urgent care, or in the emergency department. Office visit and prescription copayments do not count toward the yearly deductible. The medical assistant must make sure that the proper copayments are received and credited to patients' accounts.

A *deductible* is a set dollar amount that the policyholder is responsible for each year before the insurance company begins to reimburse the healthcare provider. The deductible amount is stated in the insurance policy.

Co-insurance means that the insured and the insurance company share the cost of covered medical services after the deductible has been met. The insurance company and the patient split the cost of the services. An 80/20 split is very common, especially for traditional insurance. This means that after the yearly deductible has been met,

the insurance company pays 80% of the fee and the insured pays 20%. The patient's deductible or co-insurance responsibility is shown on the EOB.

To help patients understand their health insurance benefits, the medical assistant must be confident in defining the terms *copayment*, *co-insurance*, and *deductible*.

The medical office can contact the insurance company on the patient's behalf to determine the amount of the deductible the patient has already paid in the calendar year. The process of precertification enables the healthcare provider to inform patients of how much the procedure will cost them.

Calculating the Co-insurance and Deductible

Consider this example: Mrs. Anita Jones' health insurance plan has a $500 annual deductible, after which the insurance company pays 95% of all charges. Mrs. Jones, therefore, has a 5% co-insurance expense, in addition to the deductible. Mrs. Jones has incurred a $10,000 charge for cardiac surgery performed by her provider.

In Fig. 18.7, Column A shows that Mrs. Jones paid the $500 deductible, and 5% of $10,000 (i.e., an additional $475). The insurance company then paid the remaining balance of $9,025.

Also in Fig. 18.7, Column B shows that Mrs. Jones' cardiac surgery cost $20,000. Mrs. Jones' total out-of-pocket expense is now $975, and the insurance company is responsible for payment of the balance of $18,525.

Allowed Amount

Another factor to be considered when determining the patient's financial responsibility is whether the provider is a PAR provider or not. To become a participating provider in an insurance network, the provider must agree to accept the insurance plan's fee schedule as payment in full for services rendered. This means that if the provider's fee is higher than the plan's allowed amount, the difference should be adjusted. For example, a provider may charge $80 for a Level I office visit; however, the insurance plan's allowable amount may be only $60. If the provider is a participating provider, he or she is obligated to adjust the difference between these two amounts – $20. The patient is not responsible for that $20. However, if the provider is not a participating provider, he or she can bill the patient for the $20 balance. Because contracts between insurance companies and providers vary greatly, it is important for the medical assistant to closely examine the EOB to ensure that the proper adjustments are done.

Let's look at how this would affect the example in Fig. 18.7. If the allowable amount for Mrs. Jones' $10,000 cardiac surgery is $8,500, the $1,500 difference between the provider's charge and the allowed amount would be either written off or passed on to the patient. Fig. 18.8 demonstrates the differences in the patient's responsibility and provider reimbursement.

TABLE 18.3 Comparing Patient Financial Responsibilities		
PATIENT'S FINANCIAL RESPONSIBILITY	**WHEN PATIENT PAYS**	**AMOUNT PATIENT PAYS**
Copayment	At the time of medical service	Fixed amount, $10 to $75 per visit
Deductible	Before the insurance company will pay	Variable amount, $250 to $5,000
Co-insurance	After the provider has been paid	Variable amount, up to 30%

CRITICAL THINKING APPLICATION 18.5

The providers in the practice where Ann works are not in-network for a preferred provider organization (PPO) that is often used in their geographic area. Many patients are confused when they have to pay a larger out-of-pocket fee for their medical services. How can Ann explain the reason for these higher fees to patients?

	Column A	Column B
Total Charge	$10,000	$20,000
Deductible (paid by Mrs. Jones)	$500	$500
Coinsurance (5% paid by Mrs. Jones)	5% of $9500 (Total charge minus the deductible) = $475	5% of 19,500 (Total charge minus the deductible) = $975
Total amount paid by Mrs. Jones	$975	$1475
Total amount paid by insurance	95% of $9500 (Total charge minus the deductible) - $9025	95% of $19,500 (Total charge minus the deductible) - $18,525

FIGURE 18.7 Deductible and Co-insurance.

	PAR	NonPAR
Total Charge	$10,000	$10,000
Allowed amount	$8,500	$8,500
$1500 difference between charged amount and allowed amount	Written off as an adjustment	Billed to the patient
Deductible (paid by Mrs. Jones)	$500	$500
Coinsurance (paid by Mrs. Jones)	$8500 − $500 (deductible) X 5% = $400	$8500 − $500 (deductible) X 5% = $400
Total amount paid by Mrs. Jones	$900	$2400
Total amount paid by insurance	$7,600	$7,600

FIGURE 18.8 PAR vs. NonPar.

Discussing the Patient's Financial Responsibility

The *guarantor* is the person legally responsible for the entire bill. It is important that the patient and the guarantor understand what the financial responsibilities are for services provided. Some patients expect insurance to pay all costs simply because they are paying a premium. Often patients do not even read their insurance policies and have no idea what is and is not covered.

The medical assistant may need to educate patients about their policies and help patients work with their insurance company to get answers to questions and make sure they are receiving all the benefits to which they are entitled. If problems come up with the insurance company, it is in the practice's best interest to actively assist the patient. The medical billing staff is usually more knowledgeable than the patient about health insurance. Helping patients with issues can help ensure that the provider is compensated for his or her services.

Medical assistants gain knowledge about the insurance industry when they actively assist patients with their concerns. The more experience a medical assistant has in working with insurance, the more helpful he or she can be to patients. As mentioned previously, medical assistants should keep a manual of medical billing policies and procedures for most of the insurance plans they handle; this can serve as an excellent source of guidance and suggestions for working with a particular payer.

Always be sure to obtain the guarantor's signature on an agreement to pay for services. Most patient information sheets have a section referring to the guarantor. A statement may be included that serves as an agreement to pay the costs of medical care. States have statutes that deal with guarantors, so be sure the office's policies comply with those laws. It is especially important to secure a written agreement to pay for services when the care will be long term or involves costly treatment or surgical procedures. Procedure 18.6 on p. 401 explains

how to inform patients of their financial obligations for services rendered.

Showing Sensitivity When Discussing the Patient's Finances

Most patients use health insurance, but they do not always recognize that they will have financial obligations after the insurance plan pays its share. This is common among Medicare patients, who often feel that they should have all their medical expenses paid because they have government insurance. It usually falls to the medical assistant to inform patients of their financial responsibilities.

Advance Beneficiary Notice (ABN)

Medicare does not cover some healthcare services, so the Advance Beneficiary Notice (ABN) is presented to patients in these circumstances. The ABN provides an option for patients to pay the provider's fee in full to receive services that Medicare does not cover. The patient decides whether he or she still wants to receive the services from the provider and completes the information on the form (Fig. 18.9).

Patients seeking medical care are not usually feeling like themselves because they may be suffering through pain and discomfort. As a result, their behavior may not be typical when the medical assistant suggests discussing their financial responsibilities.

Medical assistants should show patience and sensitivity when discussing a patient's financial obligations (Fig. 18.10). Patients should never be harassed to make a payment or forced into payment arrangements. Medical assistants should always be courteous when discussing payments with patients. In addition, the medical practice should offer a variety of payment options to meet patients' needs, including credit card and online payment options.

CLOSING COMMENTS

Accurate insurance billing practices are essential for the financial success of every healthcare facility. Medical assistants are strong assets to the healthcare facility when they can submit claims electronically, manage denied and rejected claims, and discuss financial responsibilities with patients professionally. Medical assistants should always maintain a positive attitude toward patients and keep in mind that those who are ill or facing challenges are not always at their best and may not respond in a positive way when discussing their financial responsibilities.

Patient Coaching

Patients often don't have a strong understanding of health insurance. There are so many different options out there, and their policies can change often. By explaining just what deductibles, copayment, and co-insurance are, we can help our patients understand just what their financial responsibilities are, even when they have health insurance. We can also help smooth the way for a good relationship with our patients by making sure that they understand the payment policies. No one likes to be blindsided with a request for payment. By patiently

A. Notifier: John Doe, MD, College Clinic, 4567 Broad Avenue, Woodland Hills, XY 12345 555-486-9002

B. Patient Name: Mary Judd   **C. Identification Number:** 0920XX7291

Advance Beneficiary Notice of Noncoverage (ABN)

NOTE: If Medicare doesn't pay for **D.** _B12 injections_ below, you may have to pay.
Medicare does not pay for everything, even some care that you or your health care provider have good reason to think you need. We expect Medicare may not pay for the **D.** _B12 injections_ below.

D.	E. Reason Medicare May Not Pay:	F. Estimated Cost
B12 injections	Medicare does not usually pay for this injection or this many injections	$35.00

WHAT YOU NEED TO DO NOW:
- Read this notice, so you can make an informed decision about your care.
- Ask us any questions that you may have after you finish reading.
- Choose an option below about whether to receive the **D.** _B12 injections_ listed above.
  Note: If you choose Option 1 or 2, we may help you to use any other insurance that you might have, but Medicare cannot require us to do this.

G. OPTIONS: Check only one box. We cannot choose a box for you.

☑ **OPTION 1.** I want the **D.** _B12 injections_ listed above. You may ask to be paid now, but I also want Medicare billed for an official decision on payment, which is sent to me on a Medicare Summary Notice (MSN). I understand that if Medicare doesn't pay, I am responsible for payment, but **I can appeal to Medicare** by following the directions on the MSN. If Medicare does pay, you will refund any payments I made to you, less co-pays or deductibles.

☐ **OPTION 2.** I want the **D.** _____ listed above, but do not bill Medicare. You may ask to be paid now as I am responsible for payment. **I cannot appeal if Medicare is not billed.**

☐ **OPTION 3.** I don't want the **D.** _____ listed above. I understand with this choice I am **not** responsible for payment, and **I cannot appeal to see if Medicare would pay.**

H. Additional Information:

This notice gives our opinion, not an official Medicare decision. If you have other questions on this notice or Medicare billing, call **1-800-MEDICARE** (1-800-633-4227/**TTY:** 1-877-486-2048).
Signing below means that you have received and understand this notice. You also receive a copy.

I. Signature: *Mary Judd*	J. Date: *March 20, 20XX*

According to the Paperwork Reduction Act of 1995, no persons are required to respond to a collection of information unless it displays a valid OMB control number. The valid OMB control number for this information collection is 0938-0566. The time required to complete this information collection is estimated to average 7 minutes per response, including the time to review instructions, search existing data resources, gather the data needed, and complete and review the information collection. If you have comments concerning the accuracy of the time estimate or suggestions for improving this form, please write to: CMS, 7500 Security Boulevard, Attn: PRA Reports Clearance Officer, Baltimore, Maryland 21244-1850.

Form CMS-R-131 (03/11)   Form Approved OMB No. 0938-0566

FIGURE 18.9 Advance Beneficiary Notice for Medicare patients. (From Fordney MT: *Insurance handbook for the medical office,* ed 14, St. Louis, 2017, Elsevier.)

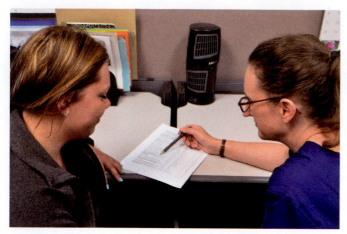

FIGURE 18.10 Medical assistants must show respect and sensitivity when discussing financial issues with patients.

explaining why a patient owes a balance, you can have a positive discussion about how to resolve that balance.

Legal and Ethical Issues

From time to time patients may ask for a reduced fee after the insurance has already paid. If the provider is a participating provider with the health insurance plan, he or she is obligated to follow the terms of the contract. This includes collecting the patient's financial responsibility detailed in the EOB. The insurance plan can penalize the healthcare facility if a concerted effort is not made to collect the patient's co-insurance and deductible amounts, thus not following the terms of the participating provider health insurance contract.

Patient-Centered Care

Most patients are unaware of their benefits and coverage through their insurance policies. The medical assistant should encourage patients to read the entire policy to become familiar with its limitations and exclusions. Inform patients that when they call the insurance company with questions, they should always write down the date, the time, and the name of the person with whom they spoke. Using email is helpful because a record of the correspondence can easily be saved or printed. Making sure that patients have a general understanding of their health insurance coverage is well worth the effort.

Often patients do not dispute the decision or question the insurance company when a claim is rejected or not paid in the expected amount. Encourage them to call the company and question rejections if they do not understand why the claim was denied.

Professional Behaviors

Medical billers must have strong organizational skills. Not only are they responsible for submitting claims electronically in a timely manner, they also must manage claim denials and rejections. Denied and rejected claims need to be adjusted and rebilled for prompt payment. An organized medical biller ensures that all medical billing activities are worked on daily.

SUMMARY OF SCENARIO

Ann realizes that the best way to keep track of all the carriers is to keep an up-to-date manual that contains the addresses, phone numbers, and medical billing policies and procedures for each insurance plan that the healthcare facility accepts. This manual can help prevent the rejection and denial of many claims because the claims will be submitted accurately the first time.

The medical assistant's understanding of how to calculate deductibles, co-insurance, and allowed amounts for procedures and services benefits both the provider and the patient. The provider's productivity, income, and losses can be easily tracked, and the patient can be educated as to the exact amounts he or she is responsible for paying.

Ann also has learned the importance of being courteous to patients when discussing their financial obligations. She has learned how to use the Assignment of Financial Responsibility form to communicate what the patient owes in a clear, straightforward manner.

SUMMARY OF LEARNING OBJECTIVES

1. **Describe the medical billing process, identify the types of information contained in the patient's billing record, and interpret information on an insurance card.**
   The medical billing process starts when a patient makes an appointment and is complete when payment has been received. Be sure to collect pertinent insurance billing information when the patient calls to schedule an appointment. Much of this information is on the patient registration form, which is completed when the patient comes to the medical office for the initial visit. (See Procedure 18.1 on p. 396 for instructions on how to interpret information on an insurance card.)

2. **Discuss managed care policies and procedures, including precertification/preauthorization and referrals, and show sensitivity when communicating with patients regarding third-party requirements.**
   Medical assistants should be aware that services provided to patients who are sponsored by an MCO plan may not be reimbursed if the policies and procedures of the specific insurance plan are not followed. To submit accurate health insurance claims, medical assistants should establish office procedures for applying MCO policies and procedures. See Procedure 18.2 on p. 396 for instructions on how to show sensitivity when communicating with patients regarding third-party requirements

SUMMARY OF LEARNING OBJECTIVES—*continued*

and Procedure 18.3 on p. 398 for information on how to perform precertification with documentation.

3. **Identify steps for filing a third-party claim.**

The medical assistant's medical billing tasks begin when the patient seeks medical services from the provider, usually when an appointment is made. Insurance billing and coding tasks typically completed by the medical assistant include collecting accurate information and submitting a complete insurance claim.

4. **Explain how to submit health insurance claims, including electronic claims, to various third-party payers.**

Medical billers should familiarize themselves with the claim submission policies and procedures of the health insurance plans commonly seen in their office. A medical assistant can successfully manage the requirements of the different insurance plans commonly seen in the practice by keeping an up-to-date manual containing the billing policies and procedures of these third-party payers. Electronic claims are insurance claims that are transmitted over the internet from the provider to the health insurance company. Most claims-processing software is designed to generate electronic claims.

5. **Review the guidelines for completing the CMS-1500 Health Insurance Claim Form and complete an insurance claim form.**

The medical assistant should follow an established list of guidelines for completing the CMS-1500 Health Insurance Claim Form, including obtaining a signed assignment of benefits. The CMS-1500 has 33 blocks; except for specific blocks that require information about the patient and the insured, the requirements for completing the form vary from payer to payer. Accuracy in completing the CMS-1500 is vital. The process for completing claim forms accurately is outlined in Procedure 18.4 on p. 398.

6. **Differentiate between fraud and abuse.**

Abuse in coding can be likened to actions that are contrary to ethical standards in the medical office. Unlike fraud, abuse is an inadvertent action that directly or indirectly results in an overpayment to the healthcare provider. Abuse is similar to fraud, except that it is unclear whether the unethical practice was committed deliberately. The term "intentional" is important in defining fraud and abuse and in deciphering whether the coding practices were ethical or not.

7. **Discuss methods of preventing the rejection of claims.**

It can be challenging for a provider to keep up with the annual changes published by Medicare, private health insurance companies, and the ICD-10-CM code set updates. Staff meetings to review third-party requirements should be conducted regularly by the medical billing supervisor.

8. **Display tactful behavior when speaking with medical providers about third-party requirements.**

Medical assistants should be respectful to the healthcare provider when discussing third-party requirements that demand more effort on the provider's part. An understanding and patient attitude goes a long way. Rejection and delay of claims cost the medical facility time and money. Proven methods of preventing rejection and delay should be established and followed; these may include reviewing electronic claims submission reports and following up on aging reports.

9. **Describe ways of checking a claim's status.**

It is important to track health insurance claims once they have been submitted electronically. A regular practice of confirming submission of a claim with the health insurance plan or the clearinghouse is essential for prompt payment. If more than 2 weeks pass after a claim submission without a response from the insurance company, it is wise to follow up either through the online insurance provider Web portal or by phone.

10. **Review and read an Explanation of Benefits.**

The EOB is sent by the insurance company to the provider who submitted the insurance claim, along with a check or a document indicating that funds were transferred electronically. The EOB breaks down each line item charge into the amount allowable, how much the insurance plan paid, and how much the patient is contracted to pay to the provider.

11. **Discuss reasons for denied claims.**

The two main reasons for denial of payment are technical errors and insurance policy coverage issues. Technical errors include incorrect or incomplete information and typographic and/or mathematical errors.

12. **Define "medical necessity" as it applies to diagnostic and procedural coding and follow medical necessity guidelines.**

To ensure correct reimbursement, accurate diagnosis codes must be submitted, and they must be linked to the medical procedure code reported. The diagnosis code is the reason the medical procedure performed was necessary. If an insurance company denies a claim on the grounds that the medical treatment provided was not medically necessary, an appeal letter should be sent (see Procedure 18.5 on p. 400). The appeal letter should not only identify the denied claim in question, but also include a statement from the provider detailing the medical reasoning for providing the billed treatment. Additional medical reports should be sent (e.g., lab reports, operative reports, H&P) if these documents support the provider's decision to treat the patient.

13. **Explain a patient's financial obligations for services rendered; also, inform a patient of these obligations, and show sensitivity when speaking with patients about third-party requirements.**

Patients must understand that the guarantor is the person ultimately responsible for the entire bill. The insurance policy is a contract between an insurance company or MCO and the policyholder, or a group of people (e.g., through an employer). The provider is not a party to this contract. Therefore, providers and their staff members are not responsible for pursuing insurance payment for the benefit of the patient. However, it is in the best interest of the staff to actively assist the patient if problems occur securing payment.

PROCEDURE 18.1   Interpret Information on an Insurance Card

Task: To identify essential information on the health insurance identification (ID) card, so as to confirm copayment obligations and obtain accurate health insurance information for claims submission.

EQUIPMENT and SUPPLIES

- Patient's health insurance ID card, both sides (see the following figure)

Front

AETNA

INSURED: Tapia, Arnold

IDENTIFICATION #: CH1197845   DEPENDENTS: Tapia, Celia B
GROUP #: 33347H   EFFECTIVE DATE: 06/26/2012

CO-PAY: $25   DRUG CO-PAY
SPECIALIST CO-PAY: $35   GENERIC: $10
EMERGENCY DEPT: $35   NAME BRAND: $50

Back

Submit claims to:

Aetna
1234 Insurance Way
Anytown, AK 12345

Member Services: 1-800-123-222

Insured: If a life threatening emergency exists, seek immediate attention.

PROCEDURAL STEPS

1. Review the patient's health insurance ID card and identify the insured on the health insurance ID card. If the patient is someone other than the insured, obtain the relationship with the insured and the insured's date of birth and gender.
   PURPOSE: To submit an accurate health insurance claim, the insured's date of birth and gender are required.
2. Identify the insurance plan.
   PURPOSE: To confirm that the provider is a participating provider for the insurance plan or the HMO network. If the provider is out of network, the patient should be informed that he or she will either have to pay more out of pocket or the medical services rendered will not be covered by the insurance plan.
3. Identify the insured's identification number and group number.
   PURPOSE: To accurately submit the health insurance claim under the correct insurance policy number and group number.
4. Identify the patient's copayment, which is due before the appointment. Collect the correct amount. (For example, if the provider is a specialist, collect the copayment listed for specialist.)
   PURPOSE: To ensure that the proper copayment is paid by the patient.
5. On the back of the health insurance ID card, make sure that a customer service phone number and medical claims address are present.
   PURPOSE: To ensure that the provider can contact customer service and has the correct mailing address.

PROCEDURE 18.2   Show Sensitivity When Communicating With Patients Regarding Third-Party Requirements

Task: Communicate in an assertive, professional manner with a third-party representative. Demonstrate sensitivity through verbal and nonverbal communication when discussing third-party requirements with a patient. Display tactful behavior when communicating with a provider regarding third party requirements.

Scenario: Ken Thomas (DOB 10/25/1961) saw Jean Burke, N.P., for his asthma today. He was prescribed a fluticasone inhaler, 220 mcg, and a refill on his Albuterol inhaler. When Ken stops at the checkout desk to make a follow-up appointment, he looks concerned. You inquire how you can help him, and he states that he is wondering if his new insurance will pick up the fluticasone inhaler. He further explains that he has used one in the past, with great results, but he recently switched insurance plans, and he is finding it doesn't have the same coverage as his old plan.

| | | |

PROCEDURE 18.2   Show Sensitivity When Communicating With Patients Regarding Third-Party Requirements—*continued*

Role-Play 1: You call the insurance company and discuss the coverage with the insurance carrier's representative. The representative tells you that the fluticasone inhaler is not covered. The representative gives you names of two other inhalers that would be covered.

When you ask if the drug would be covered through the exceptions process, the representative indicates that the provider must send a letter indicating the drug is appropriate for the patient's condition because all other drugs covered by the plan have not been effective or those drugs have side effects that may be harmful to the patient or the patient is allergic to the other drugs.

Role-Play 2: You must explain to Ken, who is upset over his insurance coverage, that he would have to cover the $250 cost of the inhaler.

Role-Play 3: Ken explains he does not have $250 for the inhaler. He asks what else he should do. You mention the exception process, and Ken requests the provider to send a letter. You need to role-play notifying the provider of the third-party requirements.

Directions: Role-play the scenarios with a peer. The peer will play the part of the insurance representative, the patient, and the provider. You need to be professional and assertive with the insurance representative. When working with the patient, you need to show sensitivity. When communicating with the provider, you need to be professional and tactful.

EQUIPMENT and SUPPLIES

- Copy of patient's health insurance ID card
- Prescription for new medication

PROCEDURAL STEPS

1. Obtain a copy of the patient's health insurance ID card and the prescription for the new medication.
   PURPOSE: Having the required documents will help you to be more efficient as you perform the task.
2. Review the insurance card for coverage information and the phone number for providers.
   PURPOSE: You will need the phone number from the ID card to call the insurance company. You will also need to provide the insurance representative with the patient's information.
3. Using role-play 1, contact the insurance company and clearly state the patient's information, the patient's question, and the name of the new medication.
   PURPOSE: The insurance representative will need the patient's information and the question to assist you. Speaking clearly as you provide the information will help the listener understand what you are asking.
4. Demonstrate professionalism in verbal communication skills by stating a respectful, clear, and organized message, pronouncing medical terminology and medication names correctly.

5. Explain to the patient the message from the insurance representative using language that can be understood by the patient.
   PURPOSE: For the patient to understand your message, you need to use language that he or she can understand.
6. Demonstrate sensitivity to the patient by paying attention and responding appropriately to his or her body language and verbal message.
   PURPOSE: Demonstrating sensitivity can be done through verbal messages and body language. Paying attention to the patient and responding appropriately to his or her message and nonverbal communication are important.
7. Demonstrate sensitivity to the patient by showing empathy and clarifying that you understand what the patient is stating. Give the patient your full attention during the conversation and reserve judgment.
8. Demonstrate sensitivity to the patient by using a pleasant, courteous tone of voice. Use body language to communicate respect (e.g., eye contact if culturally appropriate, keeping arms uncrossed and relaxed).
   PURPOSE: As the patient's frustration and anger increase, it is important to use a pleasant, courteous, and normal tone of voice. Keeping your body appearance relaxed (e.g., arms uncrossed, hands relaxed) will help to show the patient you are calm.
9. Demonstrate tactful behavior when explaining the third-party requirements to the provider.
   PURPOSE: Providing the patient with choices also shows the patient that you care.

PROCEDURE 18.3   Perform Precertification With Documentation

Task: To obtain precertification from a patient's insurance carrier for requested services or procedures.

Scenario: You are working with Dr. Julie Walden at Walden-Martin Family Medical Clinic. Erma Willis (DOB 12/09/19XX) is seen for excessive snoring, and Dr. Walden orders a sleep study. You need to complete a prior authorization/certification form for the sleep study, which will be conducted by Dr. Jim Sandman. You checked, and there is a signed release of information form.

Insurance Information
Aetna
1234 Insurance Way
Anytown, AL 112345-1234
Member ID Number: EW8884910
Group Number: 66574W

Clinic and Provider Information
Walden-Martin Family Medical Clinic
1234 Anystreet
Anytown, AL 12345
Provider: Julie Walden, MD
Fax: 123-123-5678
Phone: 123-123-1234
Provider Contact Name: (your name)

Service Information
Place: Walden-Martin Family Medical Clinic
Service Requested: Sleep study
Starting Service Date: 1 week from today
Ending Service Date: 1 week from today
Service Frequency: once
ICD-10-CM code: R06.83
CPT code: 95807
Not related to an injury or workers' compensation

EQUIPMENT and SUPPLIES

- *Paper method:* Patient's health record, prior authorization (precertification) request form, copy of patient's health insurance ID card, a pen
- *Electronic method:* Electronic health record system, such as SimChart for the Medical Office (SCMO)

PROCEDURAL STEPS

1. For the paper method, gather the health record, precertification/prior authorization request form, copy of the health insurance ID card, and a pen. For the electronic method, access the Simulation Playground in SCMO.
2. Using the health record, determine the service or procedure that requires precertification/preauthorization.
3. For the paper method, complete the precertification/prior authorization request form. For the electronic method, click on the Form Repository icon

in SCMO. Select Prior Authorization Request from the left INFO PANEL. Use the Patient Search button at the bottom to find the patient. Complete the remaining fields of the form.
PURPOSE: This provides information on the ordered procedure or service to the insurance company, which will notify the provider's representative if the procedure or service will be covered under the plan.
4. Proofread the completed form and make any revisions needed.
PURPOSE: To ensure the accuracy of the information.
5. With the paper method, file the document in the health record after it has been faxed to the insurance carrier. With the electronic method, print and fax or electronically send the form to the insurance company and save the form to the patient's record.
PURPOSE: Copies of all forms completed for the patient need to be maintained in the health record.

PROCEDURE 18.4   Complete an Insurance Claim Form

Task: To accurately complete a CMS-1500 Health Insurance Claim Form (see Fig. 18.6).

Scenario: Mr. Walter Biller had an appointment with Dr. Walden on November 16, 20XX. He came in for an influenza vaccination, and while he was there, he wanted Dr. Walden to look at his ear because he was having problems hearing. His right ear canal was impacted with cerumen; the ear canal was irrigated, and the cerumen was removed during the visit.

PROCEDURE 18.4   Complete an Insurance Claim Form—continued

Patient Demographics
Walter B. Biller (patient and insured)
87 Willoughby Lane
Anytown, AL 12345-1234
Phone: 123-237-3748
DOB: 01/04/1970
SSN: 285-77-7796
HIPAA form on file: Yes — March 19, 20XX
Signature on file: Yes — March 19, 20XX
Insurance Information
Account Number: 16611
Aetna
Policy/ID Number: CH8327753
Group Number: 33347H

Clinic and Provider Information
Walden-Martin Family Medical Clinic
1234 Anystreet
Anytown, AL 12345
123-123-1234
POS — 04 Independent clinic
Established patient of Julie Walden, MD
Federal Tax ID# 651249831
NPI# 1467253823

Diagnosis:	ICD-10-CM code	
Impacted cerumen, right ear	H61.21	

Service	CPT Code	Fee
Est. minimal OV	99211	$24.00
Cerumen removal	69210	$46.00
Vaccine — Flu, 3 Y+	90658	$24.00
Preventive — Flu Administration	G0008	$7.00

EQUIPMENT and SUPPLIES

- Patient's health record
- Copy of patient's insurance ID card or cards
- Patient registration/intake form
- Encounter form
- Insurance claims processing guidelines
- Blank CMS-1500 Health Insurance Claim Form

PROCEDURAL STEPS

Almost all medical billing is done electronically through practice management billing software. The paper CMS-1500 Health Insurance Claim Form is provided only to help students practice and develop their medical billing skills.

Complete each block (as appropriate) of the CMS-1500.

1. Gather the documents required to complete the claim form.
2. Complete the claim form using a pen. Use capital letters. Do not use punctuation (commas or dollar signs) unless indicated in the insurance manual or guidelines. Use a hyphen to hyphenate last names.
3. Using the patient's health insurance ID card, determine the type of insurance, and the insurance ID number. Enter this information into Blocks 1 and 1a.
   PURPOSE: After selecting the appropriate type of health insurance, the medical assistant can refer to the claims processing guidelines for that plan.
4. Using the ID card, the encounter form, and the registration/intake form, determine the patient's information and the insured individual's information. Accurately complete Blocks 2, 3, 5, 6, 9, and 10 a–c by entering the patient's information. Complete Blocks 4, 7, and 11 a–d with the insured's information.

PURPOSE: By distinguishing between the patient and the insured, the medical biller can determine whether the insurer requires additional information for submission of an accurate claim.

5. Complete Blocks 12 and 13 by entering "signature on file" and the date. *Note:* The Assignment of Benefits form should have been signed by the patient and/or the insured at registration. Enter the dates in either the six (6)-digit format (MM/DD/YY) or the eight (8)-digit format (MM/DD/YYYY).
   PURPOSE: To submit an insurance claim, the medical practice must be authorized to release the service information on behalf of the patient or the insured.
6. Accurately enter the physician or supplier information by completing Blocks 14 through 23. Use the eight (8)-digit format (MM/DD/YYYY) when needed.
7. Using the encounter form, complete Block 24 and the appropriate blocks from 24A through 24H. Note the following:
   - *Block 24A:* Enter the dates of service, both From and To. For ambulatory services, enter the same date in the FROM and TO fields. Enter a date for each procedure or service, or supply it in eight (8)-digit format (MM/DD/YYYY).
   - *Block 24F:* Enter the charge for the listed service or procedure. *Do not use commas when reporting dollar amounts.* The cents column is the small column to the right.
   - *Block 24G:* Enter the number of days or units. This block is usually used for multiple visits, units of supplies, anesthesia units or minutes, or oxygen volume. If only one service was performed, enter 1.

Continued

PROCEDURE 18.4   Complete an Insurance Claim Form—*continued*

8. Complete Blocks 24I through 27 by entering information on the provider, or on the healthcare facility where the service was provided, and the patient's account number. Check the correct box to indicate acceptance of assignment of benefits.

9. Complete Blocks 28 and 29 by entering the total charges, total amount paid, and the total amount due. Complete Blocks 31 through 33a by entering the provider's and facility's information.

10. Review the claim for accuracy and completeness before submitting. Correct any errors and provide any missing information.
   Note: Before sending the claim, make a copy of the form and file the copy in the patient's insurance claim file.
   PURPOSE: It is important to double-check the form for accuracy and for required information that has not been provided.

PROCEDURE 18.5   Use Medical Necessity Guidelines: Respond to a "Medical Necessity Denied" Claim

Task: To resolve the insurance company's denial of a claim for medical necessity by completing an accurate claim.

Scenario: You are working at the Walden-Martin Family Medical Clinic, 1234 Anystreet, Anytown, AL 12345 (phone: 123-123-1234). You receive a letter indicating that Medicare has denied the following claim for not being medically necessary.

Patient: Norma B. Washington   DOB: 08/07/1944   Policy/ID Number: 847744144A
Date of Service: 06/13/20XX   ICD: G43.101 (Migraine)   CPT: J3420 (B-12 injection)
Provider: Julie Walden, MD

You do some research and find that the information above was the only information sent to Medicare for that encounter. The following information was the correct information for the encounter.

Patient: Norma B. Washington   DOB: 08/01/1944   Date of Service: 06/15/20XX
ICD: G43.101 (Migraine)   CPT: J1885 (Toradol 15 mg — $15.50) and 90772 (Injection, Ther/Proph/Diag — $25.00)

ICD: D51.0 (Vitamin B_{12} deficiency anemia)   CPT: J3420 (B-12 injection — $24.00) and 90772 (Injection, Ther/Proph/Diag — $25.00)

To be billed to: Medicare, 1234 Insurance Road, Anytown, AL 12345-1234

EQUIPMENT and SUPPLIES

- *Paper method:* Patient's health record, copy of patient's insurance ID card or cards, patient registration form, encounter form, blank CMS-1500 Health Insurance Claim Form, pen
- *Electronic method:* SimChart for the Medical Office
- Insurance denial letter or scenario (see above)

PROCEDURAL STEPS

1. Review the insurance denial letter (scenario) carefully. Compare the patient's information from the denial letter to the health record, claim, and encounter form. Look for errors in the patient's name and date of birth.
   PURPOSE: Errors in patient information can be a reason for denial.

2. Compare the insurance denial letter (scenario) to the health record, claim, and encounter form. Look for errors in the date of service, the diagnosis,

and the procedure codes. The procedure must be medically necessary for the diagnosis indicated.
   PURPOSE: Errors related to the encounter must be matching for the claim to be accepted. The procedure codes must indicate an acceptable standard of treatment for the diagnosis listed. In some cases, the encounter form may contain a diagnosis that did not make it into the original claim form. Review the patient's health record to determine whether the procedure was medically necessary.

3. Complete a claim (either CMS-1500 or an electronic claim using SimChart) by entering the information about the carrier, patient, and insured.

4. Enter the information about the physician, procedures, and diagnosis. Make sure to include all the information from the encounter.

5. Proofread the claim form for accuracy before submitting the claim.

PROCEDURE 18.6   Inform a Patient of Financial Obligations for Services Rendered

Task: To inform the patient of his or her financial obligation and to demonstrate professionalism and sensitivity when discussing the patient's billing record.

Scenario 1: Mr. Walter Biller arrives for his appointment. You need to check his eligibility for services and also if he has a copayment for today's visit. His insurance information: account number — 16611; Aetna, Policy/ID Number: CH8327753; and Group Number: 33347H

Scenario 2: Christi Brown is meeting with you regarding the bill she received in the mail. She called to make the appointment, and she voiced her confusion about the bill. She stated that she thought her insurance covered everything. You check her record and see that she met her deductible and now needs to pay 20% of the billed amount. She owes $170.

Directions: Role-play the scenarios with a peer. For the first scenario, the peer will be the insurance representative and then the patient. You will be the medical assistant. You need to be professional and sensitive when working with patients regarding payments. You also need to follow the clinic's policy.

EQUIPMENT and SUPPLIES

- Facility's payment policy
- Copy of patient's insurance card (or see information in the scenario)
- Patient's account record (or see information in the scenario)

PROCEDURAL STEPS

Scenario 1: Role-play with a peer who will be the insurance representative.

1. Contact the patient's insurance company and verify the patient's eligibility for services. Provide the representative with the patient's information. Find out if the patient has a copayment for today's visit. Document the information obtained.

   PURPOSE: Understanding the patient's financial responsibility from the insurance plan will help you to explain the terms to the patient.

   Scenario 1 update: You need to provide the patient with the information that he owes a copayment for today's visit.

2. Inform the patient of his financial obligation of the copayment.
   Scenario update: He states he does not have the cash with him.

3. Inform the patient of the clinic policy regarding copayments and how the payment can be made.

4. Demonstrate sensitivity and professionalism when discussing the payment.
   Scenario 2: Role-play with a peer who will be the patient.

5. Determine the amount the patient owes by reviewing the patient's account record. Inform the patient of the amount owed for services rendered.
   Scenario update: Patient stated she does not have the money to pay the entire bill today.

6. Inform the patient of the clinic policy regarding overdue accounts and scheduling appointments. Provide the patient with options for the overdue amount based on the clinic policy.

7. Demonstrate sensitivity and professionalism when discussing the payment and the situation.

19

PATIENT ACCOUNTS AND PRACTICE MANAGEMENT

SCENARIO

Laura Casper has been working in the back office at Walden-Martin Family Medical (WMFM) Clinic for the past 3 years. Her primary job has been working with patient accounts. She has recently been asked also to take on some of the accounts payable responsibilities. This will involve banking procedures and bill paying.

While working with patient accounts, Laura has become familiar with the billing cycle and collection procedures, and she is training new employees. It can be a complicated process, but Laura finds it challenging and enjoyable.

After the addition of the banking responsibilities to her work duties, Laura met with a bank representative. They discussed some time-efficient ways to

bank with mobile depositing and online banking. Laura realizes that she still has much to learn about the daily financial duties in a healthcare facility, including working with the patient account management software, making daily deposits, reconciling bank statements, and many other banking responsibilities.

Laura wants to increase the value of the healthcare facility's bank accounts by looking for bank accounts that pay a higher interest rate and by reducing the office's operational expenses. Laura also wants to encourage patients at the healthcare facility to use debit or credit cards, instead of checks, to pay for services, because she knows that returned patient checks have created problems in the past.

While studying this chapter, think about the following questions:
- Why is it important to post charges, payments, and adjustments in a timely manner?
- What should you do when a patient wants to make payments on an outstanding patient account balance?
- What should you do when patient accounts are outstanding for more than 90 days after the date of service?
- How is online banking affecting banking in healthcare facilities?
- How can an office manager determine whether an employee can be trusted with banking procedures?
- What precautions should the healthcare facility take when accepting patient payments?
- Why is making daily deposits a good idea?
- How can the office manager reconcile the bank account, and why is this important?

LEARNING OBJECTIVES

1. Define bookkeeping and bookkeeping terms and discuss all the different transactions recorded in patient accounts.
2. Perform accounts receivable procedures for patient accounts, including posting charges, payments, and adjustments. Also, discuss payment at the time of service and give an example of displaying sensitivity when requesting payment for services rendered.
3. Describe the impact of the Truth in Lending Act on collections policies for patient accounts.
4. Discuss monthly patient account statements and list the necessary data elements on each monthly statement.
5. Do the following related to collection procedures:
   - Describe successful collection techniques for patient accounts.
   - Discuss strategies for collecting outstanding balances through personal finance interviews.
   - Describe types of adjustments made to patient accounts, including a nonsufficient funds (NSF) check and collection agency transactions.
   - Post payments and adjustments to a patient's account.
6. Do the following related to banking in today's business world:
   - Explain the purpose of the Federal Reserve Bank and the types of banks it manages.
   - Identify common types of bank accounts.
   - Discuss the importance of signature cards.
   - Explain how online banking has made standard banking processes more efficient.
7. Do the following related to checks:
   - Compare different types of negotiable instruments.
   - Identify precautions in accepting checks from patients.
   - Explain how checks are processed from one account to another.
   - Review the procedure followed when the healthcare facility receives an NSF check.
8. Identify precautions in accepting cash.
9. Discuss the use of debit and credit cards, including advantages and precautions.
10. Do the following related to banking procedures in the ambulatory care setting.

LEARNING OBJECTIVES—continued

- Describe banking procedures as related to the ambulatory care setting.
- Explain the importance of depositing checks daily.
- Prepare a bank deposit.
- Compare types of check endorsements.

- Review check-writing procedures used to pay the operational expenses of a healthcare facility.
11. Understand the purpose of bank account reconciliation for auditing purposes, and how to pay bills in order to maximize cash flow.
12. Discuss the process of employee payroll.

VOCABULARY

assets All property available for the payment of debts.

belligerent (buh LIG er ent) Hostile and aggressive.

bookkeeping The process of recording financial transactions.

cash on hand The amount of money the healthcare facility has in the bank that can be withdrawn as cash.

counterfeit (KOWN ter fit) An imitation intended to be passed off fraudulently or deceptively as genuine; forgery.

defendant An individual or a business against which a lawsuit is filed.

discretionary income Money in a bank account that is not assigned to pay for any office expenses.

emancipated minor (ih MAN suh pay tid MIE ner) A minor who has been granted emancipation by the court; the minor can assume the rights and responsibilities of adulthood.

embezzlement (em BEZ ul ment) The misuse of funds for personal gain.

EMV chip technology Global technology that includes imbedded microchips that store and protect cardholder data; also called *chip and PIN* and *chip and signature*.

executor An individual assigned to make financial decisions about the estate of a deceased patient.

expletive (EK sple tiv) An oath or a swear word.

explanation of benefits (EOB) A document sent by the insurance company to the provider and the patient explaining the allowed charge amount, the amount reimbursed for services, and the patient's financial responsibilities.

Federal Reserve Bank The central bank of the United States. The Federal Reserve system consists of a seven-member Board of Governors with headquarters in Washington, D.C., and 12 Federal Reserve banks in major cities throughout the country.

fee schedule A list of fixed fees for services.

gross The amount earned before any tax deductions or adjustments.

guarantor The person legally responsible for the entire bill. This is usually the patient, but in the case of a minor it would be a parent or legal guardian.

incurred To come into or acquire.

indigent (IN di jent) Poor, needy, impoverished.

intangible (in TAN juh buhl) Something of value that cannot be touched physically.

interest Money the bank pays the account holder, on the amount in his or her account, for using the money in the account.

negotiable (ni GOH shee uh buhl) **instrument** A document guaranteeing payment of a specific amount of money to the payer named on the document.

net The amount someone is paid after taxes and other deductions have been subtracted.

patient account A running balance of all financial transactions for a specific patient.

pegboard system A manual bookkeeping system that uses a day sheet to record all financial transactions for the date of service and maintains patient account balances by using physical ledger cards.

plaintiff An individual or a party who brings the suit to court.

reconciliation (rek uh n sill ee AY shun) To bring into agreement.

salary A fixed compensation periodically paid to a person for regular work.

small claims court A special court established to handle small claims or debts without the services of lawyers.

tickler file A chronologic file used as a reminder that something must be dealt with on a certain date.

trustee The coordinator of financial resources assigned by the court during a bankruptcy case.

unsecured debt Debt that is not guaranteed by something of value; credit card debt is the most common type of unsecured debt.

Managing the finances in a healthcare facility is an important task. Every patient encounter creates a financial transaction for the facility. Transactions generated by the patient encounter include a variety of charges, payments, and adjustments that need to be accounted for on a daily basis. Financial management is essential if the healthcare facility is to pay the business operating expenses. This includes maintaining **patient accounts** and performing collection activities and banking duties. If the expenses of operating the healthcare facility exceed the fees collected for services rendered, the business will be forced to close.

A medical assistant who works in the front office is responsible for posting charges, accepting and posting a variety of payments and adjustments, endorsing and depositing checks, writing checks for office expenses, and regularly reconciling bank and credit card statements. Mobile deposit allows healthcare facilities to deposit checks on the date payments are received, because it is conveniently done in the office. The medical assistant will have to master basic math skills (e.g., addition and subtraction) for all banking functions.

MANAGING FUNDS IN THE HEALTHCARE FACILITY

The purpose of financial management is to ensure that the healthcare facility earns enough money to cover its operating expenses. The financial records of the healthcare facility should show the following: how much money was earned in a given period, how much money was collected, how much money is owed, and the distribution of all operational expenses.

An accountant can prepare monthly and annual financial records from daily **bookkeeping** records. Periodic analyses of these reports result in improved business practices, improved time management, elimination of unprofitable services, and more efficient expense budgeting.

In order for the medical assistant to be able to properly manage finances, it is crucial that he or she understand the difference between accounts receivable and accounts payable.

- *Accounts receivable* (A/R) is money that is expected but has not yet been received. The amount charged on the encounter form is an example of accounts receivable for the healthcare facility. When a payment is made on the patient account, the received payment becomes **cash on hand**.
- *Accounts payable* (A/P) is the management of debt **incurred** and not yet paid. All invoices, statements, and operating expenses are included in accounts payable. When expenses have been paid, they are no longer categorized as accounts payable.

BOOKKEEPING IN THE HEALTHCARE FACILITY

Most healthcare facilities use practice management software for daily bookkeeping transactions. A/R transactions come from the encounter form. The charges documented on the encounter form are used to complete the health insurance claim form. *Payments* to the healthcare facility come as reimbursement from the insurance company, or from a patient payment. *Adjustments* are made to a patient's account when it is necessary to add or subtract an amount, which is not a payment, from the balance; for example, the difference between the provider's charged amount and the contracted insurance payment amount.

There are two terms used in bookkeeping that can be confusing – credit and debit. A *credit* is a bookkeeping entry that increases accounts receivable, or what is owed to the provider. Example: posting charges to a patient's account. A *debit* is a bookkeeping entry that increases accounts payable, or what is owed by the provider. Example: posting a patient payment and insurance payment to a patient's account that results in an overpayment.

A/P transactions also require bookkeeping entries. Writing checks and maintaining the checking account register are examples of A/P bookkeeping entries. Expenses are tracked by category (e.g., rent, clinical supplies, and administrative supplies).

ACCOUNTS RECEIVABLE (A/R)

The majority of the money owed to the healthcare facility comes from patient accounts. It is important for a medical assistant to understand how the patient account system works.

Patient Ledger

A patient account is created when the healthcare provider renders services. Charges are applied to the patient account when an *encounter form* (Fig. 19.1) is completed during the office visit. The *ledger* is where all the procedures and charges for services rendered are listed.

All transactions for professional services are posted to the patient's ledger daily. In this way, the ledger becomes the source for answering questions from patients about their financial obligations. The patient ledger should include all information related to collecting the balance due, such as:

- Name and address of the guarantor
- Insurance identification information
- Home, work, and cell phone numbers
- Any special instructions for billing
- Emergency or alternative contact information

The ledger (Fig. 19.2) provides a running balance, the result of all of the different financial transactions performed in the account, including charges, payments, and adjustments. This same information can be found in practice management software in an electronic format.

Entering and Posting Transactions in the Patient Ledger

When a **pegboard system** is used (Fig. 19.3), transactions are initiated before the patient goes to the exam room. The patient account ledger card is inserted under the first or next available receipt, and the first available writing line of the card is aligned with the carbonized strip on the receipt. Enter the receipt number and the date; enter the account balance in the space labeled *previous balance;* and then enter the patient's name. A copy of the receipt is detached and clipped to the patient's chart to be routed to the provider.

Posting Charges

When a practice management software system is used, charges are entered into the ledger automatically from the encounter form after the office visit (see Procedure 19.1 on p. 431). The fees for services rendered come from the **fee schedule**. Most practice management systems will automatically determine the fee based on the CPT/HCPCS code and insurance company.

Posting Payments

Payments can be received by mail, electronically, or in person. They can come from a patient or from an insurance company. All payments need to be posted to the patient's account.

Third-party payments are payments made by an insurance company. In other words, third-party payers pay the healthcare provider on behalf of the patient. The patient is one party, the healthcare provider is the second party, and the insurance company is the third party. In an electronic system, third-party payments are posted line by line, corresponding to the submitted health insurance claim. All payment amounts posted should match the total amount shown on the **explanation of benefits (EOB)** (Fig. 19.4). Once the third party pays the insurance claim, the total owed to the provider becomes the amount charged minus the payment amount and the amount adjusted by the third party. The remaining balance is still owed to the provider by the patient:

$$\text{Insurance payment amount} + \text{Adjustment amount}$$
$$+ \text{Patient responsibility} = \text{Total charged}$$

STATE LIC.# C1503X
SOC. SEC. # 000-11-0000
PIN # _____

Walden-Martin Family Medical Clinic
1234 Anystreet, Anytown, AK 12345-1234

Phone: 555-486-9002

☐ Private ☒ Bluecross ☐ Ind. ☐ Medicare ☐ Medi-cal ☐ Hmo ☐ Ppo

Patient's last name Thomas	First Ken	Account #: 11594111	Birthdate 10 / 25 / 1961	Sex ☒ Male ☐ Female	Today's date 09 / 17 / 20XX
Insurance company Blue Cross Blue Shield	Subscriber Ken Thomas		Plan #	Sub. # KT4496785	Group 55124T

ASSIGNMENT: I hereby assign my insurance benefits to be paid directly to the undersigned physician, I am financially responsible for non-covered services.
SIGNED: Patient, or parent, if minor *Ken Thomas*   Today's date 09 /17 /20XX

RELEASE: I hereby authorize the physician to release to my insurance carriers any information require to process this claim.
SIGNED: Patient, or parent, if minor *Ken Thomas*   Today's date 09 /17 /20XX

✓	DESCRIPTION	CODE NEW	EST.	FEE	✓	DESCRIPTION	CODE	FEE	✓	DESCRIPTION	CODE	FEE
	OFFICE VISITS	NEW	EST.			Venipuncture	36415			OFFICE PROCEDURES		
	Blood pressure check		99211			TB skin test	86580			Anoscopy	46600	
	Level II	99202	99212			Hematocrit	85013			Ear lavage	69210	
	Level III	99203	99213			Glucose finger stick	82948			Spirometry	94010	
X	Level IV	99204	99214	$175		IMMUNIZATIONS				Nebulizer Rx	94664	
	Level V	99205	99215			Allergy inj. X1	95115			EKG	93000	
	PREVENTIVE EXAMS	NEW	EST.			Allergy inj. X2	95117			SURGERY		
	Age 65 and older	99387	99397			Trigger pt. inj.	20552			Mole removal (1st)	17110	
	Age 40 - 64	99386	99396			Therapeutic inj.	96372			(2nd to 14th)	17003	
	Age 18 - 39	99385	99395			VACCINATION PRODUCTS				Flat warts (1st - 14th)	07110	
	Age 12 - 17	99384	99394			DPT	90701			15 or more	17111	
	Age 5 - 11	99383	99393			DT	90702			Biopsy, 1 lesion	11100	
	Age 1 - 4	99382	99392			Tetanus	90703			Addt'l. lesions	11101	
	Infant	99381	99391			MMR	90707			Endometrial Bx	58100	
	Newborn ofc		99432			OPV	90712			Skin tags to 15	11200	
	OB/NEWBORN CARE					Polio inj.	90713			Each addt'l. 10	11201	
	OB package		59400			Flu	90662			I & D abscess	10060	
	Post-partum visit N/C					Hemophilus B	90645			SUPPLIES/MISCELLANEOUS		
	LAB PROCEDURES					Hepatitis B vac.	90746			Surgical tray	99070	
	Urine dip		81000			Pheumovax	90670			Handling charge	99000	
	UA qualitative		81005			VACCINE ADMINISTRATION				Special report	99080	
X	Pregnancy urine		81025			Age: Through 18 yrs. (1st inj.)	90460			DOCTOR'S NOTES:		
	Wet mount		87210			Age: Through 18 yrs. (ea. addt'l. inj.)	90461					
	kOH prip		87220			Adult (1st inj.)	90471					
	Occult blood		82270			Adult (ea. addt'l. inj.)	90472					

DIAGNOSES **ICD-10-CM**			
Abdominal pain/unspec. . . R10.9	Colitis/unspec. K51.90	FUO R50.9	Osteoarthritis (site). . . . . M19._
Absess . . . . L02._	Confusion R41.0	Gastritis. K29.70	Otitis media . . . . H66.9_
Allergic reaction . . . . . . T78.40_	CHF I50.9	Gastroenteritis (colitis) . . . K52.9	Parkinson's disease G20
Alzheimer's disease G30	Constipation K59.00	G.I. bleed K92.2	Pharyngitis, acute. J02.9
Anemia/unspec. D64.9	COPD J44.9	Gout/unspec. M10.9	Pleurisy R09.1
Angina/unspec. I20.9	Cough R05	Headache R51	Pneumonia J18.9
Anorexia R63.0	Crohn's disease/unspec. . . K50.90	Health exam . . . . Z00._	Pneumonia, viral J12.9
Anxiety/unspec. F41.9	CVA I63.9	Hematuria/unspec. R31.9	Prostatitis/unspec. N41.9
Apnea, sleep G47.30	Decubitus ulcer. . . . . L89._	Herpes simplex. B00.9	PVD I73.9
Arrhythmia, cardiac I49.9	Dehydration. E86.0	Herpes zoster B02.9	Radiculopathy . . . . M54.1_
Arthritis, rheumatoid. M06.9	Dementia/unspec. F03	Hiatal hernia K44.9	Rectal bleeding K62.5
Asthma/unspec. J45.909	Depression, major/unsp. . . F32.9	HTN (HBP) I10	Renal failure N19
Atrial fibrillation I48.0	Diab I, no complications . . E10.0	Hyperlipidemia/unspec. . . E78.5	Sciatica. . . . . M54.3_
B-12 deficiency E53.8	Diab II, no complications . . E11.9	Hypothyroidism/unspec. . . E03.9	Shortness of breath R03.02
Back pain, low M54.5	w/kidney complic. . . . . . E11.2_	Impotentce . . . . N52._	Sinusitis, chr./unspec. . . . J32.9
BPH N40	w/ophthalmic compl. . . . E11.3_	Influenza, respiratory J10.1	Syncope R55
Bradycardia/unspec. R00.1	w/neurolog.compl. . . . . E11.4_	Insomnia G47.0	Tachycardia/unspec. R00.0
Broncitis, acute. . . . . J20._	w/circulatory cmpl. . . . . E11.5_	IBS, diarrhea . . . . K58.	Tachy., supraventric. I47.1
Bronchitis, chronic J42	Insulin use Z79.4	Lupus, systemic erythim. . M32.9	Tendinitis/unspec. M77.9
Bursitis/unspec. M71.9	Diarrhea/unspec. R19.7	MI, acute. . . . . I21._	TIA G45.9
CA, breast . . . . C50._	Diverticulitix. K57.92	MI, old. I25.2	Ulcer, duodenal/unspec. . . K26.9
CA, lung . . . . C34._	Diverticulosis. K57.90	Migraine G43.9	Ulcer, gastric/unspec. K25.9
CA, prostate C61	Dizziness. R42	Myalgia M79.1	Ulcer, peptic/unspec. K27.9
Cellulitis . . . . L03._	Dysuria R30.0	Neck pain M54.2	URI/unspec. J06.9
Chest pain/unspec. R07.9	Edema/unspec. R60.9	Neuropathy G62.9	UTI N39.0
Cirrhosis, liver/unspec. . . . K74.60	Endocarditis I38	Nausea R11.1	Vertigo R42
Cold, common J00	Esophageal reflux K21.0	X Nausea/vomiting R11.0	Weight gain R63.5
	Fatigue (lethargy) R53.83	Obesity/unspec. E66.9	Weight loss R63.4

Diagnosis/additional description: Headache	Doctor's signature/date *Dr. Martin* 09-17-20XX

Return appointment information:	-with whom	(Self)/other	Rec'd by: ☐ Cash ☐ Check ☐ Credit # _____	Total today's fee	$175
Days Wks. (Mos.) 1 month				Co-payment	$50
PLEASE RMEMBER THAT PAYMENT IS YOUR OBLIGATION, REGARDLESS OF INSURANCE OR OTHER THIRD PARTY INVOLVEMENT.				Amount rec'd. today	

INSUR-A-BILL ® BIBBERO SYSTEMS, INC. • PETULUMA, CA • © 7/90 (BM1092)   (REV. 7/11)

FIGURE 19.1 Encounter form with charges. (Courtesy Bibber Systems, an InHealth Company, Petaluma, CA (800) 242-2376 www.bibbero.com.)

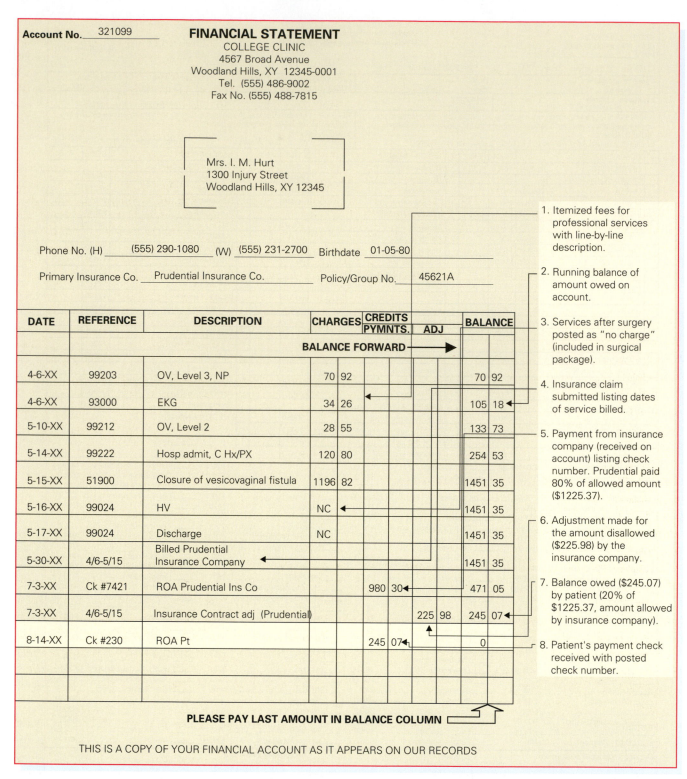

Account No. 321099

FINANCIAL STATEMENT
COLLEGE CLINIC
4567 Broad Avenue
Woodland Hills, XY 12345-0001
Tel. (555) 486-9002
Fax No. (555) 488-7815

Mrs. I. M. Hurt
1300 Injury Street
Woodland Hills, XY 12345

Phone No. (H) _____ (555) 290-1080 _____ (W) (555) 231-2700 Birthdate 01-05-80

Primary Insurance Co. _____ Prudential Insurance Co. _____ Policy/Group No. _____ 45621A

DATE	REFERENCE	DESCRIPTION	CHARGES	CREDITS PYMNTS.	ADJ	BALANCE
		BALANCE FORWARD →				
4-6-XX	99203	OV, Level 3, NP	70 92			70 92
4-6-XX	93000	EKG	34 26			105 18
5-10-XX	99212	OV, Level 2	28 55			133 73
5-14-XX	99222	Hosp admit, C Hx/PX	120 80			254 53
5-15-XX	51900	Closure of vesicovaginal fistula	1196 82			1451 35
5-16-XX	99024	HV	NC			1451 35
5-17-XX	99024	Discharge	NC			1451 35
5-30-XX	4/6-5/15	Billed Prudential Insurance Company				1451 35
7-3-XX	Ck #7421	ROA Prudential Ins Co		980 30		471 05
7-3-XX	4/6-5/15	Insurance Contract adj (Prudential)			225 98	245 07
8-14-XX	Ck #230	ROA Pt		245 07		0

PLEASE PAY LAST AMOUNT IN BALANCE COLUMN ⇧

THIS IS A COPY OF YOUR FINANCIAL ACCOUNT AS IT APPEARS ON OUR RECORDS

1. Itemized fees for professional services with line-by-line description.

2. Running balance of amount owed on account.

3. Services after surgery posted as "no charge" (included in surgical package).

4. Insurance claim submitted listing dates of service billed.

5. Payment from insurance company (received on account) listing check number. Prudential paid 80% of allowed amount ($1225.37).

6. Adjustment made for the amount disallowed ($225.98) by the insurance company.

7. Balance owed ($245.07) by patient (20% of $1225.37, amount allowed by insurance company).

8. Patient's payment check received with posted check number.

FIGURE 19.2 Patient ledger. (From Fordney WT: *Insurance handbook for the medical office*, ed 14, St Louis, 2017, Elsevier.)

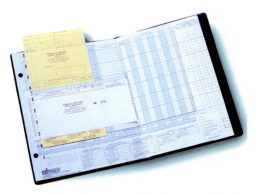

FIGURE 19.3 Pegboard billing system. (Courtesy Bibber Systems, an InHealth Company, Petaluma, CA (800) 242-2376 www.bibbero.com.)

Manual Bookkeeping

Although we live in a technology-savvy world, some providers still use a manual pegboard system. In many cases, providers who have been in practice for many years do not want to invest in a practice management software system because of the cost associated with moving to practice management software. Also, if the office computers go down, employees will have to use a manual system until the system is back up.

The medical assistant must be familiar with both manual and electronic patient account management systems. The pegboard system is the most popular manual system for this purpose. It is simple to operate and contains the same components as those of a computer system. Once a medical assistant learns the pegboard system, computer systems are much easier to understand.

The pegboard system gets its name from the board that is used. This board has a row of pegs along the side or top that holds the forms in place. The patient account ledger cards are perforated for alignment on the pegs (see Fig. 19.3). All the forms used in any system must be compatible so that they can be aligned perfectly on the board.

The pegboard system generates all the necessary financial records for each transaction (by writing once with carbonless forms) as follows:

Encounter form

Receipt

Patient account ledger card

Bookkeeping transaction entry

The system also may include a statement and bank deposit slip. It provides current accounts receivable totals and a daily record of bank deposits and cash on hand, in addition to the record of income and expenses. The need for separate posting to patient accounts is eliminated, and the chance for error is reduced.

The pegboard system allows the medical assistant to keep control over cash, collections, and receivables and ensures that every cent is accounted for and properly entered. It provides a record of every patient, every charge, and every payment, plus a daily recap of earnings — a running record of receivables and an audited summary of cash — and requires little time.

Posting Adjustments

Adjustments are used to either credit or debit a patient's account. Credit adjustments are posted to the patient ledger when an amount needs to be subtracted from a patient's balance. An example would be when the provider's fee exceeds the amount allowed stated on the EOB. The difference between the billed amount and the allowed amount would need to be adjusted (written off). Credit adjustments should always be posted to the patient account record at the same time as the payment. The patient ledger should have a column for the adjustments. Remember: payments and credit adjustments are both credits; however, payments are money that is received in the healthcare facility, and credit adjustments simply reduce the balance that the patient owes on the account. When the payments and credit adjustments are subtracted from the charged amount, the balance is either the patient responsibility or the amount billed to the secondary insurance.

Before continuing to post to the next EOB line item, confirm that the payment amount, the adjusted amount, and the patient responsibility/secondary insurance balance exactly match the amounts calculated on the EOB.

Debit adjustments are posted to the patient ledger when an amount needs to be added to the patient's balance but is not a charge for services. An example would be if a check the patient had written to the healthcare facility was returned for nonsufficient funds. The amount had initially been credited to the account, but the healthcare facility never actually got the funds. A debit adjustment must be made to add the amount of the check back to the patient's balance (Fig. 19.5).

Nonsufficient Funds Checks (NSF)

Nonsufficient funds (NSF) checks occur when a patient pays with a check without having sufficient funds in the bank to cover the payment. The bank will return the check to the healthcare practice marked NSF and will charge the practice's bank account a returned check fee. The payment posted to the patient account must be reversed. It is important to note that the original payment is not deleted; instead, a charge line item is added to the patient account record with the amount of the NSF check (see Fig. 19.5). Many medical offices add additional line items for NSF fee charges, but this is up to the discretion of the provider.

If the healthcare facility receives an NSF check, call the signer of the check immediately and ask him or her to stop by the office to pay the amount needed to cover the check and the additional fee. Most offices require that such payment be made by another form of payment, preferably credit card. Legal remedies are available for the provider if the check remains unpaid.

Many NSF problems can be cleared up quickly and easily with courtesy and tact, assuming the situation was simply a mistake or an oversight. Bad checks may be reported to several organizations, and once the writer is in their databases, the person will have difficulty writing a check to any business. Turn the account over to a qualified collection agency if you are unable to collect on the account within a short time.

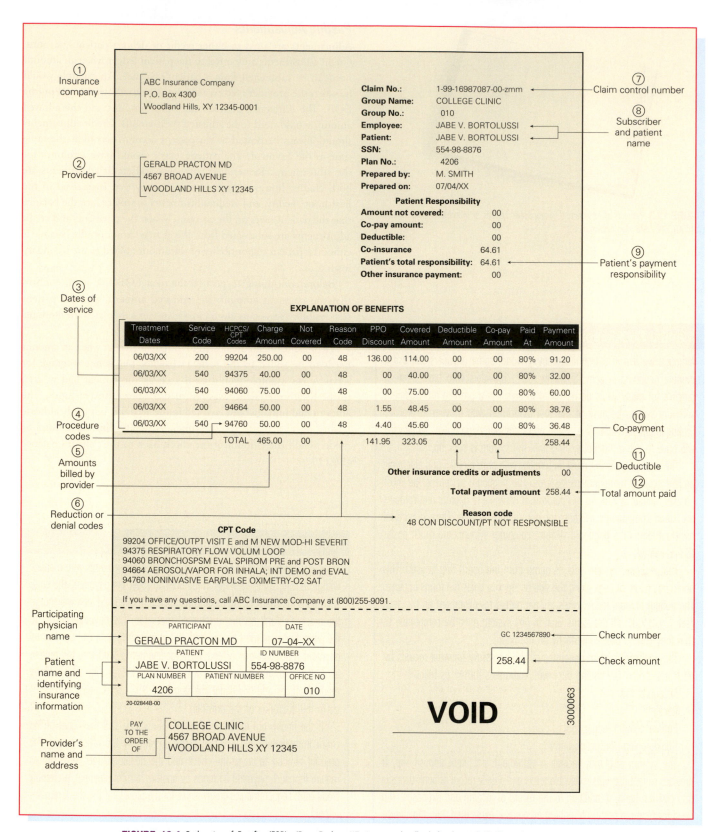

FIGURE 19.4 Explanation of Benefits (EOB). (From Fordney MT: *Insurance handbook for the medical office,* ed 14, St Louis, 2017, Elsevier.)

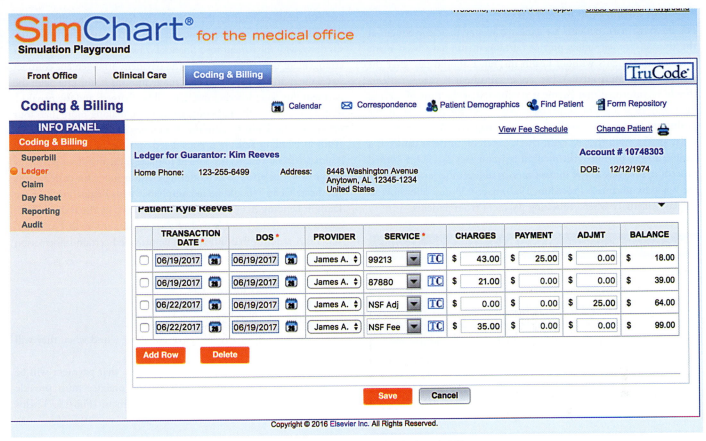

FIGURE 19.5 NSF Adjustments in SimChart for the Medical Office.

Credit Balances. A *credit balance* occurs when a patient has paid in advance, or an overpayment or duplicate payment is made. For example, an overpayment occurs if the patient makes a partial payment, and later the insurance payment is more than the remaining balance. When this happens, the patient account will show a credit balance, or an amount that the provider owes. The medical assistant should investigate to whom the credit balance is owed (i.e., the patient or the insurance company). The first place to look is the EOB from the insurance company; this document shows the exact amount of the patient's financial responsibility. The medical assistant should confirm that all the line items match the corresponding amounts on the EOB because many credit balances are created when an error is made in payment posting. If the patient's payment exceeded the amount indicated on the EOB, the provider must send a check for the balance to the patient. A credit balance creates a *debit* in the patient account, or an amount that is due by the provider to the patient or the insurance company, depending on which party made the overpayment. A debit adjustment is done showing that the patient or insurance

company was refunded. This debit adjustment should bring the account balance to zero.

Most patient account management software can enter charges, payments, and adjustments. As discussed previously, charges increase what is owed to the provider, whereas payments reduce what is owed to the provider, and adjustments can do both.

Payment at the Time of Service

For the most part, patients are expected to pay their copayment at the time of service unless previous arrangements have been made (Fig. 19.6). Patients without health insurance should pay after the visit has been completed. When an appointment is made, patients should be informed that payment is expected at the time of service. That way they are not surprised when asked for payment at the healthcare facility. The medical assistant may say, "Your charge for today is $25. Will that be cash, check, or credit or debit card?" If a patient asks to be billed, the medical assistant may say, "Our normal procedure is to pay at the time of service unless other arrangements are made in advance." Procedure 19.2 on p. 433 describes how to display sensitivity when requesting payment from patients.

Displaying Sensitivity When Requesting Payment

Informing a patient of the amount he or she will be required to pay before the person arrives for the appointment can help with the payment process. Use tact and good judgment when collecting payments. Understand that it can be uncomfortable for the patient to talk about money. Requests for payment should be made in a private setting. Do not be embarrassed to ask for payment for the valuable services that have been provided. Give each patient individual attention and personal consideration; also, be courteous and show a sincere desire to help the patient with financial problems.

CRITICAL THINKING APPLICATION   19.4

Adam Page comes to the front desk to pay his copay with a credit card. His card is declined. How can Laura handle the situation? What options could be offered to Mr. Page to make a payment at the time of service?

Payment Agreements

With the increase in high-deductible insurance plans, there has been an increase in the need for payment agreements. If the patient is having an elective procedure, payment can be made before or at the time of service. If the procedure or therapy is expensive, the patient may need to spread the payments out over time. Therefore, the medical assistant must explain to the patient the fees and the office credit policies. In most healthcare practices, the appropriate staff member sits down with the patient for a financial consultation before a payment arrangement contract is offered. The payment arrangement contract states the monthly payment; how many months it must be paid; the payment due date; whether interest will be charged; and the penalties of nonpayment. If the patient is going to be making more than four payments, the Truth in Lending Act comes into play.

Truth in Lending Act. It is considered an offer of credit when the healthcare facility allows the patient to make more than four payments on his or her balance. When offering credit options for patients, the healthcare facility should be in compliance with Regulation Z of the Truth in Lending Act (TILA). TILA is enforced by the Federal Trade Commission (FTC) and is part of the Consumer Credit Protection Act. TILA requires that individuals be provided certain information when credit is extended, including:

- The annual percentage rate (APR)
- The monthly interest rate
- The total costs to the borrower
- When payments are due
- The amount of any late payment charges and when they will be applied

If the healthcare facility and patient agree that payment will be made in more than four installments, the practice must provide a Federal Truth-in-Lending Disclosure Statement (Fig. 19.7). This

---

Walden-Martin Family Medical Clinic   DATE 2/20/2019
1234 Anystreet
Anytown, AL 12345-1234
(123) 123-1234

FEDERAL TRUTH IN LENDING STATEMENT

For Professional Services Rendered

Responsible Party: 2 Quinton Brown   Patient: 2 Quinton Brown
                   4554 Browning Street
                   Anytown, AL 12345-1234

1. Total Cash Price:	3553.00
2. Down Payment Amount:	200.00
3. Unpaid Balance of Cash Price:	0.00
4. Amount Financed:	3353.00
5. Total Finance Charge:	0.00
6. Finance Charge Expressed as Annual Percentage Rate:	0.00
7. Total of all Payments (4 + 5):	3353.00
8. Deferred Payment Price (2 + 4 + 5):	3553.00

Total of ALL PAYMENTS (item 7 above) is payable to our office at the above address in 4 monthly installments. The first 3 installments are $1,000.00 each. The first installment is payable on 2/20/2019 and each subsequent payment is due at the beginning payment period until paid in full.

The amount estimated to be covered by insurance is $0.00. Insurance coverage is only an estimation. Guarantor is responsible for all treatment not covered by insurance.

_____   2/20/2019
Signature of Patient (parent, if patient is a minor)   Date

_____   2/20/2019
Witness   Date

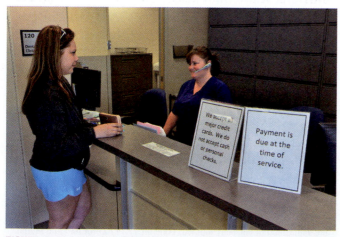

FIGURE 19.6 Most healthcare facilities display a sign informing patients that payments are due at the time of service.

FIGURE 19.7 Federal Truth-in-Lending Disclosure Statement. (Courtesy of Patterson Office Supplies, Inc.)

document should be in place even if no finance fees are charged. The statement is signed by the practice's representative and the patient.

Monthly Patient Account Statements

Healthcare facilities should send monthly statements for all patient accounts that have a balance due. A set schedule should be established for sending statements to patients. Sending them monthly is most common, but they can be sent every 2 weeks or even quarterly. When a monthly system is used, patient accounts are divided into equal segments, usually alphabetically. One segment is sent out each week of the month. This keeps an even flow of money into the healthcare facility. It can also spread out patients' calls about their statements. Statements should be printed on clean, good-quality paper. Payment options, such as check, e-check, online payments, and/or credit card, should be presented clearly. The statement should provide itemized details on the following:

- Date of service
- Services provided
- Insurance payments and adjustments
- Patient payments, including copayments

Envelopes should be printed with "Address Service Requested" in the appropriate place to maintain up-to-date mailing lists. A self-addressed return envelope included with the statement is convenient for the patient and encourages prompt payment. The statement should also indicate how old the balance is, such as 30, 60, 90, 120, or >120 days. For accounts that are more than 60 days past due, some offices apply neon-colored stickers to emphasize the need to pay the balance as soon as possible and thus avoid further collection activity.

Billing Minors

According to federal regulations, a minor cannot be held financially responsible for his or her account balance unless the individual is an **emancipated minor**. Bills for minors are usually addressed to the **guarantor**. If a bill is addressed to a minor, parents could take the stand that they are not responsible because they never received a statement.

If the parents are separated or divorced, the parent who brings the child in for treatment is responsible for payment. Whatever financial agreement exists between the parents is strictly their personal business and should not concern the healthcare practice. The responsible parent should be so informed from the first appointment.

If a minor appears in the office and requests treatment, you should determine if the person is legally emancipated. If he or she is, the minor will be financially responsible. Minors can be treated for certain conditions, such as sexually transmitted infections (STIs), pregnancy, and contraception, without parental consent. Each state has differences in the laws in these cases. Medical assistants must be familiar with their state laws and office polices to determine where the statement should be sent.

Medical Care for Those Who Cannot Pay

The medical profession traditionally has accepted the responsibility of providing medical care occasionally for individuals who are unable to pay for these services. There are government programs to help care for the medically **indigent**, but there are still patients who are not covered. In many instances, medical care for the indigent is available through social service agencies. Medical assistants should learn about local organizations and agencies that can aid patients in obtaining the necessary assistance. The provider can only provide medical services. Other agencies can help pay for hospitalization and arrange for and help pay for special therapy, rehabilitation, or medications.

Unfortunately, another segment of the population consists of uninsured or underinsured employees who are not eligible for public assistance, are not covered under a group policy, and cannot afford the high premiums for private medical insurance. Give special attention to helping these people arrange payment of their medical bills. If a provider knows in advance that a patient cannot pay for services and decides to still provide care, complete records must still be kept on the patient. The only difference in procedure is that an adjustment would be made to the account so that the balance would be zero.

Fees in Hardship Cases

Sometimes a healthcare practice is faced with the problem of deciding whether to reduce or cancel a fee in a hardship case. Before adjusting or canceling a fee, the provider or medical assistant should have a frank discussion with the patient about his or her financial situation. Find out whether the patient is entitled to or qualifies for medical assistance. If the patient's injuries are the result of a car accident, there may be medical insurance through the automobile policy. The patient may qualify for local or state public assistance, such as crime victim assistance. Maintain information about such agencies in the area and direct the patient to the appropriate one.

If the provider is aware of the hardship before services are provided, the fee can be discussed and payment arrangements made. The healthcare facility may suggest that a medically indigent patient seek care at a clinic that provides public assistance. A provider should be free to choose his or her form of charity and should not feel obligated to substantially reduce or cancel a fee when the circumstances are known in advance.

The provider and the patient may agree on a fee, but special circumstances may come up that create a hardship. If the provider agrees to reduce the fee, the patient should be told that the reduction will occur only after the adjusted amount is paid in full. For instance, if a fee of $500 is reduced to $350, the full amount of the $500 charge should appear on the ledger, and when $350 has been received, the remainder can be written off as an adjustment.

Pitfalls of Fee Adjustments

Problems can come up when a provider begins to reduce his or her fees. Patients may begin to expect fees to be reduced in all circumstances. Patients may even doubt the competency of a provider who habitually reduces fees. Make fee reductions the exception rather than the norm.

Take great care in reducing the fee for care of a patient who dies. This could be misinterpreted and result in a suit for malpractice. The family may suspect that the fee was reduced because the provider knew he or she made an error.

Collection Procedures

When to Start Collection Procedures

Collection is the process of using all legal resources available to collect payment for past due patient account balances. Sometimes a patient may have difficulty meeting all of his or her financial obligations. The patient may have lost a job or insurance coverage. An emergency could arise that depletes finances. When patients must choose between paying their medical bills and having electricity, the provider is often forced to wait for payment. Although a few patients absolutely refuse to pay for their medical care, most are honest and willing to pay but may need help with a payment plan. As discussed earlier, terms can be arranged for collecting payment in full when the office and the patient cooperate with each other. The medical assistant should attempt to work out a plan that the patient can abide by, and the patient should be expected to make promised payments. For those patients who do not pay their bill, further action is necessary.

Preparing Patient Accounts for Collection Activity

Sometimes it becomes necessary to aggressively attempt to collect the balances that patients owe. Collection procedures include telephone calls, collection reminders and letters, and personal interviews.

Before you begin collection action, it is essential to determine which accounts have a balance due and how old the account balance is. Some accounts are grouped together, or "aged," according to the dates of the last payment activity, whereas others are grouped according to the original date of service (Fig. 19.8). Common account aging categories are:

- Current
- 31–60 days
- 61–90 days
- 91–120 days
- >120 days

Most bills with balances less than 30 days old are probably waiting for the health insurance to pay, so no collection action is needed. Patient account balances more than 90 or 120 days old require a final demand letter before the account is turned over to a collection agency. Always allow the provider to review and approve the list of patient accounts being sent to a collection agency.

The medical assistant can use a variety of techniques to collect patient accounts, such as collection phone calls, collection letters, and skip tracing. Often more than one technique must be used to obtain payment. Always be courteous and kind when using all collection techniques.

Collection Telephone Calls

Whenever attempts are made to collect a debt, the Fair Debt Collection Practices Act must be kept in mind. A telephone call at the right time, with the right presentation, is more successful than notes, patient account statements, or collection letters. The personal contact call often prompts patients to mail in their payment or to make payments over the phone with a credit card. If the staff does not have enough time to make calls, the collection letter is the next best approach. If collections are a serious problem, it may be worth an extra salary to hire a person to make the phone calls.

Fair Debt Collection Practices Act

In March 1978, the Fair Debt Collection Practices Act went into effect. It was designed to eliminate abusive, deceptive, and unfair debt collection practices. The act states that collection calls cannot be made:

- at any time or place that is unusual or known to be inconvenient to the patient; before 8 a.m. or after 9 p.m.
- when the creditor is aware that the debtor is represented by an attorney with respect to the debt.
- to the patient's place of work if the patient's employer prohibits such contacts.

Always treat patients with the utmost respect on the telephone. Keep their financial record nearby in case they have questions about their bill; also, have their insurance company's phone number handy. Remember that some patients may not understand anything about insurance or third-party payers. Helping them to understand and acting as their advocate in getting as much reimbursement as possible can reduce the patient's share. Never simply insist that the insurance plan has paid, and the patient's balance is due. This puts the patient in a negative mindset. Try using phrases such as the following:

- "Mrs. Diggs, it looks as if your insurance company paid late last month. You have co-insurance for your surgery that amounts to $450. Let me review some payment options to help make that as easy as possible for you to pay."
- "Mr. Hildebrand, we're showing that you have a balance due from your surgery. Your insurance has paid, and it looks as if you owe $700. We would be happy to help you by splitting that into two or three payments. When can I schedule that first payment for you?"
- "Mrs. Crumley, it seems that you have a balance due of $450 from your surgery, and I called to see whether I could help you budget that. For example, you could pay $50 this week and split the remaining $400 into two payments over the next 2 months."

Always abide by office policy when making payment arrangements in collection situations. Never be **belligerent** with a patient. If the person becomes angry, simply state that he or she can call back when ready to discuss a solution for paying the account, say good-bye, and gently hang up the phone. Never listen to **expletives** or allow verbal abuse. Respectfully end the phone call by saying thank you and good-bye; do not slam down the phone.

Before a final demand for payment is made, a letter must be sent indicating that legal or collection proceedings will be started.

General Rules for Telephone Collections

What to do:

- Call the patient when it can be done privately.
- Call only between 8 a.m. and 9 p.m.
- Determine the identity of the person with whom you are speaking. If you ask, "Is this Mrs. Noble?" and she answers, "Yes," it could be the patient's mother-in-law or daughter-in-law, who may also be "Mrs. Noble." Use the person's full name. Include suffixes, such as "Thomas Melborn, III." This may sound too formal, but it helps to ensure that the correct person is on the phone.

Patient Account Aging Report: Walden-Martin Family Medical Clinic

Starting Date: 9/1/2020 **Ending Date: 9/30/2020** **Report Date 9/30/2020**

Jacob Abraham (3406) — Last Payment: 7/12/2020 — 15.00
Guarantor: Self — Home: 954-233-9033 — Work: NA

Date	Code	Billed	Current	31-60	61-90	91-120	>120	Total
7/12/2020	99201	45.00			45.00			45.00
7/12/2020	Cash	(15.00)			(15.00)			(15.00)
Patient Total		30.00	0.00	0.00	30.00	0.00	0.00	30.00

Frank Bullock (3412) — Last Payment: 8/20/2020 — 45.00
Guarantor: Wife — Home 954-388-0196 — Work: 954-233-5803

Date	Code	Billed	Current	31-60	61-90	91-120	>120	Total
8/20/2020	99205	195.00		195.00				195.00
8/20/2020	Check	(45.00)		(45.00)				(45.00)
Patient Total		150.00	0.00	150.00	0.00	0.00	0.00	150.00

Cynthia Dearing (3433) — Last Payment: 7/25/2020 — 10.00
Guarantor: Self — Home: 953-518-2100 — Work: 954-333-9003

Date	Code	Billed	Current	31-60	61-90	91-120	>120	Total
6/12/2020	99386	185.00				185.00		185.00
7/15/2020	BCBS	(160.00)				(160.00)		(160.00)
7/25/2020	Check	(10.00)				(10.00)		(10.00)
Patient Total		15.00	0.00	0.00	0.00	15.00	0.00	15.00

Kirsha Macken (3462) — Last Payment: 7/10/2020 — 50.00
Guarantor: Parent — Home: 954-736-7227 — Work: FT Student

Date	Code	Billed	Current	31-60	61-90	91-120	>120	Total
4/23/2020	58900	230.00					230.00	230.00
4/23/2020	Cash	(50.00)					(50.00)	(50.00)
7/10/2020	99214	90.00		3309	90.00			90.00
7/10/2020	90658	30.00			30.00			30.00
7/10/2020	Cash	(50.00)			(50.00)			(50.00)
Patient Total		250.00	0.00	0.00	70.00	0.00	180.00	250.00

Larry Nerod (3501) — Last Payment: 6/22/2020 — 15.00
Guarantor: Self — Home: 953-736-7227 — Work: 954-332-001

Date	Code	Billed	Current	31-60	61-90	91-120	>120	Total
6/22/2020	99204	140.00				140.00		140.00
6/22/2020	CCard	(15.00)				(15.00)		(15.00)
Patient Total		125.00	0.00	0.00	0.00	125.00	0.00	125.00

Emanuel Perez (3513) — Last Payment: 7/12/2020 — 46.00
Guarantor: Self — Home: 956-303-2070 — Work: 953-322-5500

Date	Code	Billed	Current	31-60	61-90	91-120	>120	Total
7/12/2020	68500	403.00			403.00			403.00
7/12/2020	Check	(46.00)			(46.00)			(46.00)
Patient Total		357.00	0.00	0.00	357.00	0.00	0.00	357.00

| Report Totals | | | 0.00 | 150.00 | 457.00 | 140.00 | 180.00 | 927.00 |
| Percent of Total | | | 0.00% | 16.18% | 49.3% | 15.10% | 19.41% | 100.00% |

FIGURE 19.8 Sample Aging Report.

- Be respectful. One can be friendly and professional at the same time.
- Ask the patient whether it is a convenient time to talk. Unless you have the attention of the patient, there is little to be gained by continuing. If you are told that it is an inopportune time, ask for a specific time to call back or get a promise that the patient will call the office at a specified time.
- After a brief greeting, state the purpose of the call. Make no apology for calling, but state the reason in a friendly, businesslike way. The provider expects payment, and the medical assistant is interested in helping the patient meet the financial obligation. Open the call with a phrase such as, "This is Alice, Dr. Walden's medical assistant. I'm calling about your account." A well-placed pause at this point in the call sometimes gets an immediate response from the debtor with regard to the nonpayment.
- Assume a positive attitude. For example, convey the impression that the patient intended to pay, and it is only a matter of working out some suitable arrangements.
- Keep the conversation brief and to the point; do not make threats of any kind.
- Try to get a definite commitment – payment of a certain amount by a certain date.
- Follow up on promises made by the patient. This is best accomplished by using a **tickler file** or a note on the calendar. If the payment does not arrive by the promised date, remind the patient with another call. If the medical assistant fails to do this, the whole effort has been wasted.
- Document the call in the patient's record.
  What *not* to do:
- Do not call between 9 p.m. and 8 a.m. To do so may be considered harassment.
- Do not make repeated telephone calls on the same day.
- Do not call the patient's place of work if the employer prohibits personal calls.
- If a call is placed to the patient at work and the person cannot take the call, leave a message asking the patient to "call Ms. Black at 951-727-9238" without revealing the nature of the call; that is, do not state that the call is from "Dr. Walden's office" or "Dr. Walden's medical assistant."
- Refrain from showing any kind of hostility. An angry patient is a poorly paying patient. Insulted patients often do not pay at all.

Collection Letters

Some experts believe that a printed collection letter or reminder enclosed with a statement is more effective than a personal letter. The idea is that a patient may be embarrassed by a personal letter and feel that he or she has been singled out for attention. An impersonal printed message will probably encourage the patient to send a payment.

Letters that are friendly requests for an explanation of why payment has not been made are effective in most cases. These letters should indicate that the provider is sincerely interested in the patient's health and well-being and wants to help resolve the financial obligation. Invite the patient to the office to explain the reasons for nonpayment so that payment arrangements can be made. To lessen the patient's embarrassment, these letters can suggest that previous statements may have been overlooked.

When receiving these letters, most patients make some effort to explain their failure to make payment. If a patient really is having financial difficulties, he or she may be able to get some type of assistance. If it is a temporary financial problem, the provider and the patient may work together to come up with a satisfactory installment plan for payment.

The medical assistant is often given a free hand in designing collection patterns and composing collection letters. Many medical assistants compose a series of collection letters using example letters they have found effective. Such a series usually includes at least five letters in varying degrees of forcefulness.

Sometimes even a person with poor paying habits will pay, as long as he or she is treated with respect and consideration. The medical assistant should never go beyond the authority granted by the provider in pursuing collections. If questions come up about special collection problems, always check with the provider or office manager before proceeding. The provider and the medical assistant should agree on general collection policies, as outlined earlier in this chapter, and the policies should be followed. In all cases when an account is to be assigned to a collection agency, make sure the provider is aware and approves.

In most healthcare facilities, the medical assistant signs collection letters using his or her title, such as "Medical Assistant" below the typewritten signature. Do not list "Collections" below the name, because the patient may assume that the account has been placed with a collection agency. Some providers want to sign these communications personally, but generally the medical assistant who handles the patient accounts also signs the collection letters.

Personal Finance Interviews

Personal finance interviews with patients can sometimes be more effective than a whole series of collection letters. Oftentimes speaking with a patient face-to-face can result in a better understanding of the problem, and an agreement about future payment plans can be reached (Fig. 19.9).

Occasionally a patient may undergo a long course of treatment and yet make no attempt to pay anything on the account. The patient may be waiting for the provider or the medical assistant to suggest that a payment be made. When it is known in advance that the

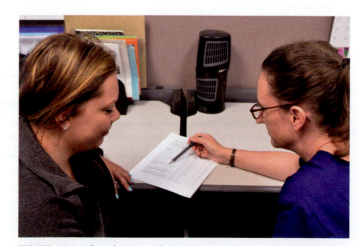

FIGURE 19.9 A face-to-face personal finance interview may motivate patients to take steps to settle their account balances.

patient requires extensive treatment, the matter of payment should be discussed early in the course of treatment. The credit policy should be explained, and some agreement should be reached on a payment plan.

Because medical services are far more **intangible** than any commercial service, collection efforts must not be delayed too long. Most responsible, sincere patients will call the provider's office after receiving a second statement and explain the delay in payment or ask for a payment plan. This is best accomplished in a private, personal interview.

If the account ultimately must be referred to a collection agency, find a good agency with a high recovery rate. All collection activity is costly. Know when to stop and call on the services of a professional agency.

Collection Situations

Tracing Skips. When a patient account statement is returned marked "Moved—no forwarding address," you may consider this account a skip. This could be an innocent error on the part of the patient, who may have forgotten to provide a forwarding address to the post office. The patient could also be attempting to avoid liability for debts. Whichever is the case, immediate action should be taken. Do not wait until the next billing cycle to attempt to trace the debtor.

The internet can be a valuable tool in tracing skips. You can use the online white pages to search for the patient's name. Patients might even be found on social networking sites, such as Facebook, and that information may provide clues about the person's whereabouts. Investigate the search results carefully so that collection efforts are directed at the right person. If all attempts fail, turn the account over to a collection agency without delay. Do not keep a skip account too long because as time passes, the trail may become so cold that even collection experts won't be able to follow it.

Suggestions for Tracing Skips

- Review the patient's original office registration card.
- Call the telephone number listed in the patient account record. Occasionally a patient may move without leaving a forwarding address but will transfer the old telephone number.
- If you are unable to contact the individual by telephone, make a few discreet calls to the references listed on the registration card to get leads.
- Check the internet to find the names and telephone numbers of neighbors or the landlord and contact these people to obtain information about the debtor's whereabouts.
- Do not inform a third party that the patient owes money. Simply state that you are trying to locate or verify the location of the individual.
- Check the guarantor's place of employment for information. If the person is a specialist in his or her field of work, the local union or similar organizations may be contacted. Although they may not give you the person's current address, they will relay the message that you are seeking to contact him or her. Often people are prompted to pay if they think their employer may learn of their failure to pay.

Claims Against Estates. The patient account for a deceased patient may be handled a little differently from regular accounts. Courtesy dictates that a bill not be sent immediately, but do not delay longer than 30 days. The **executor** will expect to receive the statements from all healthcare providers. Use the following format to address the statement:

- Estate of (name of patient)
- c/o (spouse, next of kin, or executor if known)
- Patient's last known address

A will generally is filed within 30 days of a death. The name of the executor usually can be obtained by sending a request to the Probate Department of the Superior Court, County Recorder's Office, in the county where the person lived. The time limits for filing an estate claim are determined by the state where the person resided.

An itemized statement should be sent to the executor of the estate by certified mail, return receipt requested. If no response is received in 10 days, contact the executor or the county clerk where the estate is being settled and obtain forms for filing a claim against the estate. This claim against the estate must be made within a certain time. This time frame varies from 2 to 36 months, depending on the state where it is filed.

The executor of the estate either accepts or rejects the claim. If it is accepted, the executor will send an acknowledgment of the debt. Payment can be delayed because of the legal complications involved in settling an estate. If the claim has been accepted, the provider eventually receives the payment. If the executor rejects the claim, file a claim against the executor according to state laws. The time limit in such cases starts with the date on the letter of rejection.

States have different time limits and statutes with regard to these issues. The medical assistant should contact the provider's attorney or the local court for the exact procedure to follow. Or, the provider may prefer to turn such matters over to his or her legal counsel immediately.

Bankruptcy. Bankruptcy laws were passed to ensure equal distribution of the **assets** of an individual among the individual's creditors. These are federal laws that apply in all the states. When notified that a patient has declared bankruptcy, do not send statements or make any attempt to collect on the account from the patient.

Chapter 9 bankruptcy is usually a "no asset" situation. Because the provider's charges are considered an **unsecured debt**, there is little purpose in pursuing collection. Chapter 16 is known as *wage-earner bankruptcy*, which means that the patient-debtor pays to a **trustee** a fixed amount agreed upon by the court. This money is passed on to the creditors. During this period, none of the creditors can attach the debtor's wages or otherwise attempt to collect the debt. However, the debts are paid in order, secured debts first. Consequently, the provider may never receive payment from a debtor who has filed for bankruptcy.

Using a Collection Agency

The medical assistant should try every means possible to collect on accounts before they become delinquent. An account should be sent to a collection agency as soon all collection activities have been exhausted. If the patient has failed to respond to the final letter or has twice failed to send a promised payment, the account should be considered uncollectable. Skips should be sent immediately.

Even though the collection agency will keep 40% to 60% of the amount owed, waiting only reduces the chances of recovery by the professional collector. If the agency finds that the case deserves special consideration, it will ask the provider's advice before proceeding further.

The collection agency represents the healthcare facility. Therefore, the healthcare facility should ensure that its patients are treated with as much respect and dignity as possible throughout the collection process. There are many different collection agencies. If one doesn't work out, prepare to switch to another that can better represent the healthcare practice.

A collection agency needs certain data to begin collection procedures on overdue accounts:

- Guarantor's full name
- Spouse's full name
- Last known address
- Full amount of the debt
- Date of the last entry (charge, payment, or adjustment) on the account
- Occupation of the debtor
- Employer's address and phone number

After an account has been sent to a collection agency, the healthcare facility can make no further collection attempts. Once the agency has begun its work, a number of guidelines and procedures should be followed:

- Send no more patient statements.
- The patient account should be closed for activity because the account was forwarded to a collection agency. The balance should be written off.
- Refer the patient to the collection agency if he or she contacts the office about the account.
- Promptly report any payments made directly to your office to the collection agency and pay the collection agency's fee.
- Call the agency if any information is obtained that will be of value in tracing or collecting the account.

CRITICAL THINKING APPLICATION 19.5

Laura has had several complaints about the collection agency used by the office. Patients have called to report that the collectors are threatening and unprofessional. The collection agency's supervisor has been disrespectful to patients and has said that because they owe the money, the collection agency's job is to collect the account in whatever way necessary. How should the healthcare facility approach the collection agency about these complaints?

Posting Collection Agency Transactions. Collection agencies charge the healthcare practice different percentages of the amount owed to collect delinquent accounts; the agency with the cheapest fee is rarely the most effective. Agencies pay the *net back,* which is the amount of money paid to the practice after the agency has been paid its fee. The net back is the figure that should be considered when a collection agency is used, not simply the fee percentage. If a patient sends a payment after the account has been turned over to a collection agency, the payment must be recorded in the patient account record. Because the agency charges a fee for its collection efforts, the amount sent

to the healthcare facility might be less than the actual payment amount. For instance, if the agency charges 25%, a $100 payment results in a $75 payment to the healthcare facility and the agency keeps $25. When the payment is posted, the patient account must credit the full amount paid to the collection agency. This would be done by posting a $75 payment and $25 adjustment (Fig. 19.10; see Procedure 19.3 on p. 433).

Small Claims Court

Many healthcare practices find **small claims court** a satisfactory, inexpensive means of collecting delinquent accounts. State law places a limit on the amount of debt for which relief may be sought in small claims court. This limit should be determined before the small claims court process is started.

Parties to small claims actions are not represented by an attorney at the hearing but may send another person to court on their behalf to produce records supporting the claim. Providers often send their medical assistant with records of unpaid accounts to show the judge.

If the court awards a judgment for the amount owed, the **plaintiff** in small claims court may also recover the costs of the suit. For a very small investment in time and money, the provider who uses this method saves the time of a civil court action and eliminates attorneys' fees.

After being awarded a judgment, the healthcare practice must still collect the money. The only person in a small claims action who has the right of appeal is the **defendant**. An appeal by the defendant may have the judgment set aside. The plaintiff cannot file an appeal in a small claims action; the decision of the court is final.

The necessary papers for filing action and full instructions on the course to follow may be obtained from the clerk of the local small claims court. It would be wise for a medical assistant who has never appeared in court to attend once as a spectator to preview the procedure; this should allow him or her to feel more at ease when appearing for the provider.

ACCOUNTS PAYABLE (A/P)

Managing accounts payable may be the responsibility of the medical assistant. There are many aspects of accounts payable, which will be discussed in the next section.

Banking in Today's Business World

Banks can be used to centralize all financial transactions for a healthcare facility. The bank account tracks all deposits, withdrawals, and transfers. Monthly bank account balances can help healthcare facilities establish and maintain a monthly operational budget. Banks also provide opportunities to earn **interest** and to invest for future financial gain. Overall, banks organize funds for the financial management of the healthcare facility.

Fees for banking services depend on the bank and services used (Table 19.1). The type of bank the medical practice will use is a decision made by the provider and the office manager, depending on the needs of the medical practice.

Although the **Federal Reserve Bank** (Fig. 19.11) manages all banks in the United States, healthcare facilities can choose from a number of different types of banks with which to do business.

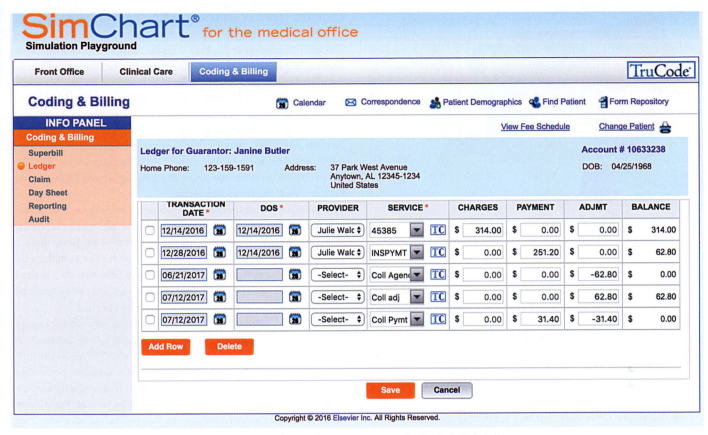

FIGURE 19.10 Posting a collection agency payment in SimChart for the Medical Office.

TABLE 19.1	Common Banking Fees		
FEE	**DESCRIPTION**	**AVERAGE FEE**	**WAIVABLE?**
Account maintenance fee	Fee for using the bank account	$5 to $25 per month	Some bank accounts waive monthly account maintenance fees if a specific balance is maintained in the account or if direct deposit is used.
Overdraft fee	Fee for the bank paying a check or debit when the balance is not in the account	$25 to $40 per occurrence	Not usually. To avoid the fee in the future, tie the checking account with an overdraft account just in case the balance is low.
Returned deposit fee	Fee charged when a deposited check is returned from the drawer's account	$5 to $10 per occurrence	Not usually. However, the practice can require the check drawer to cover this expense because the check did not clear his or her account.
Hard copy statement fee	Fee for the bank to send paper copies of bank statements	$5 to $10 per statement	This fee can be avoided by downloading all electronic bank statements when they are released.
Nonsufficient funds (NSF) fee	Fee charged when a check is written against an account with not enough funds and the check is returned unpaid	$25 to $40 per occurrence	Not usually. To avoid the fee in the future, tie the checking account with an overdraft account just in case the balance is low.
Transaction fee	Fee charged when too many transactions are made on a bank account	$.50 to $1 per transaction	Online banking is usually free, but nowadays banks are charging fees to visit bank branches and to complete transactions with customer service over the phone.

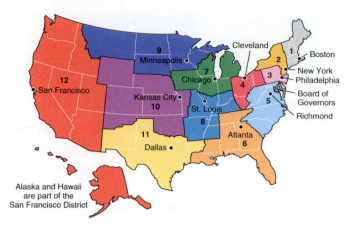

FIGURE 19.11 The 12 Federal Reserve districts.

- *Retail banks:* Offer basic banking services to the public; these banks have hundreds of branches to provide easy consumer access.
- *Commercial banks:* Offer business banking services to businesses of all sizes; they are equipped to handle large volumes of check deposits and credit card transactions.
- *Credit unions:* Nonprofit banking institutions owned by members; credit unions use the funds deposited to make loans to their members, which enables them to offer loans at lower than market rates.
- *Online banks:* Offer basic banking services at competitive rates because all banking transactions are done online; there are no branch locations to visit.

The medical assistant will most likely manage only the bank accounts set up for the income and operational expenses of the healthcare facility.

Because of their large volume of bookkeeping transactions, many healthcare facilities use accounting management software. Most online banking systems allow for the download of bank account data. These software systems can be complicated to use, so the medical assistant should be in regular contact with the accountant chosen by the provider, who can answer questions when needed.

The Federal Reserve

In 1913 Congress created the Federal Reserve Banking System. This was to provide the nation with a safer, more flexible, and stable monetary and financial system. The system consists of:

- a seven-member Board of Governors with headquarters in Washington, D.C.
- 12 Federal Reserve banks in major cities throughout the country (see Fig. 19.11)

The Federal Reserve Bank monitors the movement of money, in the form of checks, from one bank account to another. Each check has:

- a routing number
- an account number

These numbers identify which Federal Reserve Bank jurisdiction, bank location, and specific bank accounts are used in each transaction.

For additional information on the Federal Reserve System and its regional banks, visit the system's website: *https://www.federalreserve.gov.*

Common Types of Bank Accounts

Checking Accounts. By placing an amount of money in a bank, a depositor can set up a checking account. Simply stated, a checking account is a bank account against which checks can be written, or debit cards used, and funds can be transferred to the payable party. Banks typically charge a monthly account maintenance fee. In addition, there may be fees associated with banking services, such as transferring funds to other banks or using the checking overdraft (see Table 19.1).

Savings Accounts. Money that is not needed for current expenses can be deposited into a savings account. In most cases, savings accounts earn a higher interest rate than checking accounts. Interest rates fluctuate with the financial market.

A standard savings account earns interest at the lowest prevailing rate and has no minimum balance requirement and no check-writing privileges. However, penalties apply for withdrawing funds from a savings account more than six times per month. The provider may deposit a certain percentage of **discretionary income** into a savings account each month to earn interest. The money in a savings account can be transferred to a checking account when needed.

Money Market Savings Account. An insured money market savings account combines features of a checking and savings account. A minimum balance is required (anywhere from $500 to $5,000). It earns interest at money market rates (usually a higher percentage rate than for a regular savings account), and it allows only a specified number of checks (frequently three) to be written per month. Such checks are usually written to transfer funds to a checking account. Some businesses transfer excess funds from the business checking account to a money market account over the weekend, or over an extended holiday period to earn higher interest on the funds.

Signature Cards

When an account is opened at a bank branch, the account signer is required to provide his or her handwritten signature on a physical or electronic card, which is kept on file with the bank. If a check comes through and some suspicion arises that the depositor's signature has been forged, bank personnel compare the signature on the check with the original on the signature card.

The task of paying bills is often delegated to a responsible medical assistant. In this case, any staff member who has been authorized to sign the medical facility's checks must go to the bank and add his or her handwritten signature to the signature card. Only those whose names appear on the signature card are authorized to sign checks, and the bank is responsible for verifying any questionable signatures.

Online Banking

Internet banking has changed the way financial institutions manage money. People once had to fight traffic and wait in line at crowded banks; now, they can bank from their offices any time of day. A healthcare facility's banking transactions, such as paying bills and transferring funds between accounts, can be done online. In addition, staff members have access to supply companies online and can easily review costs from the office instead of driving to numerous companies to compare prices.

Online banking is a means of performing banking services electronically via the internet. All banks and credit unions have this capability, and most of them offer both basic and advanced services. With basic services, a customer usually can do the following:

- Check account balances
- Transfer funds between accounts in the same bank
- Pay bills electronically and create checks
- Determine whether a check has cleared the bank
- Download account information
- View images of transactions

More advanced services include being able to deposit checks online.

A major concern with online banking is fraud. Concern that unauthorized users may gain access to the healthcare facility's account balances is valid. Some experts believe that online banking involves a slightly greater risk of fraud than does conventional banking. Despite the disadvantages, studies show that internet banking is now mainstream.

Checks

A *check* is a bank draft, or an order to pay a certain sum of money, on demand, to a specified person or entity. When a check is presented for payment, the *drawee* (the bank on which the check is drawn or written) pays the specified sum of money written on the face of the check to the *holder* (the person presenting the check for payment).

A check is considered a **negotiable instrument**. For a check to be negotiable, it must:

- be written and signed by the *drawer* (the person who writes the check).
- contain a promise or order to pay a sum of money.
- be payable on demand or at a fixed future date.

To ensure that the amount is taken from the correct account number, the routing and account numbers are printed with magnetic ink on the bottom of the check. The check should have the amount written as a number and as text to confirm the amount. Finally, the check must be signed and dated by the drawer of the account.

Routing and Account Numbers

A *routing transit number* (RTN) is a nine-digit code printed on the bottom left side of checks. A RTN is assigned to every banking institution under the Federal Reserve Banking System. It identifies the bank upon which the check was drawn. RTNs are also used for direct deposits and the transfer of funds between banks. The first two digits indicate the Federal Reserve district where the bank is located. The third digit indicates the specific district office. And the rest of the digits represent the individual accounts that belong to the bank.

Bank account numbers are assigned to each individual account. No two account numbers in the same financial institution can be the same. *Wire transfers* and *automated clearinghouse (ACH) transfers* use the routing and account numbers to transfer funds between exact accounts. Wire transfers are between two separate banking institutions in which both accounts are verified, so funds are available quickly. ACH transfers also involve two different banking institutions, but because both accounts are not verified, a few extra days are needed for funds to be available.

Types of Negotiable Instruments

The following are different types of negotiable instruments:

- Personal check
- Cashier's check
- Money order
- Business check
- Voucher check

Personal Check. A personal check is drawn by a bank against funds deposited to a personal account in another bank. Patients typically write these checks for copayments and other financial responsibilities.

Cashier's Check. A cashier's check is a bank's own check, drawn on itself and signed by the bank cashier or other authorized official. A cashier's check is obtained by paying the bank the amount of the check, in cash. Many banks charge a fee for this service. Cashier's checks often are issued for a savings account customer who does not have a checking account.

Money Order. Money orders can be purchased at banks, some retail stores, and the U.S. Postal Service. Money orders are often used to pay bills by mail when a person does not have a checking account. The maximum face value varies, depending on the source. Cashier checks are preferable to money orders when larger amounts need to be paid.

Business Check. The checkbook most widely used in the professional office is a ledger-type book with three checks per page and a perforated stub at the left side of the check. The stubs serve as the checking account register, where the balance of the account is tracked. The checks and matching stubs are numbered in sequence and preprinted with the depositor's name and account number, along with any additional information, such as address and telephone number. Business checks can also be printed through accounting management software programs when vendors submit invoices. Today, most business checks can be prepared through online banking.

Voucher Check. A voucher check has a detachable voucher form or could be attached to an EOB. The voucher portion is used to itemize or specify the purpose for which the check was drawn. The voucher portion of the check is removed before the check is presented for deposit. The voucher is then used to post the payment in the patient account ledger (Fig. 19.12).

How Checks Are Processed from One Bank to Another

Checks received by the drawee's bank are turned over daily to a regional banking clearinghouse, which clears each one. The identifying code numbers, printed on the face of the check with magnetic ink, enable this "clearing" process to be accomplished quickly and efficiently. Checks due from and to all banks outside a specific region are settled by electronic entries. The bank keeps the canceled checks, and an electronic copy of the check is returned to the *drawer,* or the writer of the check. When the drawer needs proof of payment, a copy of the check can be requested from the bank, or the drawer can review monthly bank statements for printed copies of cleared checks. Check copies can also be obtained online through the banking portal.

Electronic Check. In an effort to prevent check fraud, many healthcare facilities accept only electronic checks. When the patient presents a personal check to the healthcare facility, the bottom of the check, which includes the routing and account numbers, is scanned. The funds are then automatically transferred from the patient's checking account and into the healthcare facility's account. Once the transaction has been approved, the paper check is returned to the patient with "VOID" printed across it to show that it has already been used. Electronic checks reduce the time involved in transferring funds from one account to another.

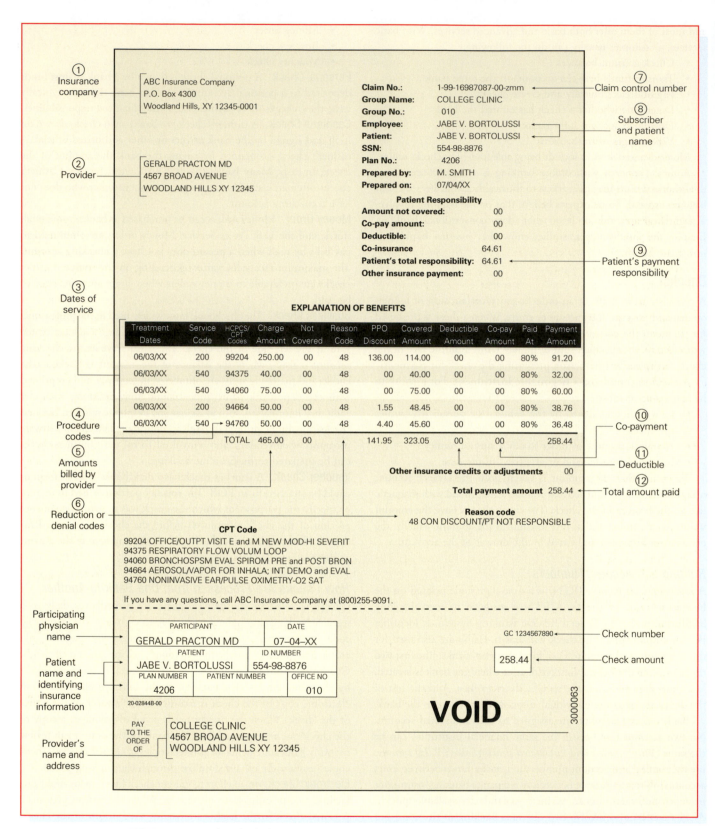

FIGURE 19.12 Sample voucher check. (From Fordney MT: *Insurance handbook for the medical office*, ed 14, St Louis, 2017, Elsevier.)

Patient Payment Management
Cash Payments

Some patients may prefer to pay in cash instead of by check or debit or credit card. Cash transactions can occur with little or no paperwork; therefore, an audit trail is harder to establish.

To prevent the mismanagement of cash, many healthcare facilities do not allow patients to pay cash for services. Healthcare facilities that have a no-cash payment policy should post a sign in the lobby to inform patients of this in advance. If a patient does not have a bank account, the medical staff can kindly refer the patient to a local money order dealer. Patients may see this as an inconvenience, but the medical assistant should explain that the policy is intended to protect the patient's account.

If the healthcare facility chooses to accept cash payments, keep in mind the following precautions:

- Make sure the cash is not **counterfeit**; use a marker or tool designed for this purpose to confirm its authenticity. If you suspect that the cash may be counterfeit, do not accept the payment and contact the local law enforcement office.
- Establish a checks-and-balance system in which the employee accepting cash must document cash payments on a register and in the patient's account to establish an audit trail.
- Inform patients that change cannot be made for larger bills.

Checks

Most payments sent through the mail are in the form of a personal check. Patients may also write a check when they are making a payment at the time of service. If it is the healthcare facility's policy to accept checks, then certain precautions need to be taken including:

- Inspect the check carefully for the correct date, amount, and signature.
- Do not accept a check with corrections on it.
- Ask for a state-issued picture ID and compare the signature on the ID to the check signature.
- Do not accept an out-of-town check, government check, payroll check, starter check, unnumbered check, or a nonpersonalized check.
- Do not accept a third-party check. For example, Mrs. Richards, a patient, receives a check written to her by her neighbor for $30. Mrs. Richards brings the check to her visit with the provider and presents it to the clinic to pay her copayment. If the check is accepted and subsequently returned by the bank, obtaining reimbursement from the patient or the neighbor may be difficult. A check from the patient's health insurance carrier is the only exception.
- When accepting a postal money order for payment, make sure it has only one endorsement. Postal money orders with more than two endorsements will not be honored.
- Do not accept a check marked "Payment in Full" unless it does pay the account in full, up to and including the date on which it is received. If a check so marked is less than the amount due, you will be unable to collect the balance on the account once you have accepted and deposited such a check. It is illegal to cross out the words "Payment in Full."
- Do not accept a check written for more than the amount due; returning cash for the difference between the amount of the check

and the amount owed is poor policy. If the check is not honored by the bank, your office suffers the loss not only of the amount of the check, but also of the amount returned in cash.

CRITICAL THINKING APPLICATION 19.6
A new patient wants to pay for his services at the end of the office visit. The charge is $75. The patient writes a check for $100 and asks Laura for $25 in currency in return. How should Laura handle the situation?

Debit Cards

Most debit cards are connected to a checking account. When the debit card is used, the amount of the transaction is immediately withdrawn from the available balance in the account. A personal identification number (PIN) is assigned to the card for cash withdrawal and point-of-sale (POS) purchases. The cards usually have a MasterCard or Visa logo and can be used wherever they are accepted. In most situations, when there are not enough funds in the account to make a purchase, the card is declined unless the account has some type of overdraft protection. Substantial fees may be charged if the bank elects to pay the debit when the account has insufficient funds.

Currently, some banks decline debit card charges at the point of sale when an account has insufficient funds. They do not charge an insufficient funds fee toward the attempted purchase. Stay abreast of recent banking legislation and always follow office policy when accepting debit cards as payment for medical services. The medical assistant may see various types of debit cards in the provider's office. Many states issue a debit card to individuals receiving child support payments or some types of state financial assistance.

Advantages of Using Debit Cards
Using debit cards for payment has many advantages:
1. Debit cards are both safe and convenient, particularly for making payments online.
2. Transactions are completed quickly.
3. The cards can be used either as debit or credit cards. For use as a debit card, the user must have a personal identification number (PIN). For use as a credit card, the user often must provide identification.
4. If stolen or lost, the debit card can be cancelled quickly with minimum liability.
5. Receipts and statements provide a permanent, reliable record of disbursements for tax purposes.
6. The debit card statement provides a summary of receipts.
7. The cards usually can be used anywhere that accepts MasterCard or Visa.

Credit Cards

Credit cards are a common method of payment from patients. Drawbacks of credit card payments include the small processing fee that is deducted from the amount deposited into the healthcare facility's bank account. There is also an increased risk of fraud with credit cards.

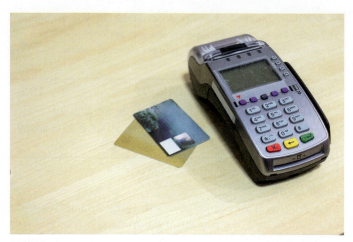

FIGURE 19.13 Card reader terminal with both EMV chip and magnetic strip readers. (mumemories/iStock/Thinkstock.)

To help reduce fraud, magnetic strip cards are being replaced with cards imbedded with **EMV chip technology**. These chip cards offer advanced security for in-person payments, but the EMV chip cards require a special terminal to read the chips. If a healthcare facility accepts credit or debit cards, it is important to have a terminal that processes the EMV chip cards. Businesses that cannot process the chip cards may be liable for fraud losses to their customers.

Many credit card processing terminals can accept both credit cards and debit cards (Fig. 19.13), and some can also process check payments electronically. Debit card transactions use a PIN but do not need a patient's signature. Credit card transactions do not need a PIN, but patients may need to sign.

Although using the credit card processing terminal incurs per-transaction charges, valuable time is saved because an office employee does not need to visit the bank branch to make the daily deposit. Credit card transactions also can reduce the chances of money mismanagement in the office, such as **embezzlement**.

Contactless Payment Systems. New technology, called *contactless payment systems,* allows payment with a phone or other device that is linked to a credit or debit card. If office policy allows this type of payment to be made, special equipment will be purchased to accommodate it.

Online Payment Options. Many offices choose to accept payment online. Patients can use their patient portal to make payments by debit or credit card, electronic check, or direct transfer. If your office uses this for payments, it should be noted in patients' bills, so they know they have this option for payments.

Precautions for Accepting Credit and Debit Cards

Just as the medical assistant must take precautions when accepting checks, care must be taken when accepting a credit or debit card as payment for medical services. Make sure that the person presenting the card is the person to whom it was issued. Always ask for a state-issued ID. Compare the name and signature to the one on the credit card. Follow the healthcare facility's policy on verifying identity if the name on the state-issued ID does not match the name on the credit card. Some patients may use a prepaid credit card, which is purchased with cash and does not have the patient's name printed

on it, to make payments on their accounts. These cards, if allowed by office policy, pay just like a normal credit card. If a patient becomes belligerent when his or her credit card is denied, refer him or her to the office manager.

Banking Procedures in the Ambulatory Care Setting

Healthcare facilities use bank accounts to deposit funds (as cash, checks, debit card, or credit card transactions) and to pay their operational expenses by check or credit card. Accounting management software can simplify the banking transactions of healthcare facilities. This type of software is compatible with many online banking portals. That means that daily transactions can be downloaded directly into the accounting program. Attentive medical assistants who download daily can manage all account balances on a regular basis. Office expenses and invoices can be entered into the accounting management software as accounts payable, and payments can be scheduled for entered invoices. Checks to vendors can be printed at any time from the accounting software, documenting the transaction – and documented transactions make bank reconciliation a snap!

How to Write a Check

Checks are written in ink or produced using software. Write or key the check by the following steps:

- Date the check using one of these formats: May 23, 20XX; 05/23/XX; or 5/23/XX.
- On the "Pay to the Order of" line, correctly write or key the person's name or the company's name.
- On the line with the dollar sign, write out the exact amount of the check starting next to the dollar sign (e.g., $135.00, not $135).
- On the line below the recipient's name, write out the amount, making sure to start at the left edge. The cents are written in a fraction. Draw a single line through the rest of the line to prevent any additions (e.g., One hundred thirty-five and 50/100—————).
- On the Memo line, indicate the purpose of the payment (optional).
- The check needs to be signed to be valid. If the provider is signing the check, clip the invoice to the check and place it on the provider's desk for a signature. If you are responsible for signing checks, your name must be on the signature card on file at the bank. For checks over a certain amount, two signatures will be needed.
- If you make a mistake when writing the check, it cannot be altered by crossing out or changing anything that was written. You will need to void the check and rewrite another check. Write "VOID" on the stub and on the check. File the voided check with other accounting documents for auditing purposes. If using accounting software, indicate the check number has been voided in the software.

Making Bank Deposits

The medical assistant should make daily bank deposits, which minimizes the risks of keeping large sums of money on hand and also makes the money available for paying expenses. Depositing checks daily is important for these reasons:

- Checks may have a restricted time payment or may be lost, misplaced, or stolen over time.
- A stop-payment order may be placed on a check, or it may be returned for insufficient funds.
- Prompt processing is a courtesy to the payer.

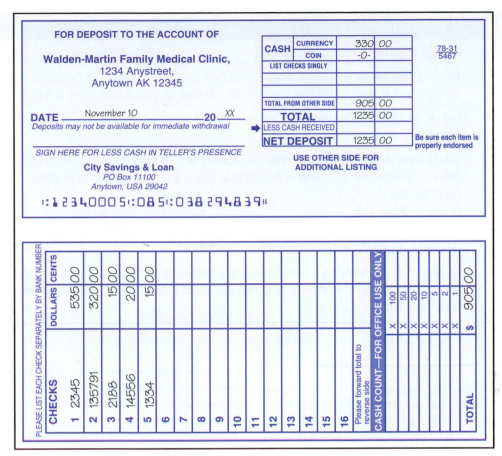

FIGURE 19.14 Front and back of a deposit slip.

Prompt check processing ensures that the money is available for the healthcare facility to use, or to be used to build interest.

Preparing the Deposit

The medical assistant must prepare a deposit slip (ticket) that accompanies the funds being deposited. The deposit slip, which can be paper or electronic, itemizes the cash or checks being deposited. It provides the information for the bank account into which the funds need to be deposited (Fig. 19.14). All details of the daily deposit should be recorded in the accounting software program; each check should be entered separately. The check number, payer, and check amount should also be recorded in the accounting software program so that the deposit amount from the software matches the bank deposit record. Many banks will not credit deposits made after 3 p.m. until the following business day (see Procedure 19.4 on p. 434).

Another option for depositing checks is using a credit card terminal that electronically processes checks at the time of payment. Also, small healthcare facilities can snap a picture of the check and use the bank's app to do a mobile deposit. Facilities receiving a high volume of checks can use a mobile check scanner (Fig. 19.15). Checks are scanned individually and documented as a bank transaction on the monthly statement. Mobile deposits can save staff time and do not require a deposit slip because the software (app) is linked to the bank account being used. When mobile deposits are used, the daily deposit amount must match the exact daily deposit amount in the accounting management software.

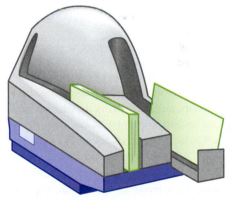

FIGURE 19.15 Mobile check scanner.

Check Endorsements

An endorsement is a signature plus any other writing on the back of a check by which the endorser transfers all rights in the check to another party. Endorsements are made with either a pen or rubber ink stamp. The medical assistant needs to endorse the back of the check in the box indicated. Regardless of how checks are deposited, they all need to be endorsed.

Types of Endorsements. Four principal kinds of endorsements can be used: blank, restrictive, special, and qualified (Table 19.2). Blank and restrictive endorsements (Fig. 19.16) are most commonly used.

TABLE 19.2	Types of Endorsements
TYPE	**DESCRIPTION**
Blank endorsement	The payee signs only his or her name. This makes the check payable to the bearer. It is the simplest and most common type of endorsement on personal checks but should be used only when the check is to be cashed or deposited immediately.
Restrictive endorsement	Specifies the purpose of the endorsement (see Fig. 19.16). It is used in preparing checks for deposit to the provider's checking account.
Special endorsement	Includes words specifying the person to whom the endorser makes the check payable. For instance, a check written to Helen Barker as the payee may be endorsed to the provider by writing on the back of the check as follows: Pay to the order of Theodore F. Wilson, M.D. Helen Barker The check is still negotiable but requires Dr. Wilson's signature or endorsement.
Qualified endorsement	The effect of the endorsement is qualified by disclaiming or destroying any future liability of the endorser. Usually the words "without recourse" are written above by an attorney who accepts a check on behalf of a client but who has no personal claim in the transaction.

Pay to the Order of
Midwest National Bank
Main Branch
For Deposit Only
ROBERT SPALDING
301-012697

FIGURE 19.16 Example of a restrictive endorsement.

Methods of Endorsement. Any endorsement should exactly match the name on the Pay To line of the check. If the name of the payee is misspelled, the payee usually must endorse the check the way the name is spelled on the face, followed by the correctly spelled signature.

A stamp can be used to endorse checks from patients and other sources. As they arrive, these checks should be recorded in the ledger and immediately stamped with the restrictive endorsement "For Deposit Only." This is a safeguard that prevents the cashing of lost or stolen checks. Most banks accept routine stamp endorsements that are restricted to For Deposit Only if the customer is well known and maintains an established account.

A signature can also be used as an endorsement. Some insurance checks or drafts require a personal signature endorsement; a stamped endorsement is not acceptable. This is stated on the back of the check. In such cases ask the payee to endorse the check, then stamp immediately below the signature the restrictive endorsement For Deposit Only.

Overdraft

When a depositor writes a check for more than the amount available in the account, the account is overdrawn. Issuing a check for more than the amount on deposit in the bank is illegal. Such a check is said to "bounce." Should this happen through error or oversight and

a check is written by an established depositor, the bank may honor the check and notify the depositor that the account is overdrawn. If the bank pays or covers the check, it issues an overdraft on the depositor's account. Considerable fees ($10 to $35) normally are charged for an overdraft. If the bank does not cover the amount of the check, it will be returned as NSF.

Stop-Payments

A depositor or check writer who wants to take back the check has the right to request that the bank stop payment on it. Stop-payment orders should be used only when absolutely necessary; as with overdrafts, most banks charge a fee for this service. Reasons for stop-payment requests include:

- Loss of a check
- Disagreement about a purchase
- Disagreement about a payment

Bank Statements and Reconciliation

The bank creates a statement at the end of each month. The medical assistant can download the bank statement directly into the accounting management software, which has a **reconciliation** feature. The purpose of reconciliation is to start with the beginning balance, add all deposits, and subtract all checks and other debit transactions. This will then leave the ending statement balance. The ending balance should match the ending balance on the bank statement. If it does, the account has been reconciled. Bank statement reconciliation is used as an audit, or to ensure that the bank is managing the funds in the account accurately. It can also help to locate any errors made in the checking account register. Any errors on the bank statement should be immediately reported to the bank. Bank statements typically contain the following elements (Figs. 19.17 and 19.18):

- Beginning balance
- Deposits made
- Checks paid (including images of all cleared checks)
- Transfer transactions

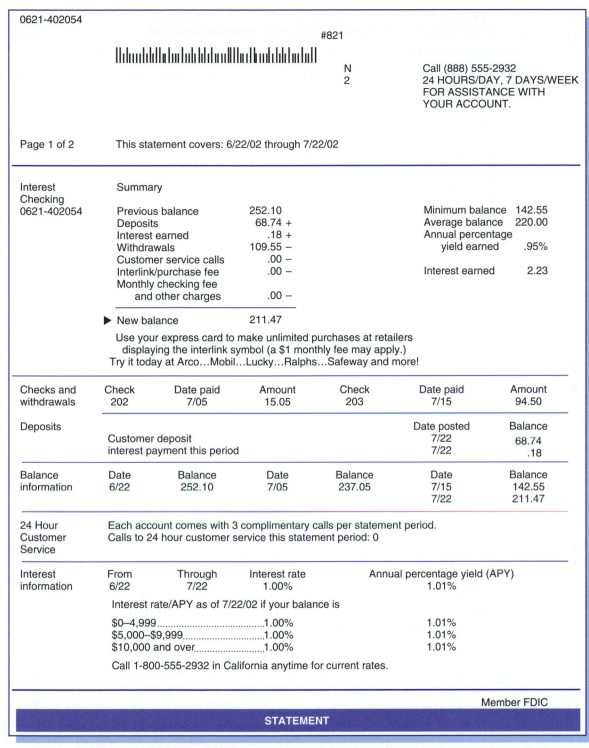

0621-402054

#821

N
2

Call (888) 555-2932
24 HOURS/DAY, 7 DAYS/WEEK
FOR ASSISTANCE WITH
YOUR ACCOUNT.

Page 1 of 2   This statement covers: 6/22/02 through 7/22/02

Interest Checking 0621-402054

Summary

Previous balance	252.10	Minimum balance	142.55
Deposits	68.74 +	Average balance	220.00
Interest earned	.18 +	Annual percentage	
Withdrawals	109.55 −	yield earned	.95%
Customer service calls	.00 −		
Interlink/purchase fee	.00 −	Interest earned	2.23
Monthly checking fee and other charges	.00 −		
▶ New balance	211.47		

Use your express card to make unlimited purchases at retailers
displaying the interlink symbol (a $1 monthly fee may apply.)
Try it today at Arco...Mobil...Lucky...Ralphs...Safeway and more!

Checks and withdrawals

Check	Date paid	Amount	Check	Date paid	Amount
202	7/05	15.05	203	7/15	94.50

Deposits

	Date posted	Balance
Customer deposit	7/22	68.74
interest payment this period	7/22	.18

Balance information

Date	Balance	Date	Balance	Date	Balance
6/22	252.10	7/05	237.05	7/15	142.55
				7/22	211.47

24 Hour Customer Service

Each account comes with 3 complimentary calls per statement period.
Calls to 24 hour customer service this statement period: 0

Interest information

From	Through	Interest rate	Annual percentage yield (APY)
6/22	7/22	1.00%	1.01%

Interest rate/APY as of 7/22/02 if your balance is

$0–4,999	1.00%		1.01%
$5,000–$9,999	1.00%		1.01%
$10,000 and over	1.00%		1.01%

Call 1-800-555-2932 in California anytime for current rates.

Member FDIC

STATEMENT

FIGURE 19.17 Example of a regular checking account statement.

- Online payment transactions
- Bank charges
- Ending balance

What to Do When the Balances Do Not Match

When there is a large number of transactions from check deposits and bill payment activities, it can be challenging to match the closing balance of the bank statement with the closing balance indicated in the accounting management software. Keeping accurate records of deposits and bill payment activities makes the bank reconciliation much smoother. All deposit copies should be maintained with a copy of the calculator tape totaling the day's deposit. Every online bill pay transaction should be recorded accurately in the accounting management system.

If you have carefully recorded every transaction and the balances still do not match, ask yourself the following questions:

This worksheet is provided to help you balance your account

1. Go through your register and mark each check, withdrawal, Express ATM transaction, payment, deposit or other credit listed on this statement. Be sure that your register shows any interest paid into your account, and any service charges, automatic payments, or Express Transfers withdrawn from your account during this statement period.

2. Using the chart below, list any outstanding checks, Express ATM withdrawals, payments or any other withdrawals (including any from previous months) that are listed in your register but are not shown on this statement.

3. Balance your account by filling in the spaces below.

ITEMS OUTSTANDING		
NUMBER	AMOUNT	
TOTAL	$	

Enter

The new balance shown on
this statement .... $_____

Add

Any deposits listed in your register $_____
or transfers into your account which $_____
are not shown on this statement. $_____
      +$_____

Total .... + $_____

Calculate the subtotal .... $_____

Subtract

The total outstanding checks and
withdrawals from the chart at left .... – $_____

Calculate the ending balance

This amount should be the same
as the current balance shown in
your check register .... $_____

If you suspect errors or have questions about electronic transfers

If you believe there is an error on your statement or Express ATM receipt, or if you need more information about a transaction listed on this statement or an Express ATM receipt, please contact us immediately. We are available 24 hours a day, seven days a week to assist you. Please call the telephone number printed on the front of this statement. Or, you may write to us at United Trust Company, P.O. Box 327, Anytown, USA.

1. Tell us your name and account number or Express card number.

2. As clearly as you can, describe the error or the transfer you are unsure about, and explain why you believe there is an error or why you need more information.

3. Tell us the dollar amount of the suspected error.

You must report the suspected error to us no later than 60 days after we sent you the first statement on which the problem appeared. We will investigate your question and will correct any error promptly. If our investigation takes longer than 10 business days (or 20 days in the case of electronic purchases), we will temporarily credit your account for the amount you believe is in error, so that you may have use of the money until the investigation is completed.

FIGURE 19.18 Reverse side of a bank statement, which is used for reconciling a checking account.

- Is your math correct? Could a deposit, check, or online bill pay amount be transposed?
- Did you forget to include one of the outstanding checks?
- Did you fail to record a deposit or did you record one twice?

Most banks ask to be notified within a reasonable time (e.g., 10 days) of any error found in the statement. The bank statement should be reconciled as soon as it is received. Most banks provide a form for reconciliation (bank statement reconciliation formula) on the last page of the bank statement:

Bank statement balance	$ _____
Minus outstanding checks	$ _____
Plus deposits not shown	$ _____
Corrected bank statement balance	$ _____
Checkbook balance	$ _____
Minus any bank charges	$ _____
Corrected checkbook balance	$ _____

If the two corrected balances agree, stop there. If they do not agree, subtract the lesser figure from the greater figure; the difference usually provides a clue to the error. For instance, if the shortage is $35, examine all the transactions for $35 on the statement and checkbook register and determine whether one of them has a posting error. Check the math and make sure all figures were added and subtracted correctly. Look at each figure and make sure none has been transposed. These tips usually catch the mistake.

Preventing Check Fraud in the Healthcare Facility

The National Check Fraud Center suggests the following steps to minimize the chance of check fraud in the healthcare facility:

- Check bank statements immediately after receiving them. If check fraud is not reported within 30 days of receipt of a monthly statement, the bank usually does not have to reimburse the loss.
- Make sure all extra checks, deposit slips, bank statements, and records are stored securely (e.g., locked in a file cabinet or a secure electronic folder).
- Bank statements and records should be maintained for up to 7 years and then shredded before disposal.

For more information on how to prevent check fraud or what to do if fraud occurs, consult the National Check Fraud Center's website: *http://ckfraud.org.*

Petty Cash

Petty cash is a small amount of money kept on hand for small, miscellaneous expenses, such as:

- parking money for a conference
- postage due
- lunch for the provider
- deliveries
- minor office supplies

Although it is a small amount of money, records still need to be kept and expenses tracked. If an employee is being reimbursed for expenses, a receipt should be written out and the disbursement tracked in the petty cash log. Periodically the petty cash fund should be balanced, much like the checking account reconciliation.

If funds are running low in the petty cash fund, a check should be written and the addition of the new funds noted on the petty cash register.

Paying Bills to Maximize Cash Flow

It is important to establish a systematic plan for paying bills. Some offices use an online bill paying system and pay bills as soon as they are received. Some pay bills monthly. In establishing the procedure for accounts payable, a medical assistant should keep in mind that most vendors allow 30 days to pay. When each invoice is received, check the "terms," which are usually located at the top of the document. Sometimes a bill will be discounted if it is paid within a specified time, such as 10 days. Such discounts usually are indicated at the bottom of invoices or billing statements. If the terms say, "Net 30," this means the total amount of the bill is due within 30 days.

Remember to allow a certain number of days for mailing (2 to 5, depending on where the payment is sent). If the business checking account is an interest-bearing one, do not pay bills before their due date. This way, the funds in the account continue to earn interest until the check is cashed. Also, if the practice has a weekly service (e.g., a laundry or cleaning service) that bills several times a month, accumulate the invoices and issue only one check per month.

Invoices and Statements

The vendor usually includes an *invoice* for payment with delivery of the merchandise. An invoice describes the products delivered and shows the amount due. Always verify that the items listed on the packing slip and invoice are included in the delivery.

Invoices should be placed in a designated accounts payable folder until paid. The healthcare facility may make more than one purchase from the same vendor during the month and send only a single payment at the end of the month for all deliveries.

CRITICAL THINKING APPLICATION   **19.7**

Laura does not recall ordering a certain item from the office supply company. However, it was included in her last shipment and was shown on the packing list. How can she determine whether the item was ordered?

Online Bill Pay

Online banking is a common practice for personal and business accounts. The healthcare facility can set up the account so that bills are paid automatically. This results in debiting the customer's account and crediting the merchant's account. This works well for those bills that occur every month or on a regular cycle, such as insurance premiums, rent payments, and utility bills. All banking transactions can be downloaded into an accounting management program for efficient money management. Online banking also is an excellent way to research the checks that have cleared the bank and to compute accurate bank balances.

Direct Deposit

Direct deposit, also known as *electronic funds transfers* (EFT), is the electronic payment of payroll, money owed to vendors or business establishments, and payments from government agencies. Direct deposit payments are safe, secure, efficient, and less expensive than paper checks. Their greatest advantage is the cost savings: the U.S. government pays $1.03 to issue each check payment, but only $0.105 to issue a direct deposit. Electronic processing becomes more common each day, and business transactions are processed faster and more efficiently through electronic means.

EMPLOYEE PAYROLL

A medical assistant is oftentimes responsible for processing employee payroll for the healthcare facility. Employees can be paid either on an hourly basis or with a **salary**. If the employee is salaried, his or her **net** paycheck will always be the same dollar amount. If the employee is paid hourly, the net paycheck will depend on how many hours the person worked during the pay period. The hourly rate is multiplied by the number of hours worked to determine these individuals' **gross** pay. In either situation, the gross amount earned is used to determine how much is withheld for taxes.

Each employee must complete a W-4 form, Employee's Withholding Allowance Certification. This form indicates the person's tax status and how many allowances he or she is claiming. This information is used to determine how much money is withheld for income taxes.

Other deductions from an employee's paycheck could be for insurance premiums, retirement savings, health savings accounts, or flexible spending accounts.

All employers are required to provide their employees with a W-2 form on a yearly basis. This must be sent to employees by January 30. This form lists the amounts that were withheld for income tax purposes. The employee needs this information to compute his or her taxes for the year.

It is important for the healthcare facility to keep exact records regarding payroll, withholding, and deductions. The employer is responsible for submitting the withheld tax amounts to the federal and state governments in a timely fashion. These are usually submitted on a quarterly basis (i.e., every 3 months).

CLOSING COMMENTS

Patient accounts management and collections are critical responsibilities in the healthcare facility, and a responsible medical assistant is a great asset in this important area. Always maintain a positive attitude with patients when discussing financial matters. Remember that people who are ill or facing challenges are not always cordial, so they may not respond positively to discussion of their patient account balances. Make every attempt to work with each patient to develop a financial plan for settling the account balance. The healthcare facility works hard to collect every dollar, so effective financial management is essential for practice success.

An equally important financial aspect for the healthcare facility is accounts payable. This must also be handled in an efficient manner. Being aware of the different banking options can help with depositing funds and paying bills. Making sure that there are policies in place

for patient payment methods is crucial. Patients should also be made aware of those policies.

Patient Coaching

In some cases, patients may not fully appreciate all the costs involved in providing high-quality health care. The medical assistant may need to respectfully educate the patient about the basic costs associated with the services provided by the healthcare facility. Patients may not need a lengthy explanation, but they should be informed that the provider does not set his or her fees arbitrarily. The healthcare facility office is a small business, and like thousands of other small businesses, it should collect enough money to cover its operating expenses.

Legal and Ethical Issues

A patient who has filed for bankruptcy cannot be contacted or billed further. Another legal concern is that a threat to send a patient's account into collections should not be made unless this is the provider's intention. Never tell a patient that the provider intends to act if the provider does not plan to follow through.

Because collection laws vary greatly from state to state, medical assistants should review the statutes pertaining to billing and collecting in the area of the healthcare facility's address. Develop a strong understanding of what is required of small businesses in collecting fees and billing patients for their financial responsibility. Remember that laws change often, so it is important to update the healthcare facility's policies on billing and collecting to reflect current statutes.

Patient-Centered Care

It should be emphasized that patients are financially responsible for balances on their accounts. Patients should be informed of the healthcare facility's payment policy at the very first appointment. If a patient submits an NSF check, the medical assistant should call the patient and explain the problem, requesting that he or she correct the matter as soon as possible. It is important to remember that most overdrafts are simply the result of mathematical errors or a delay in deposited funds being available for withdrawal. Therefore, the medical assistant should be patient and courteous when discussing NSF issues with patients. However, patients need to know that overdrafts are costly not only to them but also to the medical facility.

Professional Behaviors

The medical assistant is responsible for coordinating communication between the patient and the provider about financial issues. Some patients may act belligerently toward or try to bully the medical assistant in an effort to reduce their financial obligation. Be sure to inform the patient that the provider's decision about the patient's financial responsibility is not based on the medical assistant's discretion. Also, explain that the medical assistant represents the provider in his or her financial decision making. If the patient's behavior is out of control, politely excuse yourself and consult with the office manager. Inform the manager of all the details of the encounter, including the healthcare provider's instructions regarding the patient's account. The more information you give the office manager, the better able he or she will be to represent you in discussing the matter with the patient. During the entire encounter, remember to remain professional and treat the patient with respect, even though that respect may not be reciprocated.

SUMMARY OF SCENARIO

Laura has learned a lot about the different types of bookkeeping transactions performed daily in the healthcare facility. As she has gained more experience, she has come to appreciate the important role of patient accounts collection in the practice's cash flow and ability to cover its operating expenses.

After the visit with the bank representative, Laura implemented a few changes in bank account management, which have increased productivity in the office. For one, Laura requested that the bank send a mobile deposit machine, so this could be done in-house, which has saved Laura a lot of time.

Laura has also set up an online bill pay system and manages all invoice payments through the banking portal online. She sits down once a month and sets up all payments for the month. In this way, she can budget the office expenses for the month and can transfer unused funds to a money market account that pays a higher interest rate.

Laura is working closely with the providers at WMFM to make some financial policy changes in the office to streamline banking processes. As of January 1 of the new year, the sign at the healthcare facility's lobby window will explain that cash will no longer be accepted for services and that a $35 fee will be charged for NSF checks.

SUMMARY OF LEARNING OBJECTIVES

1. **Define bookkeeping and bookkeeping terms and discuss all the different transactions recorded in patient accounts.**

   Bookkeeping is the recording of financial transactions in the patient account records. Charges, payments, and adjustments can all be recorded in patient accounts.

2. **Perform accounts receivable procedures for patient accounts, including posting charges, payments, and adjustments. Also, discuss payment at the time of service and give an example of displaying sensitivity when requesting payment for services rendered.**

   Practice management software systems automatically calculate the correct fees or charges when a CPT/HCPCS code is entered (see Procedure 19.1 on p. 431). All insurance payment amounts posted should also match the total amount paid on the Explanation of Benefits (EOB). The patient account record should have a column for the adjustment to be posted as a credit.

   The medical assistant must believe that the provider and the facility have a right to charge for the services provided. Do not be embarrassed to ask for payment for the valuable services the clinician provides. When tact and good judgment are used in billing and collecting, patients appreciate the service they receive and the help the medical assistant provides. Procedure 19.2 on p. 433 discusses how to inform a patient of financial obligations for services rendered.

   Give each patient individual attention and personal consideration; also, be courteous and show a sincere desire to help the patient with financial problems.

3. **Describe the impact of the Truth in Lending Act on collections policies for patient accounts.**

   If credit options are offered for patients, the healthcare facility should be in compliance with Regulation Z of the Truth in Lending Act (TILA). If an agreement exists between provider and patient that the healthcare facility will accept full payment in more than four installments, the healthcare facility must provide a Federal Truth in Lending Statement, even if no finance fees are charged, and it should be signed by the healthcare facility representative and the patient.

4. **Discuss monthly patient account statements and list the necessary data elements on each monthly statement.**

   Patient account records should include all information pertinent to collecting the account, such as the name and address of the guarantor, insurance identification, home and business telephone numbers, name of employer, any special instructions for billing, and emergency or alternative contact information.

5. **Do the following related to collection procedures:**

   - *Describe successful collection techniques for patient accounts.*

     The medical assistant can use a variety of techniques to collect patient accounts, such as collection phone calls, collection letters, and skip tracing. Often more than one technique must be used to obtain payment. Always be courteous and kind when using collection techniques.

   - *Discuss strategies for collecting outstanding balances through personal finance interviews.*

     Personal finance interviews with patients sometimes can be more effective than a whole series of collection letters. By speaking with a patient face to face, the medical assistant can come to an understanding of the problem more quickly, and an agreement about future payment plans can be reached.

   - *Describe types of adjustments made to patient accounts, including a nonsufficient funds (NSF) check and collection agency transactions.*

     With a check drawn on an account with insufficient funds, the bank returns the check to the healthcare facility marked "NSF" and charges the healthcare facility bank account a returned check fee. The payment posted to the patient account must be reversed. Note that the original payment is not deleted; rather, a charge line item is added with the amount of the NSF check; the transaction description should read "NSF Date 02/23/20XX." Many medical offices add additional line items for NSF fee charges, but this is up to the discretion of the provider. Because collection agencies charge a fee for their collection efforts, the amount credited to the patient's account might be less than the actual payment amount.

   - *Post payments and adjustments to a patient's account.*
     See Procedure 19.3 on p. 433.

Continued

6. **Do the following related to banking in today's business world:**
   - *Explain the purpose of the Federal Reserve Bank and the types of banks it manages.*
     The Federal Reserve Bank manages all banks in the United States. Healthcare facilities have a choice among different types of banks with which to do business, such as retail and commercial banks, credit unions, and online-only banks.
   - *Identify common types of bank accounts.*
     The bank accounts most commonly used by healthcare facilities are checking, savings, and money market accounts.
   - *Discuss the importance of signature cards.*
     When an account is opened at a bank branch, the depositor is required to provide a handwritten signature on a physical or electronic card, which is kept on file with the bank. If a check comes through and some suspicion arises that the depositor's signature has been forged, bank personnel compare the signature on the check with the original on the signature card.
   - *Explain how online banking has made standard banking processes more efficient.*
     Online banking allows healthcare facilities to perform mobile deposits, thereby reducing the number of times a staff member visits the bank branch. Online banking also provides up-to-the-minute account balances, online bill pay, and easy account balance transfers so that the healthcare facility's manager can spend less time managing the bank account.

7. **Do the following related to checks:**
   - *Compare different types of negotiable instruments.*
     The different types of negotiable instruments used to transfer funds from one bank account and deposit them in another are the personal check, cashier's check, money order, business check, and voucher check.
   - *Identify precautions in accepting checks from patients.*
     When accepting a check, compare the name and address on the check to the name and address in the patient's health record. Scan the check carefully for the correct date, amount, and signature. Do not accept a check with corrections on it. If you do not know the person presenting a personal check, ask for identification and compare signatures.
   - *Explain how checks are processed from one account to another.*
     Local branches are assigned a routing number, which is printed on the bottom left side of the check. The check also has the specific account number assigned by the branch, which specifies the account from which funds are taken. When a check is presented to the bank, the check is sent to a regional banking clearinghouse, which requests funds from the check-sponsoring financial institution. Then the funds are moved from the payer's account to the payee's account. The endorsement on the back of the check includes the number of the account into which the funds are to be deposited.
   - *Review the procedure followed when the healthcare facility receives an NSF check.*

     When the healthcare facility is informed that a patient's check has been returned for nonsufficient funds, the patient should be contacted immediately. Inform the patient that the balance plus the overdraft fee is payable by money order or debit or credit card immediately. The patient should also be informed that he or she can no longer pay by check for any future services.

8. **Identify precautions in accepting cash.**
   Many healthcare facilities refuse to accept cash from patients to prevent employees from being tempted to embezzle. In addition, cash cannot be deposited by mobile deposit, and maintaining records for accepting cash can be difficult.

9. **Discuss the use of debit and credit cards, including advantages and precautions.**
   The advantages of debit cards include their safety and convenience, in addition to the availability of receipts and statements. The most important precaution in accepting credit cards is to verify the patient's identity by asking to see the person's state-issued ID. Patients must know the debit card's PIN, so this is considered a verification of identity.

10. **Do the following related to banking procedures in the ambulatory care setting:**
    - *Describe banking procedures as related to the ambulatory care setting.*
      Banking procedures include withdrawals, deposits, writing checks, reconciling bank statements, paying bills, and other transactions, most of which can be done conveniently in the healthcare facility through online banking or through accounting management software.
    - *Explain the importance of depositing checks daily.*
      Deposits should be made daily for these reasons: a stop-payment order may be placed; the check may be lost, misplaced, or stolen; delay may cause the check to be returned because of insufficient funds; the check may have a restricted time for cashing; prompt processing is a courtesy to the payer; and the accounts receivable may be inflated because payments have not been deposited daily.
    - *Prepare a bank deposit.*
      Bank deposits should be made daily. The process for preparing a bank deposit is outlined in Procedure 19.4 on p. 434.
    - *Compare types of check endorsements.*
      Endorsements include (1) a blank endorsement, in which the payee simply signs his or her name on the back of the check; (2) a restrictive endorsement, which specifies in which bank and which specific account the funds are to be deposited; (3) a special endorsement, which names a specific person on the back of the check as payee; and (4) a qualified endorsement, which disclaims future liability. This type of endorsement is used when the person who accepts the check has no personal claim in the transaction.
    - *Review check-writing procedures used to pay the operational expenses of a healthcare facility.*

Writing checks is a routine and basically simple function; however, certain guidelines should be followed to prevent potential problems. The bank account should have a check signer that is on file with the bank, and correction fluid for errors should not be used on checks.

11. **Understand the purpose of bank account reconciliation for auditing purposes, and how to pay bills in order to maximize cash flow.**

    The procedure for reconciliation starts with the beginning balance; then, all deposits are added, and all checks and other debit transactions are subtracted — the ending statement balance should be left. It is extremely important to make sure that the ending balance is achieved at the end of reconciliation. The bank statement reconciliation is used to audit the account; that is, to ensure that the bank is managing the funds in the account accurately. Any errors on the bank statement should be reported to the bank immediately.

12. **Discuss the process of employee payroll.**

    When working with employee payroll, the medical assistant must understand the differences between salary, net pay, and gross pay in order to ensure that the proper amount for taxes is withheld. There are also a number of forms involved with employee payroll, including W-4 and W-2.

PROCEDURE 19.1   Post Charges and Payments to a Patient's Account

Task: To enter charges into the patient account record manually and electronically.

Scenario: Ken Thomas is a returning patient of Dr. Martin. He makes his $50 copayment at the time of the office visit.

EQUIPMENT and SUPPLIES

- Patient account ledger card
- SimChart for the Medical Office software
- Encounter form/superbill
- Provider's fee schedule

PROCEDURAL STEPS

Posting Charges Manually

1. For new patients, create the patient account by entering the following information on a patient account ledger card:
   - Patient's full name, address, and at least two contact phone numbers
   - Date of birth (DOB)
   - Health insurance information, including the subscriber number, group number, and effective date
   - Subscriber's name and date of birth (if the subscriber is not the patient)

   PURPOSE: To keep all insurance and collection information available with the patient account record balance for reference.

2. For returning patients, review the account record to see whether a balance is due. If there is a balance, bring this to the patient's attention when he or she comes for the appointment. Respectfully explain that the provider would appreciate a payment on the previous balance before he or she can see the patient. Use the following dialogue:

   Laura: Good morning, Ken. How are you feeling today?

   Ken: Not so good, I really need to see Dr. Martin again because my headaches have been getting worse.

   Laura: I'm sorry to hear that. Let's get you in to see the doctor right away. I can collect the $50 copayment for today's visit, and here is a statement for your previous balance of $214. How would you like to take care of that today?

   Ken: Oh, I didn't know about the previous balance. Can I just pay the copayment today?

   Laura: Dr. Martin would like at least half of this previous balance paid before seeing you today, please. I know that medical bills can pile up pretty quickly, but Dr. Martin would like to continue to provide you with quality care so you can feel back to yourself really soon.

   Ken: Yes, I know you're right. I need to keep coming to see Dr. Martin. I can pay half of the $214 today, along with the copayment.

   Laura: Thanks, I know Dr. Martin really appreciates you as a patient. Would that be check or credit card?

   Ken: Credit card, please.

   Brenda: Okay, here is the credit card receipt and a copy of the updated statement. By the way, I'd like to document on your patient account when you will be able to pay the rest of this statement amount.

   Ken: I'll pay the balance next month; is that okay?

   Laura: I'll let Dr. Martin know and put a note in your account. Thanks; you'll be called in shortly.

   PURPOSE: To respectfully inform the patient of his or her financial obligations and the provider's intention of having the previous balance paid in full.

   After seeing the patient, the provider completes the encounter form, which includes all procedures and the associated fee schedule. Using the completed encounter form in Fig. 19.1, enter the charges manually on the ledger card for the patient's account record. Total all the charges on the encounter form for the services rendered. Then subtract the copayment made from the total charges. The previous balance, if any, is added to this new total. Use the following worksheet to calculate the new balance. The new balance-due amount should be presented to the patient before he or she leaves the healthcare facility.

TOTAL CHARGES	$_____
Amount paid (copayment)	$_____
+ Previous balance (if any)	$_____
= New Balance Due	$_____

Continued

PROCEDURE 19.1   Post Charges and Payments to a Patient's Account—*continued*

Posting Charges in SimChart for the Medical Office

1. After logging into SimChart, locate the established patient by clicking on Find Patient; enter the patient's name, verify the DOB, and click on the radio button. This will bring you to the Clinical Care tab. If there is no encounter shown, create an encounter by clicking on Office Visit under Info Panel on the left, select a visit type, and click on Save. Once an encounter has been created, return to the Patient Dashboard and click on the Superbill link on the right (or click on the Coding and Billing tab). (See the following figure.)

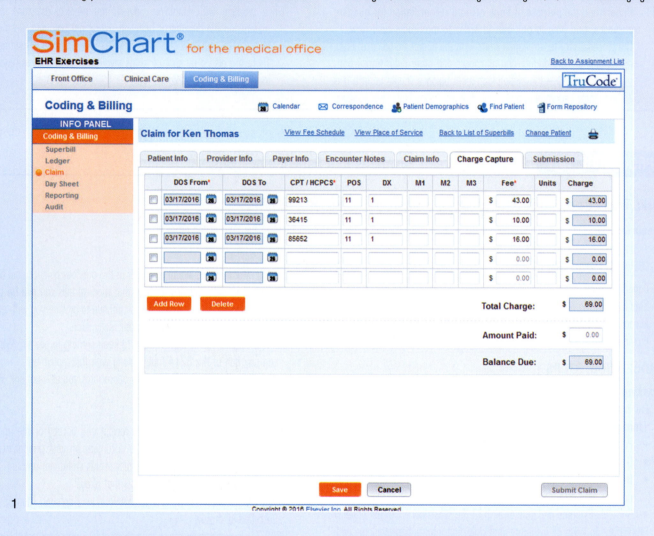

2. From the Superbill area, in the Encounters Not Coded section, click on the encounter (in blue). On page 1 enter the diagnosis in the Diagnosis field and document the services provided (additional services are found on pages 2 and 3 of the Superbill).

3. Complete the information needed on page 4 of the Superbill and submit.
4. Click on Ledger on the left and search for your patient. Once your patient has been located, click on the arrow across from the name in the ledger.
5. Enter the payment received. The balance will be autocalculated for you.

PROCEDURE 19.2   Inform a Patient of Financial Obligations for Services Rendered

Task: To inform a patient of his or her financial obligation and to demonstrate professionalism and sensitivity when discussing the patient's billing record.

Scenario: During this role-play, Christi Brown is meeting with you regarding the bill she received in the mail. When she called to make the appointment, she voiced her confusion about the bill, stating she thought her insurance covered everything. You check her record and see that she met her deductible and now needs to pay 20% of the billed amount. She owes $170.

EQUIPMENT and SUPPLIES

- Patient's account record
- Copy of patient's insurance card

PROCEDURAL STEPS

1. Determine the patient's financial responsibility under the insurance plan by reviewing the copy of the patient's insurance card.
   PURPOSE: Having an understanding of the patient's financial responsibility from the insurance plan will help you to explain the terms to the patient.
2. Determine the amount the patient owes by reviewing the patient's account record.
   PURPOSE: It is important when working with a patient that you are familiar with the facts of the situation.
3. Discuss the situation with the patient. (Role-play the above scenario.)
4. Demonstrate professionalism when discussing the situation with the patient. Verbal and nonverbal communication should demonstrate patience, understanding, and sensitivity. The medical assistant should refrain from inappropriate and unprofessional behavior, including eye rolling, harsh words, disrespectful comments, and similar behaviors.
5. Demonstrate professionalism by respectfully providing the patient with payment options based on the clinic's policies and what the patient can pay on a monthly basis.
   PURPOSE: The medical assistant should not force or harass the patient into paying. The medical assistant will be more successful if the communication with the patient is respectful.

PROCEDURE 19.3   Post Payments and Adjustments to a Patient's Account

Task: To post payments and adjustments to patient accounts accurately.

Scenario: Monique Jones (06/23/1985) was seen 6 months ago for a wellness visit and lab work. Her insurance had lapsed, and she is completely responsible for the bill. She did not make any payments and resisted all attempts at collection of the balance of $172. Her account was turned over to a collection agency, which was able to collect the balance in full. The collection agency retains 50% of what it collects as payment. Post the collection agency payment and adjustment to Ms. Jones' account.

EQUIPMENT and SUPPLIES

- Patient account ledger card, or SimChart for the Medical Office software

PROCEDURAL STEPS

1. Look up the ledger card for the patient account (or the patient ledger in SimChart). Confirm that you have the correct patient account.
   PURPOSE: All transactions need to be posted to the correct account.
2. Post an adjustment to reverse the adjustment done when the account was turned over to the collection agency.

PURPOSE: The account should show a zero balance. If the reverse adjustment is not done, the account will have a credit balance.

3. Post the payment and adjustment that reflects the actual dollar amount received from the collection agency and the amount that was retained as payment (see the following figure).
   PURPOSE: Both the payment amount and adjustment must be posted, to give the patient credit for the full payment that was sent to the collection agency.

Continued

PROCEDURE 19.3 | Post Payments and Adjustments to a Patient's Account—*continued*

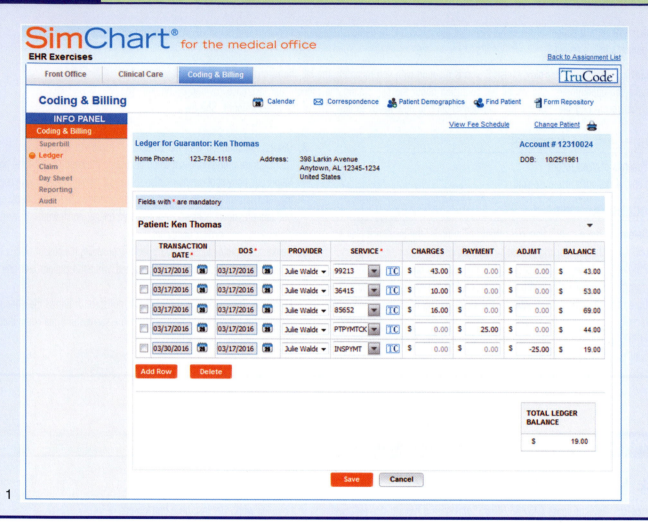

1

PROCEDURE 19.4 | Prepare a Bank Deposit

Task: To prepare a bank deposit for currency and checks.

Scenario: The following checks need to be deposited: #3456 for $89; #6954 for $136; #9854 for $1366.65; #8546 for $653.36; and #9865 for $890.22. The following currency and coins need to be deposited: (19) $20 bills; (10) $10 bills; (46) $5; (73) $1. The healthcare facility's name is Walden-Martin Family Medical Clinic, account number 123-456-78910, and the bank is Clear Water Bank, Anytown, Anystate.

EQUIPMENT and SUPPLIES

- Checks and currency for deposit (see Scenario)
- Check for endorsement
- Calculator
- Paper method: bank deposit slip
- Electronic method: SimChart for the Medical Office (SCMO)

PROCEDURAL STEPS

1. Gather the documents to be used. For the electronic method, enter the Simulation Playground in SCMO. Click on the Form Repository icon. On the INFO PANEL, click on Office Forms and then select Bank Deposit Slip.
2. Enter the date on the deposit slip.

PROCEDURE 19.4 | **Prepare a Bank Deposit**—*continued*

3. Using the calculator, calculate the amount of currency to be deposited. Enter the amount in the CURRENCY line, completing the dollar and cent boxes.

4. Enter the total amount in the TOTAL CASH line.

5. For each check to be deposited, enter the check number, the dollars, and cents. List each check on a separate line.
   PURPOSE: The bank requires that each check be listed separately; this also helps when verifying the checks before the deposit.

6. Calculate the total to be deposited and enter the number in the TOTAL FROM ATTACHED LIST box.

7. Enter the number of items deposited in the TOTAL ITEMS box.

8. Before completing the deposit slip, verify the check amounts listed and recalculate the totals. For the electronic method, click on SAVE.
   PURPOSE: It is crucial to verify the accuracy of check amounts and totals.

9. Place a restrictive endorsement on the check(s).
   PURPOSE: To prevent cashing of checks in case of loss or theft.

SCENARIO

Kate Gilliam is the office manager for Walden-Martin Family Medical (WMFM) Clinic. The clinic has a full appointment schedule each day. Kate encourages the medical office staff to communicate and work as a cohesive team to meet the goal of providing exceptional care to the practice's patients. Kate knows that positive motivation will encourage the office team to meet this goal. At weekly staff meetings, employees are free to offer their suggestions on office procedures. Kate regularly consults her team members and always asks for their thoughts on how the office can function more effectively. She recognizes that employees need to feel that they are part of the team, and by implementing some of the procedures her team members suggest, she creates a forward-thinking and empowered work environment for the office staff.

Kate has been praised by the providers as a transformational manager because she has implemented new and efficient health information systems and technologies in the clinic. In addition, when an office position becomes vacant, Kate is careful about whom she hires. She always checks at least three references per applicant and verifies each previous place of employment. She also always requests a background check, a credit check, a drug test, and a bond if the applicant will be assigned to manage office money matters.

Kate trains each new employee herself, using the office's policies and procedures manual. She makes sure the employee knows that this manual also contains a detailed job description, so the employee knows the duties expected of his or her job. Kate regularly reviews employee performance and keeps checklists that reflect that new employees are trained accurately. All new employees are probationary until they have been evaluated by Kate at 90 days after hire. She works hard to improve the types of benefits offered to her team, to improve employee satisfaction and retention.

Kate makes sure each employee has the tools needed to do his or her job effectively. She also trains the team in ways to reduce expenses and waste in the medical office. Major office changes are presented to the entire staff, and although providers make the final decision, Kate seeks the suggestions of other employees. The cooperative attitude between management and employees of the healthcare facility provides a great atmosphere for teamwork, and Kate and the providers are pleased with the team-building atmosphere they have implemented.

While studying this chapter, think about the following questions:

- How friendly should office managers become with staff members?
- Why are checking references and a background check important when considering a new staff member?
- How should negative employee evaluations be handled?
- How can the office manager promote a teamwork atmosphere in the medical office?

LEARNING OBJECTIVES

1. Define the qualities and responsibilities of a successful office manager in a healthcare facility.
2. Explain how to conduct a staff meeting with an agenda.
3. Identify several ways in which employees are motivated.
4. Do the following related to creating a team environment:
   - Discuss strategies to create a team environment in the healthcare facility.
   - List communication barriers and how to overcome them.
5. Do the following related to finding the right employee for the job:
   - Identify the need to find the right employee for an opening in the medical office.
   - Review a general job description for medical assistants.
   - Explain how to search through resumes and applications for potential candidates.
   - List and discuss legal and illegal interview questions.
   - Explain how to select the most qualified candidates.
   - Identify follow-up activities the office manager should perform after an interview.
6. Review new employee orientation, including paperwork, training, and development.
7. Discuss strategies for determining fair salaries and raises, addressing a problem employee, and terminating an employee.
8. Identify the information that should be included in a personnel policy manual.
9. Describe how office policies and procedures are different from personnel policies.
10. Explain the office manager's role in regulatory compliance.

VOCABULARY

cohesive (koh HEE siv) Sticking together tightly; exhibiting or producing cohesion.

compliant (kum PLIE unt) Obeying, obliging, or yielding.

consensus (kun SEN sus) General agreement

credential (kri DEN shul) Evidence of authority, status, rights, entitlement to privileges.

delegate To appoint a person as a representative.

disparaging (di SPAR a jing) Slighting; having a negative or degrading tone.

human resources file (HR file) Contains all documents related to an individual's employment.

incentive Things that incite or spur to action; rewards or reasons for performing a task.

matrix (MAY triks) The environment where something is created or takes shape. A base on which to build.

mentor A steady employee whom a new staff member can approach with questions and concerns.

rapport (ra PORE) A relationship of harmony and accord between the patient and the healthcare professional.

retention A term referring to actions taken by management to keep good employees.

solvent (SOL vent) Able to pay all debts.

The management of a professional healthcare facility can greatly influence the success of the business. Good management allows the provider to see and treat patients in a functional environment with the confidence that the business side of the facility is operating as it should be. A well-managed office is not something that just happens. Great effort and teamwork are necessary to ensure that the day-to-day activities are carried out efficiently and that the many details needing attention are handled urgently.

Although most medical assistants do not enter medical office management right after graduation, they can look forward to advancing their careers as they gain experience. The information in this chapter can help the medical assistant understand what it takes to become a good manager. Many of these traits can be developed as a new employee after graduation, such as punctuality, respect, and responsibility. Additionally, the medical assistant will learn the employment process from the office manager's point of view. This information also is valuable to a new medical assistant who is applying for a position. By studying office management, the medical assistant prepares for future management positions, but also learns to see both the employee side and the manager side of the operating healthcare facility.

MEDICAL OFFICE MANAGEMENT

Choosing Healthcare Management as a Profession

There are many aspects to healthcare. Some people are attracted to the clinical side, with direct patient care. Some people are attracted to the administrative side, with some patient contact. What everyone who works in healthcare has in common is the desire to help others. There can be many different routes to becoming a manager in a healthcare setting. Some will pursue an educational route that is solely aimed at healthcare management, such as a degree in Healthcare Administration. Another educational route could include a degree in Business Administration. Yet another route could be a healthcare worker, such as a medical assistant or registered nurse, who has worked in his or her field for a period of time and has developed an interest in the management side of healthcare.

For those who come from a clinical care background, some additional education may be needed in the healthcare administration area. Those who come from more of a business background may need to call on others with clinical expertise in certain situations. For example, if there is a complaint about the care given to a patient by a certain provider, the manager with a business background may ask another provider or clinical staff member to review the care that was given.

Traits of a Successful Medical Office Manager

Successful medical office managers have excellent communication and organizational skills. These skills are very useful when you are working with patients, staff, and providers. A manager will have to deal with situations involving hiring and firing, disciplinary actions, and irate patients. The office manager is often the liaison between the staff and providers. If the staff are having an issue with the provider or vice versa, the issue will come to the office manager, who will be expected to work toward a solution. Proper professional communication is needed in all aspects of managing a medical office.

It is necessary to have an understanding of budgeting and financial reports. Those with an educational background in management will have that knowledge. Someone moving into management may need to take some courses in those areas.

In addition, an office manager must possess good leadership skills. The office staff will look to the manager for direction and will follow the example set by the manager. When possible, the manager should seek out the opinions of the staff when a major decision is going to be made. That decision will likely impact how many people do their jobs, and they would like to contribute to the decision-making process. If **consensus** is used to reach a decision, the staff will feel more invested in the decision. They will also feel more valued as an employee and will develop a sense of loyalty to the organization.

Keeping the Management Relationship Professional

When people work together for an extended period of time, the relationship sometimes develops into a close friendship. This is a normal occurrence, but the office manager must be careful about becoming too close to his or her employees. When the relationship is too friendly, reprimanding an employee when needed can be difficult. Some employees take advantage of a good relationship with the office manager and may begin to arrive late or call in sick more than usual. A healthy respect for each other must be maintained. The manager can have a good **rapport** with employees without becoming overly friendly, and this is the best policy. Some facilities have strict rules about socializing with employees outside the work facility. It is advisable to keep the relationship on a professional level at all times.

OFFICE MANAGEMENT RESPONSIBILITIES

Personnel Management

There are many aspects to personnel management, including performance evaluation and salary review, maintaining employment records, and recruitment and selection of new staff members.

Performance evaluations typically occur on an annual basis. Salary review usually occurs at the same time, with a merit increase given if appropriate. Disciplinary actions are also part of the office manager's responsibilities. Performance evaluations and the disciplinary process will be discussed in more detail later in the chapter.

The performance evaluation is part of the employment record, but an office manager will also be responsible for employees' Social Security numbers, the number of tax exemptions claimed, wages, and the deductions associated with payroll. The employment record will also include **credential** documentation for the providers and staff — that is, making sure that licenses and certifications are kept up to date.

Financial Management

In order to keep the healthcare facility **solvent**, the office manager is responsible for tracking all of the income. This involves billing, collections (patient and insurance), and banking procedures. Having some accounting knowledge is helpful in this area.

Scheduling

There are several types of scheduling that occur in a healthcare facility. The most obvious is patient scheduling. Getting the **matrix** established (see Chapter 11) can be the responsibility of the office manager, working in conjunction with the provider, in addition to developing the scheduling policies and procedures. An office manager can also be responsible for setting the staff schedule. If these schedules are not handled properly, it can affect employee morale and patient satisfaction.

Facility and Equipment Management

Overseeing the inventory of equipment and supplies is part of the office manager's responsibilities. Having adequate supplies and equipment that works properly will help to ensure that things flow smoothly and efficiently. Making decisions about equipment replacement usually falls to the office manager. Arranging for the maintenance of the facility is also the responsibility of the office manager.

Risk Management

Risk management involves identifying, planning, and implementing strategies to minimize the provider's risk of a lawsuit. Creating policies

and procedures is part of this process and will be discussed in more detail later in this chapter. Reviewing incident reports (see Chapter 4) to see if changes need to be made to procedures and/or facility management will also help with risk management. The office manager is very involved in this process.

OFFICE MANAGER ROLE

Communication

Effective communication is a vital skill for anyone working in healthcare. An office manager will be communicating with employees, patients, vendors, insurance companies, and providers. This communication can happen in person or in written format. Good office managers will be able to communicate professionally with anyone they come in contact with. Using the 5 Cs of good communication is an excellent place to start.

5 Cs of Good Communication

- Clear — Use words that accurately convey your meaning and are presented in a logical order.
- Concise — Get to the point and do not wander off topic.
- Consistent — Provide the same message day to day, so that people can rely on what you say.
- Correct — Use technical terms correctly. Make sure you do not make any grammatical or spelling errors.
- Courteous — Be friendly, open, and honest.

It is also important to keep in mind some basic communication guidelines:
- Speak slowly and clearly to ensure that your message is received, and misunderstanding does not occur.
- Do not interrupt when someone is speaking. This can convey that what the speaker is saying is not important.
- Use a respectful tone of voice.
- Ask for feedback to ensure that the correct message was sent.

Active Listening

A large part of the communication process is actually listening. Active listening is discussed in Chapter 2 as it relates to working with patients, but the same concepts apply when working with staff, providers, vendors, and insurance companies. Active listening means that the listener is concentrating on what is being said and how it is being said. The words are important, but so is the nonverbal communication that accompanies it. Distractions should be eliminated so that you can really focus on what the person is saying. This may mean taking the individual somewhere other than your office, where the phone can ring or others can interrupt. A conference room or an empty exam room can be used. The office manager should also be aware of who might overhear a conversation. The Health Insurance Portability and Accountability Act (HIPAA) considerations must be kept in mind. Whether the office manager is talking with an employee about an issue with a co-worker, a patient with a treatment concern, or a provider about a billing issue, active listening will help to ensure that all parties receive the correct message.

Characteristics of a Good Listener

- Remain nonjudgmental and neutral.
- Refrain from interrupting with a comment or question.
- Allow for periods of silence.
- Smile and nod your head to show you are listening to the message.
- Use appropriate eye contact so the speaker is not intimidated.
- Lean slightly forward or sideways toward the speaker.
- Avoid distractions (e.g., fidgeting, looking at the clock, doodling).

CRITICAL THINKING APPLICATION   **20.2**
A situation with an upset patient came up. The patient was visibly upset and asked to speak with the office manager. What steps should Kate take to minimize distractions and protect the patient's privacy?

Time Management

Time management is a skill that is invaluable for an office manager. Not only are you responsible for getting your own tasks done, but you need to make sure that the staff is also able to complete their tasks. Prioritization is the key to good time management.

Goal setting is the first step in prioritization. If you know what the goals are for the week, month, and year, you can then develop a plan to reach those goals. There will be goals for the healthcare facility, the staff, patient care, and personal goals. Determining the goals for the whole facility will determine some of the goals for the office manager and the staff. Once the goals have been defined, determining how to achieve those goals will become the task.

Once the tasks have been defined, they can be prioritized. One way to prioritize is to use an ABC system. The most urgent or important task is given an A; less urgent or important tasks are given a B; those that are the least urgent or important are given a C. Within those categories the tasks can be ranked by importance, such as A1, A2, B1, B2, etc. (Fig. 20.1). An office manager does not have to do

FIGURE 20.1 ABC system of prioritization.

all of the tasks; some can be **delegated** to others who are qualified to do them. The tasks can be tracked on a To-Do list that is kept either on paper or electronically. Another method for prioritization can be found in Chapter 1.

Monthly Planning

Keeping track of the activities that occur in the healthcare facility can be a daunting task. Laying out the office schedule for the month is one way to do that. Noting all of the providers' vacations and conferences, vendor meetings, and accountant meetings will help you to stay on track and to avoid double-booking.

The office manager is also in charge of approving staff vacations. By having a calendar in place that shows when everyone is on vacation, including the providers, the office manager can make sure the approval process moves forward more smoothly. Part of time management for the healthcare facility is making sure that there is adequate staff coverage at all times, keeping in mind that someone may call in sick or have a family emergency during that time.

Staff Meetings

Staff meetings are a formal channel used to keep the office manager and other team members current and communicating on a regular basis. One of the most common complaints from office personnel is that they are unable to discuss problems with the providers. The solution to this problem may be to hold regular staff meetings, which may be scheduled as frequently as weekly but should be held no less often than quarterly. Some of the best ideas on improvement come from the staff; the expression and exchange of good ideas should be encouraged.

Set aside a specific time for regular meetings at an hour when most people can attend with the least disruption. The meetings need not be long or overly formal, but to be effective, they must be planned and organized. There must be a leader, often the office manager, and someone should be appointed to take notes. All members of the staff should be encouraged to submit ideas for discussion.

Draw up a simple agenda listing the issues to be discussed and prepare any supporting data needed for the meeting. The agenda can be distributed to the team members ahead of the meeting so everyone can prepare and participate.

There are many kinds of staff meetings; they may be purely informational, problem-solving, or brainstorming meetings. They may be work sessions for updating manuals, training seminars, or whatever is necessary to the individual practice. Meetings also may be scheduled to discuss new ideas and any changes in office procedures. Some meetings are held simply to resolve specific problems. The staff meeting must not be allowed to deteriorate into a gripe session. Individual complaints should be handled privately.

The meeting's agenda might be similar to that of any business meeting:

1. Reading of the last meeting's minutes
2. Discussion of any unfinished business
3. Discussion of any problems in the clinical area
4. Discussion of any problems in the administrative area
5. Discussion of any problems in common areas
6. Adjournment

Some providers like to combine the staff meeting with breakfast or lunch. The time or place is not important as long as it meets the needs of the practice. Meetings should be conducted democratically, and without interruption. Meetings should be kept as brief as possible. Always follow up on the items discussed, otherwise, the only result will be frustration and a reluctance to discuss problems at future meetings. The status of action items from the staff meeting should be introduced in the next staff meeting as *minutes*.

Motivation

Managers have a great deal of influence over the staff they supervise. Successful managers must be interested in people they work with on a daily basis. It is said that if one helps others get what they want in life, the individual usually also gets what he or she wants.

Successful managers learn that their employees should be encouraged to perform at optimum levels, and managers should be confident enough in their own skills to give credit to employees who develop ideas and concepts for the team. These managers know how to let their employees help them "look good." A manager with a group of outstanding employees usually is looked on as an effective leader.

Frederick Herzberg, known as the Father of Job Enrichment, stated, "Quality work that fosters job satisfaction and health enjoys top priority in industry all over the world." In his book, *The Motivation to Work,* Herzberg stated three points:

1. Jobs must be satisfying and must motivate employees to grow and reach their full capabilities.
2. Employees who show greater ability should be given more responsibility.
3. If the job does not allow the employee to use his or her full ability, a different employee who can grow and find motivation in the work should be placed in that position.

Effective medical office managers, or office team leaders, recognize that employees are more than static workers. Therefore, motivation is a key component in developing successful employees.

The Power of Motivation

A number of factors can motivate a person to reach a goal, including:

- Challenging work
- Money
- Recognition
- Satisfaction
- Freedom
- Fear
- Family
- Insecurity
- Competition
- Fulfillment
- Integrity
- Honor
- Reputation
- Responsibility
- Prestige
- Needs
- Love

Any of these motivators can prompt an employee to action. There are two general types of motivation. *Intrinsic motivation* is internal, or originates within a person. Intrinsic motivation is long term and can be focused toward a lifelong goal. *Extrinsic motivation* is external and more material in nature. Generally, extrinsic motivation is short-lived and less satisfying than intrinsic motivation.

Use of Incentives and Employee Recognition

The staff of the provider's office should feel satisfaction with the working conditions and atmosphere in the facility. The office manager plays a part in ensuring that this happens.

Incentives give employees reasons to perform over and above the level expected of them. An important element in incentive success is that management establishes clear and attainable goals. If the staff meets or exceeds a goal that has been set, the provider may elect to provide tickets to a sports or entertainment event for the entire staff. Some providers have an incentive program for outstanding patient account collection for a given period. These ideas provide a goal for the employees to work toward and an opportunity to expand their efforts as a team.

Incentives and employee recognition should reward employees for a job well done; also, they will motivate staff members to keep up the great work. Here are some sensible incentives and employee recognition opportunities:

- After an office accomplishment, take the office out to lunch, order lunch into the office, or schedule a potluck lunch.
- Recognize an employee for his or her exceptional work during a team meeting with a personalized certificate and modest award.
- Set aside a specific time to play office games, trivia, or bingo for modest prizes at the end of a workweek.
- Schedule a weekend activity, such as a company picnic, to which employees can invite their families.

Recognition is a strong method of improving employee morale and encouraging outstanding performance. Certificates for peak performance are a great way to motivate employees. For instance, the office manager may decide to award a certificate each month to the employee who provides the highest rated customer service. Patients could even be involved by allowing them to nominate employees for this honor. When an award is at stake, most employees enjoy participating and striving to accomplish the goals that have been set.

CRITICAL THINKING APPLICATION   20.3

Kate has noticed that the medical coding department has been running behind more than usual. As a result, health insurance reimbursements have been lagging. What can Kate do to motivate her employees?

CREATING A TEAM ENVIRONMENT

Teamwork is critical in the medical profession. Communication improves when staff members collaborate as a team in the healthcare workplace, and improved communication can reduce medical errors and increase patient satisfaction. Therefore, the manager must promote an atmosphere in which employees are willing to work together toward common goals. Morale in the office may be low because of recent changes in policies or procedures, changes in staff or management, recent terminations of employees, lack of business, or for any number of other reasons. Some managers try to shield employees from negative information, but this practice can cause rumors to circulate and worsen morale.

One of the most effective ways to improve employee morale is to communicate openly and honestly. Regular staff meetings, emails,

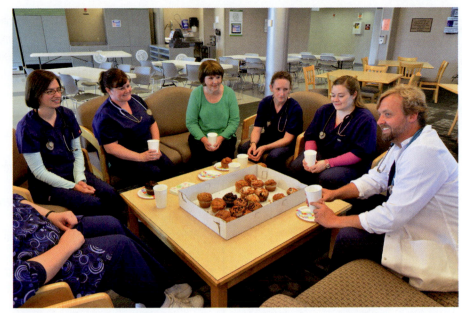

FIGURE 20.2 Communication is vital when building a team. Employees appreciate good communication with management. Sharing good and bad news openly with employees leads to fewer rumors and eases workers' concerns.

and memos are critical for good communication and the smooth operation of a healthcare facility (Fig. 20.2). Communicating changes and developments that affect employees helps to improve morale. Morale can also be improved by scheduling activities that involve the families of employees.

Recognize and Overcome Barriers to Communication

Effective communication is important to increase efficiency and improve teamwork. Recognizing barriers to communication in the workplace is critical to the health of the team. The following are five barriers that can occur in a healthcare agency. It is important for the medical assistant to recognize the barriers and help the team overcome them.

- **Physical separation barriers** In large healthcare facilities, employees can be separated by departments, or even by distance if they are in different buildings. Communicating via email can be difficult, and communication cues can be missed, leading to misinterpretation of the message. Using technology (e.g., video conferencing and webcams) can help employees interact and strengthen communication.
- **Language barriers** Our workplaces are becoming more diverse. Employees live and train in different areas, learning different communication styles and different words for the same thing. For instance, a surgical instrument may be known by several names, as a result of providers training in different parts of the world. Supervisors who encourage awareness and acceptance of everyone's language and culture differences will strengthen the team's communication.
- **Status barriers** People may perceive that only those in higher ranking positions in a healthcare organization are important. This can lead to communication barriers and malfunctioning teams. It is important for the supervisor to promote awareness and acceptance that everyone counts and every position on the team is important.

- **Gender difference barriers** Males and females communicate differently, with females typically preferring a closer, more personal communication style than males. In some situations, the minority gender in an organization may not be as comfortable in communicating with peers. It is important for the supervisor to ensure that all employees, regardless of gender, feel empowered to communicate openly with others.
- **Cultural diversity barriers** Behaviors, words, and gestures have different meanings from one cultural group to another. How persons of different cultural groups communicate can also be different. For instance, some cultural groups do not believe in eye contact, whereas other groups may perceive a person to be lying or uncomfortable if eye contact is minimal. It is important for the supervisor to help the team embrace the cultural differences among the members, and educating the team on the differences can help promote understanding and cohesion.

FINDING THE RIGHT EMPLOYEE FOR THE JOB

The most important asset of any healthcare facility is a staff that genuinely cares for patients. From providers to the receptionist, all play a vital role in the quality of the healthcare delivered. Hiring staff members who can be molded into a **cohesive** team is not an easy task. Care should be taken to choose employees who have the necessary skills and the right personality for the ambulatory care facility.

When the need for a new employee arises, the office manager should discuss with the providers the type of employee needed and the job description for that individual. Ask what qualities the providers desire for the position and the tasks for which the person will be responsible. Once the need has been established and the duties confirmed, the office manager can begin the recruiting process.

One of the most effective methods of finding new employees is allowing medical assistant students to complete their practicum at the healthcare facility. This provides the student the opportunity to learn about the facility, staff, providers, and for the supervisor to see how the student interacts with others. Even if no openings exist, supervisors can ask the students for a resume to keep on file until a position opens up. Another effective method for finding new employees is advertising on local job boards. Larger facilities will post the job on their employment website page and link to other job boards. Smaller agencies will usually advertise on local free or low-cost job boards and advertise in local newspapers.

When creating an online ad or a job posting on an employment website, the office manager should list the basic responsibilities and expectations for the position. Briefly describe the office, location, and the qualifications needed. Some offices also list a few of the benefits offered to attract applicants and also may disclose a salary range.

Job Description

The job description is a tool designed to inform job candidates about the duties they would be expected to perform. Well-written and detailed job descriptions list the essential functions of the job and reveal the chain of command the employee should follow when questions or concerns arise. These documents provide a good guideline for potential employees so that they will understand exactly what is expected of them and their responsibilities at work.

Job descriptions are essential in the search for the perfect candidate. They highlight the specific educational background and skill set needed to be successful in the position. A clear job description in the hiring process increases the chance that an applicant with the required skills will apply for the open position. If a job description is too vague, many unqualified applicants may apply, and sorting through all the applications to find the right person for the position will be difficult.

The job description should include a statement that says the employee must perform any additional duties as assigned by the supervisor. With this statement in place, the employee cannot say, "That's not my job." All employees should be willing to pull together and assist with any tasks, but this statement gives added weight to assignments that are not specified in the written job description.

An effective manager understands the phrase "inspect what you expect." When duties are assigned, the manager should ensure that the tasks were completed correctly and in a timely manner. New employees should be monitored to make sure their delegated tasks are being done and done right. Without inspection, the manager cannot know whether the new employee is meeting expectations. Once employees have earned a degree of trust, inspecting their work is not as necessary as in the beginning. Some managers practice a skill called "management by walking around." By strolling through the areas where subordinates work, managers can observe and hear about issues that might be brewing, and at the same time improve morale by offering encouragement and praise.

Job Description for a Medical Assistant

Medical assistants are qualified for a variety of tasks in the ambulatory care site. To fill any open medical assisting positions, the manager must determine which specific experience meets the facility's needs. With experience, professional skills can develop in specific aspects in the medical assisting profession. The website https://www.monster.com provides the following general job description for medical assistants.

Medical Assistant's Job Responsibilities

Helping patients through information, services, and assistance.

Medical Assistant's Job Duties

- Interviews patient to collect health data; records medical history and confirms purpose of the visit.
- Collects vital patient data by taking blood pressure, weight, and temperature; reports patient history summary.
- Secures patient's private information and preserves patient confidentiality according to HIPAA standards.
- Performs diagnostic and procedural coding, medical billing, and collection procedures for all patient accounts.
- Schedules patient appointments in the medical office and for surgery. Prepares the health record, pre-admit paperwork, and all required consent forms.
- Counsels patients on following provider's orders and answers patients' questions about follow-up care.
- Manages biohazard waste and infection control to protect patients and medical office staff.
- Works with the medical care team to create a safe, secure, and healthy work environment by following office policies and procedures.
- Maintains inventory for medical supplies in the office by taking stock, placing orders, and verifying receipts.
- Supports healthcare facility equipment maintenance by following operating instructions, troubleshooting equipment failure, conducting preventive maintenance, and calling for repairs.
- Displays exceptional customer service to all patients, regardless of age, race, gender, religion, or socioeconomic background.

Medical Assistant's Skills and Qualifications

Customer service, clinical skills, written and verbal communication, infection control management, time management, scheduling, professionalism, confidentiality, working on a team.

Reviewing Applications

Depending on the situation, the manager may look at the applications as they come in or at the closing date. With today's technology, many agencies have applicants submit cover letters, resumes, and applications online, although some still use paper documents. The first step in reviewing resumes is to separate the applications that meet the minimal qualifications from those that do not. Typically, the minimal qualification includes successful completion of a medical assistant program and/or a medical assistant credential.

Applicants who meet the minimal qualifications are divided into three stacks: individuals to call for an interview; candidates, but not the strongest; and those who will not be called for an interview. Usually, the manager makes these decisions after reviewing the resumes. Those with related experience, strong related skill sets (e.g., customer service), no unexplained employment gaps, and customized, error-free resumes and cover letters are more apt to be moved to the top of the pile.

Online Job Applications

Many healthcare facilities request job applicants to complete their employment application online. The online job application portal is beneficial for the job applicant and the health facility. The health facility can provide specific details about the open medical assisting positions, including the job responsibilities, a brief description of the benefits package, and a description of the company, including its mission statement. For the healthcare facility employer, online medical assisting applicants can be filtered by each individual professional experience, skills, certifications, and educational background. These portals allow employers to ask for more information specific to the job description; they can reduce the pool of applicants to just a few skilled candidates.

Once the original stack of applications has been reviewed, the office manager can return to the qualifying applications to determine which candidates to interview. Careful judgment and objectivity must be used in the search for an employee suitable for the healthcare facility. The manager should review the final applications with the following questions in mind:

- Does the applicant's grammar meet the office's standards? Can the applicant write a business letter?
- Does the applicant have basic computer skills?
- Has the applicant been employed previously in an ambulatory care facility? What were some of his or her responsibilities? Is this experience in line with the job description of the open position?
- If the applicant was previously employed, how long was he or she in the last position? Why did the applicant leave?
- Does the applicant seem to accept and enjoy responsibility? Does he or she have any professional goals that the medical office can train the individual to achieve?
- What is the applicant's formal education? Is he or she registered or certified?
- Is the applicant a member of a professional organization? Does he or she attend meetings?

Arranging the Personal Interview

In many of the larger healthcare facilities, a human resources representative will conduct a prescreening interview either over the phone or using technology such as Skype. At this time, basic questions can be asked by the representative to gauge the interest of the applicant. That information is then forwarded to the office manager. In other agencies, the office manager may conduct the prescreening interview, to evaluate the person's telephone voice, attitude, and communication skills. In addition, the manager may want to ask several questions about the person's education, skills, and professional experience. Because the employee probably will speak with patients on the telephone, a qualified candidate should speak with ease. Those who perform well during the prescreening phone call should be scheduled for an interview.

TABLE 20.1   Legal and Illegal Interview Questions

LEGAL QUESTIONS	ILLEGAL QUESTIONS
• Why did you leave your last job?	• How long have you been working?
• What are your strengths and weaknesses?	• When was the last time you used drugs?
• What motivates you to succeed?	• Do you have any children?
• What are some of your hobbies?	• What religion do you practice?
• Are you willing to work more than 40 hours a week?	• Are you married?

CRITICAL THINKING APPLICATION   20.4

Kate was impressed with Carol Limpken's resume and application, but when scheduling an interview on the telephone, she noticed that Carol's grammar was not as professional as Kate would like. Should this influence Kate's decision whether to hire Carol?

Why is speech such an important issue in a healthcare facility?

Should Kate be concerned about a candidate's grammar and spelling errors on the resume or application? Why or why not?

Set a time for the personal interview when the applicant can be given undivided attention. An applicant who is being considered for employment should have an opportunity to see the facility during a period of fairly normal activity. The candidate who is interviewed in a peaceful, quiet office may not be prepared for the activity on a normal working day.

Before interviewing any applicant, become thoroughly familiar with the federal, state, and local fair employment practice laws affecting hiring practices. The Equal Employment Opportunity Act of 1972 prohibits inquiries into an applicant's race, color, gender, religion, and national origin. Inquiries about medical history, arrest records, or previous drug use also are illegal. Office managers must research the laws that pertain to employment in their own states or work with the human resources team, who are more familiar with these laws. It is important to develop a list of questions that will be asked of all interviewees. Creating a question list before the interviews helps to ensure no illegal questions are asked and that all interviewees are fairly evaluated (Table 20.1).

Laws Affecting Employment

Numerous laws affect the way employees are treated, from the interview through the end of employment. The office manager should be familiar with these laws and how they affect the practice.

Fair Labor Standards Act

- State standards for minimum wage and overtime pay; employees must be paid minimum wage and time and a half for overtime hours, as they apply
- Prohibits those under age 18 from performing certain kinds of work and restricts the hours of workers under age 16

Occupational Safety and Health Act
- Regulates conditions affecting employees' safety and health in the workplace

Workers Compensation
- Regulates the benefits of employees who have been injured on the job
- Determines pay for employees who are not working because of an on-the-job injury

Family and Medical Leave Act
- Requires employers of 50 or more employees to offer up to 12 weeks of unpaid, job-protected leave to eligible employees for the birth of a child, an adoption, or a personal or family illness

Pregnancy Discrimination Act
- Forbids employers to refuse to hire a woman based on pregnancy, childbirth, or related medical conditions
- Requires employers to hold open a job for a pregnancy-related absence the same length of time that a job would be held open for employees on sick or disability leave

Americans With Disabilities Act
- Prohibits discrimination against individuals with disabilities

Age Discrimination Act
- Prevents discrimination in hiring on the basis of age
- Prevents discrimination in promoting, discharging, and compensating employees

The Interview

The interview is usually conducted by the office manager or with a panel of employees. If a panel is being used, the members should meet before the interview to create a list of interview questions and discuss the flow of the interview. Each interviewee should be asked the same questions. Additional questions may be asked of individual candidates to clarify responses to the standard set of questions.

The interview typically starts with an introduction of the interviewers and a review of the job description. Usually, the first question (e.g., "Tell us about yourself") is meant to put the person at ease and get a summary of the person's professional and educational background. As the interview progresses, different types of questions will be asked to explore the person's past experiences and personality. Straightforward questions relate to the position duties. Behavioral questions are given to explore how the person behaved during a difficult past situation to anticipate how he or she might handle future issues. Situational questions help the interviewers understand how the person would handle a hypothetical situation. The interviewers use the questions to explore the person's personality and past experiences and to gauge how the person might fit into the existing team.

After the questions are completed, the manager should give the interviewee an opportunity to ask questions. Some interviews conclude with a discussion of the benefits and pay, but many times this occurs when the job is being offered to the applicant, because the human resources representative is the best resource for this information. Last, the office manager should give the interviewee an idea of the next steps in the process and when the decision will be made. If the person hasn't completed an application form, it is important to have that completed before the person leaves. References should also be collected from the interviewee.

Once the applicant leaves, the interviewers should rate or summarize their impressions of the applicant, listing the strengths and weaknesses on the interview question form. Be objective and professional and do not write **disparaging** information. The form will be kept on file in case of discrimination claims in hiring practices.

Usually, discussions of the candidate among the interview team are not encouraged until after all the interviews are completed. After all the interviews are conducted, the interviewers as a group should rank the candidates and finalize the top choices.

Follow-up Activities

Always carefully check all references and follow through on any leads for information. Contact all listed references. When speaking with a candidate's former employer, be sure to "listen between the lines." Note the tone of the replies to the questions. Do not ask questions that might incriminate the person answering them. The following questions are effective as an introduction:

- When did (the applicant) work for you? For how long?
- What were his or her duties and responsibilities? Did the employee assume responsibility well?
- Did the employee work well in a team environment? Did any conflicts arise that we should know about?

Some employers provide information only on the date of hire, job title, and date of termination of the employment. However, if the employer states, "She worked in our office from May, 2018, to July, 2019, and is not eligible for rehire," the reasonable assumption is that the employee did not perform well. The tone of voice and emphasis on the word "not" should be clues that this person is probably not right for the job. Still, if all other references are glowing, call and ask the applicant about the facility that gave the negative response. There could be a reasonable explanation for what might have been a bad experience. Respect the company's policy and do not press for further information.

After the applicant list has been narrowed to two or three candidates whose references have been checked thoroughly, a second interview may be arranged. The providers may want to participate in these interviews.

Selecting the Right Applicant

Once the final interviews have been conducted, it is time to choose the best candidate. Never rely strictly on a "gut instinct" about a potential employee. Base hiring decisions on logical conclusions drawn from all contacts with the applicant, including:

- Grammar and enunciation
- Office manners and customer service skills
- Professional appearance
- Work history
- Match to required job skills
- Friendly, personable attitude

When a decision has been reached to hire someone, either a human resource representative or the office manager will contact the person. This is the most common time to discuss wages and benefits. The applicant may request 2 to 3 days to think over the offer. Make sure you have a firm date when the applicant will make his or her decision.

When the position is filled, the human resources representative or the office manager needs to contact all the applicants and explain the job has been filled. This notification can occur through email, a letter, or a phone call. Be courteous in the notification and thank the individual for applying.

Paperwork for New Employees

The office manager should develop a checklist of the paperwork needed for newly hired staff members and all the information that should be covered with the new employee at the start of the job. Basic new employee paperwork often includes:

- HIPAA confidentiality statement
- Computer passwords and agreement statement
- Job application
- Form I-9 (Employment Eligibility Verification)
- W-4 Form (Employee's Withholding Allowance Certificate)
- Notice of Workers Compensation coverage
- Consent for background check, drug testing, and search (if applicable)
- Acknowledgment of receipt of company handbook or policy manual
- Agreements regarding pay, wage deductions, benefits, schedule, work location, and so on
- Notices of at-will employment status
- Direct deposit application
- Occupational Safety and Health Administration (OSHA) compliance acknowledgement or checklist

All of these forms, once completed and signed, should be kept in the employee's personnel file. Other forms and paperwork may be necessary that vary from state to state and company to company. The Form I-9 (Employment Eligibility Verification) is required by the federal government (Fig. 20.3). This form must be completed for all newly hired employees to verify their identification and authorization to work in the United States. The most current form is available at *http://www.uscis.gov*, along with training materials. The newly hired employee should complete the first section of the form and provide it to the human resource representative or office manager on the first day of work. The remaining information is completed by the representative or manager. Specific documents need to be shown to prove the person's identification and authorization to work in this country. A person who cannot provide the required documentation should not be allowed to remain as an employee.

Employees should also understand the *at-will employment* status. Under the at-will employment principle, the employer can terminate the employment at any time, for any reason/cause and without notice. Unless the employer violated labor laws or the employee rights, the employee has little recourse. Only a few states protect employees from termination without good cause. At-will employment also means that the employee can leave the employment at any time, but professionally it is important to give the employer the required notice.

Orientation and Training

The hiring process does not end with hiring a new employee. Orientation and training help new employees understand what is expected and develop to their full potential (Fig. 20.4). A critical error made when bringing new staff members aboard is failing to provide them with a fair orientation and training period.

Some managers assign a **mentor** to assist the new employee during the initial probationary period. This type of "buddy" system is a good practice because the new person does not feel isolated and alone during the first few weeks on the job.

Acquaint the new employee with the following:

- Staff members and their names
- Physical environment and layout of the office
- Nature of the practice and specialty
- Types of patients seen in the office
- Office policies and procedures
- Employee benefits
- Short- and long-range expectations
- HIPAA and computer training

Types of Employee Benefits

- *Employer-sponsored health insurance:* The employer pays a percentage of the employee's health insurance premium.
- *Dental and vision benefits:* The employer may offer dental and vision benefits for employees but may choose not to sponsor any of the premium.
- *Cafeteria plan:* A tax-free account in which employees can invest some of their paycheck and from which they can withdraw amounts for qualified health and/or child day care expenses.
- *401k retirement account matching:* The employer matches the exact amount or a percentage of the investment the employee makes every pay period (2% to 3%), up to a specific amount ($1,500).
- *Life insurance:* The employer pays for a small life insurance policy (usually up to $15,000) for minimal after-death expenses.
- *Disability insurance:* A benefit employees pay for that pays them if they are disabled and unable to work.

All new employees should be required to familiarize themselves with important office policies and procedures by reviewing the policies and procedures manual. It is advisable for the manager to require the employee to sign a statement verifying that the manual has been read.

Make sure the employee's file is complete before allowing the person to work even 1 hour. Also, make sure all federal and state regulations that apply to new employees have been met.

Using Performance Evaluations Effectively

A new employee should be granted a probationary period. The traditional period is 60 to 90 days, but many employers believe that 2 weeks is sufficient to determine whether the employee will be able to learn and adapt to the position. Set a specific date for a performance evaluation covering the probationary period when the new employee is hired. This evaluation should not be squeezed in between patient visits or be given a token few minutes at the end of a day. Schedule a time that provides the opportunity to relax and talk. Tell the new employee how well expectations have been met and whether there are any deficiencies; then give the employee an opportunity to ask questions. Sometimes an employee fails to perform because he or she was never told what was expected. Although the probationary period does not always allow time to train an individual fully for a specific

Department of Homeland Security
U.S. Citizenship and Immigration Services

Form I-9, Employment Eligibility Verification

Read instructions carefully before completing this form. The instructions must be available during completion of this form.

ANTI-DISCRIMINATION NOTICE: It is illegal to discriminate against work-authorized individuals. Employers CANNOT specify which document(s) they will accept from an employee. The refusal to hire an individual because the documents have a future expiration date may also constitute illegal discrimination.

Section 1. Employee Information and Verification (To be completed and signed by employee at the time employment begins.)

Print Name: Last	First	Middle Initial	Maiden Name

Address (Street Name and Number)	Apt. #	Date of Birth (month/day/year)

City	State	Zip Code	Social Security #

I am aware that federal law provides for imprisonment and/or fines for false statements or use of false documents in connection with the completion of this form.

I attest, under penalty of perjury, that I am (check one of the following):

☐ A citizen of the United States

☐ A noncitizen national of the United States (see instructions)

☐ A lawful permanent resident (Alien #) _____

☐ An alien authorized to work (Alien # or Admission #) _____

until (expiration date, if applicable - *month/day/year*)

Employee's Signature	Date (month/day/year)

Preparer and/or Translator Certification *(To be completed and signed if Section 1 is prepared by a person other than the employee.) I attest, under penalty of perjury, that I have assisted in the completion of this form and that to the best of my knowledge the information is true and correct.*

Preparer's/Translator's Signature	Print Name

Address (Street Name and Number, City, State, Zip Code)	Date (month/day/year)

Section 2. Employer Review and Verification (To be completed and signed by employer. Examine one document from List A OR examine one document from List B and one from List C, as listed on the reverse of this form, and record the title, number, and expiration date, if any, of the document(s).)

	List A	OR	List B	AND	List C
Document title:					
Issuing authority:					
Document #:					
Expiration Date (if any):					
Document #:					
Expiration Date (if any):					

CERTIFICATION: I attest, under penalty of perjury, that I have examined the document(s) presented by the above-named employee, that the above-listed document(s) appear to be genuine and to relate to the employee named, that the employee began employment on *(month/day/year)* _____ **and that to the best of my knowledge the employee is authorized to work in the United States. (State employment agencies may omit the date the employee began employment.)**

Signature of Employer or Authorized Representative	Print Name	Title

Business or Organization Name and Address (Street Name and Number, City, State, Zip Code)	Date (month/day/year)

Section 3. Updating and Reverification (To be completed and signed by employer.)

A. New Name (if applicable)	B. Date of Rehire (month/day/year) (if applicable)

C. If employee's previous grant of work authorization has expired, provide the information below for the document that establishes current employment authorization.

Document Title:	Document #:	Expiration Date (if any):

I attest, under penalty of perjury, that to the best of my knowledge, this employee is authorized to work in the United States, and if the employee presented document(s), the document(s) I have examined appear to be genuine and to relate to the individual.

Signature of Employer or Authorized Representative	Date (month/day/year)

Form I-9 (Rev.) Y Page 4

FIGURE 20.3 The I-9 Form (Employment Eligibility Verification) is designed to help the employer gather the documents necessary to prove that an employee is eligible to work in the United States.

LISTS OF ACCEPTABLE DOCUMENTS
All documents must be unexpired

LIST A	LIST B	LIST C
Documents that Establish Both Identity and Employment Authorization	**Documents that Establish Identity**	**Documents that Establish Employment Authorization**
	OR ... **AND**	
1. U.S. Passport or U.S. Passport Card	1. Driver's license or ID card issued by a State or outlying possession of the United States provided it contains a photograph or information such as name, date of birth, gender, height, eye color, and address	1. Social Security Account Number card other than one that specifies on the face that the issuance of the card does not authorize employment in the United States
2. Permanent Resident Card or Alien Registration Receipt Card (Form I-551)		2. Certification of Birth Abroad issued by the Department of State (Form FS-545)
3. Foreign passport that contains a temporary I-551 stamp or temporary I-551 printed notation on a machine-readable immigrant visa	2. ID card issued by federal, state or local government agencies or entities, provided it contains a photograph or information such as name, date of birth, gender, height, eye color, and address	3. Certification of Report of Birth issued by the Department of State (Form DS-1350)
4. Employment Authorization Document that contains a photograph (Form I-766)	3. School ID card with a photograph	4. Original or certified copy of birth certificate issued by a State, county, municipal authority, or territory of the United States bearing an official seal
	4. Voter's registration card	
5. In the case of a nonimmigrant alien authorized to work for a specific employer incident to status, a foreign passport with Form I-94 or Form I-94A bearing the same name as the passport and containing an endorsement of the alien's nonimmigrant status, as long as the period of endorsement has not yet expired and the proposed employment is not in conflict with any restrictions or limitations identified on the form	5. U.S. Military card or draft record	
	6. Military dependent's ID card	5. Native American tribal document
	7. U.S. Coast Guard Merchant Mariner Card	
	8. Native American tribal document	6. U.S. Citizen ID Card (Form I-197)
	9. Driver's license issued by a Canadian government authority	
	For persons under age 18 who are unable to present a document listed above:	7. Identification Card for Use of Resident Citizen in the United States (Form I-179)
6. Passport from the Federated States of Micronesia (FSM) or the Republic of the Marshall Islands (RMI) with Form I-94 or Form I-94A indicating nonimmigrant admission under the Compact of Free Association Between the United States and the FSM or RMI	10. School record or report card	8. Employment authorization document issued by the Department of Homeland Security
	11. Clinic, doctor, or hospital record	
	12. Day-care or nursery school record	

Illustrations of many of these documents appear in Part 8 of the Handbook for Employers (M-274)

Form I-9 (Rev.) Y Page 5

FIGURE 20.3, cont'd

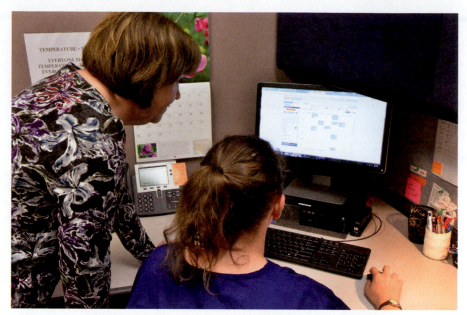

FIGURE 20.4 The training of successful employees begins with the job orientation.

position, it is fair to assume that the potential for being a satisfactory employee can be judged at this time. Now is the time to talk about any problems and make suggestions for improvement. Sometimes the employee is released after an unsuccessful probationary period.

The formal performance appraisal usually occurs at the end of the probationary period and then at the hiring date anniversary. A typical appraisal includes feedback on teamwork, punctuality and attendance, motivation, accuracy with skills, customer service, professionalism, and potential continuing education and future goals. In many facilities, the appraisal relates to the pay increase the person will receive. Agencies do performance appraisals differently, yet one of the more common methods is for the supervisor to gather input from peers that work with the employee. The 360-degree evaluation is a process in which the supervisor, peers, and those who interact with the employee outside of the department provide feedback for the performance appraisal. If an employee works well with peers in the department yet is rude and unprofessional to employees in other areas of the facility, the 360-degree evaluation will provide that information. This evaluation process holds the employee accountable for all his or her interactions in the facility.

When negative information is to be relayed to the employee during a performance appraisal, sandwich the negative comment between two positive ones whenever possible. For instance, tell the employee, "Jewel, you are a pro at greeting patients and making them feel at home. I would like to see you improve your time management skills, however, because I feel you are spending too much time with individual patients. I must confess that they feel a part of the clinic family. Let's work on some time management issues and keep making them feel so welcome!"

Managers also may use the "feel, felt, found" approach when talking with employees about their performance. For example, "Jewel, I feel the same way you do about patients taking up a lot of our time. I know there are some who want to talk with us for hours, and I have felt the pressure of wanting to make them feel comfortable but having so much to do, too. I have found that if I explain that I have a meeting or another patient to assist, they are very understanding and not offended. Perhaps you can try that approach, too."

No supervisor enjoys giving an evaluation (Fig. 20.5) that is not a positive one. It is difficult to know exactly where to begin when the employee has not performed as expected or hoped. Perhaps the best way to open the conversation is to say, "Rebecca, your review today is not going to be a positive one. It seems that we do not have a meeting of the minds about your duties and our expectations of you. Let's talk about your performance and discuss whether this position is a good match for you." Having detailed documentation of performance issues leaves little room for argument and places the manager on the offensive. The employee may be apprehensive or even defensive at this point, but the phrasing will certainly get his or her attention, and the discussion should produce either the motivation to improve or the clarity that termination is in order.

Fair Salaries and Raises

Medical office managers should recruit employees who want to remain with the office for a long time. There are always situations such as a part-time worker returning to college, or a summer worker going back to school. However, good employee **retention** is the goal.

To retain good employees, the practice must pay them a fair salary with regular raises if they perform as expected. The office manager can find information about salary comparisons on the internet. Periodically review job descriptions and salary analyses online to see whether the salary the medical facility offers is comparable to that for similar jobs in the area.

Merit raises are increases based on an employee's commendable performance. Cost of living increases are given when earned, usually after specific periods or annually, and are based on national statistics and trends. An employee who is promoted should also be awarded a salary increase. When the office pays a fair salary for work done, the facility retains happy employees.

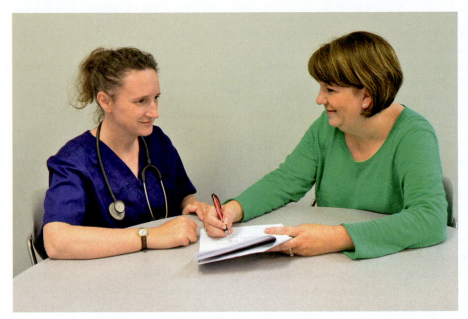

FIGURE 20.5 Performance Evaluation and Development Plan. Performance evaluations should be considered tools that help employees reach their personal goals and the goals of the organization.

Problem Employees

Occasionally, employees do not perform at the expected level or demonstrate unprofessional behaviors. Counseling these employees to determine the source of their difficulties is the first step toward resolution. Many employees can be redirected to become productive staff members with a little patience and understanding on the manager's part. Employees who display a willingness to improve their attitude are worth the investment the office manager makes to help them succeed.

Many offices allow one verbal warning before written reprimands go into the employee's file. It is important that the manager document the specific times, dates, and descriptions of incidents, even issues such as tardiness. If the manager does not make a habit of writing a formal warning in the employee's **human resources file (HR file)**, there may be insufficient documentation of problems. The manager should never be in a position in which the termination of an employee cannot be justified through documentation.

CRITICAL THINKING APPLICATION   20.5

Kate has two employees who have never seemed to get along. One of the employees has a history of being vindictive and manipulative, but never in an obvious enough way for Kate to have sufficient proof to reprimand her in writing. One day, one of the employees comes to Kate's office to report that she saw the other employee, who has an exemplary record, taking drugs from the supply cabinet. How does Kate handle this situation? What steps should Kate take from here?

Terminating Employees

Terminating an employee is unpleasant at best, but if the ground rules are decided in advance, written into the office policies and procedures manual, and explained to all employees, the problem is partially solved. The policies must be applied equally and impartially to all employees. The providers of the healthcare facility will most probably make the final decision on dismissal, but it may be based on the recommendation of the office manager. Unless there are mitigating factors that suggest otherwise, the person who does the hiring should do the firing.

A probationary employee who does not prove satisfactory should be dismissed at the end of the probationary period, with tact and a full explanation of the reasons for dismissal. In all fairness, an individual should be told why the employment is being ended and not be given weak excuses or untruths that do not help correct deficiencies. If the manager is not straightforward in giving the reason for dismissal, the employee will not have the opportunity to grow and improve his or her performance.

An employee who has been in service for some time and is not performing satisfactorily should be warned and given an explanation of the specific improvements expected. If a second chance does not produce improvement in performance or attitude, dismissal must follow. It should be done privately, with tact and consideration.

Most practice consultants believe that firing should come close to the end of the day and end of the workweek, after all other employees have left, and that the break should be clean and immediate. A dismissed employee should never be allowed to train or influence a replacement.

The exit meeting should be planned just as carefully as the employment interview. Be honest with the employee. Discuss both the employee's assets and liabilities and give the reasons for the termination. There is no need to dwell on the employee's deficiencies. These should have been thoroughly discussed at the warning interview, and the employee need only be told that the necessary improvements have not been made. Listen to the employee's feedback, unless it becomes lengthy or abusive. This may reveal some important administrative problems that need correction.

After dismissing an employee, do not leave that person in the office unattended. Request the office keys and any other equipment in the employee's possession immediately, before the dismissed employee leaves the building, and block all access to the healthcare facility's electronic health records (EHRs). Most states have strict payday laws that do not allow holding the final paycheck for any reason. Do not offer to give the employee a good reference unless it can be done sincerely.

If there is any indication that an employee may become abusive or violent once told about the termination, the supervisor should bring a representative from the human resources department or security to the final interview. It is possible that an employee can "snap" and suddenly become violent; however, more often it is the warning flags raised by an employee's behavior before termination that justify care in the termination interview. This is why supervisors should always document any strange or suspicious employee behavior and any breach of office policy or procedures in the employee's personnel file, according to office policy. Documenting everything creates a clear picture of the employee's actions throughout the time of employment. Of course, the supervisor must be willing to confront an employee about his or her negative actions in the workplace.

Some specific employee behaviors in the workplace, such as embezzlement, insubordination, and violation of patient confidentiality, are grounds for immediate dismissal without warning. These behaviors display a lack of respect for the healthcare facility and can lead to the mistreatment or endangerment of patients if the employee is not terminated immediately.

Occasionally an employee voluntarily leaves a position without giving a valid reason. The provider or office manager may want to follow up with a letter to the former employee to determine whether a problem prompted the resignation. The employee may reveal serious issues with other personnel or with the office that need to be addressed and corrected.

CRITICAL THINKING APPLICATION   20.6

While Kate is explaining to a particularly poor employee why she plans to terminate her, the employee begins screaming and accusing Kate of discrimination and harassment. How should Kate handle this situation? What are Kate's options if the employee does not stop the inappropriate behavior?

POLICIES AND PROCEDURES

Personnel Policy Manual

Information about the employer-employee relationship is found in the personnel policy manual, sometimes referred to as the employee handbook. It spells out the healthcare facilities rules regarding things such as:

- Health benefits
- Vacation time
- Sick leave
- Holidays
- Overtime
- Performance evaluations
- Termination of employment

- *Grievance* (complaint) process
- Dress code
- Office safety
- Employee's role in case of an emergency

Some agencies will give each new employee a copy of the personnel policy manual, and others keep a copy in a central location. More commonly, the manual will be found electronically on the agency's intranet. The personnel policy manual should be updated on a regular basis. This can easily be done when it is in an electronic format, but employees should be notified when an update occurs.

Workplace Sexual Harassment

The U.S. Equal Employment Opportunity Commission states that sexual harassment is unwelcome sexual advances, requests for sexual favors, and other verbal or physical harassment of a sexual nature. Sexual harassment is against the law. Both the victim and the harasser can be either a woman or a man, and victim and harasser can be the same sex. The harasser can be the victim's supervisor, a supervisor in another area, a co-worker, or someone who is not an employee of the employer, such as a client or customer.

A medical office manager will need to make all employees aware of what conduct is considered sexual harassment. When an employee feels that he or she is being sexually harassed the employee should report it to the supervisor or the office manager. Once a report has been made, the manager must investigate the allegation. Actions must be taken to protect all employees, because the healthcare facility is at risk for a lawsuit.

The office manager wants to ensure that the healthcare facility is a comfortable place for all employees to work without being the target of unwanted sexual advances. There are no laws against two employees dating each other, but it is a good idea to have a policy in place regarding supervisors dating subordinates. It can be hard to determine whether the subordinate felt pressured to date the supervisor in order to keep his or her job.

Employees should keep in mind that it can be considered sexual harassment to have an explicit calendar or poster. If another employee finds it offensive, he or she can make a claim of sexual harassment. Some organizations will have a policy regarding office decorations.

Workplace Bullying

Workplace bullying is defined by the Workplace Bullying Institute as repeated mistreatment of an employee by one or more employees; abusive conduct that is threatening, humiliating, or intimidating; work sabotage; or verbal abuse. The institute's 2017 survey showed that 19% of Americans are bullied, and 60.4 million people are affected by workplace bullying. Only 29% of those who are bullied report it. It is likely that these workers will leave their jobs to get away from the bullying. It is the office manager's responsibility to take all accusations seriously and to also create an environment in which employees will freely come to the manager when there is an issue, whether the person is the victim or a witness. It has to be made clear that bullying will not be tolerated.

Office Policies and Procedures

Office policies and procedures differ from personnel policies in that they provide direction on the ways to complete tasks within the healthcare facility.

Clinical Procedures

Clinical procedures will vary from one healthcare facility to another, depending on the type of facility. A family practice facility will have different procedures than a plastic surgery facility. All procedures should have a list of instruments and supplies needed, along with step-by-step instructions on how to complete the procedure. Having a standard procedure that everyone follows ensures consistency in patient care.

Administrative Procedures

Administrative procedures can also vary, depending on the type of medical practice, but they usually cover topics such as opening and closing the office, appointment scheduling, patient account processing, insurance claim processing, and eligibility verification.

Regulatory Compliance

It is important for an office manager in a healthcare facility to stay current with all changes in legislation at both the state and federal levels. This will ensure that the facility is working within the legal boundaries. There can be severe consequences when a healthcare facility is noncompliant.

Health Insurance Portability and Accountability Act (HIPAA)

The office manager is responsible for making sure that the healthcare facility is **compliant** with all aspects of HIPAA (see Chapter 4). All employees should be trained in HIPAA compliance, such as protecting patient information. Violations of HIPAA can result in fines and possible jail time. The Office for Civil Rights (OCR) is responsible for enforcing the HIPAA Privacy and Security Rules. The fines were increased when the Health Information Technology for Economic and Clinical Health Act (HITECH) was enacted.

Health Information Technology for Economic and Clinical Health Act (HITECH)

HITECH includes provisions that allow for increased enforcement of the privacy and security of electronic transmission of health information. HITECH expanded on HIPAA by:

- Making business associates directly liable for compliance with HIPAA.
- Prohibiting the sale of protected health information (PHI) without the patient's authorization.
- Creating a tiered violation category: unknowing, reasonable cause, willful neglect–corrected, and willful neglected–uncorrected. Violation penalties range from $100 for each "unknowing" violation to $1.5 million per calendar year. The greater the violation, the greater the penalty amount. Individuals, healthcare agencies, and business associations could be penalized and fined.
- **Breach** notification requirements were increased. Individuals must be notified of the breach via mail or email. If the facility does not have up-to-date contact information for 10 or more patients, then a notice must be posted on the company's website for at least 90 days. If more than 500 individuals were impacted, then the media and the OCR secretary must be notified. A list of breaches reported is published on the OCR website (*https://ocrportal.hhs.gov/ocr/breach/breach_report.jsf*).

Table 20.2 describes the possible penalties that could be imposed by OCR.

On June 1, 2018, a $4.3 million fine was imposed on the University of Texas MD Anderson Cancer Center. There were three separate data breaches that involved the theft of an unencrypted laptop and the loss of two unencrypted thumb drives that contained unencrypted electronic protected health information (ePHI) of more than 33,500 individuals. HIPAA compliance should not be taken lightly.

You can see why compliance with HIPAA and HITECH is very important. It is one of the responsibilities of an office manager to make sure that the healthcare facility is completely compliant with all regulations.

Occupational Safety and Health Act

The Occupational Safety and Health Act of 1970 (OSH Act) created and is enforced by the Occupational Safety and Health Administration (OSHA). OSHA sets workplace standards and inspects employers to ensure employee safety. The standards related to healthcare include

TABLE 20.2 HIPAA Penalties		
HIPAA VIOLATION	**MINIMUM PENALTY**	**MAXIMUM PENALTY**
Unknowing	$100 per violation, with an annual maximum of $25,000 for repeat violations	$50,000 per violation, with an annual maximum of $1.5 million
Reasonable cause	$1,000 per violation, with an annual maximum of $100,000 for repeat violations	$50,000 per violation with an annual maximum of $1.5 million
Willful neglect but violation is corrected within the required time period	$10,000 per violation, with an annual maximum of $250,000 for repeat violations	$50,000 per violation, with an annual maximum of $1.5 million
Willful neglect and is not corrected within the required time period	$50,000 per violation, with an annual maximum of $1.5 million	$50,000 per violation, with an annual maximum of $1.5 million

bloodborne pathogens, hazard communication, occupational exposure to hazardous chemicals in laboratories, ionizing radiation, nonionizing radiation, and means of egress. Employers must be compliant with all of OSHA's regulations. More information on the OSHA standards can be found in Chapter 4. Employers with more than 10 employees are required to keep a record of serious work-related injuries and illnesses. Each year employers must post a summary of the injuries and illnesses recorded for the previous year. This tracking and reporting would be the responsibility of the office manager.

CLOSING COMMENTS

Medical assistants are not likely to go into office management immediately after graduation. The goal of this chapter is to introduce and discuss further professional opportunities in office management and the supervision of the healthcare facility staff. Successful office managers care about their employees and the vision for the healthcare facility. The areas of authority and responsibility must be clearly defined to prevent management problems. A detailed office policies and procedures manual helps the healthcare manager run an efficient facility.

Legal and Ethical Issues

Office managers must stay abreast of current employment laws and regulations for all the different agencies that govern the medical office. Joining a local office managers' association can help the manager keep the office up to date and in compliance. Periodic online checks of the websites of various organizations (e.g., OSHA) are a good way for the office manager to keep up with the most recent changes in policies and rules.

HIPAA compliance training should be required for all healthcare facilities. The facility's office manager should be knowledgeable not only about all HIPAA provisions, including those affecting the privacy and security of patient health information, but also about the penalties associated with information breaches.

Patient-Centered Care

Office managers who diligently complete all of the responsibilities associated with their position ensure that patient care will be the best it can possibly be. A good office manager will make sure that the staff is more than competent and that they have the tools needed to provide that care. They will ensure that there are policies and procedures in place that will protect both the patients and the staff. A good office manager will look at the whole picture and take the appropriate actions to safeguard the healthcare facility by ensuring compliance with all state and federal regulations. A good office manager understands that if there are no patients, there is no need for the healthcare facility to exist; he or she takes the appropriate measures to provide the means for patient-centered care.

Professional Behaviors

Managers who encourage their staff create a strong team in the healthcare facility. By focusing on team building, office managers can accomplish more tasks efficiently, delegate some of their workload, and promote high-quality patient care. Office managers can become immersed in their daily office responsibilities; however, they must keep in mind that slacking off on staff training and team development meetings results in lower office productivity. Staff meetings should be scheduled in advance, and attendance should be mandatory for all staff members.

SUMMARY OF SCENARIO

Kate has had a positive effect on her team at WMFM. She treats her employees well and is fair about administering office policies and procedures. Her staff appreciates her flexibility and professionalism as she manages the day-to-day operations of the facility. Kate treats her employees as team members, never speaking to them as if she were superior to them. She shares vital information with the staff so that they feel a part of the whole team, and she believes that even negative information should be relayed to the staff so that everyone is aware of the challenges the office faces. She makes strong hiring decisions and firmly believes in a good orientation and training program. Dr. Walden has placed a great deal of trust in Kate, and she has performed well, proving to be a reliable office manager.

Kate knows that she should display a friendly attitude toward her staff members when it is appropriate to do so. She is kind and considerate and treats the staff as individuals. She does not fraternize with them but is open to having lunch with the staff at various times and participates in all casual office activities. She maintains a healthy distance so that she can be an effective manager, but she listens to those who are experiencing difficulty and is compassionate about helping whenever possible.

Kate knows that when hiring for a vacant position, she must be diligent in checking references so that she brings reliable, qualified individuals on board as staff members. Unless she receives acceptable references, she will not hire a medical assistant to become a part of her team. Once she hires someone, she conducts a thorough training program and takes special care to share the experience and skills of the new staff member with the rest of the team.

When Kate must give a negative employee evaluation, she states that fact at the beginning of the meeting. Although she is compassionate, she is able to point out a staff member's shortcomings in a detailed, fair way. She usually is willing to give an employee time to improve, but if he or she fails to perform, Kate does not hesitate to end the employment.

Kate leads a group of cooperative team members who function well together every day, and this results in an efficient office and a pleasant work environment.

SUMMARY OF LEARNING OBJECTIVES

1. **Define the qualities and responsibilities of a successful office manager in a healthcare facility.**

   The provider counts on the office manager to run the business aspects of the office so that he or she can focus on providing good patient care. A high degree of trust is placed in the office manager. A good office manager is fair and flexible. Good communication skills are necessary, as is attention to detail. The manager should care about the employees and have a sense of fairness. The ability to remain calm in a crisis is important, as are the use of good judgment and the ability to multitask. Successful medical office managers work to promote a positive team environment to facilitate cohesion.

2. **Explain how to conduct a staff meeting with an agenda.**

   Staff meetings are an opportunity to communicate with the staff of the healthcare facility. This will allow the staff to discuss any problems that have come up with the office manager and the providers. Issues to be discussed should be solicited from all employees and then an agenda can be put together. Having an agenda will help to make sure that all concerns are addressed.

3. **Identify several ways in which employees are motivated.**

   Employees are motivated by various factors, including money, praise, insecurity, honor, prestige, needs, love, fear, satisfaction, and many others. An effective manager attempts to discover what motivates an employee to do a good job. Employees can also be motivated by incentives and recognition.

4. **Do the following related to creating a team environment:**

   - *Discuss strategies to create a team environment in the healthcare facility.*

     Teamwork is critical in the medical profession. In the healthcare facility, the manager must promote an atmosphere in which employees are willing to work together toward common goals. Morale in the facility may be low because of recent changes in policies or procedures, changes in staff or management, recent terminations of employees, lack of business, or any number of other reasons. The wise manager takes steps to improve employee morale continuously, including scheduling frequent meetings and keeping employees abreast of changes and developments that affect them.

   - *List communication barriers and how to overcome them.*

     It is important for the medical assistant to recognize the barriers and help the team overcome them. Physical separation barriers can be reduced by using technology (e.g., video conferencing and webcams). Language barriers can be addressed by encouraging awareness and acceptance of everyone's language and cultural differences. Status barriers can be reduced by promoting awareness and acceptance that everyone counts and every position on the team is important. Gender difference barriers can be addressed by helping all employees feel empowered to communicate openly with others. Cultural diversity barriers can be reduced by helping the team embrace the cultural differences among the members and educating the team on the differences.

5. **Do the following related to finding the right employee for the job:**

   - *Identify the need to find the right employee for an opening in the medical office.*

     From the providers to the receptionist, all play a vital role in the quality of healthcare delivered to patients. Hiring staff members who can be molded into a cohesive team is not an easy task. Care should be taken to choose employees who have the necessary skills and the right personality for the ambulatory care facility. When the need for a new employee arises, the office manager should discuss with the providers the type of employee required and the job description for that individual.

   - *Review a general job description for medical assistants.*

     Medical assistants are qualified for a variety of tasks in the healthcare facility. To fill an open medical assisting position, the manager must determine the specific experience that meets the facility's needs. Management should summarize the educational and skills sets needed to be successful at the position in the job description.

   - *Explain how to search through resumes and applications for potential candidates.*

     Resumes and applications should be reviewed for accuracy and completeness. Gaps in employment dates should be explained fully, and the office manager should verify any references. Documents should be legible, and the information should be consistent and without oversights.

   - *List and discuss legal and illegal interview questions.*

     The interviewer should be aware of various federal and state laws protecting the interviewee. Title VII of the Civil Rights Act of 1964, as amended by the Equal Employment Opportunity Act of 1972, prohibits inquiries into an applicant's race, color, gender, religion, and national origin. Inquiries about a person's medical history, arrest record, or previous drug use also are illegal. Most states have laws designed to protect the rights of job applicants, and these laws may impose additional restrictions. Office managers must research the laws that pertain to employment in their own states.

   - *Explain how to select the most qualified candidates.*

     The first step in reviewing resumes includes separating applicants who meet the minimal qualifications from those who do not. Then, divide those that meet the minimal qualifications into three stacks: applicants to call for an interview, possible candidates but not the strongest, and applicants who will not be called for an interview. Applicants with related experience, strong related skill sets (e.g., customer service), no unexplained employment gaps, and customized, error-free resumes and cover letters are more apt to be moved to the top of the pile.

   - *Identify follow-up activities the office manager should perform after an interview.*

     When the interview is over, the office manager or interview team should immediately take a few moments to rate or summarize

Continued

SUMMARY OF LEARNING OBJECTIVES—*continued*

the applicant's strengths and weaknesses. After all the interviews have been conducted, the team then rates the interviewees and identifies the top candidates. References are checked, and a second interview may occur before the final person has been selected.

6. **Review new employee orientation, including paperwork, training, and development.**

   The office manager should develop a checklist of the paperwork needed for newly hired staff and all the information that should be covered with the new employee at the start of the job. Basic new employee paperwork often includes a job application; Form I-9 (Employment Eligibility Verification); W-4 Form (Employee's Withholding Allowance Certificate); Notice of Workers Compensation coverage; consent for a background check and drug testing; acknowledgement of receipt of the company handbook or policy manual; agreements regarding pay, wage deductions, benefits, schedule, work location, and so on; notices of at-will employment status; acknowledgement of ethics statement; direct deposit application; and the OSHA compliance acknowledgement or checklist. Orientation and training help new employees to understand what is expected and to develop to their full potential.

7. **Discuss strategies for determining fair salaries and raises, addressing a problem employee, and terminating an employee.**

   When negative information is to be relayed to an employee during a performance appraisal, the office manager should sandwich the negative comment between two positive ones whenever possible. Counseling these employees to find the source of their difficulties is the first step toward resolution. Many employees can be redirected to become productive staff members with a little patience and understanding on the manager's part. The manager should have

good documentation of the problems that led to the poor evaluation. An employee who has been in service for some time and is offering unsatisfactory performance should be warned and given an explanation of the specific improvements expected. If a second chance does not produce improvement in performance or attitude, dismissal must follow. It should be done privately, with tact and consideration.

To keep good employees, the practice must pay a fair salary with regular raises if the staff member performs as expected. The office manager can find information about salary comparisons on the internet. The manager should periodically review job descriptions and salary analyses online to see whether the salary the medical facility offers is comparable to those for similar jobs in the area.

8. **Identify the information that should be included in a personnel policy manual.**

   The personnel policy manual should include information related to health benefits, vacation time, sick leave, holidays, overtime, performance evaluations, termination policies, grievance process, dress code, office safety, and the employee's role in case of an emergency.

9. **Describe how office policies and procedures are different from personnel policies.**

   The personnel policies are related to the employer-employee relationship. Office policies provide step-by-step instructions for completing the tasks that are done in the healthcare facility.

10. **Explain the office manager's role in regulatory compliance.**

    The office manager must stay up to date with current changes in state and federal legislation. The office manager is also responsible for complying with all reporting that is required by that legislation. It is also important to make sure that the staff is trained in all of the requirements to remain in compliance.

MEDICAL EMERGENCIES

SCENARIO

Gabe Garcia, CMA (AAMA), has worked for Walden-Martin Family Medical (WMFM) Clinic for 4 years. He was hired right after he completed his medical assistant program. Gabe has learned a lot through the years. He has impressed his supervisor with his dedication, attention to detail, punctuality, and patient care skills. Gabe was just promoted to a medical assistant lead position. In this new position, Gabe has additional responsibilities. He will now oversee the crash carts in the clinic, and he will train staff on emergency procedures.

The current emergency procedures need to be revised, and the crash cart procedures need updating. Gabe is excited to take over his new responsibilities. He looks forward to what he will learn in this new role.

While studying this chapter, think about the following questions:
- How are emergencies handled in ambulatory care settings?
- What are common emergency equipment and supplies found in the ambulatory care settings?
- What are first aid actions for cold and heat illnesses, burns, poisonings, anaphylaxis, bites, and foreign bodies in the eye?
- What are first aid actions for diabetic emergencies?
- What are first aid actions for musculoskeletal emergencies?
- What are first aid actions for neurological emergencies, including vertigo, concussion, seizure, and stroke?
- What are first aid actions for respiratory emergencies, including hyperventilation, asthmatic attack, and choking?
- What are first aid actions for cardiovascular emergencies, including syncope, bleeding, shock, and heart attack?

LEARNING OBJECTIVES

1. Discuss emergencies in healthcare settings and possible roles each team member has during an emergency.
2. Describe emergency equipment and supplies.
3. Explain first aid procedures for environmental emergencies, including temperature-related emergencies, burns, poisonings, anaphylaxis, bites and stings, and foreign bodies in the eye.
4. Discuss diabetic emergencies and provide first aid for a patient in insulin shock.
5. Discuss musculoskeletal and neurological emergencies and provide first aid for a patient with seizure activity.
6. Discuss respiratory emergencies and provide first aid for a choking patient.
7. Discuss cardiovascular emergencies and provide first aid for a patient with a bleeding wound, fracture, or syncope; a patient in shock; and a patient in need of rescue breathing or cardiopulmonary resuscitation (CPR).

VOCABULARY

cardiopulmonary resuscitation (ri sus i TAY shun) **(CPR)** The application of manual chest compressions and ventilations (also called *rescue breathing*) to patients who are not breathing or do not have a pulse; also known as *basic life support* (BLS).

code A term used in healthcare settings to indicate an emergency situation and to summon the trained team to the scene.

concussion (kuhn KUSH uhn) A traumatic brain injury caused by a blow to the head.

endotracheal (en doe TRAY kee al) **(ET) tube** A catheter that is inserted into the trachea through the mouth; provides a patent airway.

erythema (er ee THEE mah) Redness.

intraosseous (in tra OS ee us) Within bone; route for delivery of fluids and medications through a needle inserted into the marrow of certain bones (e.g., humerus, tibia, and femur).

nasopharyngeal (nae zoe fah RIN jee ahl) **airway (NPA)** A soft flexible tube that is inserted in the nose and provides a patent airway; also known as a *nasal trumpet*.

necrosis (neh KROH sis) Tissue death.

patent (PAY tent) Open.

pocket face mask A device used to deliver a rescue breath.

pruritus (proo RIE tuss) Itching.

recovery position A position on the person's side that helps to keep the airway open and clear.

VOCABULARY—continued

retractions (re TRAK shuns) The sucking in of tissues between the intercostal spaces and neck due to respiratory distress; classic sign of severe asthma.

standard of care The level and type of care an ordinary, prudent healthcare professional with the same training and experience in a similar practice would have provided under a similar situation.

triage (tree AHZH) To sort out and classify the injured; used in the military and emergency settings to determine the priority of a patient to be treated.

triaging flow map A written flow map to make triage decisions; based on answers to questions, the person moves through the map until a triage decision is made.

vasoconstriction Contraction of the muscles, causing narrowing of the inside tube of the vessel.

vertigo (VER ti goe) Sensation that causes someone to feel as though everything is spinning.

Emergencies happen everywhere. As a medical assistant, it is important for you to know how to handle emergencies because you may need to respond to one:

- *Outside of your job, in the community.* You may be one of the first people on the scene and need to provide first aid to the victims.
- *In the healthcare setting.* You may need to provide first aid as the provider assesses the injured person. Additional treatments, such as oxygen and medications, are provided in the healthcare setting.
- *Over the phone.* You may need to obtain information from someone involved in an emergency and provide first aid coaching. The medical assistant asks screening questions and provides the information to the provider. The provider instructs the medical assistant what to tell the caller.

This chapter starts by discussing emergencies in the healthcare setting and the medical assistant's role. Next, common emergency medical equipment, supplies, and medications are explained. Lastly, emergency conditions are described, along with the first aid procedures to perform.

EMERGENCIES IN HEALTHCARE SETTINGS

Every employee in a healthcare setting should know how to get help in an emergency. This process will vary. Healthcare facilities use special phrases for emergencies. For instance, "Code Blue Urgent Care" may indicate that an emergency is occurring in Urgent Care. Sometimes the **code** words indicate the age of the person. For instance, "Code Pink Family Practice" may mean that an emergency is occurring in Family Practice and "pink" indicates a child.

Once the call goes out for help, staff members respond to the scene. In small settings, most members of the staff may be needed. In large facilities, only certain staff members respond. Usually, medical assistants, licensed practical nurses (LPNs), registered nurses (RNs), and providers attend the emergency. Possible roles for each team member include:

- *Provider:* Assesses the patient, orders treatments and procedures, performs advanced procedures, may administer intravenous (IV) medications, and indicates when 911 needs to be called.
- *Nurse:* Registered nurses (RNs) administer intravenous (IV) medications and fluids. Licensed practical nurses (LPNs) may do the same if permitted by the state's scope of practice. RNs and LPNs assist with treatments and procedures, perform **cardiopulmonary**

resuscitation (CPR), call 911, and document the code activities as they occur.

- *Clinical medical assistant:* Assists with treatments and procedures, performs CPR, documents the code activities as they occur, and calls 911. He or she may hand supplies to staff members and assist with caring for the family (moving them to a private area away from the emergency).
- *Administrative medical assistant:* Performs CPR and hands supplies to the staff (in small agencies), calls 911, escorts the emergency responders to the patient, and assists with caring for the family.

Importance of Documentation

In a code situation, it is important that at least one team member document everything that occurs. This is a stressful job because many things are occurring during an emergency. There are several reasons why accurate documentation is critical.

- The information is used during the code. For instance, CPR was started, and the team member documented "1413 CPR initiated." As the code progresses, the provider may want to know when the CPR was started.
- Emergency responders will need to know what occurred during the code. (What medications were given? When were they given? How much was given?)
- The documentation will provide evidence that the **standard of care** was met in the treatments given to the patient. Many lawsuits have originated from emergencies. The lawyers review the documentation. They look for delays in emergency care and lack of appropriate treatment. Complete and accurate documentation may make a difference between a lawsuit surviving and being dismissed in favor of the healthcare team.

If you are new to codes and if given the option, perform a role other than documenting. Observe what occurs during a code as you complete your task. Study the code documentation form during noncode times. As you become more comfortable with codes, assist the documenter if you can. A second pair of eyes is always helpful. Lastly, become the documenter and have a seasoned team member assist you.

EMERGENCY EQUIPMENT AND SUPPLIES

The emergency supplies available at healthcare facilities will vary based on the size and location of the facility. Some practices have a small box that contains a few supplies and medications. Other practices place many crash carts throughout the building (Fig. 21.1). A *crash cart* is a rolling supply cart that contains emergency equipment.

The crash cart should be checked monthly. This can be done by the supervisor or by two qualified employees (e.g., medical assistants, LPNs, or RNs). Expiration dates on the supplies are checked. Old supplies are replaced with new supplies. All the equipment and supplies are inventoried. When the inventory is completed, a plastic lock (or locking tag) is placed on the cart. The crash cart is used only in emergencies. You should never break the lock and use something from the crash cart unless it is an emergency. The plastic locks should be kept safe and used only when the cart is inventoried monthly or after an emergency. Many of the locks are numbered, and the number is written on the inventory document. Keeping the locks safe minimizes the number of people going into the crash cart for nonemergency reasons.

This section will focus on the equipment and supplies typically found on a crash cart. The medical assistant should be familiar with the supplies and their location within the crash cart.

Oxygen and Airway Supplies

Oxygen and airway supplies are common items found on crash carts. If the patient needs oxygen, the provider will order oxygen to be applied via a mask or a nasal cannula. (Refer to Chapter 40 in the main text for additional information on oxygen delivery systems.)

If the patient has difficulty breathing or if an airway constriction may be occurring, the provider will insert a **nasopharyngeal airway** or an **endotracheal (ET) tube** to create a **patent** airway (Fig. 21.2). Providers also use the following to maintain airways:

- *Esophageal tracheal tubes*, which are placed in the trachea or esophagus
- *Laryngeal mask airways*, which are inserted through the mouth and advanced to the hypopharynx
- *Laryngeal tubes*, which are also inserted through the mouth and placed in the hypopharynx

Endotracheal Tube Intubation

The medical assistant should be aware of the equipment required during an ET tube intubation. During an endotracheal intubation, the provider will need the following:

- *Laryngoscope* with either a curved (MacIntosh) or straight (Miller) blade. The sizes of blades are indicated on the side or back of the blade (Fig. 21.3A). The medical assistant must hand the laryngoscope with the blade attached to the provider (Fig. 21.3B).
- ET tube in the appropriate size. Cuffed ET tubes come in a variety of sizes for adults and older children (e.g., 7.5, 8, and 8.5). Uncuffed ET tubes come in a variety of sizes for children (e.g., 2.5, 3, and 3.5) (Fig. 21.4). A syringe is used to inflate the cuff with air once it is in place.
- *Stylet* is a metal or flexible plastic wire inserted into the ET tube to create a firm, curved tube (see Fig. 21.4). After the ET tube is in place, the stylet is removed.
- Ambu-bag, which is attached to the ET tube and used to administer room air or oxygen (Fig. 21.5). An Ambu-bag can cover the mouth or be attached to an airway tube (e.g., endotracheal tube). Ambu-bags can come with oxygen tubing

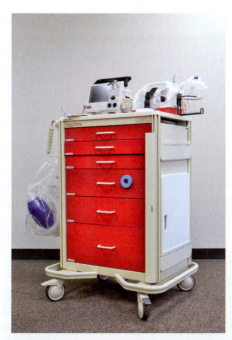

FIGURE 21.1 Crash carts are used in an emergency. The drawers should be labeled to allow speedy retrieval of supplies.

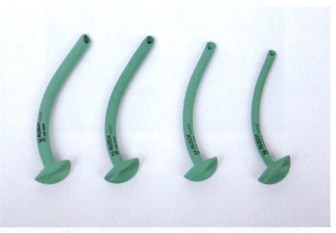

FIGURE 21.2 Nasopharyngeal airways come in a variety of sizes.

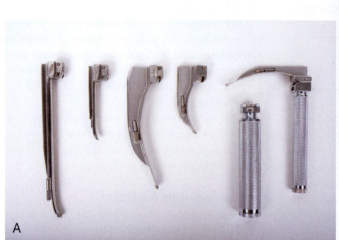
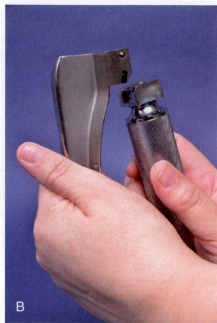

FIGURE 21.3 **(A)** *Left to right:* Two different sizes of straight blades and curved blades; adult laryngoscope handle and an assembled pediatric laryngoscope. A curved or straight blade must be attached to the laryngoscope handle. **(B)** To attach the blade, hold the blade parallel to the handle and attach.

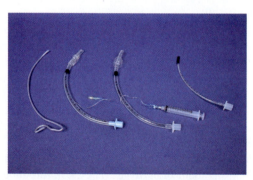

FIGURE 21.4 *Left to right:* A stylet is threaded into the endotracheal (ET) tube to help maintain the tube's curve. ET tubes for adults are cuffed (or have a balloon that is inflated using a syringe). ET tubes for children are uncuffed *(far right)*. ET tubes come in a variety of sizes.

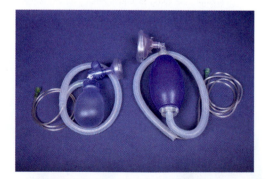

FIGURE 21.5 *Left to right:* Pediatric and adult Ambu-bags.

attached, which can be connected to an oxygen tank. Oxygen can be administered during the ventilation.
• Stethoscope. Once the tube is in place, a team member will provide ventilation with the Ambu-bag. The provider must ensure the ET tube is in the correct location by listening over

the lung field for air movement. If the ET tube is in the wrong location, the abdomen will become bloated with air. The patient is then not being ventilated. (A provider will usually state that breath sounds are heard bilaterally. This is important to document on the code form. This verifies the ET tube is in the correct location.)

CRITICAL THINKING APPLICATION   **21.2**
Gabe has decided that the crash carts must be inventoried monthly. He will have two medical assistants inventory each cart. Gabe feels it is important that all medical assistants have an opportunity to inventory the crash cart at least every 4 months. Why would this be important for the medical assistants? Besides checking expiration dates, what else could they do to increase their skills and knowledge for emergencies?

Defibrillator

A *defibrillator* is a device that delivers an electrical shock to the heart muscle in an attempt to restore a normal heartbeat. The defibrillator's shock causes the heart to momentarily stop. When it restarts, the hope is the heart will beat at a normal rhythm. The quicker a defibrillator can be used, the better the person's chances of survival.

Typically, a defibrillator or an automated external defibrillator (AED) is used in healthcare facilities.
• A defibrillator consists of two handheld paddles that are placed on gel pads located on the patient's chest (Fig. 21.6). Gel pads are required to prevent burns. They provide better electricity conduction from the paddles to the patient. The provider indicates how many joules at which to set the machine, and someone

announces "All clear" to ensure no one is touching the patient. The provider pushes the button to give the shock.

- An *automated external defibrillator* is a portable, lightweight machine (Fig. 21.7). Sticky pads that contain electrodes (sensors) are attached to the patient's chest. The AED checks the heart rate and determines if a shock is required. If a shock is needed, the AED gives audible directions to the user to administer a shock.

Medications

The medications in crash carts can vary. Common medications used in emergencies are listed in Table 21.1. Most crash carts and emergency supply boxes include intravenous (IV) supplies. An IV is usually inserted into the hand, wrist, or arm of the patient. If an IV line cannot be inserted, the provider may insert an **intraosseous** needle that can be used to give IV fluids and medications (Fig. 21.8). The intraosseous needle can be inserted into the humerus, tibia, femur,

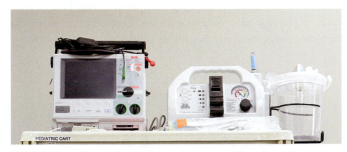

FIGURE 21.6 *Left to right:* The defibrillator usually sits on top of the crash cart. Other equipment, such as a suction machine, can also be found on the top of the crash cart.

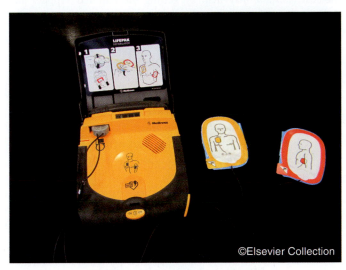

©Elsevier Collection

FIGURE 21.7 Automated external defibrillator.

TABLE 21.1	Common Medications Used in Emergencies	
MEDICATION	**ACTION**	**USED FOR**
amiodarone (Cordarone, Pacerone)	Slows the heart rate and allows blood to fill in the ventricular chambers.	Ventricular tachycardia, ventricular fibrillation
atropine	Increases the heart rate.	Bradycardia
calcium chloride	Increases the calcium levels in the serum.	Hyperkalemia and *hypocalcemia* (too little calcium in the blood)
diazepam (Valium)	Affects the chemicals in the brain.	Seizures, agitation
diphenhydramine (Benadryl)	Antihistamine that reduces the effects of histamine.	Allergic reactions, second-line drug for anaphylaxis (used after epinephrine has been given)
dopamine (Intropin)	Increases the stimulation of the heart muscle	Hypotension, heart failure
epinephrine (Adrenalin)	Increases the stimulation of the heart muscle; vasoconstrictor and bronchial relaxant	Anaphylaxis, cardiac arrest, severe asthma, bronchospasms
glucagon	Hormone that stimulates the liver to release glucose into the blood	*Hypoglycemia* (below-normal glucose in the blood)
lidocaine	Helps to restore the regular heart rhythm	Ventricular arrhythmias
magnesium	Electrolyte that helps maintain a normal heart rhythm	Arrhythmias
naloxone (Evzio, Narcan)	Blocks or reverses opioid medication effects	Opioid (narcotic) overdose
nitroglycerin	Vasodilator	Congestive heart failure, angina
sodium bicarbonate	Decreases the pH of the serum	Metabolic acidosis, *hyperkalemia* (excessive potassium in the blood)

sternum, or iliac crest. The provider must be specially trained to insert the intraosseous needle.

Administering IV medications is outside the scope of practice for the medical assistant. In many states, inserting an IV and giving IV fluids are also outside the medical assistant's scope of practice. The medical assistant may help by getting the required supplies and documenting what was given.

Other Supplies

Various other supplies can be found in the crash cart. Some items not already mentioned include:

- Personal protective equipment (PPE), such as gloves, a sharps disposal container, and a **pocket face mask**
- *Algorithms,* or step-by-step instructions for reference
- Clipboard with documents for charting the code
- Backboard, which is placed under the patient to provide a firm surface for compressions
- Extra batteries for the laryngoscope

Pediatric Supplies

In the 1980s, James Broselow, a family practice doctor working in an emergency department, came up with an idea for simplifying pediatric medication doses administered during emergencies. Medications for children are based on weight. Rescue personnel spent critical moments during emergencies calculating medication doses for children. Broselow's idea was to measure the child's length and come up with

a suggested dose. After much research, the Broselow tape was created (Fig. 21.9A).

A healthcare professional measures a child using the tape. The tape is placed from the top of the head to the child's heel. The length is measured as a specific color (see Fig. 21.9B). Based on the "color" of the child, the tape lists common medication dosages and emergency equipment sizes that should be used for that size of child. This system has sped up the response time for treating children during emergencies. It eliminates the use of reference guides and calculators for medication dosages.

Many ambulatory care settings that routinely see sick children use the Broselow tape. In addition to the tape, pediatric crash carts (Broselow ColorCode Carts) have been created (Fig. 21.10). Each color on the tape has a matching drawer. Each drawer contains the right-sized equipment for that size of child.

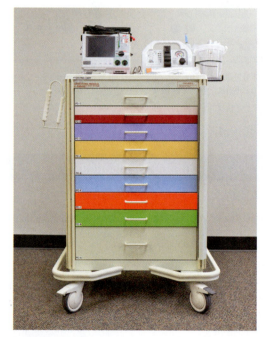

FIGURE 21.10 Each drawer in the Broselow ColorCode Cart is color coded.

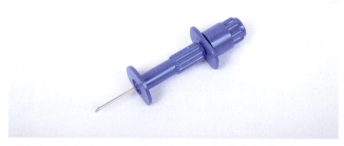

FIGURE 21.8 An intraosseous needle may be used to give IV fluids and medications in an emergency.

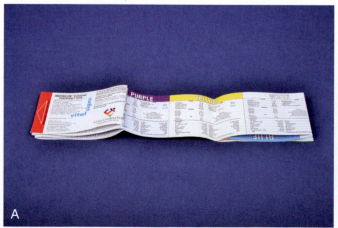

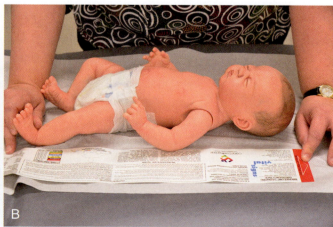

FIGURE 21.9 **(A)** Broselow tape. **(B)** Measure the child with the Broselow tape. Measure from the head to the heel and identify the color by the child's heel. This is the color to use during the emergency.

HANDLING EMERGENCIES

In the ambulatory care setting, many different types of emergencies can occur. Some of the more common emergencies include these:

- A patient who is being seen and treated has a life-threatening occurrence (e.g., an allergic reaction to a medication).
- A person (e.g., employee, visitor, or patient) has an accident or health issue that results in an emergency.
- A *walk-in patient* (a patient without an appointment) comes to the facility with a critical health issue.
- An individual calls about an emergency.

How these are handled can differ greatly among ambulatory care facilities. Factors that affect how emergencies are handled include:

- Facility's size and distance from emergency medical services
- Available equipment and supplies
- Providers' training and scope of practice
- Number and type of clinical care employees (medical assistants, licensed practical nurses, and registered nurses) and their scopes of practice

Some facilities only have minimal staff, whereas others have specific employees who respond to emergencies.

In small facilities, the medical assistant may be responsible for screening emergency calls and walk-in patients. The medical assistant must follow the facility's screening protocols. She or he cannot assess the patient or give advice. The information collected must be reported to the provider. The provider tells the medical assistant what should be done. Examples of screening questions are provided later in the chapter.

In larger facilities, registered nurses (sometimes called **triage** nurses) gather information from walk-in patients and emergency calls. Using a **triaging flow map** or triaging software, the nurse identifies how quickly the patient needs to be seen and where the patient needs to be seen (Fig. 21.11).

Sometimes patients come to the ambulatory healthcare setting with life-threatening conditions. The provider sees these patients immediately and assesses their conditions. The provider will order 911 to be called if needed. Treatment is provided as the team waits for the emergency responders to transport the patient to the emergency department. The following sections explain the first aid given for different types of emergencies.

Environmental Emergencies

Environmental emergencies arise from an exposure to a harmful environmental agent rather than a traumatic injury or medical condition already present in the patient. For instance, the outdoor temperature can cause a life-threatening condition. A bite from certain reptiles can cause death if not treated immediately. A flying piece of metal in a factory can cause blindness. Many environment-related emergencies are severe enough that the affected person seeks medical care.

Temperature-Related Emergencies

Overexposure to hot or cold temperatures can cause mild to life-threatening issues. Environmental temperatures affect the body's temperature.

Cold-Related Conditions. Cold-related conditions include frostbite and hypothermia. In cold weather, our bodies tend to lose heat faster than we can produce it. This results in a lowered body temperature. Uncovered skin can result in injuries faster than covered skin. It does not take long for frostbite to occur. For instance, with a 10-mile-per-hour (mph) wind speed and a temperature of −5°F (−20.6°C), a person can get frostbite in 30 minutes. With the same wind speed and a temperature of −25°F (−31.7°C), a person can get frostbite in 5 minutes.

Possible screening questions for cold-related conditions include:

- What is the person's age?
- How long was the person exposed to the cold temperature?
- What symptoms does the person have? What color is the exposed skin?
- What is the person's medical history?

Table 21.2 describes frostbite and hypothermia. With severe hypothermia, an individual can develop arrhythmias. Medical attention is critical. Warming a patient with hypothermia too quickly can also lead to cardiac issues and additional tissue damage. Because of this, the emergency department gradually warms all patients with hypothermia.

Heat-Related Conditions. Heat injuries occur most often on hot, humid days. Heat-related conditions include cramps, exhaustion, and stroke (Table 21.3).

Possible screening questions for heat-related conditions include:

- What is the person's age?
- How long was the person exposed to the hot temperature?
- What symptoms does the person have? Is the person sweating? What does the skin look like? Is the person alert or confused?

It is important to treat heat-related illnesses immediately. An untreated condition can progress to become a more severe situation.

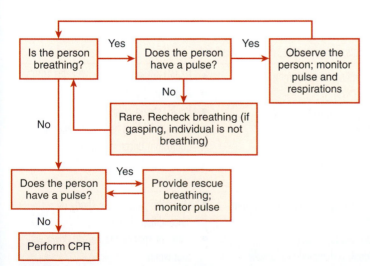

FIGURE 21.11 Example of a flow map. Similar flow maps can be used when triaging or treating emergencies.

TABLE 21.2	Cold-Related Conditions	
CONDITION	**FROSTBITE**	**HYPOTHERMIA**
Description	Occurs when the skin and body tissues are exposed to cold temperatures. Susceptible areas include cheeks, nose, ears, fingers, toes, and chin.	Core body temperature drops to below 95°F (35°C). In severe hypothermia, the body temperature drops to 82°F (27.8°C), causing a life-threatening condition.
Etiology and Risk Factors	Caused by exposure to cold temperatures. Risk factors include: • Smoking or taking a beta-blocker medication (e.g., atenolol) • Having diabetes or poor blood circulation • High winds, wet clothes	Caused by exposure to cold temperatures or immersion in cold water for a long period of time. Risk factors include those for frostbite; also dehydration and exhaustion.
Signs and Symptoms	Pins-and-needles sensation followed by numbness; hard, pale, cold skin; aching or lack of feeling in area; blisters.	Slurred speech; slow, shallow breathing and weak pulse; clumsy, drowsy, confused, loss of consciousness; bright red, cold skin (seen in infants).
First Aid Procedures	• Move the person to a warmer location. • Remove all wet clothing and cover with warm dry clothing. • Observe for signs of hypothermia. • Seek medical care; if not available, then rewarm the area by soaking in warm water (104°–108°F [40°–42.2°C]) for 20–30 minutes. Do not rub the area. Apply sterile dressing to area. • Give the person a warm drink to replace lost fluids; do not give alcohol.	• Move the person to a warmer location. • Remove all wet clothing and cover with warm dry clothing. • Seek medical care. • Give the person a warm drink to replace lost fluids; do not give alcohol.

TABLE 21.3	Heat-Related Conditions		
CONDITION	**HEAT CRAMPS**	**HEAT EXHAUSTION**	**HEAT STROKE**
Description	Mild heat-related illness that causes muscle pains and spasms due to electrolyte imbalance. Usually occurs with strenuous activities or in those who sweat a lot.	Milder form of heat-related illness. Due to exposure to high temperatures and inadequate fluid and electrolyte replacement.	Most serious heat-related illness. Body is unable to sweat and thus cannot cool down.
Etiology and Risk Factors	Caused by prolonged heat exposure. With high humidity, sweat, which cools the skin, does not evaporate as quickly. Risk factors include: • Age (older adults and children age 4 and younger) • Fever, dehydration, heart disease, poor blood circulation • Mental illness, sunburn; using alcohol • Prescription drugs (e.g., antidepressants, anticonvulsants, antipsychotics, and diuretics)		
Signs and Symptoms	• Muscle pains or spasms in the abdomen, arms, or legs.	• Heavy sweating, muscle cramps • Cool, moist skin • Fast, weak pulse; fast, shallow respirations • Tired, weak, pale • Dizzy, headache, fainting • Nausea, vomiting	• Body temperature over 103°F (39°C) • Red, hot, dry skin • Rapid, strong pulse • Dizzy, throbbing headache, nausea • Confusion, unconsciousness
First Aid Procedures	• Rest for several hours in a cool place. • Drink cool electrolyte (sports) beverages to replace electrolytes lost. • Do not drink caffeinated or alcoholic beverages, which can cause dehydration.	• Move to a shady or air-conditioned area and rest. • Drink cool sports beverages. • Do not drink caffeinated or alcoholic beverages. • Take a cool shower or sponge bath.	• Move the person to a shady or air-conditioned area. • Spray or sponge the person down with cool water. • Seek medical attention immediately.

An effective way to lower the person's temperature is to apply cool, wet cloths and then fan the moist skin. This will lower the person's body temperature by the evaporation process.

Burns

Heat, freezing cold temperatures, chemicals, sunlight, radiation, and electricity can cause burns to the body tissue. Hot liquids, fires, and flammable products are the most common causes of burns. Breathing in smoke can also cause inhalation injuries. Table 21.4 describes the different degrees of burns.

Possible screening questions for burns include:
- What occurred? Where was the person burned? What caused the burn?
- What symptoms does the person have? What does the person's skin look like?
- If the face or chest is affected: Is the person experiencing any breathing issues?

Providers estimate the percent of total burn surface area (%TBSA) by using the rule of nines diagram (Fig. 21.12). Table 21.5 shows the difference between the rule of nines for an adult and for a child.

TABLE 21.4 Types of Burns

CONDITION	FIRST-DEGREE BURN	SECOND-DEGREE BURN	THIRD-DEGREE BURN	FOURTH-DEGREE BURN
Also Known As	Superficial burn	Partial-thickness burn	Full-thickness burn	Deep full-thickness burn
Description	Damage to epidermis	Damage to the epidermis and part of the dermis	Damage to the epidermis, dermis, and subcutaneous tissue	Damage beyond the subcutaneous tissue into the muscle and bone (not universally accepted)
Signs and Symptoms	Redness (erythema), tenderness, physical sensitivity No scar development	Redness, blisters, and pain. Possible scar development.	No pain because nerve endings are destroyed. Skin appears deep red, pale gray, brown, or black. Scar formation is likely.	
First Aid Procedures	For minor burns: • For unbroken skin, soak in cool water (not ice water) for at least 5 minutes. • Cover with sterile dressing. • (For second-degree burns 3 inches or larger or located on hands, feet, groin, buttock, or over joint – treat as major burn.)		For major burns: • Seek immediate medical attention (call 911). • Do not remove burned clothing stuck to skin. • Monitor breathing. Perform rescue breathing or CPR as needed. • Raise burned body part above heart level. • Separate burned fingers or toes with dry, sterile dressing.	

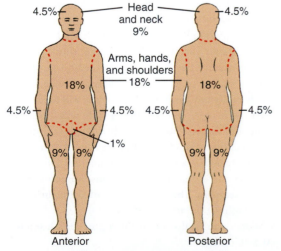

FIGURE 21.12 Rule of nines for adults. (From Callen JP, Greer KE, Saller AS, et al: *Color atlas of dermatology*, ed 3, Philadelphia, 2003, Saunders.)

TABLE 21.5 Rule of Nines for Adults and Children

AREA BURNED	ADULT	CHILD
Head and neck	9%	18%
Front of torso	18%	18%
Back	18%	18%
Arm, hand, and shoulder	9% (LA) 9% (RA)	9% (LA) 9% (RA)
Leg and foot	18% (LL) 18% (RL)	13.5% (LL) 13.5% (RL)
Genital	1%	1%
Total	100%	100%

LA, Left arm; *RA*, right arm; *LL*, left leg; *RL*, right leg.

Poisonings

Poison can enter the body through swallowing, inhaling, injecting, or absorbing it through the skin. Common poisons include:

- Medications (prescription or over the counter) taken in high doses
- Overdoses of illegal drugs
- Household products (e.g., laundry detergent, furniture polish, and cleaning products)
- Indoor and outdoor plants
- Pesticides and fertilizers
- Metals (e.g., mercury and lead)

American Association of Poison Control Centers are national poison resources with 55 centers around the country. This resource is available online (PoisonHelp.org) and via a hotline (1-800-222-1222). Medical assistants should have the phone number and website available for reference. If the medical assistant receives a call regarding a poisoning, the call must be handled according to the facility's protocols. Many times, the medical assistant must contact Poison Control while keeping the patient on the phone. The medical assistant then relays the information from Poison Control to the patient.

Signs and symptoms of poisoning can develop over time. They can also vary based on the poison. Some examples of symptoms include:

- Bluish lips, cough, difficulty breathing
- Heart palpitations, chest pain
- Confusion, dizziness, double vision, drowsiness, irritability, headache
- Nausea, vomiting, abdominal pain
- Numbness, tingling, seizures
- Unconsciousness, stupor, weakness, unusual odor

First aid includes checking and monitoring the person's airway, breathing, and pulse. If required, rescue breathing and cardiopulmonary resuscitation (CPR) are provided. Call 911 for medical help. If the person vomits, clear the airway. Monitor the person until help arrives. If poisoning is suspected, it is important to identify what the toxin is and how much was taken.

Do not have the person vomit unless you are instructed to do so by the Poison Control staff. If the person has swallowed a corrosive substance, it will cause additional injury as it is vomited. In this type of situation, a tube must be passed into the stomach to remove the substance. This is usually done in the emergency department.

Poisoning Facts

- Children younger than 6 years of age make up about half of the poisoning exposures reported.
- Children ages 1 to 2 have the greatest risk of poisoning.
- Cosmetics and personal care products, followed by cleaning products, are the most common substances involved in childhood poison exposures.
- About 20% of adult poisonings and 40% of teen poisonings are suspected suicides.
- Analgesics, followed by sedative/hypnotics/antipsychotic medications, are the top substances in adult poisonings.

From Poison Control. *http://www.poison.org/poison-statistics-national.* Accessed October 23, 2018.

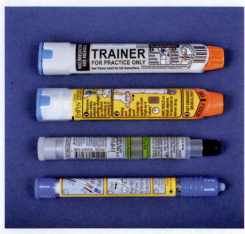

FIGURE 21.13 *Top to bottom:* Trainer that comes with the EpiPen, adult EpiPen, EpiPen Jr., and a generic adult epinephrine pen.

CRITICAL THINKING APPLICATION   **21.4**

Where might Gabe post the Poison Control numbers around the clinic? Describe places where this number will be useful.

Anaphylaxis

Anaphylaxis is a severe allergic reaction that can be life-threatening. Food, insect stings, and medications are the top allergens that cause anaphylaxis (Table 21.6). Allergic reactions that affect breathing are life-threatening.

First aid for severe allergic reactions includes:

- Do the 3Cs: Check the scene for safety. Call 911. Care for the victim.
- Give *epinephrine* (EpiPen) if the person has it available (Fig. 21.13).
- Stay with the individual and try to keep the person calm.
- If the person has a bee sting, scrape the stinger off the skin if it is visible. Use a fingernail or credit card to scrape it. Don't use tweezers, which can squeeze the stinger, releasing more venom.
- Monitor the individual's airway, breathing, and pulse. Perform rescue breathing or CPR if needed.
- Have the person lie flat and raise the feet 12 inches. Keep the person warm. This will help to prevent shock.

In the ambulatory care facility, if the medical assistant suspects the patient is starting to have an allergic reaction, he or she should immediately notify the provider. The provider will order epinephrine to be given and oxygen to be administered. Research has shown that epinephrine administered intramuscularly (IM) into the vastus lateralis absorbs quicker than that given IM in the deltoid or subcutaneously in the arm. If ordered, repeat every 5 to 10 minutes. Do not administer repeated injections in the same site, because **vasoconstriction** may cause tissue **necrosis**. The typical dose of epinephrine injectable solution (1 mg/mL) for anaphylaxis is:

- Children and adults (66 lb [30 kg] or more): 0.3 to 0.5 mg (0.3–0.5 mL)
- Children (under 66 lb [30 kg]): 0.01 mg/kg (0.01 mL/kg) with a maximum dose per injection of 0.3 mL

TABLE 21.6 Common Allergens and Anaphylaxis Symptoms

COMMON ALLERGENS	MOST COMMON ALLERGENIC FOODS	ANAPHYLAXIS SYMPTOMS
• Animal dander • Insect bites and stings (especially bee stings) • Medicines • Plants • Pollens • Foods	• Eggs • Fish • Milk • Tree nuts (hazelnuts, walnuts, almonds, Brazil nuts) • Peanuts (groundnuts) • Shellfish (crab, mussels, shrimp) • Soy • Wheat	• Warm feeling, flushing • Shortness of breath • Dyspnea (difficulty breathing), wheezing • Throat tightening, difficulty swallowing • Cough • Anxiety • Pain or cramping • Vomiting or diarrhea • Unconsciousness • Shock • Palpitations, dizziness

The 3 Cs Are Important When Responding to Emergencies

If you are the first to arrive at the scene of an emergency, it is important to follow the 3 Cs:

- **Check** the scene of the emergency. Is it safe for you? Are there any toxic or electric hazards? What occurred? How many victims are involved? Where did it occur (so you can tell the 911 dispatcher)?
- **Call 911** or the local emergency number. Provide all the details you know.
- **Care** for the victims if it is safe to do so.

Always make sure you are safe before you assist others. If it is not safe for you, then wait for the emergency responders to arrive.

Insect Bites and Stings

Insect bites and stings can cause immediate skin reactions, including pain, burning, **erythema,** numbness, swelling, and **pruritus**. In some cases, the venom can cause severe illness and death. Some people have anaphylactic reactions to stings and bites (e.g., bee stings). Anaphylaxis symptoms were addressed in the prior section. If the medical assistant receives a phone call regarding a bite or sting, it is important to gather additional information for the provider, such as:

- What bit you?
- Do you have any allergies?
- How does the wound look? Describe the wound to me.
- Are you having any problems breathing? Any wheezing, shortness of breath, or difficulty breathing?
- Is there any swelling in the mouth or lips?

First aid for severe reactions includes all the steps indicated in the anaphylaxis section. Additional steps include removing any nearby constricting items, such as rings and clothing. The affected area may swell, and constricting items can cause additional problems. First aid for mild reactions includes:

- Move to a safe location.
- Remove the stinger if it is visible.
- Wash the affected area with soap and water.
- To reduce pain and swelling, apply a cool cloth and elevate the extremity.
- For pain, apply hydrocortisone or lidocaine cream to the area. An over-the-counter pain reliever can also be taken.
- Calamine lotion or a similar product can be applied to the area to reduce the pruritus.

Patients may also call for advice on removing ticks.

Removing Ticks

Ticks can spread diseases, including Rocky Mountain spotted fever, Powassan virus, *Babesia* infection, Lyme disease, and ehrlichiosis. If a person has a tick embedded, it needs to be removed. Wear gloves and use a fine-tipped pointed tweezers. Get as close to the head as possible. Do not squeeze the abdomen, because it may inject secretions into the person's body. Slowly pull the head out. Do not twist. Do not burn it or use petroleum jelly or nail polish. Once the tick is removed, place it in a container of rubbing alcohol to kill it. Clean the site with antiseptic soap and water. Apply an antibiotic ointment. Monitor the site for infections or other complications.

CRITICAL THINKING APPLICATION 21.5

Gabe realized that there were no patient education pamphlets in the exam rooms. He would like to talk with his supervisor about getting brochure racks for each room. His thought was to include procedures on home emergencies/first aid for patients. If you were Gabe, describe the talking points you could make to your supervisor in favor of placing patient education materials in the exam rooms.

Animal Bites

Patients who have animal bites will typically seek care or call their providers. It is important for the medical assistant to ask some screening questions before talking with the provider, such as:

- What type of animal bit you? Do you know the animal? If so, are the shots up to date?
- How does the wound look? Is it bleeding, dirty, or deep? Was it a puncture wound?
- Have you had the rabies vaccine series?
- When was your last tetanus vaccine?

Frequently, the bites are caused by domestic pets (e.g., dogs and cats). First aid for minor bites that only break the skin includes washing the area with soap and water. Then the person should apply over-the-counter antibiotic cream and cover the area with a clean bandage.

It is important to seek medical attention in the following situations:

- *For fang punctures:* For instance, cat bites. Bacteria are left deep in the puncture wound. Initially the wound may not look bad, but in a few hours the entire area could be hot and swollen.
- *For bleeding wounds*: Apply pressure with a clean cloth or bandage and seek help.
- *For dirty or deep wounds*: The person may require a tetanus vaccine booster if the last injection was given 5 or more years earlier.
- *For wounds that look infected*: The wound may look swollen, red, painful, or oozing.
- *For questions about the rabies risk*: Any wild or domestic mammal can get rabies and pass it on to people. Animals commonly seen with rabies include raccoons, skunks, bats, woodchucks (groundhogs), foxes, coyotes, cats, dogs, and cattle.

In the ambulatory care facility, the wound is examined, cleaned, and bandaged. The medical assistant should gather information on the patient's last tetanus booster. A tetanus immunization may be given. If there is a chance of rabies exposure, the provider will discuss the treatment options. Treatment for rabies can be costly, and the treatment time window is narrow. Table 21.7 describes the medications that can be given as treatment.

Foreign Body in the Eye

It is common for people with "something in the eye" to call or visit the ambulatory healthcare facility. This condition is known as a *foreign body in the eye*.

First aid for a foreign body in the eye is eye irrigation. Washing your hands before starting is important. Flush the eye with clean, warm water or with saline eye drops. Saline eye drops will be less irritating than water. If the foreign body cannot be removed through irrigation, the person should seek immediate medical care. It is important not to rub the eye, which may cause further damage.

In the ambulatory care facility, the medical assistant needs to ask the patient how the injury occurred. Further irrigation may be ordered after the provider examines the patient. It is important to check the date of the patient's last tetanus booster. The provider may order an updated tetanus booster, along with additional treatments.

Diabetic Emergencies

Diabetic emergencies occur when the person's blood glucose level is too low or too high. When a person eats carbohydrates (starches and sugars [e.g., breads, candy]), the blood glucose level rises. The pancreas makes insulin, and some people with diabetes mellitus must take insulin injections. Insulin is the only thing that moves the glucose out of the blood and into the cells, where it is used for energy. Without enough insulin, the blood glucose level rises. With too much insulin, the blood glucose level drops (Table 21.8).

If the blood glucose gets too high or too low, the person can go into a diabetic coma. Permanent brain damage and death can occur. If you come across an unresponsive person, check to see if the individual has a medical alert bracelet or necklace. (Some individuals have tattoos instead of wearing the medical alert jewelry.) The medical alert information may provide clues to what is occurring.

First aid for hypoglycemia includes:

- Test the blood glucose level if possible.
- *If the individual is conscious and able to swallow*: Give 4 ounces of fruit juice or regular (not diet) soda or three glucose tablets. Test the blood glucose every 15 minutes. If the blood glucose is under 70, give additional glucose. Continue until the glucose level is 70 or above (see Procedure 21.1, p. 477).
- *If the individual is unconscious*: Place the patient in the **recovery position** (Fig. 21.14). Call 911 and get medical help. Monitor

TABLE 21.7	Rabies Postexposure Treatment for Nonimmunized Individuals	
MEDICATION	**PURPOSE**	**ADMINISTRATION**
Rabies immune globulin (RIG)	Antibodies specifically for rabies. Provides rapid (immediate) passive immune protection against rabies.	Dose based on weight. Administer only once between day 0 (day of the bite) to day 7. Provider injects RIG around the bite wound if present. Remaining RIG is administered IM in the vastus lateralis or deltoid muscle (most distant from the wound). *If required, live virus vaccines (varicella, measles) must be either given with or spaced out 4 months after RIG.*
Rabies vaccine	Helps to provide long-term active immune protection against rabies.	Administer 1 mL IM in the deltoid muscle for adults and the vastus lateralis for children. Administer one dose on days 0, 3, 7, and 14. A fifth dose may be recommended on day 28 for immunocompromised individuals

TABLE 21.8 Diabetic Emergencies

CONDITION	INSULIN SHOCK	DIABETIC KETOACIDOSIS (DKA)
Alternative Names	Severe *hypoglycemia* (low blood glucose); insulin reaction	Severe *hyperglycemia* (high blood glucose)
Why Does It Occur?	Imbalance between insulin and blood glucose. Too little glucose is in the blood because the individual: • Took too much insulin • Ate too few carbohydrates • Engaged in too much physical activity • Drank alcohol (may occur up to 2 days after drinking)	Imbalance between insulin and blood glucose. Too much glucose is in the blood because the individual: • Took too little insulin • Ate too many carbohydrates • Is ill, has an infection, trauma, or surgery • Used an illegal drug (e.g., cocaine, Ecstasy)
Symptoms	**Hypoglycemia** • Double or blurry vision • Fast pulse, palpitations • Irritable, aggressive, nervous • Headache, unclear thinking • Shaking, tired • Sweaty, cold skin • Hunger **Severe Hypoglycemia** • Disorientation, unconsciousness • Seizures • Shock • Diabetic coma and death	**Hyperglycemia** • Thirsty, hungry, stomach pain • Nausea, vomiting • Frequent urination • Fatigue • Shortness of breath • Very dry mouth • Rapid pulse **Diabetic Ketoacidosis** • Fruity odor on breath • Diabetic coma and death

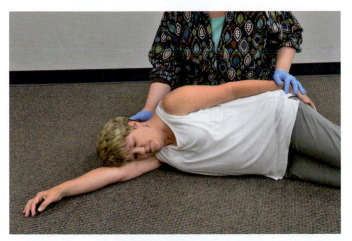

FIGURE 21.14 Recovery position.

How to Place a Person in the Recovery Position

- While kneeling at the person's side, place the lowermost arm next to the head with the palm facing up. Take the other arm and place it next to the person's side.
- Bend the lowermost leg up.
- You want to roll the person as one unit in case of head, neck, or spinal injuries. To do this, carefully slide one arm under the person's shoulder closest to you and the other under the arm and hip. Roll the person away from you and onto his or her side.
- Bend the top leg at the knee and place on top of the other knee. Place the upper arm near the person's hip.

the airway and pulse. Perform rescue breathing and CPR as needed. For an unconscious adult patient, glucagon 1 mL is given subcutaneously or IM (Fig. 21.15). Repeat dose in 15 minutes if patient is unconscious. (Children younger than 6 years of age get 0.5 mL.) Monitor the blood glucose. Once the patient is alert and able to swallow, give additional food (e.g., sandwich).

First aid for hyperglycemia includes:

- Call 911 and get medical help. Monitor the airway and pulse. Perform rescue breathing and CPR as needed.
- The patient will need IV fluids, insulin, and monitoring to bring down the blood glucose level.

Musculoskeletal Emergencies

Without a diagnosis, it is hard to tell if an injury is a strain, sprain, fracture, or dislocation. It is important always to treat the injury as a fracture until the provider diagnoses the injury. A few symptoms will indicate if the injury is more severe (e.g., dislocation), including:

- The person has difficulty or is not able to move the extremity normally.
- The extremity is deformed.
- Bone is exposed through the skin.
- There is heavy bleeding.

If a person has any of these symptoms or the injury was related to major trauma, call 911 and get medical help. Additional first aid steps involve:

- *For bleeding*: Apply pressure to the wound with a clean cloth or sterile bandage.
- *Immobilize the injured area*: Do not push the bone back. Do not move the area affected by the injury. Apply a splint beyond the joint above and the joint below the injury (Figs. 21.16 and 21.17).

- *To limit swelling*: Apply a cold pack to the area. Make sure to cover the cold pack with a towel. Do not apply the cold pack directly on the skin (Fig. 21.18).
- *If the person is going into shock*: Make sure the person is lying down with the head slightly lower than the abdomen and elevate the legs. Monitor the person's breathing and pulse rate. Provide rescue breathing and CPR if needed.

Many times, patients will contact their provider regarding musculoskeletal injuries. The medical assistant should screen the patient and relay the information to the provider. Possible screening questions for musculoskeletal emergencies include:

- What happened?
- What does the injured body part look like? Is it deformed? Is it bleeding?
- Can the person move the injured part? Is there pain?
- How does the skin look over and near the injury?

Typically, the provider will need to examine the patient; then an x-ray will be taken before a final diagnosis is made. Depending on the diagnosis, the medical assistant may need to help apply a splint, cast, sling, or another device. Good patient education is required. The medical assistant should coach the patient on checking the circulation on the affected extremity. Coaching the patient on how to handle the protective device (e.g., cast, splint) while doing basic hygiene

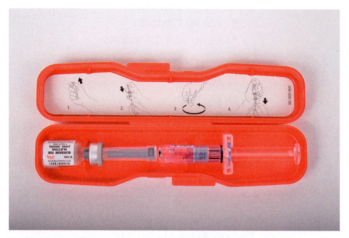

FIGURE 21.15 Glucagon is given to unconscious patients with diabetes. This hormone stimulates the liver to release glucose into the bloodstream, thus increasing the blood glucose level.

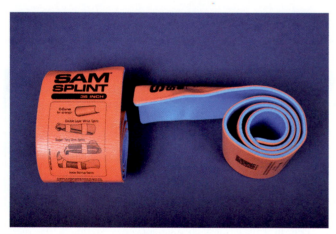

FIGURE 21.16 SAM Splint is a reusable splint that can conform to the extremity affected by the injury.

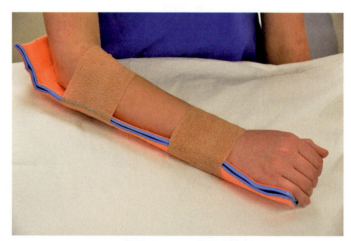

FIGURE 21.17 Splint beyond the joint, above and below the injury.

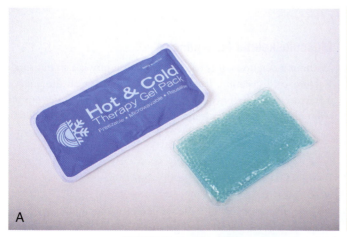

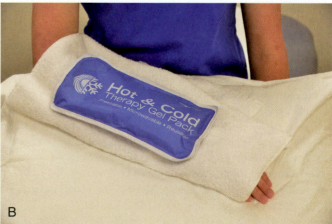

FIGURE 21.18 **(A)** A cold or hot pack cannot be applied directly to the skin. **(B)** Place a towel between the pack and the skin.

activities (e.g., showering) is important. Typically, musculoskeletal injuries require rest, ice, compression, and elevation (RICE).

First Aid and Applying a Splint

- Splint the body part in the position it is in. Do not attempt to readjust the area or straighten it.
- Use a commercial splint or create a splint. Use sticks, a board, or rolled up magazines, newspaper, or clothing as a splint.
- Make sure the splint extends below and above the injury.
- Secure the splint with ties (e.g., belt, cloth strips).
- Check the injured area for swelling, paleness, or numbness, which may indicate the ties are too tight. Loosen ties if needed.

Neurological Emergencies

Neurological emergencies can range from minor conditions, such as dizziness, to serious conditions, such as stroke. The medical assistant should know how to handle neurological emergencies.

Vertigo and Dizziness

Peripheral **vertigo** is caused by a problem in the inner ear (i.e., vestibular labyrinth, semicircular canals, and vestibular nerve). This issue affects the sense of balance. *Central vertigo* is caused by a brainstem or cerebellum disorder. It can be caused by certain drugs (e.g., aspirin, anticonvulsants, and alcohol), migraines, multiple sclerosis, stroke, and tumors.

With *dizziness*, people may feel lightheaded or lose their balance. Many people get dizzy if they move too quickly from a sitting or lying position to a standing position. Their blood pressure drops, causing dizziness. People may feel as if they will pass out. Usually dizziness resolves on its own, but it could be a symptom of another disorder.

First aid for vertigo and dizziness involves sitting or lying down. The affected person should gradually resume activities when the episode passes. In addition, he or she should avoid sudden position changes and bright lights and should drink more fluids. The patient should contact the provider if any of the following apply:
- This is the first episode of vertigo or dizziness.
- The episodes are increasing in number.
- The episodes are getting worse.

Concussion

A **concussion** is a traumatic brain injury caused by a blow to the head. Violently shaking the head can also cause a concussion. Concussions can occur with sports injuries, falls, physical assaults, and traffic accidents. Concussion symptoms may be slow to develop and could last for weeks. Symptoms include:
- Head pressure or headache
- Temporary loss of consciousness right after the incident
- Confusion, amnesia, disorientation, irritability, personality changes
- Dizziness, ringing in the ears
- Nausea and vomiting; taste and smell issues
- Slurred speech, delayed response to questions

- Listlessness, tiredness, sleep disturbances, concentration and memory issues
- Loss of balance, unsteady gait (walk)

First aid for moderate to severe head injuries involves immediately calling 911. Monitor the person until help arrives. Check the breathing and pulse. Provide rescue breathing and CPR as needed. If the person is breathing and has a pulse, treat the condition as a spinal injury. Stabilize the head and neck by placing your hands on both sides of the person's head. Prevent any movement of the head and keep the head in line with the spine until help arrives. If the person vomits, roll the person to the side and move the head, neck, and body as one unit. Moderate to severe head injuries are often seen in the emergency department.

Patients will call or come to ambulatory care facilities if they have a possible concussion or a mild head injury (see Procedure 21.2, p. 478). Possible screening questions include:
- What happened?
- Did the person lose consciousness? If so, for how long?
- Any bleeding?
- How is the person doing? Any vomiting? Are the pupils dilated, or is one larger than the other?
- Does the person remember what happened? Is the person confused or slurring his or her speech?

For mild head injuries, usually a person should seek medical treatment if these occur:
- Loss of consciousness lasting longer than 30 seconds after the initial injury
- Repeated vomiting
- Worsening headache
- Changes in behavior or coordination (irritable, stumbling, or falling)
- Changes in orientation and speech (disoriented, confused, or slurred speech)
- Neurological changes (seizures, visual disturbance, recurrent dizziness, difficulty with concentration, one pupil larger than the other or both pupils dilated)

The patient may need to undergo radiologic testing to check for skull fractures and internal bleeding. If there are no fractures, the provider will educate the patient about other symptoms that would require follow-up and postconcussion care. Athletes need to refrain from playing sports until the concussion symptoms are gone. Another hit on the head can cause additional damage.

CRITICAL THINKING APPLICATION 21.6

Gabe has a 12-year-old son who plays middle school football. Before the season started, Gabe and his wife had to sign an acknowledgment form discussing concussions. What are the benefits of informing parents of school athletes about concussion symptoms?

Seizures

A *seizure* is a sudden increase of electrical activity in one or more parts of the brain. *Epilepsy* is a disorder that causes recurring seizures. Seizures are classified based on how the abnormal brain activity begins. The three major classifications of seizures are:

- *Generalized onset seizure*: Affects both sides of the brain at the same time. Includes several types of seizures, such as tonic-clonic and absent. Symptoms may include jerking, rigid or twitching muscles, and staring spells.
- *Focal onset seizure*: Affects one area of the brain. This type of seizure used to be called a partial seizure. There are two subgroups of focal onset seizures:
  - *Aware seizure*: The person is awake and alert during the seizure.
  - *Impaired awareness seizure*: The person is confused during the seizure. This type of seizure was known as a complex partial seizure.
- *Unknown onset seizure*: When the seizure began is not known.

In most situations, seizures last 30 seconds to 2 minutes. Usually, they do not cause lasting issues. It is a medical emergency if the seizure lasts longer than 5 minutes or if a person has multiple seizures without becoming conscious between them.

Parents commonly call when their child has had a seizure. According to the facility's protocol, the medical assistant may need to ask some screening questions and relay the information to the provider. Possible screening questions for musculoskeletal emergencies include:

- What did the patient do during the seizure? How long was the seizure?
- Did the person lose consciousness?
- How is the patient now after the seizure?

If a person has a seizure in the healthcare facility, the medical assistant must also notify the provider immediately (see Procedure 21.3, p. 479). First aid for seizures focuses on the safety of the individual:

- Move the person to the floor and place the patient in the recovery position. Gently raise the chin to tilt the head back slightly to open the airway. Monitor the person's breathing and pulse. Perform rescue breathing after the seizure has stopped if the patient does not resume breathing. Provide CPR if needed.
- Protect the patient from harm. Clear the area of anything hard or sharp. Place a soft, folded towel under the head.
- Do not place anything in the patient's mouth.
- Remove any glasses and loosen any constrictive clothing around the neck (e.g., ties).
- Time the length of the seizure. Call 911 if the seizure lasts longer than 5 minutes.
- Stay with the person until he or she is fully awake and alert.

Cerebrovascular Accident

A cerebrovascular accident (CVA), also called a *stroke*, is a medical emergency. There are three types of strokes:

- *Ischemic stroke*: Occurs when the arterial blood flow to part of the brain is blocked. The brain cells start to die after a few minutes. This is the most common type of stroke. Two common types of ischemic stroke are:
  - *Thrombotic stroke*: A blood clot forms in an artery, blocking the blood to part of the brain.
  - *Embolic stroke*: A blood clot or other debris forms elsewhere in the body and moves into the brain arteries, blocking the blood flow.
- *Hemorrhagic stroke*: Occurs when an artery in the brain leaks or ruptures. The leaked blood puts pressure on the surrounding brain cells, causing damage. Two types of hemorrhagic stroke include:

- *Intracerebral hemorrhage*: The most common type of stroke; it occurs when a cerebral aneurysm ruptures.
- *Subarachnoid hemorrhage*: Bleeding occurs in the subarachnoid space, usually as a result of small aneurysms.
- *Transient ischemic attack (TIA)*: Also called a "mini-stroke" because it lasts for only a few minutes. The blood supply to a part of the brain is briefly blocked. Symptoms are similar to stroke symptoms but do not last as long (e.g., 1 to 24 hours).

The symptoms of a CVA relate to the part of the brain affected. The individual may not have all the symptoms. Possible symptoms of CVAs include:

- Confusion or mental changes; sudden severe headache
- Speech problems (difficulty forming words, difficult to understand, or using words that do not make sense)
- Numbness of the face, arm, or leg, usually on one side of the body
- Problem seeing in one or both eyes; facial drooping
- Trouble walking, lack of coordination or balance, or arm weakness

First aid for stroke-type symptoms involves getting help (calling 911) immediately. The emergency department (ED) is the best place for a patient to go. There is a small window of time during which clot-dissolving medications (e.g., a tissue plasminogen activator) can be given to help the body break down the clot that is blocking the artery. If a bleeding artery has caused the stroke, the ED providers can detect this on radiologic studies.

If a patient comes to the ambulatory care facility with stroke-like symptoms, it is important for the provider to see the patient immediately. Be ready to call 911 when the provider orders you to do so. Also, monitor the patient's vital signs for changes.

FAST

The American Stroke Association promotes FAST to spot stroke signs and encourages calling 911:

- **F**: Face drooping. Is one side of the face drooping or numb? Ask the person to smile to see if the smile is uneven or drooping on one side.
- **A**: Arm weakness. Is one arm weak or numb? Raise both arms and watch for an arm to drift downward.
- **S**: Speech difficulty. Is the person slurring his or her words? Is the person having problems speaking? Do the words not make sense, or are they hard to understand? Give the person a simple sentence to say and see if it is repeated correctly.
- **T**: Time to call 911. If the person is showing any of these symptoms, call 911 immediately. Let the emergency responders know you think it might be a stroke. Watch the person's respiration rate and pulse rate. Do not give the person anything to eat or drink. Have the person sit upright if possible.

American Stroke Association, http://www.strokeassociation.org/STROKEORG/WarningSigns/Stroke-Warning-Signs-and-Symptoms_UCM_308528_SubHomePage.jsp. Accessed October 23, 2018.

Respiratory Emergencies

Respiratory emergencies can create a number of different signs and symptoms. For example:

- *Skin*: Unusually moist, flushed, pale, bluish or ashen
- *Respirations*: Slow, rapid, deep, or shallow; trouble or no breathing
- *Audible breathing sounds*: Gasping, gurgling, high-pitched noises (e.g., whistling sound), wheezing
- *Patient complaints*: Shortness of breath, dizziness, lightheadedness, chest pain, tingling in extremities, fearful

It is important to get help immediately with respiratory emergencies. After calling 911, help the conscious individual into a comfortable position and monitor the respirations and pulse. Be ready to provide rescue breathing and CPR if required.

Common respiratory emergencies are discussed in the following sections. It is important for the medical assistant to recognize when a patient is having a respiratory emergency and get help immediately.

Hyperventilation

Hyperventilation, or overbreathing, is rapid and deep breathing. This leads to a low carbon dioxide level in the blood. This gas imbalance creates symptoms that can mimic those of a heart attack, thus increasing the person's anxiety, in addition to the hyperventilation. Symptoms of hyperventilation include:

- Dry mouth, belching, and bloating
- Lightheadedness, weakness, dizziness, and difficulty concentrating
- Shortness of breath and breathlessness
- Chest pain and heart palpitations
- Numbness and tingling in the arms or around the mouth
- Muscle spasms

Hyperventilation can be caused by many things, including panic attacks, stress, anxiety, bleeding, heart attack, drugs, and infections.

First aid treatments focus on raising the carbon dioxide level in the blood. This can be done by relaxing and using pursed lip breathing or slowly blowing out through the lips. A person should seek medical care if the hyperventilation episodes get worse. After diagnosing the condition, the provider may have the patient breathe slowly into a paper bag. This helps to restore the carbon dioxide and oxygen balances in the blood.

Asthmatic Attack

Asthma affects the airway and the lungs. During an asthmatic attack, the airway constricts, reducing the air moving into and out of the lungs. Mucus clogs up the airway, making airflow more difficult. Asthma causes wheezing, breathlessness, chest tightness, and coughing. Typically, asthmatic attacks occur at night or in the early morning hours.

If a patient or family member calls about an asthma attack, it is important to gather information quickly and talk with the provider. Possible questions to ask include:

- What symptoms is the person experiencing?
- Was medication given? What was the medication, and how much was administered?
- Did the medication ease the symptoms?
- Is the person having severe respiratory distress (e.g., unable to talk, blue lips, or **retractions**)? (This would be a medical emergency and calling 911 is critical.)

In the ambulatory healthcare setting, an asthmatic attack is an emergency. The provider needs to see the patient immediately. First aid actions for an asthmatic attack include:

- Helping the person into a comfortable sitting position. Usually sitting upright allows for easier breathing.
- Giving short-acting inhalers (e.g., albuterol), which will lessen the asthma attack within minutes.
- Monitoring the pulse oximetry and vital signs

Choking

Choking can occur in all age groups. Most choking cases relate to swallowing large pieces of food or doing an activity (e.g., running) while eating. Other causes are denture-related issues and eating too fast. Children under 5 tend to choke on candy, grapes, and large pieces of food. They are also more likely to put nonfood items in the mouth. Plastic, balloon pieces, coins, and buttons are extremely dangerous to children. Objects smaller than 1.75 inches (the diameter of a golf ball) can be caught in the throat and cause choking.

Any object caught in the throat is considered a foreign body obstruction. Signs of a partial airway obstruction include:

- Can still speak
- Forceful or weak coughing
- Labored, noisy, or gasping breathing
- Panicked appearance, extreme anxiety, or agitation

Signs of a total airway obstruction include:

- Clutching the throat with one or both hands
- Unable to breathe, cry, cough, or speak
- Bluish skin color (e.g., lips)

Do not give the person any liquids until the obstruction is cleared.

First aid for choking includes asking the individual if he or she is choking. If the person is forcefully coughing, stand by and see if the person can clear the airway without assistance. Procedure 21.4 on p. 479 describes the *abdominal thrusts* used on a conscious adult with a total airway obstruction. Treat children older than 1 year of age the same as adults (Fig. 21.19). If a person is pregnant or obese, wrap your arms around the person's chest. Place your fist in the middle of the breastbone between the nipples. Give firm, backward thrusts.

Conscious Choking Infant

Do the 3 Cs after gaining consent from the parent or guardians. Check the scene, call 911 (or have someone else call), and care for the infant. Hold the child with the head below the chest for the entire procedure. This allows gravity to help move the obstruction. Support the chin with your hand and the infant's body with your arm.

Have the child facing downward and give five back blows between the shoulder blades with the heel of your hand (see Fig. 21.19A). Flip the infant and place two or three fingers below the nipple line on the chest. Give five chest thrusts (see Fig. 21.19B). Do a mouth check, and insert a finger only to pull a loose object out. Doing a finger sweep is not recommended because it can push the item in farther. Continue until the object is out or the child becomes unconscious. If the child is unconscious, then place the child on a hard surface and begin CPR, starting with chest compressions.

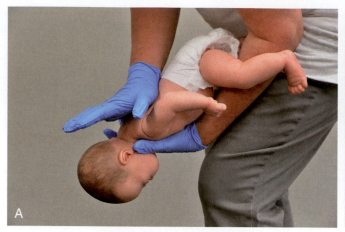
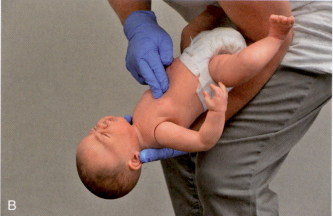

FIGURE 21.19 **(A)** Support the infant with your arm and thigh while giving back blows. **(B)** Chest thrusts are administered in the same position as for cardiac compressions.

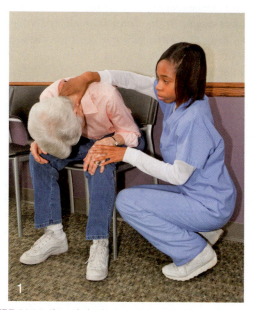

FIGURE 21.20 Placing the head between the legs helps to reduce the faint feeling.

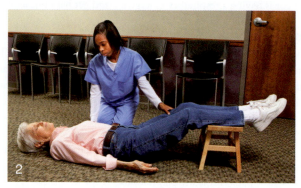

FIGURE 21.21 Elevate the legs about 12 inches using pillows, blankets, or a small stool.

Cardiovascular Emergencies

Syncope

Syncope means fainting, passing out, or having a temporary loss of consciousness. When people are about to faint, they may feel dizzy, nauseous, or lightheaded. The skin may be cold and clammy. People may experience a "black out" or "white out" in their visual field. Muscle control is lost. Fainting occurs when the blood pressure drops suddenly and the blood flow to the brain is reduced.

First aid actions for people who feel faint include having them sit and place their head between their knees (Fig. 21.20). For people who faint, position them on their back. Check their airway and make sure it is clear. Check for a pulse. If the pulse is not present, start CPR. Additional first aid actions include:

- Loosen any constrictive clothing.
- Raise the legs above the heart level (about 12 inches) (Fig. 21.21).
- Get help/call 911 if the person does not regain consciousness within 1 minute.

Possible Causes of Syncope

- Too hot
- Dehydrated and alcohol use
- Standing up too quickly
- Drop in blood glucose
- Certain medications: Diuretics, antihistamines, levodopa, calcium antagonists, angiotensin-converting enzyme (ACE) inhibitors, nitrates, antipsychotics, and narcotics
- Neurological conditions: Parkinson disease, postural orthostatic tachycardia syndrome (POTS), and diabetic neuropathy
- Heart problems
- Vasovagal syncope: Emotional stress, trauma, pain, reaction to the sight of blood, prolonged standing
- Carotid sinus syncope: Constriction of the carotid artery in the neck (occurs with turning the head, shaving, or wearing tight clothing around the neck)
- Situational syncope: Occurs during defecation, urination, and coughing

Bleeding

Bleeding can occur with and without trauma. First aid for bleeding involves stopping the bleeding and calling for help (see Procedure 21.5, p. 480). Nosebleeds are common in certain people. If a person has a nosebleed, have him or her sit upright and lean forward to prevent the person from swallowing the blood. Pinch the nostrils for 5 to 10 minutes, which helps to stop the bleeding. Continue to pinch the nostrils until the bleeding stops. The individual should refrain from blowing the nose for several hours to prevent rebleeding.

In the ambulatory care facility, always wear gloves and the required personal protective equipment (PPE) before assisting patients. Follow these steps to stop the bleeding:

- For bleeding wounds, remove any obvious debris. Do not remove any large objects embedded in the wound.
- Place a sterile gauze or clean cloth over the wound and press firmly to control the bleeding. Do not put direct pressure over an embedded object, an eye, or displaced organs.
- For severe bleeding, help the person lie down and cover him or her with a blanket. This will keep the person warm and conserve body heat.
- If the bleeding seeps through the gauze, apply another layer on top of the initial gauze. Do not move the initial gauze.
- To slow the bleeding or if the bleeding is spurting from an artery:
  - Elevate the bleeding extremity above the heart level. Hold direct pressure over the site.
  - If the bleeding does not stop with the elevation and direct pressure, apply pressure to the artery above the wound by pushing the artery against a bone. Continue to apply direct pressure on the wound. To see if the bleeding has stopped, slowly lift your fingers from the pressure point over the artery. Check to see if the wound is still bleeding. If so, continue to apply pressure. Do not hold pressure at the pressure point for longer than 5 minutes after the bleeding stops.

Shock

Shock occurs when the body is not getting enough blood flow. The vital organs (e.g., heart, brain) do not get enough oxygen and nutrients for the cells to function properly and survive. Organ damage can occur. Shock is a life-threatening condition. There are many types of shock, such as:

- *Cardiogenic shock*: Due to heart muscle damage caused by a *myocardial infarction* (also known as MI, heart attack); the heart cannot pump enough blood to the other organs.
- *Hypovolemic shock*: Due to heavy bleeding (i.e., accident or internal bleeding) or dehydration; blood volume is too low to provide nutrients and oxygen to the organs.
- *Anaphylactic shock*: Caused by a severe allergic reaction (*anaphylaxis*); blood pressure drops and the airway narrows. Not enough blood gets to the vital organs, and the narrowed airway prevents adequate oxygenation.
- *Septic shock*: Caused by a severe infection (severe sepsis) that affects the functioning of vital organs (e.g., heart, brain, kidneys). The blood pressure falls, and major organs can fail.
- *Neurogenic shock*: Due to a central nervous system injury (e.g., spinal cord injury). Leads to vasodilation (not enough blood can return to the heart) and low blood pressure.
  Possible signs and symptoms of shock include:
  - Anxiety, agitation, dizziness, feeling faint, lightheadedness, confusion, and unconsciousness
  - *Cyanosis* (blue lips, fingernails) and shallow respirations
  - Chest pain and a rapid, weak pulse

- Moist skin and *diaphoresis* (profuse sweating)
- Poor or no urine output

Shock requires immediate treatment for the person to have a chance of survival.

First aid actions for shock include calling 911 immediately. Check the person for responsiveness. Monitor the airway, breathing, and pulse. If needed, perform rescue breathing and CPR. If the person is breathing and has a pulse, monitor the vital signs at least every 5 minutes. If the person does not have any injuries to the head, neck or back, or legs, raise the legs 12 inches. This helps the blood to move back to the vital organs of the body. If the person has pain with raising the legs, keep him or her flat. Make sure the person's head is flat. Loosen clothing and provide the appropriate first aid for the person's injuries (see Procedure 21.6, p. 481).

If a person goes into shock in the ambulatory healthcare facility, the provider will order that 911 be contacted. Oxygen and IV fluids are given. The vital signs are monitored, and the person's legs are elevated. Based on the medications available and the person's blood pressure, the provider may give IV medications that will increase the blood pressure. The goals are to keep the blood pressure high enough to sustain life, and to get the patient to the emergency department as quickly as possible.

Myocardial Infarction

Myocardial infarction (MI) is more commonly known as *heart attack*. Coronary arteries that bring blood to the heart muscle are blocked by a clot or narrowed by plaque. When the blood flow to an area of the heart is limited or stopped, the heart cells die, and an MI occurs. Chest pain (*angina pectoris*), cold sweats, and heartburn are the most common symptoms. Chest pain can be described as mild or severe; sharp, burning, heaviness, squeezing, pressure; and constant or *intermittent* (comes and goes). Additional symptoms include:

- Upper body discomfort or pain in one or both arms, shoulders, neck, jaw, upper part of the abdomen, or back
- Arrhythmia, palpitations, tiredness without a reason, nausea, and vomiting
- Shortness of breath with activity or rest, cold sweats, dizziness, and lightheadedness
- Women may have back pain

First aid for a heart attack includes these measures:

- Have the person sit down and rest; keep the individual calm and loosen any tight clothing on the chest and neck area.
- Have the person take nitroglycerin if prescribed.
- Call 911 within 5 minutes of the onset of pain.
- Chew an aspirin (if not allergic).
- Monitor the person's respirations and pulse. Perform rescue breathing and CPR if needed (Figs. 21.22–21.24, Table 21.9, and Procedure 21.7 on p. 482).

If a patient arrives at the ambulatory care facility with chest pain or other MI-type symptoms, bring the patient to a procedure or exam room immediately. Notify the provider at once. Usually the provider will give these orders:

- One aspirin chewed and nitroglycerin administered sublingually
- Call to 911
- Vital signs, pulse oximetry, ECG, oxygen to be administered while waiting for the ambulance

The goals are to limit the damage to the heart muscle and transport the patient to the emergency department.

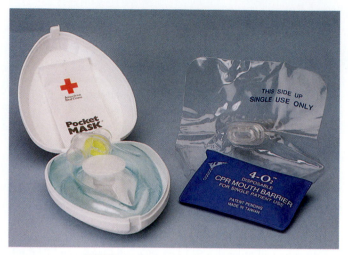

FIGURE 21.22 Rescue breathing mouth barriers.

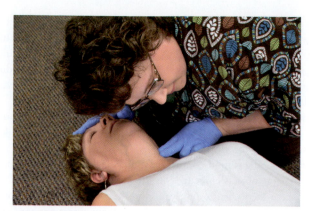

FIGURE 21.23 Use the head-tilt position to open an adult's airway while checking the carotid pulse.

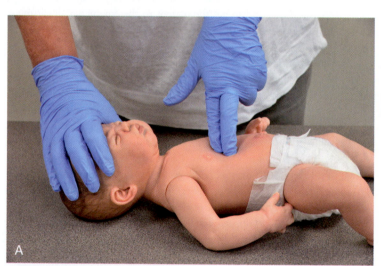

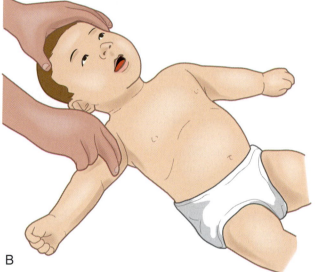

FIGURE 21.24 (A) Open an infant's airway by tilting the head to a neutral position. For chest compressions, place two fingers below the nipple line. **(B)** In an infant, check for a brachial pulse.

TABLE 21.9	Summary of Rescue Breathing and Cardiopulmonary Resuscitation Differences		
	ADULT	**CHILD**	**INFANT**
Check Responsiveness	Shout, "Are you all right?"		Tap infant's foot.
Open Airway	Head-tilt or if spinal injury is suspected, use the jaw thrust without head extension (see Fig. 21.23).	Tilt head slightly past the neutral position.	Tilt head to the neutral position (see Fig. 21.24A).
Assess Pulse	Feel for a carotid pulse near the middle of the throat (see Fig. 21.23).		Feel for brachial pulse on inside of upper arm (see Fig. 21.24B)
Give Rescue Breathing (Ventilation) Only	One rescue breath every 5–6 seconds; deliver each breath for 1 second.	One breath every 3 seconds; deliver each breath for 1 second.	
Chest Compression Hand Position	Heel of a hand is placed on the lower part of the chest (below the nipple line), and other hand is placed on top so that it overlaps the first hand.		Place two fingers just below the nipple line

TABLE 21.9   Summary of Rescue Breathing and Cardiopulmonary Resuscitation Differences—*continued*

	ADULT	CHILD	INFANT
Compressions	2–2.4 inches deep; 100–120 per minute	2 inches deep; 100–120 per minute	1.5 inches deep; 100–120 per minute
Compression-to-Ventilation Ratio	One or two rescuers: 30 compressions and two ventilations.	One rescuer: 30 compressions and two ventilations. Two rescuers: 15 compressions and two ventilations.	
Automated External Defibrillator (AED) Pads	Use only adult pads. Place one pad on the upper right chest and the second on the left side of the chest.	Use pediatric pads for children younger than 8 years; if not available use adult pads. If pads touch, place one on the back between the shoulder blades.	Use pediatric pads; if not available use adult pads. Place one pad on the chest and the other on the back.

Nitroglycerin and Angina

Nitroglycerin is used for *angina* (chest pain). It dilates the coronary arteries, allowing more blood to move into the heart muscle. Nitroglycerin can be given as an oral spray, a sublingual (SL) powder, or sublingual tablets.

- Do not shake the spray. Prime (or release a test spray) 5 to 10 times for new bottles, up to 5 times for bottles not used within 3 months, and 1 to 2 times for bottles that have not been used in more than 6 weeks. Prime the bottles away from everyone. When administering the dose, spray onto or under the tongue. One or two sprays can be taken at the start of the pain. Then, if the pain is not relieved in 5 minutes, give the third spray. Call 911 if the pain continues for an additional 5 minutes.
- Empty the pack of powder under the tongue. Allow the powder to dissolve without swallowing. Make sure the patient does not eat or rinse the mouth for 5 minutes.
- Tablets cannot be chewed or swallowed. Place a tablet under the tongue and let it dissolve. Usually it starts providing relief within 1 to 5 minutes. If the pain is not relieved in 5 minutes, give another tablet. If the pain continues after 5 minutes, give a third tablet. Call 911 if the pain is not relieved 5 minutes after taking the third tablet. (Do not give more than three tablets within 15 minutes.)

Nitroglycerin works fast. The patient may feel dizzy, lightheaded, or faint after taking the medication.

CRITICAL THINKING APPLICATION   21.7

Gabe is thinking of having a rescue breathing mouth barrier in each exam room and procedure room. He is also thinking of adding one to each of the first aid kits located in other parts of the clinic. Why is it important to make mouth barrier devices more available in the clinic?

CLOSING COMMENTS

Patient Coaching

Many ambulatory care facilities are coaching patients on what types of emergencies can be addressed in their facilities and what conditions need to be addressed in emergency departments. People seeking care in emergency departments for possible strokes, heart attacks, and other similar conditions will receive timely care, whereas such services in the ambulatory care facilities are limited and require the patient to be transported to the hospital. Educating patients through voice mail messages, websites, and flyers can help the public understand the limitations of ambulatory care services.

Legal and Ethical Issues

Lawsuits related to care provided during emergencies in healthcare settings are prevalent. Ambulatory care facilities need to have procedures in place to handle emergencies. Staff members need to be trained in handling emergencies. Many agencies have mock codes to help prepare staff. These are training events that allow staff members to practice their skills. Often after mock events, the supervisors assess how the training went. They identify processes and procedures that need refinement and additional training.

Another method of improving processes comes after a real-life code situation. Usually a few days after a code, the staff involved will gather to debrief or discuss what occurred. They will usually talk about:

- How the code progressed, from the time the patient had symptoms to the time the patient was transported to the emergency department
- What went well and what went not so smoothly
- Where more training is needed

These debriefings are extremely important after an emergency situation.

Patient-Centered Care

Medical emergencies are scary for patients and their families. We may be focused on providing emergency care, but we need to remember to communicate with the patient. Being sensitive to what patients are feeling is important. Remember to explain what you are doing. Ask the patient how he or she is doing.

Families of patients are often forgotten. In emergencies, often the family is moved to another room to allow more room for those helping with the code. It is helpful for the family to have a staff person wait with them. If this is not possible, then a staff person needs to report to the family and provide updates. It is important to remember that the rules of the Health Insurance Portability and Accountability Act (HIPAA) still apply in emergency situations.

Professional Behaviors

Code situations can be anxiety-inducing and stressful for staff members. It is important to talk through what occurred, taking confidentiality into account. Besides talking, it is critical to manage one's stress by maintaining a healthy diet and getting adequate sleep and exercise.

An employee assistance program (EAP) is also helpful after stressful code situations. EAP is a work-based program designed to help employees resolve issues. These issues can be personal (e.g., financial, marital, or involving substance abuse) and professional (e.g., communication issues with co-workers and stress-related issues). The EAP services are confidential and designed to help the employee's work performance. EAP counselors help employees to deal with the aftereffects of an emergency.

SUMMARY OF SCENARIO

Gabe has been in his new position for only 2 weeks. Already he has a list of concerns and possible solutions he wants to address with his supervisor. Gabe also wants to discuss forming an emergency response team. This team would respond when a code is called throughout the building.

He hopes to begin quarterly mock codes within the next 3 months. He wants to rotate the types of emergencies addressed by the mock codes. Gabe hopes that with additional training and more exposure to emergency supplies, the medical assistants will feel more comfortable with emergencies.

SUMMARY OF LEARNING OBJECTIVES

1. **Discuss emergencies in healthcare settings and possible roles each team member has during an emergency.**

   Healthcare facilities use special phrases for emergencies. Once the call goes out for help, staff members respond to the scene. In small settings, most members of the staff may be needed. In large facilities, only certain staff members respond. Usually, medical assistants, licensed practical nurses (LPNs), registered nurses (RNs), and providers attend the emergency. Refer to the section in the text for specific roles of each healthcare team member.

2. **Describe emergency equipment and supplies.**

   The emergency supplies available at healthcare facilities will vary based on the size and location of the facility. Some practices have a small box that contains a few supplies and medications. Other practices place many crash carts throughout the building. Equipment and supplies include:
   - Oxygen and airway supplies (includes endotracheal tube intubation supplies and equipment)
   - Defibrillator or an automated external defibrillator (AED)
   - Medications and IV supplies
   - Other supplies: Personal protective equipment, a sharps disposal container, pocket face mask, algorithms, clipboard with documents for charting the code, backboard, and extra batteries for the laryngoscope
   - Pediatric supplies

3. **Explain first aid procedures for environmental emergencies including temperature-related emergencies, burns, poisonings, anaphylaxis, bites and stings, and foreign bodies in the eye.**
   - Temperature-related emergencies: Tables 21.2 and 21.3 discuss first aid for temperature-related emergencies. Hypothermia and heat stroke are emergencies, and the person needs to be transported to the hospital.
   - Minor burns can be treated at home; however, people with major burns need to seek immediate medical attention.

   - First aid for severe allergic reactions and severe reactions related to bites and stings includes giving epinephrine and monitoring the patient's airway, breathing, and pulse.
   - First aid for poisonings includes monitoring the patient's airway, breathing, and pulse. Call 911. The Poison Control staff can be a resource.
   - First aid for a foreign body in the eye is to try to irrigate it out. Flush the eye with clean, warm water or with saline eye drops. Saline eye drops will be less irritating than water. If the foreign body cannot be removed through irrigation, the person should seek immediate medical care.

4. **Discuss diabetic emergencies and provide first aid for a patient in insulin shock.**

   First aid for hypoglycemia includes:
   - Test blood glucose if possible.
   - If the individual is conscious and able to swallow: Give 4 oz. of fruit juice or regular (nondiet) soda or three glucose tablets. Test blood glucose every 15 minutes. If the blood glucose is under 70, give additional glucose. Continue until the glucose level is 70 or above (see Procedure 21.1, p. 477).
   - If the individual is unconscious: Place the patient in the recovery position. Call 911 and get medical help. Monitor the airway and pulse. Perform rescue breathing and CPR as needed. For an unconscious adult patient, administer glucagon 1 mL, given subcutaneously or IM.

   First aid for hyperglycemia includes:
   - Call 911 and get medical help. Monitor the airway and pulse. Perform rescue breathing and CPR as needed.
   - The patient will need IV fluids, insulin, and monitoring to bring down the blood glucose level.

5. **Discuss musculoskeletal and neurological emergencies and provide first aid for a patient with seizure activity.**
   - First aid for major musculoskeletal injuries involves calling 911.

SUMMARY OF LEARNING OBJECTIVES—continued

- Other first aid actions include applying pressure for bleeding, immobilizing the injury, and applying a cold pack to minimize swelling.
- If the person goes into shock, make sure he or she is lying down with the head slightly lower than the abdomen and elevate the legs. Monitor the person's breathing and pulse rate. Provide rescue breathing and CPR if needed.
- First aid for vertigo and dizziness involves sitting or lying down.
- First aid for moderate to severe head injuries involves immediately calling 911. Monitor the person until help arrives. Provide rescue breathing and CPR as needed. If the person is breathing and has a pulse, treat the condition as a spinal injury. Stabilize the head and neck by placing your hands on both sides of the person's head.
- First aid for seizures focuses on the safety of the individual. Move the person to the floor and into the recovery position.
- First aid for stroke-type symptoms involves getting help (calling 911) immediately.

6. **Discuss respiratory emergencies and provide first aid for a choking patient.**
   - First aid treatments focus on raising the carbon dioxide level in the blood. This can be done by relaxing and using pursed lip breathing or slowly blowing out through the lips.
   - First aid actions for an asthmatic attack include helping the person into a sitting position, giving short-acting inhalers, and monitoring the pulse oximetry and vital signs.
   - Procedure 21.4 on p. 479 discusses first aid for choking.

7. **Discuss cardiovascular emergencies and provide first aid for a patient with a bleeding wound, fracture, or syncope; a patient in shock; and a patient in need of rescue breathing or cardiopulmonary resuscitation (CPR).**
   - Refer to Procedure 21.5 on p. 480 for first aid steps for a patient with a bleeding wound, fracture, or syncope.
   - First aid actions for shock include calling 911 immediately. Check the person for responsiveness. Monitor the airway, breathing, and pulse. If needed, perform rescue breathing and CPR. If the person is breathing and has a pulse, monitor the vital signs at least every 5 minutes. If the person does not have any injuries to the head, neck or back, or legs, raise the legs 12 inches.
   - Refer to Procedure 21.7 on p. 482 for the steps to provide rescue breathing and CPR and for using the AED.

PROCEDURE 21.1   Provide First Aid for a Patient in Insulin Shock

Task: Provide first aid to an individual with hypoglycemia.

Scenario: You are working with Dr. Martin, a family practice provider. Maude Crawford arrives for her appointment.

EQUIPMENT and SUPPLIES

- Sugary drink (4-oz fruit juice or regular soda) or three glucose tablets
- Patient's health record

PROCEDURAL STEPS

1. Wash hands or use hand sanitizer.
   PURPOSE: Hand sanitization is an important step for infection control.
2. Greet the patient. Identify yourself. Verify the patient's identity with full name and date of birth.
   PURPOSE: It is important to identify the patient in two different ways to ensure that you have the correct patient.
   Scenario update: Mrs. Crawford has diabetes and states that she thinks she has low blood sugar. She has blurry vision, tremors, and a headache. She asks you for something to eat. According to the facility's policy, you check her blood glucose level and it is 48 mg/dL.
3. Obtain a sugary drink or a fast-acting sugary food. Indicate how much to give to the patient.
   PURPOSE: Consuming a sugary food or drink will help to increase the blood glucose. Do not give a drink or food that contains fat or protein, which can slow the absorption rate.

Scenario update: After 15 minutes, her blood glucose level is 59 mg/dL. You notify the provider while a co-worker stays with the patient.

4. Describe follow-up care for the patient.
   PURPOSE: A blood glucose test should be done to find out how low the patient's level is. After 15 minutes of her eating/drinking the sugary food, the glucose test should be done. If her level is below 70 mg/dL, give her additional sugary food/drink and repeat the glucose test in 15 minutes. Continue until the blood glucose level is 70 or higher.
   Scenario update: After 15 minutes, her blood glucose level is 82 mg/dL. You notify the provider.
5. Document the situation. Include the blood glucose levels, your actions, the provider who was notified, and the patient's response.
   10/04/20XX 1023 Pt c/o blurry vision, tremors, and a headache. She stated she thought she had low blood sugar. Four oz. of orange juice given to pt. After 15 minutes her blood glucose was 59 mg/dL. Dr. Martin notified and ordered additional orange juice and to recheck blood glucose until 70 mg/dL or more. Four oz. of orange juice given and after 15 minutes her blood glucose was 82 mg/dL. Provider notified. _____ Gabe Garcia, CMA (AAMA)

| PROCEDURE 21.2 | Incorporate Critical Thinking Skills When Performing Patient Assessment |

Tasks: Use critical thinking skills while performing a patient assessment regarding a neurological emergency.

Scenario: You are working with Dr. Martin, a family practice provider. Maude Crawford's daughter calls, concerned about her mother. She states that Maude fell and hit her head. She was "knocked out" for about a minute. She has been acting differently since the fall. You need to follow the "Emergency Phone Protocol" for your clinic.

Directions: Role-play the scenario with a peer. The peer will be the daughter, and you will be the medical assistant. The peer can make up information regarding the scenario. Your instructor will be the provider.

WMFM – Neurological Emergency Phone Protocol

Obtain the patient's name, date of birth, signs/symptoms, and the history of the situation. After call, document situation, symptoms, and action in the patient's health record.

With the following neurological concerns, send the patient to the emergency department via the ambulance immediately.

- Seizure lasting 3 or more minutes
- Passing out or fainting; dizziness or weakness that doesn't go away
- Sudden or unusual headache that starts suddenly
- Unable to see or speak; sudden confusion
- Neck or spine injury
- Injuries that cause loss of feeling or inability to move
- Head injury with passing out, fainting, or confusion

With the following concerns, schedule a visit for the same day. If no appointments are available, consult the triage nurse or the provider regarding the situation.

- Headache/migraine
- Nonemergent neurological concern

EQUIPMENT and SUPPLIES

- Patient's health record
- Paper and pen
- Emergency Phone Protocol for clinic

PROCEDURAL STEPS

1. Write five questions that can be asked to obtain additional information on the patient's signs and symptoms.
   PURPOSE: It is important to ask open and closed-ended questions to obtain information about the patient's condition.
2. Obtain the patient's name and date of birth.
   PURPOSE: Obtaining the patient's information is important for any patient-related phone call.
3. Write down the patient's information obtained.
   PURPOSE: Writing down the information will help when you discuss the situation with the provider and when you document the call.

4. Using critical thinking skills, ask appropriate questions to obtain information about the patient's condition.
   PURPOSE: Thoughtful questions related to the situation and the patient's condition must be asked to gather the appropriate information.
5. Follow the protocol to determine what actions to take.
   PURPOSE: Protocols are approved and signed by the providers. They need to be followed by the staff.
6. Instruct the caller on what should be done.
   PURPOSE: The caller needs clear directions on what to do.
7. Document the call in the patient's health record. Include the caller's name, the patient's condition (e.g., signs, symptoms, and concerns), name of the protocol used, information given to the caller, and the provider who was notified.
   PURPOSE: Legally it is important to document all patient interactions.

PROCEDURE 21.3 Provide First Aid for a Patient With Seizure Activity

Tasks: Provide first aid to an individual having seizure activity and document it in the health record.

Scenario: You are working with Dr. Martin, a family practice provider. Walter Biller arrives for his appointment.

EQUIPMENT and SUPPLIES

- Watch
- Folded towel, blanket, or coat
- Patient's health record
- Gloves and other personal protective equipment (as required)

PROCEDURAL STEPS

1. Wash hands or use hand sanitizer.
   PURPOSE: Hand sanitization is an important step for infection control.
2. Greet the patient. Identify yourself. Verify the patient's identity with full name and date of birth.
   PURPOSE: It is important to identify the patient in two different ways to ensure that you have the correct patient.
   Scenario update: While you are getting Mr. Biller's health history, he starts to have seizure activity.
3. Lower the patient to the floor and note the time when the seizure started. Gently raise the chin to tilt the head back slightly to open the airway.
   PURPOSE: The patient needs to be on the floor for his safety. It is important to time seizures.
4. Yell for help while moving the patient into the recovery position.
   PURPOSE: The recovery position will help to open up the person's airway. Yelling for help in the ambulatory care facility is reserved for emergencies. You need to notify the provider as soon as possible.
5. Check his pulse rate and respiration rate.
   PURPOSE: You need to make sure he is breathing and has a pulse. If not, rescue breathing and CPR must be started.
6. Put on gloves and other personal protective equipment as needed.
   PURPOSE: Wearing personal protective equipment will protect you if the patient vomits or becomes incontinent of urine or stool during the seizure.
7. Clear any hard or sharp items away from the patient. Place a soft folded towel, blanket, or coat under the patient's head.
   PURPOSE: It is important to protect the patient from harm.
8. Remove the patient's glasses (if on) and loosen any constrictive clothing around the neck. Stay with the person until he or she is fully awake and continue to monitor the respiration and pulse rates.
   PURPOSE: Tight clothing can restrict breathing.
9. Document the first aid measures you provided in the order that they occurred. In addition, document the seizure activity you witnessed, the length of the episode, and the provider notified.
   PURPOSE: Specifying the care provided, along with details of the seizure activity, will help the provider.
   10/05/20XX 1423 While rooming pt, he started to jerk his arms. He became unresponsive. Pt was moved to the floor and placed in the recovery position. P: 86 regular, thready; R: 18 regular, normal. Dr. Martin arrived. Pt's clothing was loosened. The seizure activity lasted for 4.5 minutes.
   —————————————————————————— Gabe Garcia, CMA (AAMA)

PROCEDURE 21.4 Provide First Aid for a Choking Patient

Tasks: Provide first aid to a conscious adult who is choking. Document it in the health record.

Scenario: You are working with Dr. Martin, a family practice provider. As you return from lunch, you notice that an adult visitor is having an issue. It appears that she had been eating fast food and now she is holding her neck with both hands. She appears to be panicking.

EQUIPMENT and SUPPLIES

- Patient's health record
- Gloves
- Mannequin

PROCEDURAL STEPS

1. Approach the person and ask, "Are you choking?"
   PURPOSE: If the person can speak and is coughing forcefully, then let her cough and try to dislodge the obstruction. If the person is not able to speak, then assist the patient.
   Scenario update: She nods her head yes but cannot speak. She is standing.
2. Yell for help. Put on gloves if available. Stand behind the victim with your feet slightly apart. Reach your arms around the person's waist.
   PURPOSE: With an obstructed airway, the person may lose consciousness at any time. The rescuer must be prepared to lower the unconscious individual to the floor safely. If the person in distress is a child, the rescuer may need to kneel when providing assistance.
3. Make a fist and place it just above the person's navel. Make sure your thumb side is next to the person. Grasp the fist tightly with your other hand (see the following figure).
   PURPOSE: Correct hand position is important as you do abdominal thrusts.

Continued

| PROCEDURE 21.4 | Provide First Aid for a Choking Patient—*continued* |

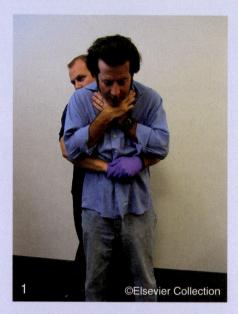

1   ©Elsevier Collection

Scenario update: The next steps must be done on a mannequin.

4. With the correct hand position, make quick, upward and inward thrusts with your fist. Do 5 abdominal thrusts before doing back blows.
   PURPOSE: The fist should be placed in the soft tissue of the abdomen to avoid injury to the sternum or rib cage. If the person is supine, straddle and face the person's head. Push your grasped fist upward and inward.

5. Stand behind the person and wrap one arm around the person's upper body. Position the person so he or she is bent forward with the chest parallel to the ground.
   PURPOSE: This position helps objects to dislodge.

6. Use the heel of your other hand to give a firm blow between the shoulder blades. Check to see if the object dislodges. If not, continue by giving another 4 back blows.
   PURPOSE: Back blows can help dislodge the item.

7. Continue to give 5 abdominal thrusts followed by 5 back blows until the object is dislodged or the person loses consciousness.
   PURPOSE: Repeated abdominal thrusts and back blows can help dislodge the item.
   Note: If the person faints or loses consciousness, lower the person to the floor. Call 911 (or the local emergency number) or have someone else call. Begin CPR, starting with chest compressions. Check to see if the item is in the airway. Remove it only if it is loose.
   Scenario update: After two sets, she coughs out a piece of food. She can now talk.

8. Arrange for the person to be seen by the provider. Document the first aid measures you provided in the order that they occurred.
   PURPOSE: Specifying the care provided, along with details of the situation, will present the provider with a full picture of what happened.
   10/06/20XX 1223 Pt was found in reception room with her hands on her throat. She appeared to be panicky. She could not speak but indicated with a nod of her head that she was choking. After being given 2 sets of back blows and abdominal thrusts, she was able to cough out some undigested food. R: 22 regular, normal. Pt is alert. She agreed to see Dr. Martin immediately.
   _____ Gabe Garcia, CMA (AAMA)

| PROCEDURE 21.5 | Provide First Aid for a Patient With a Bleeding Wound, Fracture, or Syncope |

Tasks: Provide first aid to an individual with a suspected fracture, a bleeding wound, and syncope. Document the first aid you provide.

Scenario: You are returning from lunch and see a person fall at the entrance of the healthcare facility. He is an older man and complains of pain in his right lower arm. His arm looks deformed and is bleeding. You call for help. A provider comes, and co-workers bring supplies. The provider tells you to care for the wound and splint the arm before moving the individual. You have a co-worker helping you.

EQUIPMENT and SUPPLIES
- Gloves
- Sterile gauze
- Bandage
- Splinting material (e.g., SAM Splint)
- Coban wrap or gauze roll

PROCEDURAL STEPS

1. Wash hands or use hand sanitizer if possible. Identify yourself to the patient. Obtain the patient's name and date of birth as you put on gloves.

PURPOSE: It is important to wear gloves when working with a wound. Obtaining the patient's name is important because the patient will be seen and you need to document the first aid provided.

2. Using sterile gauze, apply direct pressure over the wound to stop the bleeding. Make sure to immobilize the injured arm as you apply pressure. If possible, elevate the arm to help slow the bleeding. If the blood seeps through the gauze, apply another layer of gauze on the initial one. Continue with the direct pressure until the bleeding stops.
   PURPOSE: Applying pressure and elevating the arm will slow the bleeding.

PROCEDURE 21.5   Provide First Aid for a Patient With a Bleeding Wound, Fracture, or Syncope—continued

3. Once the bleeding has stopped, cover the dressing with a bandage. Remember to immobilize the injured arm as you work.

   PURPOSE: It is important to cover the wound with a bandage in case the bleeding restarts. Immobilizing a suspected arm is important until the splint can be applied.

   Scenario update: As you apply the bandage to the injured arm, the patient states he does not feel good. He says he feels dizzy and thinks he is going to pass out. Your peer takes over by supporting his arm, and the man faints. He is still breathing and has a pulse.

4. Position the patient on his back. Continue to check his respirations and pulse rates.

   PURPOSE: If the patient is not breathing or does not have a pulse, administer rescue breathing and begin CPR.

5. Loosen any constrictive clothing around the neck and chest. Raise the legs above the heart level (about 12 inches).

   PURPOSE: Raising the legs allows the blood to return to the vital organs.

   Scenario update: After a few minutes, he starts to come around. He jokes that blood makes him faint. As he is lying on his back talking with you, you need to splint his injured arm.

6. Use the splint material and shape it to the injured arm. Do not straighten the arm. Apply the splint beyond the joint above and the joint below the injury.

   PURPOSE: It is important to keep the arm in the same position until the provider examines the arm and x-rays are taken.

7. Use Coban or a gauze roll to secure the splint in place. Encourage the patient to hold the injured arm against his chest as he moves.

   PURPOSE: If the patient can hold the arm, this will reduce the pain.

8. Document the first aid measures you provided in the order they occurred. Note that the provider was at the scene.

   PURPOSE: Specifying the care provided, along with details of the seizure activity, will help the provider.

   10/07/20XX 1215 Pt fell at the clinic entrance. He c/o pain in his lower right arm. Dr. Martin ordered wound care and splinting of the arm before moving the pt. Using sterile gauze, applied direct pressure over the wound until the bleeding stopped. Wound was covered with a bandage while arm was manually immobilized. Pt stated he felt dizzy and fainted. P: 68 regular, thready; R: 16 irregular, normal. Pt was positioned on his back with his feet elevated. Within a few minutes patient came to and started talking. SAM Splint applied to right arm and Coban applied to hold the splint. Pt held arm while transferring into wheelchair. Pt to see Dr. Martin immediately. _____

   _____ Gabe Garcia, CMA (AAMA)

PROCEDURE 21.6   Provide First Aid for a Patient in Shock

Tasks: Provide first aid to an individual who is in shock. Document the first aid you provide.

Scenario: You are working with Dr. Julie Walden. The administrative medical assistant at the reception desk notifies you that Robert Caudill (date of birth [DOB] 10/31/1940) is here and looks very ill. You bring the patient and his wife immediately back to the procedure room, because it is the only available room. He asks to move to the exam table, and you assist him as he transfers to the table. You obtain his vital signs, which are P: 92, R: 26, BP 72/48, and T: 103.2.

EQUIPMENT and SUPPLIES

- Stethoscope
- Watch
- Pen
- Sphygmomanometer (blood pressure cuff)
- Pillows, blankets, or small stool to help elevate the feet
- Exam table

PROCEDURAL STEPS

1. Call for help. Monitor the patient's breathing and pulse until the provider arrives.

   PURPOSE: It is important to have the provider see the patient immediately.

   Scenario update: The provider examines the patient and suspects septic shock. You administer 2 L of oxygen per nasal cannula as the provider ordered. The triage RN inserts an IV and administers IV fluids. The provider directs another medical assistant to call 911.

2. Raise the patient's legs 12 inches.

   PURPOSE: Raising the person's legs helps the blood to return to the heart. Some tables will allow you to elevate the foot section. If this is not possible, use things such as pillows, blankets, or a small stool.

3. Make sure the patient's head is flat on the bed.

   PURPOSE: This helps the blood to flow to the head.

4. Loosen the person's clothing. Make sure the clothing does not restrict the neck and chest area.

   PURPOSE: Clothing that is tight can affect the breathing.

5. Obtain a pulse rate, respiration rate, and blood pressure. Continue to monitor the patient's airway, pulse rate, and respiration rate.

   PURPOSE: Monitor vital signs. If the person is not breathing, provide rescue breathing. If the person has no pulse, start CPR.

6. While monitoring the patient, speak calmly with him. Use a gentle tone of voice. Demonstrate calming body language (e.g., do not appear scared, rushed, or out of control).

Continued

PROCEDURE 21.6   Provide First Aid for a Patient in Shock—*continued*

PURPOSE: It is important to keep the patient calm during the crisis. Anxiety can be a symptom of shock.

7. Talk calmly with the patient's wife and explain what is occurring. Answer any questions the wife may have.

   PURPOSE: In an emergency, it is important to keep the family in the room updated on what is occurring. Depending on the emergency, sometimes a staff person will take the family members to another room.

8. Document the first aid measures you provided in the order they occurred. Indicate which provider examined the patient. In addition, document the administration of oxygen and the vital signs obtained.

   PURPOSE: Specifying the care provided, along with the vital signs, will help the provider and the emergency responders.

10/07/20XX 1525 P: 92 irregular, thready; R: 26 regular, shallow; BP: 72/48 RA lying; T: 103.2 (TA). Notified Dr. Walden. Pt resting on table with his wife at his side. _____ Gabe Garcia, CMA (AAMA)

10/07/20XX 1535 Administered 8 L of oxygen per mask per Dr. Walden's order. Raised legs about 12 inches, and head is flat. P: 98 irregular, thready; R: 32 regular, shallow; BP: 70/42 RA lying. _____ Gabe Garcia, CMA (AAMA)

PROCEDURE 21.7   Provide Rescue Breathing, Cardiopulmonary Resuscitation (CPR), and Automated External Defibrillator (AED)

Tasks: Perform rescue breathing and CPR. Use the AED machine.

Scenario: You are out jogging and find a person on the ground. No one is around.

EQUIPMENT and SUPPLIES

- AED machine with adult pads
- Barrier ventilation device
- Mannequin
- Gloves (if available)

PROCEDURAL STEPS

1. Check the scene for safety. Is it safe to approach and provide help to the victim?

   PURPOSE: It is important to look for toxic or electrical hazards. Also, look for other hazards that make the scene unsafe for you. If you find something, call 911 and wait for the emergency responders.

2. Check the person's response. Tap the individual on the shoulder and shout, "Are you all right?" Pause for a few moments for a response.

   PURPOSE: If the patient is responsive, the individual will talk, moan, move, or do something that indicates responsiveness.

   Scenario update: There is no response from the individual. A bystander comes up and you direct that person to find an AED machine.

3. Call 911 and answer the questions from the dispatcher.

   PURPOSE: The dispatcher needs to know what is occurring and the location of the emergency.

4. Put on gloves if available. Roll the person over if the person is face down. Roll the person as an entire unit, supporting the head, neck, and back. Open the airway and assess the respirations and the pulse for 5 to 10 seconds.

   Note: Occasional gasping is not considered breathing.

- Person is breathing and has a pulse: If no head, neck, or spinal injury is suspected, then place the patient in the recovery position.
- Person is not breathing and has a pulse: Give ventilations and monitor pulse.
- Person is not breathing and has no pulse: Give CPR starting with compressions.

   PURPOSE: Before you initiate rescue breathing or CPR, you need to know if the person is breathing or has a pulse.

   Scenario update: The individual has a weak pulse and is not breathing. (Use a mannequin for the following steps.)

5. Use a barrier device if available. Pinch the person's nose and give each rescue breath over 1 second. Watch for the chest to rise. Give the appropriate amount of ventilations for the person's age (see Table 21.9). Continue to monitor the pulse as you give rescue breaths.

   Note: For a situation in which a person had been choking, look in the mouth before giving a rescue breath. If you see the object, sweep it out with your finger. You can also provide nose ventilation, if the mouth is injured. Stoma ventilation must be done if the person has a stoma (in the throat area).

   PURPOSE: Adults get a rescue breath every 5 to 6 seconds. Children and infants get one every 3 seconds. If the chest does not rise, reposition and open the airway.

   Scenario update: When you check the pulse again, there is no pulse.

6. Place your hands at the correct location on the chest (see the first of the following figures). Bring your shoulders directly over the victim's sternum as you compress downward. Keep your elbows locked (see the second of the following figures).

PROCEDURE 21.7	Provide Rescue Breathing, Cardiopulmonary Resuscitation (CPR), and Automated External Defibrillator (AED)—*continued*

PURPOSE: The correct position will allow you to do the compressions at the depth they need to be.

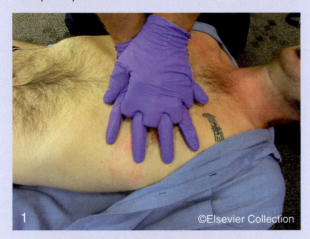

1 ©Elsevier Collection

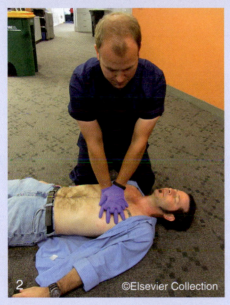

2 ©Elsevier Collection

7. Give 30 compressions at the appropriate depth (see Table 21.9). Give 100 to 120 compressions per minute.
PURPOSE: The appropriate depth is required to help compress the chambers of the heart.

8. Give two ventilations and watch for the chest to rise. Continue with the cycle.
PURPOSE: It is important to continue to provide ventilations and compressions until you are too exhausted, the person is breathing, an AED arrives, or emergency responders arrive.

Scenario update: After two cycles, a bystander brings an AED but does not know how to use it. The bystander also does not know CPR. You need to stop the CPR and use the AED.

9. Turn on the AED and follow the directions. Attach the AED pads to the individual's bare dry chest (see Table 21.9 and the following figure). Attach the pads to the machine if required.
Note: Make sure to remove any medication patches and medication residue from the chest before applying the pads.
PURPOSE: The pads need to be placed on the bare, dry chest for the AED to work correctly.

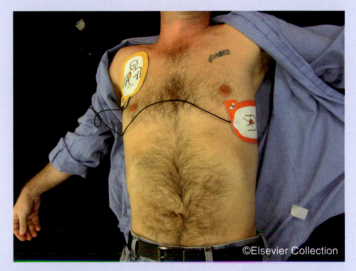

©Elsevier Collection

10. Have everyone stand back from the patient by announcing, "Stand clear." Push the analyze button and allow the machine to analyze the heartbeat.
PURPOSE: "Stand clear" tells everyone to not touch the patient during this step.

11. Follow the prompts on the AED machine.
- If a shock is advised, announce, "Stand clear" and make sure no one is touching the individual. Press the shock button. After the shock, do CPR for 2 minutes, starting with compressions. Continue following the prompts until the emergency responders arrive.
- If a shock is not advised, continue doing CPR for 2 minutes, starting with compressions. Continue following the prompts until the emergency responders arrive.
PURPOSE: The AED will prompt you as to what to do next.

22

SKILLS AND STRATEGIES

SCENARIO

Michelle, Krysia, and Zacarias (or "Zac" to his friends) met during their first semester of college. They have developed a great friendship over the past few months. They will be graduating from the medical assistant program in less than 6 weeks. Michelle just graduated from high school a year ago. Krysia entered the military just after her high school graduation. She spent 10 years in the Marines. Zac has been out of high school for several years and worked in a factory. He started as a line worker and gradually advanced to supervisory positions. Due to downsizing, his position was eliminated. He went back to school. These friends are looking forward to graduation and getting jobs as medical assistants.

As these three friends discuss finding a job, Michelle is hesitant about the job search experience. Her only work experience is 2 years as a waitress at a local restaurant. She has never created a resume or a cover letter. She only had a very informal interview with the restaurant owner before she was given the job. Krysia is concerned about her military career. The positions she held were not related to healthcare. She managed inventory and supervised others. She was also deployed to many hot spots around the world. Zac has a lot of experience in the factory setting, but he feels that that world is so different from healthcare. As they talk with each other, it is clear that each person has a unique situation, and they all must take a closer look at their past experiences as they prepare for their job search adventure.

While studying this chapter, think about the following questions:
- What personality traits are important to employers?
- What are the best job search methods?
- How do you develop a resume and cover letter?
- How do you complete a job application?
- How do you prepare for an interview?

LEARNING OBJECTIVES

1. Describe personality traits important to employers.
2. Discuss personality traits, technical skills, and transferable job skills.
3. Describe how to develop a career objective and identify your personal needs.
4. Explain job search methods.
5. Create a resume and cover letter.
6. Complete an online profile and job application.
7. Describe how to create a career portfolio.
8. Practice interview skills during a mock interview.
9. List legal and illegal interview questions.
10. Create a thank-you note for an interview.
11. Explain common human resource hiring requirements when starting a new job.

VOCABULARY

clarification Allows the listener to get additional information.

collaboration (kuh lab uh RAY shun) The act of working with another or other individuals.

counteroffer Return offer made by one who has rejected an offer or a job.

dignity The inherent worth or state of being worthy of respect.

interpersonal skills The ability to communicate and interact with others; sometimes referred to as "soft skills."

job boards Websites where employers post jobs; they can be used by job seekers to identify open positions.

mock Simulated; intended for imitation or practice.

reflecting Putting words to the patient's emotional reaction, which acknowledges the person's feelings.

reverse chronologic order The most recent item is on top and the oldest item is last.

paraphrasing Rewording a statement to check the meaning and interpretation; also shows you are listening to and understanding the speaker.

proofread To read and mark corrections.

skill set A person's abilities, skills, or expertise in an area.

summarizing Allowing the listener to recap and review what was said.

As you move toward graduation, you may be experiencing many emotions. You might be excited about finishing your medical assistant program. You might be scared of the future changes. The thought of finding a job might be overwhelming. These are common feelings of all graduates. The important step before graduation is to prepare for the next phase: getting a job.

Preparing for the job-seeking phase is very important. This chapter will help you:

- Understand the characteristics that employers want
- Identify your strengths, experiences, and skills
- Develop your career objectives

When you have done these things, you are ready to market yourself to potential employers. You will market yourself through your resume and interview experiences. Remember that an early job search, even before graduation, can be the key to landing a job soon after graduation.

UNDERSTANDING PERSONALITY TRAITS IMPORTANT TO EMPLOYERS

It is important to understand what employers are looking for in employees. Employers spend money and time training new employees. It is critical that they initially find the right employees. Many employers will agree that they can help refine technical skill proficiencies. It is more difficult to help grow or change personality traits. We will examine the five personality traits that are most important to employers. These include collaboration, interpersonal skills, professionalism, compassion, and a sincere interest in the job.

Collaboration and Interpersonal Skills

Collaboration and **interpersonal skills** are crucial to the efficiency of the healthcare environment. Employers look for people who can blend well with the current staff. New employees need to be flexible, dependable, supportive of peers, and remain calm under pressure. Employers want employees who will provide excellent customer service by having outstanding interpersonal skills, including the following:

- *Effective verbal communication*: Involves using clear, thoughtful, and easily understood language.
- *Professional nonverbal communication*: Relays more information to patients and peers than any words you could use. Eye contact, posture, voice, and gestures provide insights into a person's attitude. Being focused, calm, polite, and interested in the other person are traits of effective nonverbal communication.
- *Good listening skills*: Critical when working with peers and patients. For effective communication to occur, listening must occur. Appropriate questions can draw others into the conversation and show others you are listening and care. Communication techniques such as **reflecting**, **paraphrasing**, **summarizing**, and asking for **clarification** are also excellent ways of demonstrating active listening skills.
- *Good manners*: Are essential, along with a basic understanding of the diversity of your patient population.

Professionalism

A person's professionalism is being evaluated from the cover letter to the interview and beyond. Employers are looking for employees who project a professional image in all situations. Professionalism includes a person's appearance (i.e., dress and grooming habits) and behaviors. The behaviors include a person's flexibility, punctuality, honesty, attention to detail, time management skills, ability to following directions, and ability to prioritize.

Compassion

Compassion is another trait employers look for. *Compassion* means to have a deep awareness of another's suffering and the desire to lessen it. **Dignity** and respect are part of providing compassionate care to others. Many people go into healthcare to help others. They may like the technical skills involved with patient care. Providing dignity and respect during patient care is just as important. Compassion and respect help healthcare employees connect to patients and their families. Acts of kindness and thoughtfulness that lessen stress are welcomed by patients.

Dignity and Respect Example

Imagine being a patient in your 70s. You have a walker. You spent 4 months in a wheelchair recovering from a stroke. You are proud to be walking today, even if you are slow. You know that walking is important, so that you do not get stiff and then cannot walk.

The medical assistant calls you in for the visit. You slowly walk to her and then she takes you down the hall. She is far ahead of you as you slowly make your way. It appears the room is at the end of the long hall. You hear the medical assistant calling to a peer to get a wheelchair. She looks back at you and states, "We have a wheelchair for you to speed things up." How do you feel? Do you feel that she values you? Is she showing you respect?

If you reverse the roles, how could you, as a medical assistant, show that you respect and value the patient?

Genuine Interest

Employers also look for people genuinely interested in the job. This trait can be seen during the interview. Does the person ask thoughtful questions regarding the position and the facility? Genuine interest in the job extends beyond the hiring phase into day-to-day operations. Being interested in one's job is critical. Looking for ways to improve procedures and provide better patient care is an important behavior to demonstrate to the employer. This genuine interest is reflected in your attitude and performance in the workplace. It helps ease your transition into a new job and promotes your success.

CRITICAL THINKING APPLICATION   22.1

Think of the three friends in the Scenario. Michelle just graduated from high school and has 2 years of waitressing experience. Krysia has 10 years in the military, where she managed inventory, supervised others, and was deployed to many hot spots around the world. Zac has been working in a factory, advancing to supervisory positions. Now think about the personality traits that employers want. What personality traits might each friend possess? Explain your answer.

- Create your own list of the personality traits that employers want, and you possess.

ASSESSING YOUR STRENGTHS AND SKILLS

As you prepare to market yourself to potential employers, you need to examine your strengths and skills in three different areas. What personality traits do you possess? What technical skills are your strengths? What are the transferable job skills that you possess?

Personality Traits

In addition to the typical personality traits required by employers, the job posting may list extra traits, including personality traits. Which of these skills and strengths do you possess? Many people will tell potential employers what they think employers want to hear. They claim to be "a team player," to "communicate well," to be "dependable," and so on. Listing these phrases on your resume or during the interview is not enough to convince the potential employer that you truly have those characteristics. They like "supporting evidence"!

Early on in the preparation phase, make a list of the qualities that you believe you possess. For each quality provide one or two pieces of "evidence" to support your claims. Your "evidence" may be a past job review or practicum evaluation in which the author indicates your strengths and characteristics. These are excellent documents to include in your portfolio, which will be discussed later in the chapter. Using stories of situations in which you portrayed those characteristics is another way to illustrate your qualities. It is important to share these during the interview, if pertinent to the questions asked.

Technical Skills

Employers are also interested in your technical skills. Technical skills for medical assistants can be related to clinical procedures, such as phlebotomy, injections, electrocardiograms (ECGs), and obtaining vital signs. Technical skills can also be related to administrative procedures, including software proficiency, keyboard speed, reception duties, and coding procedures.

You may be able to provide supporting documentation of your technical skills through the use of practicum skill checklists or through a portfolio. Technical skills might also include skills that you developed outside the medical assistant program but that still relate to your chosen career. For instance, if you worked as a pharmacy technician at a local hospital, several of the technical skills you acquired may relate to a clinic position.

Transferable Job Skills

Transferable job skills are the last area to examine. A person develops these skills in one job or experience. The skills can be "transferred" to another job. This means the person will use these skills in other jobs. Many of these skills may sound familiar. They are also characteristics employers are looking for.

Potential Transferable Skills

- Customer service
- Compassion and empathy
- Strong communication and listening skills
- Computer skills
- Leadership skills
- Organizational skills
- Teamwork
- Time management and prioritizing skills
- Creativity
- Grace under pressure
- Problem-solving skills

Identifying transferable job skills can be difficult for many people. Job descriptions for past experiences can be very useful. To start, make a list of your past jobs, military experience, and volunteer opportunities. Make a list of potential transferable skills you developed and used for each experience. Some examples of transferable skills for different jobs and situations include:

- Wait staff jobs: Strong communication and listening skills, prioritizing, and customer service skills
- Factory jobs: Communication skills, teamwork, and problem solving
- Military experience: Strong communication skills, grace under pressure, and prioritizing
- Stay-at-home parent: Organization, prioritizing, budgeting, time management, and problem solving

This list of transferable job skills will be used as you create your resume and prepare for your interview.

CRITICAL THINKING APPLICATION   22.2

What might be some transferable skills that the three friends, Michelle, Krysia, and Zac, possess? Explain your answer.

- Using the list you have already started, add on the personality traits, technical skills, and transferable job skills that you possess. Also, indicate why you believe you have these skills (e.g., which job or experience helped you develop the skill).

DEVELOPING CAREER OBJECTIVES

Each medical assistant has a reason for entering the healthcare field. This basic desire should influence decisions concerning his or her career choices. Because medical assisting is such a versatile profession, a medical assistant has numerous options after graduation.

Medical assistant students should take some time to think about what they want from their careers. While the medical assistant is attending school and subsequently completing the practicum, ideas may surface about the area of healthcare or a specific facility in which she or he most wants to work.

When developing career objectives, the medical assistant should start by asking several questions:

- What areas and skills did I enjoy in practicum?
- Where do I want to be in 5 years?
- Where do I want to be in 10 years?
- What additional skills do I need to get where I want to go?

Write down the questions and answers and go into specific detail. Set realistic goals and develop a plan as to how and when they will be reached. Remember, career objectives are reached over time. It is important to know where you want to be, so you can start down the right path to reach your goals. Keep your list of goals available and visible so you can revisit it frequently.

CRITICAL THINKING APPLICATION   22.3

For the following four questions, write down your answers and explain them. These answers will help you as you start the job search process.

- What areas and skills did I enjoy in practicum?
- Where do I want to be in 5 years?
- Where do I want to be in 10 years?
- What additional skills do I need to get where I want to go?

IDENTIFYING PERSONAL NEEDS

The next step in the process is to identify personal needs. What do you need in a job? Do you need a specific wage to meet your living expenses? What benefits do you need? What hours do you need to work? Some people need to consider day care and school hours for their children. How far are you willing to travel for a job? Do you have a reliable mode of transportation? Evaluating your personal needs will help you find a job that matches your requirements.

> **CRITICAL THINKING** APPLICATION   22.4
> What are your personal needs? Make a list identifying your needs that must be considered when seeking a new position.

FINDING A JOB

Finding employment and staying employed in healthcare are typically not difficult. Usually healthcare employment needs remain high, even in a poor economy. However, graduation from a medical assisting program does not guarantee employment. Completion of the program gives the medical assistant the job skills needed to work. A good attitude and positive outlook are essential for success in the job search. The medical assistant should always be open to new and better opportunities.

Some job seekers assume that potential employers will not interact with students until they have passed a credential examination. However, searching for a job before graduation is a smart idea. Some employers do not require credentialing examinations. Others may hire a medical assistant before the exam is taken. They may have an agreement that the medical assistant obtain the credential within a specified period of time. Many employers are interested in hiring new graduates. They consider new graduates "teachable." This means they can train and "mold" them into the employee they require. Employers recognize that new graduates have more current knowledge and skills.

> ### Certification Exams
>
> - Certified Medical Assistant (CMA) through the American Association of Medical Assistants (AAMA)
> - Registered Medical Assistant (RMA) through the American Medical Technologists (AMT)
> - Certified Clinical Medical Assistant (CCMA) through the National Healthcareer Association (NHA)
> - National Certified Medical Assistant (NCMA) through the National Center for Competency Testing (NCCT)
> - Clinical Medical Assistant Certification (CMAC) through the American Medical Certification Association (AMCA)

Two Best Job Search Methods

There are many ways to find employment. Networking and checking **job boards** are the best and most effective methods.

Networking

Networking is the exchange of information among others in your field. For medical assistant graduates or students searching for a

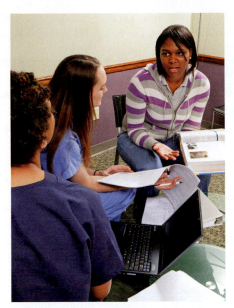

FIGURE 22.1 Stay in touch with classmates. They are excellent networking contacts and may be able to provide job leads.

job, networking involves meeting individuals in healthcare. It also involves sharing information on available opportunities. Through the medical assistant program, a student forms a network of friends and acquaintances (Fig. 22.1). Staying in contact with these people allows for networking opportunities. Email, LinkedIn, Facebook, Twitter, and other social networking advances make staying in touch very easy.

The practicum experience gives medical assistant students opportunities to network. During the practicum (externship), you will be working with many healthcare professionals. It is crucial that you look at the practicum as a continuous job interview. It is important to be professional, follow the guidelines, and strive to do your very best. It is not uncommon that, when staff members find a student who portrays the characteristics of a professional medical assistant, they are willing to help the student find a job.

> ### Strategies Medical Assistants Can Use in Practicum to Assist With Job Seeking
>
> During practicum, medical assistant students can:
> - Inquire about potential job openings, either through their mentor, supervisor, or the facility's human resource department.
> - Ask their mentors if they would be willing to provide a reference or a letter of recommendation.
> - Show their gratitude by formally thanking their mentors for the opportunity. In most cases, the practicum agencies provide assistance to help train the medical assistant student. It is important to send a thank-you note to the mentor, the supervisor, and to the department.
> - Provide the supervisor with a resume and cover letter.

Another networking technique is to join a medical assistant organization. The members who attend regular meetings often know about job leads in the area. Creating connections with currently employed medical assistants can be helpful in the job search process.

CRITICAL THINKING APPLICATION   22.5

Michelle, Krysia, and Zac know that networking is a great way to find employment. They make a list of people with whom they can share their resume or whom they can inform that they are now ready to seek employment as a medical assistant.

- Who among your relatives would be good prospects for networking?
- Who among your professional contacts would be good prospects for networking?

Job Boards

Job boards are websites where employers post job openings. There are two types of job boards:

- *Facility job boards*: Larger healthcare facilities post job openings on their websites. The employment website can use different tools that make the process easier for the job seeker and the employer. Some sites allow the job seeker to register for a specific type of job. The software will generate emails to job seekers when new jobs are posted. Some websites allow job seekers to complete online profiles or applications and upload a resume and cover letter. These tools are useful to both the job seeker and the facility.
- *Public job boards*: These job boards include jobs from a variety of employers. The job boards can be local, state, or national. Local job boards may be found through your school or your community's media (i.e., newspaper, television, radio) agencies. These websites target the local audience. They are usually cheaper for employers. Smaller healthcare organizations tend to advertise using these boards. The Department of Workforce Development in each state addresses unemployment. It provides a job board for job seekers. National job boards, such as Monster, Indeed, alliedhealthjobcafe.com, and glassdoor.com, provide job seekers the ability to search for openings across the country. Medical assistant jobs available in the federal government can be found at the website *http://www.usajobs.gov*.

Many positions for medical assistants use alternative job titles. Some agencies may use "technician" or "coordinator" for medical assistant jobs. It is important to research the local job titles that are used for medical assistants. If you do not know the local job title, try looking at the allied health positions. Look at a job posting. What are the educational requirements? Are the duties skills you have? Make a list of job titles related to medical assisting and search by those as you identify potential openings.

CRITICAL THINKING APPLICATION   22.6

Michelle, Krysia, and Zac make a list of possible job boards to review frequently for medical assistant postings. They know that sometimes the postings are only available for a short time, so they develop a schedule to review the sites.

- Make a list of five job boards you would like to check for potential jobs.
- What might be other titles that are used for medical assistants in your area?

Additional Job Search Methods

Besides using networking and checking job boards, the medical assistant can find job postings by other, more traditional methods. The school's placement office resources, newspaper ads (online and print), and employment agencies also can have medical assistant job postings.

School Career Placement Offices

Students usually have lifetime access to their school placement offices. Students and graduates should take advantage of the opportunities offered. Many schools offer resume building, job search classes, and interviewing assistance. School placement offices may also work with local employers to advertise their openings online to graduates. The school has a vested interest in helping you find employment. The placement office should be the first resource for the student's job search.

Newspaper Ads

Smaller healthcare facilities usually use newspaper ads to find potential employees. Many newspaper companies post their ads online. This allows more job seekers to view those positions.

Employment Agencies

Employment agencies hire staff to fill in at healthcare facilities. The employment agency is paid by the facility to staff different positions. Some employment agencies hire and pay the medical assistant. The medical assistants work in a healthcare facility as employment agency employees. After a period of time, if the medical assistant proves to be a good employee, the healthcare facility then hires that person. This allows the employment agency to do the hiring, firing, and managing of employees until the employees "prove themselves" to the healthcare facility.

Being Organized in Your Job Search

As you submit your resume and cover letter for various positions, it is important that you stay organized and track the jobs you applied for. You should also keep the original electronic files of your customized documents.

Create a handwritten or an electronic log of the jobs you apply for. Include the job title, number, and facility name. When you submit your resume and cover letter, update the log with the date of those activities. As you are notified about an interview, add the interview information (e.g., date, time, location, interview team members) to your log. Continually update the status of each job in the log.

It is important for you to save the customized documents for each job position. If you are called for an interview, it is important to bring copies of your customized resume and cover letter. The easiest method is to create a job-seeking folder on your computer. For each job you apply for, create a subfolder in the job-seeking folder. Save your customized resume and cover letter in the subfolder. Save any other documents related to that job in that subfolder, including the job posting. If you get called for an interview, print the customized resume and cover letter for your interview portfolio and for the interviewer(s). You may also want to print the job posting as a reference during the interview.

One of the most important things to remember with job searching is that it takes time, stamina, and persistence to find a job. Do not expect to get a job with the first resume and cover letter you send or with the first interview you have. By keeping good records, you will not apply for the same job twice or overlook job opportunities because you thought you had applied for them already.

DEVELOPING A RESUME

The purpose of a resume is to "market" yourself. You want an employer interested in you. You want your resume to be included in those selected for an interview. A resume summarizes your qualifications, education, and experience. Medical assistants must determine what to include in the resume. The resume should be developed before the cover letter is written. Strengths for the posted job must be identified and emphasized on all documents. These documents include the resume, cover letter, and application.

Resume Formats

There are three commonly used resume formats: chronologic, combination, and targeted resumes. The resume format used will depend on the medical assistant's situation.

A *chronologic resume* is the most popular format used. It is useful when people are seeking employment in the same field as their education or previous experience. The chronologic resume focuses on the person's employment history. Job duties for each position are bulleted out (Fig. 22.2). See Procedure 22.1 on p. 506 for the steps in creating a chronologic resume.

Michelle Marison

1234 Cedar Way, Mytown, OH 45458
Home phone: 715.555.1899
Cell phone: 715.555.1355
mmarison@elsevier.net

Education
Community College, Mytown, OH
Medical Assistant Diploma, 20XX
- GPA 3.6

Health Care Experience
Family Practice Associates, Mytown, OH
Medical Assistant Practicum, April 20XX to May 20XX (220 hours)
- Performed injections, electrocardiogram, wound care, phlebotomy, throat swabs, and waived tests.
- Obtained vital signs and measurements on children and adults.
- Utilized an electronic health record to document patients' histories, test results and treatments.
- Answered calls, checked-in patients, and updated patients' demographic and insurance information.

Mytown Hospital, Mytown, OH
Volunteer, January 20XX to May 20XX
- Provided hospital information to visitors.
- Maintained confidentiality of patients.
- Assisted with deliveries of mail and flowers to patients.
- Assisted nursing staff as needed.

Work Experience
Mytown Family Diner, Mytown, OH
Waitress, June 20XX to present
- Provide efficient, accurate, and timely service to customers.
- Prioritize duties to meet customer needs.
- Provide exceptional customer service.

Special Skills
Fluent in Spanish.
Keyboarding speed: 73 wpm
Proficient in word processing and spreadsheet software

Credentials
Certified Medical Assistant, American Association of Medical Assistants (expires May 20XX)
BLS for Healthcare Providers, American Heart Association (expires March 20XX)

FIGURE 22.2 Chronologic resume.

The *combination resume* is sometimes confused with a functional resume. A true functional resume showcases a person's **skill sets**. It does not include a work history. A combination resume is preferred over a functional resume. A combination resume:

- Lists a person's abilities and skill sets, as does the functional resume
- Includes the person's employment history, as does the chronologic resume (Fig. 22.3)

A combination resume may be used if a person is switching careers. Transferable skills related to the new position will be emphasized. It can also be used by applicants who have a gap in their work history. The focus is on the person's skills and ability, rather than the employment history.

The third type of resume is the *targeted resume*. This type of resume is customized to a unique job posting (Fig. 22.4). Targeted resumes:

- Detail key skills required for the position
- Indicate how the applicant has demonstrated those skills
- Take longer to create, but can be the most effective format

---

Zacarias Garcia
523 River Way, Mytown OH 45459

Cell phone: 715.555.5472
ZacGarcia@elsevier.net

Education
Community College, Mytown, OH
Medical Assistant Diploma, 20XX
- Medical Assistant Practicum at Mytown Orthopedic and Massage Center, Mytown, OH
  o Obtained and charted history and vital signs in electronic health record.
  o Assisted providers with tests and treatments.

Credentials
Certified Medical Assistant, American Association of Medical Assistants, expires May 20XX.
BLS for Healthcare Providers, American Heart Association, expires March 20XX.

Skills and Achievement
Strong communication skills
- Supervised 60 employees in a factory setting for over 3 years.
- Initiated procedures to improve communication between employees and management.
- Promoted in union to assist with negotiations with upper management.
- Fluent in Spanish.

Excellent problem-solving skills
- Problem-solved factory issues that delayed shipments to customers.
- Initiated solutions to expedite shipments and increased the profit margin of the company.

Excel in Teamwork
- Assisted team on assembly line, helping fill in when others were absent.
- Promoted to Team Lead within 6 months of hire.
- Received "Outstanding Employee" award in 20XX, 20XX, and 20XX.

Work Experience
Mytown Doors, Mytown, OH
Supervisor, (March 20XX – January 20XX)
Team Lead – Door Assembly, (January 20XX – March 20XX)
Door Assembler, (August 20XX – January 20XX)

FIGURE 22.3 Combination resume.

Krysia Debski
111 Mall Drive • Mytown, OH 45457
Cell phone: 715.555.6956 • Email: KDebski@elsevier.net

Education
Community College, Mytown, OH
A.S. in Medical Assisting, 20XX
- Medical Assistant Practicum at Mytown Associates, Mytown, OH
  o Obtained and charted patients' histories and vital signs in the electronic health record.
  o Assisted providers with tests and treatments in a busy internal medicine practice.
  o Performed injections, throat swabs, and phlebotomy.

Skills
ORGANIZATION SKILLS
- Organized supplies to expedited restocking procedures and decrease financial loss .
- Exceptional organizational and filing skills utilized to maintain purchase and delivery records from over 300 suppliers.
- Assisted with the install and training for inventory tracking software for warehouse.

TEAMWORK
- Refined teamwork skills with over ten years in the U.S. Marines.
- Taught teambuilding courses.
- Promoted teamwork among staff by incorporating incentives.

COMMUNICATION SKILLS
- Assertive when working with suppliers to meet deadlines.
- Utilized excellent listening skills to identify needs of various teams that impact the warehouse.
- Composed frequent emails and letters for supervisors.
- Fluent in Spanish and Polish

Credentials
Certified Medical Assistant, American Association of Medical Assistants, (expires May 20XX)

BLS for Healthcare Providers, American Heart Association (expires March 20XX)

Work Experience
United States Marines
Supply Administration and Operations Specialist (May 20XX – September 20XX)
Warehouse Clerk (August 20XX – May 20XX)

FIGURE 22.4 Targeted resume customized for a medical assistant posting. The medical assistant should possess strong organizational skills, experience with teamwork, and exceptional communication skills. The posting indicated it required a person with a Certified Medical Assistant (CMA) credential and a current Basic Life Support (BLS) certification.

Resume Content

Between the resume formats, there are similarities and differences in the information presented. The following discussion will describe the content found in the different sections of a resume. See Procedure 22.1 on p. 506 for the steps in creating a chronologic resume.

Header

The person's contact information is found in the header of the document. This includes the person's name, mailing address, professional email address, phone number, and personal websites (e.g., LinkedIn).

This information or a variation of the information should appear on each sheet if the resume is more than one page long.

Professional email addresses may include your first and last name or first initial and last name. Email addresses that include expressions such as "one_hot_chick" or "party_dude" are not professional and are not used on resumes. An old email format may indicate that you are not knowledgeable about the current technology. If you do not have a professional email address or have an old email address, free email sites are available (e.g., gmail.com). Like professional emails, personal websites should be professional and contain a professional image of you.

Education

The education section includes information on the schooling that the person has received after high school. The information should appear in **reverse chronologic order**. Information should include:

- *If a diploma was obtained:* List the school's name, city, and state, the degree, and the year it was obtained.
- *If no degree was obtained:* Summarize the coursework completed. List the school's name, city, and state, and the years of the coursework.
- *Practicum (externship) information:* Include the location, dates, and duties (optional; some will include this information in the Healthcare Experience section, discussed later in the chapter).
- *Academic recognition:* Include academic awards, scholarships, and overall GPA if greater than 3.0.

The location of the education section can differ based on the person's situation. For new graduates, the education section should appear toward the top of the resume. If the degree is not related to the position or the degree is older, the education section would come toward the end of the resume. Moving education to the end allows the person's achievements and work history to be emphasized.

Work Experience

This section can be titled several different ways. If a person is strictly including job information, then "Work Experience" or "Job Experience" can be used. Using the word "job" or "work" implies the person got paid for the position. If a person wants to include volunteer positions with job positions, then the section should be titled "Related Experience" or "Other Experience." "Related" means it relates to the position the person is applying for. If the section contains unrelated experience, then use "Other Experience." For those with military experience, it is recommended to add a special section to discuss the military experience.

If you have prior healthcare experience, you may want to separate your volunteer and job experiences into two sections. First, use "Healthcare Experiences." Include any healthcare jobs and volunteer positions you have had. Some students may opt to include their practicum in this section. Second, use a topic header, such as "Other Experience" or "Additional Experience." Include all of your non-healthcare jobs and volunteer positions. Do not repeat information you included in prior sections.

The information in this section should be presented in reverse chronologic order. All three resumes discussed require the following elements for each position:

- Name of the facility
- City and state of the facility
- Title of position or positions held at that facility
- Dates in that position (include start date [month and date] and end date [month and date]; for a current position, include the start date and use "to present")

For those in the workforce for 10 years or longer, employers want to see 10 years of employment information. For those working at the same facility for over 10 years, it is important to list changes and advancements in the position over the duration of employment. Any gaps in the employment history should be explained to the potential employer during the interview or discussed in the cover letter.

For the chronologic resume, the most relevant job duties need to be listed. For instance, if you worked as a housekeeper in a motel, making beds is not related to medical assisting. Providing customer service would be relevant.

The statements regarding the duties should be bulleted and begin with an active verb. For present positions, use active verbs in the present tense (e.g., administer, provide). For past positions, use active verbs in the past tense (e.g., administered, provided) (Fig. 22.5).

The position of the work experience section is dependent on the resume format. Chronologic resumes typically have work experience near the top, whereas combination and targeted resumes list it toward the end of the resume.

Summary and Skills

A "Summary" section appears at the top in the targeted resume. This section summarizes why the applicant is the best candidate for the job. It is helpful to use key words from the job posting when describing skills one possesses. This helps to make the connection of why the person is the best candidate for the job.

A "Skills" or "Skills and Achievements" section is found in combination resumes. It showcases specific transferable skills that relate to the new position. These transferable skills may have been obtained in the military, by a stay-at-home parent, or by a person switching careers.

A "Special Skills" section is found in a chronologic resume. Information that may appear in this section includes:

- Fluency in another language (e.g., fluent in Spanish)
- Keyboarding speed (e.g., keyboarding speed: 85 wpm)
- Computer skills and experiences (e.g., used electronic health records during practicum)

Certifications

Many employers may require specific certifications or credentials for a job position. It is important to include those that relate to the job position. When listing the information, include these items:

- Title of the certification or license
- Awarding agency
- Expiration date

An example for all resume formats would be: "BLS for Healthcare Providers, American Heart Association, expires 10/2022."

Appearance of the Resume

As you create your resume, keep in mind the eye appeal or interest the resume will create for the reader. It is recommended to bold-face only important information. A job title should be bold, whereas the facility should not be bold. Simple bullets help organize information and provide a neat appearance to the resume. Changing the font size in certain areas can emphasize more important elements and help keep content on one page.

Spacing is crucial to the appearance of a resume. A lot of spacing creates too much "white space." This can give the reader a negative impression of the resume. Too little spacing creates a busy, text-heavy

Administered	Copied	Performed
Advocated	Developed	Posted
Aided	Distributed	Prepared
Answered	Documented	Processed
Arranged	Established	Provided
Assigned	Filed	Purchased
Assisted	Guided	Reconciled
Balanced	Helped	Restocked
Calculated	Instructed	Reviewed
Cared	Listened	Scanned
Coded	Logged	Scheduled
Collected	Mailed	Sorted
Compiled	Maintained	Supported
Composed	Monitored	Taught
Computed	Operated	Trained
Contacted	Ordered	Wrote
Coordinated	Organized	

FIGURE 22.5 Action verbs in the past tense.

resume that is difficult to read. Make sure to use the same spacing between the sections. Use less spacing, but be consistent between subsections (e.g., different employment positions).

It is important to have resume paper available. Even if you submit your resume online, you should bring copies of your resume on resume paper to the interview. Use a light solid-colored resume paper (e.g., cream, light gray). The light colors will duplicate better than a pattern or dark-colored paper.

Before submitting your resume, have another person review it. Obtain the person's initial impression of the resume's appearance. Is there too much white space? Does the resume look too wordy? Does it look too plain? Does it look too busy? Then have the person read the content in the resume and provide you with feedback. Use the feedback to revise your resume.

Tips for creating a resume include:

- Do not add clipart or other pictures.
- Do not include personal information (e.g., married, children, and religious affiliation).
- Do not lie or exaggerate the truth.
- Do not add unrelated content, such as hobbies and interests.
- Do not include "References available upon request" or a similar statement, because it is understood references will be requested and required.
- Do not use personal pronouns, such as "I."
- Do not repeat content.
- Do not include any pay/salary information.
- Always keep the resume to one page, unless you have been in the workforce for multiple years. Then use an additional page, but your content must fill both pages.
- Be concise and clear.
- Use key terms found in the job posting or job description in your resume.
- Put important details first.
- Perform a grammar and spelling check on your resume.
- Limit abbreviations to only the abbreviations used in the job posting (e.g., BLS for basic life support, CPR for cardiopulmonary resuscitation).

CRITICAL THINKING APPLICATION   **22.8**

Zac, Michelle, and Krysia drafted their resumes. They read each other's and provided feedback. Who else might they give their resumes to for proofreading and feedback?

- Think of your circle of family and friends. List three people who might be great candidates to provide feedback on your resume.

DEVELOPING A COVER LETTER

A cover letter must always accompany the resume (Fig. 22.6). The cover letter is a critical tool that gains the reader's attention. The goal is to have the cover letter create enough interest that the reader wants to look at the resume. The cover letter gives the reader more information on the applicant's personality than the factual resume. Cover letters allow applicants to express themselves.

Strategies When Writing a Cover Letter

To create a professional cover letter, it is important to follow these strategies:

- *Match the appearance of the cover letter and resume*
  - Headers on both documents should be identical.
  - Font type and margins should be identical.
  - If using paper, use the same paper for both documents.
- *Address the inside address and the salutation (greeting) to a specific person*
  - Address the letter to the person who is hiring the new employee. This shows that you took time to find out the details.
  - Use the person's name and job title in the inside address.
  - Use a formal salutation (e.g., *Dear Mr. Jones:*).
  - Call the healthcare facility or use online resources, such as LinkedIn, to find out the information.
- *Start the body of your cover letter off with a bang!*
  - In the first paragraph: Show enthusiasm as you summarize why you believe you are the best candidate for the job. Also include the job title and the number for easy reference for the reader.
  - For example: "Having a strong customer service background and a degree in medical assisting, I am confident that I can fulfill your expectations for the family practice medical assistant position (#123)."
- *Sell yourself to the reader*
  - In the second paragraph: Provide a snapshot of your experiences.
  - Weave in the key "requirement" words from the job posting. Address the requirements first, followed by the lesser requirements or "would like" qualities. Some experts recommend using bold font for these key words.
  - You can bullet your qualifications and abilities but limit the bullets to four or five points.
  - Be concise, yet clear. Do not repeat the resume. You want the reader to move onto the resume for the details.
- *Reaffirm that you are an excellent match for the job*
  - In the final paragraph: Use such phrases as "I believe I have the qualities you require" or "I am confident I will meet your expectations."
  - If you include an action you will take (e.g., "I will call the week of…"), do not be overly aggressive in your tone.
  - Finish the paragraph by expressing your interest in and enthusiasm for an interview (e.g., "I am very excited about this opportunity and would enjoy meeting with you to explore how my qualifications could meet your needs.").
- *Be professional*
  - Express your thanks to the reader for his or her consideration.

Proofreading the Cover Letter

After writing the cover letter, review it for inaccuracies. Use the spell-check tool in your word processing software to help identify errors. Also **proofread** your letter. Make sure your spelling, punctuation, grammar, and sentence structure are correct. Common cover letter weaknesses include:

Michelle Marison

1234 Cedar Way, Mytown, OH 45458
Home phone: 715.555.1899
Cell phone: 715.555.1355
mmarison@elsevier.net

May 15, 20XX

Ms. Alex Brown
Medical Assistant Supervisor
Mytown Medical Clinic
555 Clover Drive
Mytown OH 45457

Dear Ms. Brown:

I was excited to see the posting on the Mytown Telegram job board for the medical assistant position (#1243) and would like to be considered for that position. I am graduating from Community College on May 30, 20XX and will be taking my AAMA CMA exam June 2, 20XX.

With two years of customer service experience and five months of being a hospital volunteer, I have learned the importance of prioritizing, teamwork, and communication. During my medical assistant practicum, I have utilized these skills along with my attention to detail and my medical assistant knowledge, as I assist providers with procedures and treatments. The knowledge and skills I am learning in practicum combined with the skills I have developed as a waitress and volunteer will help me provide the best care to my future patients.

I have heard excellent things about Mytown Medical Clinic and would love to be a part of the staff of such a caring agency. I am available for interviews whenever it is convenient for you. I am available either by phone or email.

Thank you so much for considering me for this position.

Sincerely,

Michelle Marison

Enclosure: 1

FIGURE 22.6 Basic cover letter.

- Starting a majority of sentences with "I"
- Introducing yourself in the first sentence (for instance, "*Hi, I am Sally Green.*")
- Spelling, grammar, punctuation, and sentence structure errors
- Missing parts of the letter (e.g., date, inside address)
- Not including the position title and posting number
- Too busy (overuse of font styles), too wordy, or too much white space
- Inappropriate spacing that leads to the body of the letter being too high or too low on the page. Remember, the body should be centered vertically on the page.
- Creating a generic letter that does not contain the key requirement words from the job posting. (Many larger employers use software to screen letters and resumes for key words. Those with key words are reviewed more closely. Those that lack the key words are discarded.)

Create an error-free cover letter. It must have a professional tone and appearance. Also, have a few people proofread your letter. Use their advice as you make your changes. Refer to Chapter 9 if you need assistance with composing a business letter. Procedure 22.2 on p. 507 will help guide you in writing a professional cover letter.

COMPLETING ONLINE PROFILES AND JOB APPLICATIONS

Many healthcare agencies use the internet during the employment process. The online human resource software may require applicants to create a profile before applying for open positions. The online profile collects the information that previously was collected by paper applications.

Online profiles have many advantages over paper applications for both the employer and the applicant. An applicant completes the profile once and updates the information as needed. Typically, the agencies keep the profiles active for years. Employers can:

- Track the activities of applicants
- Easily read a person's information
- Advertise new postings to potential applicants whose profiles meet certain requirements

If a healthcare facility does not use online profiles, then the applicant will need to complete a job application (Fig. 22.7). Some organizations require the application to be submitted with the cover letter and resume. Others have applicants arriving for interviews complete the application. If you need to complete an application before an interview, come prepared with your information. Arrive at least 20 minutes before the interview so you can complete the application. See Procedure 22.3 on p. 507 for the steps in completing a job application.

Regardless of whether you need to complete a profile or an application, you will need to provide the same information. Even if you have the information on your resume, you still need to add it to the application or profile. Having the reference information in a word-processed document will save you time. If you are providing the information online, the copy and paste feature will speed up completion time. Table 22.1 contains the information you should include in the word-processed document.

When filling out the application or profile, answer the questions carefully. When addressing your current and past employment, keep these points in mind:

- When giving your availability date, make sure you know how long you have to give notice at your current position. Most employers have a 2-week notice policy. If you are hired, your new employer will understand that you need to give a 2-week notice.
- When giving the reason you left prior positions, make sure to write the reason using a positive tone. For instance, "Obtained a

---

APPLICATION FOR EMPLOYMENT

Date:_____

Name: (First, Middle Initial, Last)_____

Social Security No.:_____   Phone: _____

Address:_____

EDUCATION

	Name, City, State	Graduation Date	Degree Obtained
High School:			
College:			
Other:			

LICENSURE/CERTIFICATION/REGISTRATION

Type of Certification, License or Registration	Agency/State	Registration Name

List any special skills or qualifications which you possess and feel are relevant to health care and the position for which you are applying._____

_____

EMPLOYMENT HISTORY

May we contact and communicate with your present employer? ☐ Yes ☐ No

Employer:	Phone:
Address:	Supervisor:
Employed	Hourly Pay:
Position title and responsibilities:	
Reason for leaving:	

FIGURE 22.7 Application for employment.

TABLE 22.1 Information Required for Online Profiles and Applications

INFORMATION	DETAILS NEEDED
Education	Institution's name and address; dates and titles of coursework or diploma
Past and present jobs	Facility name and address; supervisors' names, titles, and contact information; job title, duties, start and end salary, start and end dates; and reason for leaving
Certifications and credentials	Certifying agency's name and address; certification/credential; expiration date (a copy of your certification and BLS card may be required by the employer)
References	Name, title, facility, address, phone number, and email address

Typical Items Found in Career Portfolios

Using a three-ring binder with plastic sheet protectors and divider tabs, include the following:

- Table of contents at the beginning with identified tabbed sections
- Cover letter and resume (a copy of what was sent to that facility)
- References
- Certifications (e.g., copy of BLS card, copy of credentials [e.g., CMA or RMA card])
- Education-related documents
  - Copies of letters of recommendation
  - Copies of transcripts, awards, and honors
  - A list of the courses successfully completed with a short description of each course (optional, but consider if you are moving to another location where your institution may not be known)
  - Copies of practicum evaluation forms and skill document form
  - Scholarships awarded
  - Copies/details of school-related activities (e.g., officer in student medical assistant group, athlete, volunteer activities)
- Prior employment documents
  - Copies of past employment evaluations
  - Copies of letters of recommendations
- Documentation showing the student balancing work and education (this can help exhibit a strong work ethic, organizational skills, and prioritizing skills)
- Examples of work or summaries of projects that can provide evidence of abilities and skills
- Criminal background documentation, blood titers, vaccination history, and current tuberculosis (TB) skin or blood tests results (optional)

position that would advance my skill set" or "Resigned to focus on my education" sounds more professional than "I hated the job."

If you have a unique situation (e.g., sick parent, new baby), ask the advice of your school's placement counselor if you are unsure what to say in these sections. Most employers require an explanation for time not employed.

As you complete the online profile or paper application, you will be required to read important legal statements and add your signature (or electronic signature). This is a legal document. It should be filled out accurately and completely.

CREATING A CAREER PORTFOLIO

Many job seekers claim to have the skill sets required by the potential employer. Very few actually show the employer evidence of those qualifications. A career portfolio is a fantastic tool to show that you have the skills required for the job.

The portfolio should be developed along with the cover letter and resume. Creating a different portfolio for each type of job applied for is a great strategy. A receptionist portfolio would look different from a phlebotomy portfolio. There will be similarities in the information for all portfolios, but different "evidence" of skills will be in each. The medical assistant should be prepared to leave the portfolio with the interviewer, so no originals should be included.

The documents placed in the career portfolio binder should be positive and helpful to you in your mission of getting a job. You may want to consider adding the following:

- *A transcript*: Some experts state that a B average GPA or better is considered appropriate to add to a resume for an entry level position. Thus, you may want to add your transcript to the portfolio if you have a B average GPA or higher. Some employers require a higher GPA, and in these situations, only include your transcript if you meet their GPA requirement.

- *Performance evaluations*: Include positive employment or school-related performance evaluations.
- *Projects*: Include projects that provide evidence of personal characteristics or specific skills mastered.

Be creative as you prepare your portfolio, keeping the appearance professional and neat.

Just before an interview, the medical assistant should customize the portfolio for that employer (see Procedure 22.4, p. 508). A copy of the cover letter and resume sent to the employer should be in the portfolio. A list of references should also be included. All three of these documents should be printed on the same type of resume paper. The medical assistant should do additional customization of the portfolio. The examples of work or the summary of projects should reflect the skills required and key words in the job posting.

JOB INTERVIEW

Interviewers can consist of one or two people or a panel of employees. The job seeker may interview with a human resource employee, the office manager, the provider, and/or potential peers. The job seeker may have a number of interviews before the actual decision is made.

For many people, the interview is a stressful part of the job search. Some individuals dread job interviews and become extremely nervous at the prospect of interviewing. Others are very comfortable and consider the interview to be as much for their own purposes as for the employer's. The more interviews people do, the more comfortable they become with each subsequent interview.

We will examine the four phases of an interview. These include preparation for the interview, the interview itself, the follow-up, and the negotiation.

Preparation for the Interview

When preparing for an interview, the job seeker needs to:
- Research the facility
- Practice answering potential questions
- Select interview attire
- Prepare for the day of the interview

We will discuss each of these in depth. The better prepared the job candidate is, the more comfortable he or she will be during the interview.

Research the Healthcare Facility

The job seeker should learn everything possible about the employer. The organization's website is an excellent source of information. A job seeker should research the following topics:
- Mission and value statements
- Size of the organization
- Size of the department with the open position
- Names and types of providers in the department

It is important to ask questions at the interview. Possible questions can relate to your research on the facility:
- "I see that there are two providers in this department. Would I be working with both of them?"
- "There are three locations for your clinic on your website; how will I interact with the other locations?"
- "Given the size of your organization, is there an opportunity to interact with the other departments?"

Questions that relate to your research show the interviewer you are truly interested in the position. They also show that you prepared for the interview.

Practice Answers to Questions

Organizations need to follow federal and state hiring laws. The agencies cannot discriminate. During the interview phase, most organizations use a preset list of questions. All candidates are asked the same questions. You will not know the exact questions that will be asked. It is important to practice answering some standard interview questions (Fig. 22.8). This practice will help you prepare for the interview and also appear more confident during the actual interview.

When practicing your answers to standard interview questions, start by writing down your answer. Review your answer. Does it answer the question? What perception might you be giving to the interviewers by your answer? Is it the perception you want to be giving? How might you strengthen your answer? Is it really short or does it ramble on? Be clear and concise. Expand on the topic, but do not get too wordy. Provide examples to support what you say. When you have refined your answers, practice your answers before the interview.

Decide on Your Interview Attire

Prior to the interview, it is important to select an interview outfit. Be conservative with wardrobe choices. For example:
- Females: Business suit; skirt or dress pants and blouse. Skirt or dress should be of modest length (i.e., at the knee or longer). Blouse should not be sheer or show cleavage.
- Males: Business suit; dress pants and shirt. Conservative tie.

Be sure clothing is clean, wrinkle free, and well fitting, and that shoes are clean and shined. For a medical assistant, scrubs may be acceptable for an interview. (It is appropriate to ask the person arranging the interview if scrubs can be worn.) Take care in washing and pressing your scrubs, and use a lint roller on them, before wearing them on an interview.

Pay particular attention to other aspects of appearance. Make sure your hair is clean and styled attractively, your teeth are clean, and your breath is fresh. Nails should be clean and well-groomed. Nails should not be excessively long or painted in highly visible colors. Do not wear perfumes or colognes. Do not wear excessive jewelry or makeup. Do not chew gum during the interview. Do not smoke in your interview attire. Remember the appearance guidelines that applied to the practicum. Some employers will react negatively to tattoos, piercings, extravagant hairstyles, unnatural hair colors, or other excessive wardrobe choices. Always dress appropriately and conservatively for an interview. Once hired, the new employee may be allowed to wear more diverse styles that comply with the employee handbook or procedures manual.

Prepare for the Interview Day

Do a test run before the day of the interview to identify the travel time. Always arrive 15 minutes early for the interview. Never take anyone along on a job interview, especially children. Expect to be a little nervous. Any interview can be a stressful situation. If necessary, practice stress-relieving strategies (e.g., deep breathing) that you can use before the interview. The better prepared a person is, the more successful the interview will be.

You should also prepare what you need to bring for the interview. These items include:
- An interview portfolio
- A copy of your cover letter and resume for each interviewer
- A notepad and pen to take notes
- A list of references on resume paper
- A list of questions for the interviewer

If you will be completing an application, bring the information discussed in the prior section regarding completing online profiles and applications.

During the Interview

During the interview it is important to be professional. Your professionalism may be tested if the interviewer asks illegal questions. We will discuss how to answer interview questions. We will also discuss professionalism during the different types of interviews.

Answering Interview Questions

It is important to give the interviewers a good impression of you. As discussed in a prior section, it is important to practice answering questions before the interview. This will help you to prepare and to feel more confident during the interview.

1. Tell me about yourself.	16. What do you know about this facility and our competitors?
2. Why do you want to work for this company?	17. What has been your most rewarding experience at work?
3. Why should I hire you?	18. What was your single most important accomplishment for the company on your last job?
4. How do you work under pressure?	19. What was the toughest problem you have ever solved and how did you do it?
5. How do you handle criticism?	20. How do you see yourself fitting in with our company?
6. What do you think your co-workers think about you?	21. What skills did you learn on your last job that can be used here?
7. Describe your last supervisor.	22. What immediate contribution could you make if you came to work for us today?
8. What would you like to change about yourself?	23. Do you prefer working with others or by yourself?
9. What is your best asset?	24. Can you take instructions or criticism without being upset?
10. What adjectives would you use to describe yourself?	25. What job in this company would you choose if you could?
11. How would you describe the perfect job?	26. What have you done that shows initiative and willingness to work?
12. Why did you leave your last job?	27. What will previous supervisors say about you?
13. Why did you choose this type of profession?	28. Why would you be successful in this job?
14. What are your strongest and weakest personal qualities?	29. Can you explain the gap in your employment history?
15. What personal characteristics are necessary for success in your chosen field?	30. Are you a member of any professional organizations?

FIGURE 22.8 Top 30 interview questions.

Tips for All Interviews

- For simple, straightforward questions, do not pause before you answer. Any pause would be hinting at insincerity.
- For complex questions, pause for a few seconds as you think about your answer. Write down some key words to help you focus and answer the question.
- Refrain from saying "um."
- Do not volunteer any negative information.
- Be honest and do not exaggerate experiences or lengths of employment.
- Never speak negatively about former employers.

- Write down the names of the interviewers to help you as you follow up after the interview.
- Avoid a "know-it-all" attitude, which indicates overconfidence and reluctance to take direction.
- Express a sincere interest in the employer and his or her projects, rather than in what the employer can do for the employee.
- Ask intelligent questions at the end of the interview if given the opportunity. Your first question should never be, "How much will I be paid?" Money, although important, cannot appear to be your primary concern.

Many times, the interview will start with a question such as, "Tell me about yourself." The temptation is to answer the question focusing on your personal life. For example, "I'm a recent graduate, and I am married and have two children." The answer to this question should not reflect information about personal issues. Answer instead with, "I am a recent graduate and completed a 6-week practicum in a family practice." Focus all answers on your career, your strengths and attributes, and what skills you have to bring to the healthcare setting. Be able to prove the skills you claim. You can provide examples either by relating professional situations you have handled well, or by using your interview portfolio. Before the interview ends, the medical assistant should ask when a decision will be made and if it would be acceptable to call to follow up (see Procedure 22.5, p. 509).

Illegal Interview Questions

The interviewer should not ask any illegal questions. Table 22.2 lists such topics and potential illegal questions. Employers may either intentionally or accidentally ask illegal questions. The way that the medical assistant answers the questions can influence the employer's hiring decision. Here are some points to consider:

- If the medical assistant is openly offended: Employers may negatively conclude that the applicant will be offended by abrasive comments from patients.
- If the illegal question is answered: Discrimination may occur in the hiring process. The employer may use the information to weed out the medical assistant as a candidate.

The best approach is to politely address the question. Either answer the question or redirect the interviewer back to the job requirements. For example, an interviewer asks if the candidate plans to put his or her children in day care. This may be a way of determining the age of the dependent children. It could also provide information on the likelihood of absenteeism because of the children's illnesses. The medical assistant could answer, "I will be able to meet the work schedule and the responsibilities that this job requires."

Some questions that might normally be considered illegal, such as, "What organizations are you a member of?" might be job related. The employer may be interested in knowing if the medical assistant is a member of various professional organizations, such as the AAMA or the AMT.

CRITICAL THINKING APPLICATION   **22.9**

Krysia is enjoying a good interview when the interviewer, a male supervisor, asks her if she is married. When Krysia replies that she is not, he asks if she has a steady boyfriend.

- What might the supervisor's motive be with this line of questioning?
- How should Krysia respond?
- Are these questions inappropriate or do they serve a purpose?

Phone Interview

Phone interviews are usually done by the supervisor or the human resource representative. A phone interview may be done to:

- Screen applicants and narrow the candidate pool
- Provide additional information (e.g., benefits, job description) and verify the applicant wants an interview
- Replace a face-to-face interview, especially if the candidate is from out of town

It is important to treat a phone interview as a regular interview. Make sure to thank the interviewer at the end of the call.

Tips for Phone Interviews

- Prepare for the interview just as you would for a face-to-face interview.
- Take the call in a quiet environment. Make sure no dogs or children are in the room. Be alone in the room.
- Pay attention to the caller. Do not use other electronic devices or use the bathroom during the call.
- Have a copy of your resume and cover letter.
- Have your list of questions.
- Have a glass of water available should you need it.

TABLE 22.2	Illegal Versus Legal Interview Questions	
TOPIC	**EXAMPLES OF ILLEGAL QUESTIONS**	**EXAMPLES OF LEGAL QUESTIONS**
Birthplace, ancestry, or national origin	When did you move to the United States?	Are you eligible to work in this state?
Marital status, children, or pregnancy	Who will look after your child when he or she is born?	Are you able to work an 8 a.m. to 5 p.m. schedule?
Physical disability, health or medical history	What medications are you on?	Can you perform the essential job functions of a medical assistant with or without reasonable accommodation?
Religion or religious days observed	Where do you attend church services?	Can you work on weekends?
Age, race, ethnicity, gender, or color	How old are you?	Are you 18 or older? (or whatever the minimum age is for the facility)
Criminal record	Have you ever been arrested?	Have you ever been convicted of a crime?

Face-to-Face Interview

When you meet the interviewers, greet each person and shake hands. A firm handshake is recommended. Ensure each person has a copy of your resume and cover letter before the interview begins.

During the actual interview, maintain good eye contact. Many supervisors refuse to hire people who seem uncomfortable looking them directly in the eyes. Never take control of the interview. Allow the supervisor or panel members to ask questions at their own pace. Do not fidget in the chair or display any nervous habits (e.g., tapping your pen) (see Procedure 22.5).

Video Interview

A third interview possibility is a video interview using technology such as Skype. As with a phone interview, a video interview works well when the candidate is from out of town. There is a certain amount of technology needed for a video interview. Your school's placement office may be able to help you with that. The organization may have contacts for you to arrange your end of the interview. The benefit of a video interview over a phone interview is that the interviewers can actually see the interviewee. This allows the interviewers to assess the body language and the verbal message being presented. You should dress as you would for a face-to-face interview. You should have the same materials ready to access during the interview process. As with the face-to-face interview, you need to refrain from nervous habits.

Follow-Up After the Interview

Follow-up is critical after an interview. Always send a thank-you note, letter, or email to the person who conducted the interview (see Procedure 22.6, p. 509). It can be challenging to figure out what to send to the interviewer.

- *Send an email if:* the decision is going to be made quickly. Send an email later the day of the interview.
- *Send a written thank-you note or a letter if:* the facility is more conservative and formal. Also, it can be sent if the decision is going to be made in a week or two. Send the thank-you note within 24 hours of the interview.

Many employers see the thank-you as an expression of gratitude and professionalism. Even if you don't see yourself in that position, it is still important to send a thank you. This may be their last perception of you, and it may help you in the future at that facility.

Typically, at the end of the interview, there will be a discussion of how quickly the decision will be made. Many agencies using online hiring software will indicate the status of the job on the posting. Candidates not selected for the position usually receive an email or letter.

After the initial interviews are completed with all the candidates, several things can occur. With some employers, the list of interviewed candidates will be narrowed. The top two or three may be asked to come back for a second interview with additional team members (e.g., providers, medical assistants). With other employers, the top candidate is selected and references are checked. These processes take time, and the deadline may be extended if vacations or out-of-office times occur.

If the interviewer indicates a decision would be made in 2 weeks, wait to hear from the facility. Give a few days after the deadline before you follow up. At that time you can call and ask the status of the job. Remember, following up prior to the deadline may not be in your best interest. The employer may perceive that you do not follow directions if you make extra phone calls. If you receive a job offer from another facility but are waiting for a decision on your favorite position, it is appropriate to contact the interviewer. Explain that you were offered another position and wondered about the status of this position. Many employers will let you know if you are in the running for the position.

Never place all your hope in one job. Make sure to continue to search and interview until an offer is made and accepted. In addition, always be on the lookout for the next job opportunity.

Negotiation

The negotiation stage of job acceptance can be as stressful as the actual interviews. The salary and benefits must be considered when determining whether to accept a position or not. When a job offer is made, there should also be a discussion of the other benefits. If the salary offered is a bit lower than expected, but the employee's share of the health insurance premium is less than expected, the salary offer becomes more attractive. Medical assistants should know the lowest salary/benefit combination they can afford. They should ask for a little more than that figure.

Bracket salary requests are often helpful in this. Instead of asking for $13 per hour, ask for a salary in the "mid to high twenties." Let the employer mention a figure or a range of salary first. Usually the person who mentions a salary range first has the disadvantage. For example, if the medical assistant requests $13 per hour, but the facility was willing to pay $16 per hour, the medical assistant probably will get $13.

Many organizations have a starting pay level for new medical assistants. If you hope to get a higher pay level, you may need to:

- Obtain a national medical assistant credential (e.g., CMA [AAMA] or RMA)
- Show an advanced skills level acquired from previous work experience in healthcare. Having a well-designed interview portfolio will allow you to show the interviewer all that you have accomplished.

Never say "no" to a job offer on the spot. Request at least 24 hours to consider the offer. Before accepting or rejecting a job offer, consider whether the position carries any authority, the benefits, the hours, the distance from home, and the potential for advancement. People accept jobs for reasons other than the salary; remember the value of experience.

CRITICAL THINKING APPLICATION   **22.10**

Michelle has been on several interviews and likes the prospect of working for three different physicians. If an offer is made at each office, how can Michelle decide which to accept? What will help Michelle make this decision?

IMPROVING YOUR OPPORTUNITIES

We will examine ways to improve your opportunities for finding a job.

Finding Job Postings

Some students and graduates may not find job postings. This can be stressful, but it is important not to give up. Those who are not having success with the job search may want to re-evaluate their search methods. Consider these questions:

- *Am I looking for a very selective opportunity?* For instance, are you looking for a dermatology medical assistant position in a specific facility? Those positions may be very limited. Try to broaden your search to other possible opportunities.
- *Am I looking for the correct job title?* Remember, employers may use a wide range of titles for a medical assistant.
- *Am I looking at all agencies that potentially could hire a person with my skill sets?* Depending on your area, medical assistants can be in many agencies besides a medical clinic, including a nursing home, hospital, school, assisted-living facility, and insurance company.
- *Can I increase the geographical search area for employment opportunities?* Can I relocate to an area with greater employment opportunities?
- *Where can I network to increase my awareness of job openings?*
- *What job boards are being used by local employers?*

Increasing Interview Opportunities

For people who apply for jobs but never get calls for interviews, it is important to re-evaluate their information given to employers. Consider these questions:

- *Is your cover letter, resume, online profile, or application negatively affecting the job search?* It may be important to get another opinion on the content and presentation. Often the school career placement officer will provide improvement tips.
- *Do you have spelling and grammar errors in your information?* Some employers may perceive that details are not important to you, and so they may not be interested in hiring you.
- *Do your cover letter and resume need to be reformatted or revised?* Applicants need their letter and resume to stand out from the crowd. People get very creative in how they make this occur.
- *Are your cover letter and resume customized to the job posting?* Do your documents reflect the key words in the posting? Or do your documents look "generic"? With generic-looking documents, employers perceive that the person is not into details and wasn't interested enough to spend the time to customize the documents.
- *Are you following the directions in the job posting?* For instance, an employer may want a handwritten cover letter to be included. Sometimes the employer provides a mailing address and states that no calls or visits will be allowed. If applicants do not follow the directions, they may not be considered for the job.
- *Are you providing a professional image with your email address and on social media sites, such as Facebook?* Graduates struggling to find positions may want to review their social media sites. Consider tighter security settings to limit outside viewers. You may want to remove any questionable content and pictures.

Increasing Job Offers

If you are getting interviews but no job offers, re-evaluate your interview strategies. Again, the school's career placement office may have interview assistance. **Mock** interviews can help you refine your interview skills and behavior.

The following is a ranked list of reasons interviewers do not hire job candidates, as expressed by surveyed career consultants and reported on the website *http://careers.workoplis.com*:

- Not sufficiently differentiating themselves from others
- Failure to successfully transfer past experience to the current job opportunity
- Not showing enough interest and excitement
- Focusing too much on what they want and too little on what the interviewer is saying
- Feeling they can "wing" the interview without preparation
- Not being able to personally connect with the interviewer
- Appearing overqualified or underqualified for the job
- Not asking enough or the right questions
- Not researching a potential employer/interviewer
- Lacking humor, warmth, or personality during the interview process

It is always important to prepare for the interview, show enthusiasm for the position, and ask the right questions. Other factors that may have negatively affected the decision include:

- *Inappropriate interview attire and grooming*: The outfit was too tight, neckline was too low, pants dragged on the ground, or the shoes were too casual (e.g., flip-flops). The perfume or cologne was too strong. The hairstyle or color was too extreme.
- *Didn't fit in the environment*: Each facility has a corporate environment. The interviewer looks to see which candidate would fit best. If a person is too shy, too talkative, or too loud, he or she might not be the best fit. Or, a person may have worn too many piercings, or too many tattoos were visible.
- *Used poor grammar*: Some employers correlate good grammar with intelligence. Employers look for candidates who sound intelligent and who will positively represent their facility.

If you have heard or feel that your resume lacks skills needed for specific positions you want to obtain, you may want to improve your skill sets. This can occur through education and experience. Some people improve their job history and skill sets by obtaining temporary employment through temp agencies. Temporary jobs can provide experience and also help you refine your skills. Another way to better your skill sets through experience is by volunteering at a healthcare facility or free clinic. Depending on the volunteer position, it may help enhance your skill sets and also provide you with potential job leads. Volunteer activities should be added to the resume, because these valuable experiences often can be used in a healthcare setting. It does not matter that the position was not a paid job; experience counts, whether paid or not.

YOU GOT THE JOB!

Human Resource Requirements

When you obtain a job, you will be required to complete a number of documents (Table 22.3). You will be asked to bring in proof of identity and employment authorization (e.g., US passport, Social Security account number card, and driver's license). These documents are required for the employer's portion of the Form I-9. Form I-9 must be completed within the set time period to meet governmental regulations. Make sure to complete all the required forms in a timely manner. Meet the deadlines given to you by the human resource representative.

TABLE 22.3 Forms to Complete When Hired

FORM	DESCRIPTION
Form I-9: Employment Eligibility Verification Form	Form I-9 is used to verify a person's identity and employment authorization. All US employers must ensure the form is completed by both the new hire and the employer. The form requires the new hire to provide the employer with documents that prove identity and employment authorization proof.
Form W-4: Employee's Withholding Allowance Certificate	New hires must provide their tax status (e.g., single) and how many allowances they are claiming. This information is used when the employer withholds money from their paycheck for income taxes.
Insurance benefit form	Most agencies have health and life insurance benefits that the new hire can participate in. Completion of paperwork is required as part of the enrollment activities.
Background check form	Many healthcare providers will pay for background checks on new hires. Some hiring may be contingent based on a clean background check. Some types of background checks include criminal, sexual offender registry, and caregiver.
Emergency contact form	The new employee gives the employer information on whom to contact in case of an emergency.
Handbook acknowledgement form	Some agencies have handbooks for each employee. They may require that the employee sign a form to acknowledge receiving the handbook.
Direct deposit form	Most healthcare agencies will pay the employees using the direct deposit method. Funds are transferred into the employee's bank account instead of the employee receiving a paper paycheck.
Agreement forms	The newly hired employee must sign agreement forms related to the Health Insurance Portability and Accountability Act (HIPAA) and computer security.

Getting Started

When you get your first job, it can be an exciting and scary time. You may feel excited for the new opportunities yet scared of the new responsibilities. With any job, it takes time to learn the position. Most healthcare agencies have *probationary periods* for new employees. This time frame can vary. The purpose of the probationary period is to see if the new employee is the right fit for the job. If the employee is not able to do the job or is not the right person for the job, the employer can terminate the employee during the probationary period.

It is important for the medical assistant to do well during the probationary period. The first weeks to months of the job are usually devoted to orientation. The new employee learns the processes and becomes efficient and confident in the role. To be successful it is important for the medical assistant to:

- Arrive 10 to 15 minutes prior to the start of the day. Limit absences, especially during the probationary period.
- Be groomed appropriately according to the facility's dress code.
- Be honest, trustworthy, and respectful in all interactions with peers, patients, and providers.
- Be willing to try new things and ask questions.
- Take feedback professionally and with a positive attitude.
- Be motivated to do a good job and be willing to keep learning.
- Be a team player and be willing to help others.
- Provide safe care to patients, always working within the medical assistant scope of practice.
- Be open to new ideas, concepts, and procedures.

- Attempt to resolve simple differences with peers before involving the supervisor.
- Work with the supervisor to improve oneself and the department.
- Finish all assigned tasks in a timely manner and look for additional duties if time is available.

Maintaining Your Job

For the medical assistant to continue with the facility, it is important to be a reliable employee. It is also important to improve one's weaknesses. The medical assistant will get regular feedback from supervisors through performance appraisals. The performance appraisals inform employees of their strengths and weaknesses on the job. These appraisals are done after the probationary period and annually thereafter. Types of performance appraisals include:

- *180-degree style*: Supervisors evaluate their employees based on their observations of job performance over a given time period.
- *360-degree style*: Supervisors gather input from your co-workers and others whom you interact with on a regular basis.

Do not expect to receive a perfect appraisal. Employees are seldom perfect in all aspects of their jobs. If the supervisor gives perfect scores to an employee, there is no room for growth or improvement. The areas for growth are usually discussed during a meeting with the supervisor. You may be asked where you want to grow or improve and your goals for the coming year. It is important to consider these topics prior to the meeting with the supervisor.

Professional development is also important in maintaining one's job. Medical assistants must keep updated and current in the healthcare industry. It is important to meet the continuing education units (CEUs) needed to maintain your certification or registration. Information on the requirements can be found on the credentialing agency's website.

Leaving a Job

Always offer at least 2 weeks' notice when resigning from a job. Prepare a written notice of resignation and take it to the supervisor in person. Do not just leave it on a desk or place it in the interoffice mail.

Resigning from a job just as an attempt to get a salary increase is a dangerous practice. Once the employer doubts the employee's loyalty, the future is not usually bright for the employee at that facility. Resign only after a final decision has been made. If the medical assistant is resigning to take another position, the current employer may be expected to make a **counteroffer**. However, be wary about accepting counteroffers. What led you to look for a new job in the first place? Has the situation been resolved? Ask yourself these questions before agreeing to stay with the current employer. Often employees who accept a counteroffer and stay at their original job find that few changes are made, and the employee ends up leaving the position in the long run.

CLOSING COMMENTS

As you finish your medical assistant program, embrace the challenge of finding a job. Spend time preparing for the search. Design a professional resume and cover letter that positively set you apart from the other graduates. Network and check job boards for job openings. Apply for any jobs that interest you. Keep organized in your search so you don't overlook opportunities. Work with employment resources at your school to increase your confidence in interviewing. Your preparation and hard work will help you find your first medical assistant job!

Legal and Ethical Issues

Always be completely honest when completing a job application and offering information on a resume. Most facilities stipulate that if an individual is not truthful on these documents, his or her employment can be terminated when the deception is discovered. Employers are more interested in honesty and a forthright explanation than in minor problems that affect the job performance.

If a medical assistant has had some brush with the law that requires disclosure on the job application, the best policy is to be honest and to deal with the ramifications of telling the truth. Most businesses can verify whether a potential employee has any type of criminal record. A solid explanation of the facts, admission of a past mistake, and excellent current references often prompt an employer to have faith and make a positive decision about offering employment.

Professional Behaviors

The development of professional behaviors must begin before the start of a new job. Use your time in school to develop those behaviors that employers are looking for: collaboration and interpersonal skills, professionalism, and compassion. By developing these behaviors in school, your teachers and practicum mentors will be able to give a recommendation that stresses those skills. By being on time and prepared for class, you are showing that you will be on time and prepared for work. By being diligent and self-directed in the classroom, you demonstrate that you have a strong work ethic, which is an important characteristic to employers.

SUMMARY OF SCENARIO

Before graduation, Michelle was offered a job at Walden-Martin Family Medical (WMFM) Clinic. She took her instructor's advice and sent a thank-you note to those who interviewed her. When she was offered the job, the supervisor mentioned how thoughtful the note was. During the call, the supervisor summarized the benefits and the starting salary. She mentioned to Michelle that all medical assistants start at the same wage, but after they pass the CMA (AAMA) certification examination, they get a raise. Michelle took 2 days to consider the position and decided to accept the job offer. The wage was lower than what she was hoping for, but the benefits were much better.

Krysia interviewed for several medical assistant positions over the past few weeks. She found that employers respected her service to her country and valued the skills she learned in military service. She just received her third job offer within the last few days and has decided to accept the position at the local Veterans Affairs (VA) clinic. It is a full-time position with great benefits. The higher wage will help offset the extra mileage that she will be driving to work. She is very excited to be working with other veterans.

Zac has struggled identifying what type of clinic he wants to work for. With his strong leadership skills, he hopes to find a position where he can advance to a supervisory position. He has interviewed for job positions at small and large clinics. He is finding that he is more interested in working with surgeons than with family practitioners. He likes the complexity involved with surgical patients. He is hoping to receive a job offer shortly after graduation. He has decided that if his "dream job" is not offered to him, he will pursue a position in family medicine or internal medicine. This will give him a solid foundation for his new career and then someday he can move into orthopedics or surgery.

SUMMARY OF LEARNING OBJECTIVES

1. **Describe personality traits important to employers.**

   With the cost of training new employees, employers must find the best person to hire. Many employers struggle with assisting new employees to evolve or change personality traits. Thus, employers seek people who already have collaboration and interpersonal skills, professionalism, compassion, and a sincere interest in the job. Collaboration and interpersonal skills allow the new employee to blend well with the current staff. Being flexible, dependable, supportive of peers, remaining calm under pressure, listening, and having good manners are just some of the characteristics of a person with great collaboration and interpersonal skills. Being professional includes proper dress and grooming habits, punctuality, honesty, attention to detail, and the abilities to follow directions, prioritize, and manage time efficiently. Providing compassionate and respectful care and supporting the patient's dignity are crucial to good patient care. Lastly, being genuinely interested in the position positively affects the person's attitude and performance in the job.

2. **Discuss personality traits, technical skills, and transferable job skills.**

   A medical assistant must identify the personality traits, technical skills, and transferable job skills that he or she possesses. Using a portfolio will help the interviewee showcase the qualities that he or she has. Technical skills consist of administrative and clinical skills the person has developed during his or her medical assistant program. Transferable job skills are skills that were used in an unrelated position but relate or transfer to the new position.

3. **Describe how to develop a career objective and identify your personal needs.**

   Medical assistants should take some time to think about what they want from their career and develop a career objective. Your personal needs (e.g., wage, benefits, hours, locations) help you determine what job might be right for you, so you can focus your job search.

4. **Explain job search methods.**

   The two best methods to identify jobs are through networking and using job boards. Networking involves the medical assistant exchanging information with other professionals and family members in hopes of obtaining possible job leads. Job boards are online sites that list positions posted by employers. They can be specific to the healthcare facilities or they can be managed by local media organizations. National job boards can be very helpful for those who want to relocate to another part of the country. Traditional job search methods include school career placement offices, newspaper ads, and employment agencies.

5. **Create a resume and cover letter.**

   The three commonly used resume formats are chronologic, combination, and targeted resumes. Procedures 22.1 and 22.2 describe the steps involved with preparing a resume and cover letter. As you create your resume, keep in mind the eye appeal or interest the resume will create in the reader. A cover letter should always accompany a resume, and much attention to detail is necessary.

6. **Complete an online profile and job application.**

   Many healthcare agencies use the internet during the employment process, and an online profile can have many advantages over paper applications. However, not every employer uses online profiles, and students also may have to fill out job applications. Procedure 22.3 describes the steps involved in completing a job application.

7. **Describe how to create a career portfolio.**

   Procedure 22.4 describes the steps involved in creating a career portfolio.

8. **Practice interview skills during a mock interview.**

   Refer to Procedure 22.5.

9. **List legal and illegal interview questions.**

   See Table 22.2 for examples of illegal and legal interview questions that address the following topics: birthplace, ancestry, or national origin; marital status, children or pregnancy; physical disability, health or medical history; religion or religious days observed; age, race, ethnicity, gender, or color; and criminal record.

10. **Create a thank-you note for an interview.**

    Writing a thank-you note for an interview is a way to make you stand out from the other people who have interviewed for the same position. It shows that you are a courteous and conscientious person and also gives you another opportunity to show why you are the right person for the job. Refer to Procedure 22.6.

11. **Explain common human resources hiring requirements when starting a new job.**

    When you obtain a job, you will be required to complete a number of documents, including Form I-9, Form W-4, insurance benefit form, background check form, emergency contact form, handbook acknowledgement form, direct deposit form, and agreement form. You will be asked to bring in proof of identity and employment authorization (e.g., US passport, Social Security account number card, and driver's license). These documents are required for the employer's portion of Form I-9.

PROCEDURE 22.1   Prepare a Chronologic Resume

Task: Write an effective resume for use as a tool in obtaining employment.

EQUIPMENT and SUPPLIES

- Computer with word processing software and a printer
- Current job posting
- Resume paper
- Paper and pen

PROCEDURAL STEPS

1. Apply critical thinking skills as you create a list of the personality traits (wanted by employers), technical skills, and transfer job skills that you possess. Also write down your career goal(s).

   PURPOSE: To determine the strongest aspects of your abilities so that they can be emphasized on the resume.

2. Using the current job posting, identify the required and recommended qualifications and credentials needed for the position.

   PURPOSE: Identifying what the employer requires and would like will help you tailor your resume to address these qualifications and credentials.

3. Using the computer with word processing software, create a professional-looking header for your document. Include your name, address, telephone number(s), and email address. Select an appropriate font style for your name and a smaller font size for your contact information.

   PURPOSE: To make sure potential employers have a means of contacting you. Using a font style that is bold and a larger size for your name will help your name stand out. Make sure to have your contact information in a smaller, nonbold style so it will not detract from your name.

4. Create a section header for "Education." For the learning institution(s) you attended, list the school's name, city and state, degree obtained, or coursework successfully completed, and the year. Include any additional educational information, such as grade point average (GPA), awards, and practicum information.

   PURPOSE: It is important to provide the school's name, city, and state, along with the degree. Some employers may need to verify the information.

5. Create a section header for "Healthcare Experience" and/or "Work Experience." Provide details about your work experience, including the facility's name, city and state, title of your position, start and end date (month and year), and job duties. The job duties must start with an active verb using the appropriate tense (e.g., a past job would have past tense verbs and a current job would include present tense verbs).

   PURPOSE: The potential employer will need to know your employment history and all the details.

6. Create a section header for "Special Skills" and list your special language skills, computer proficiencies, and other unique skills you possess that relate to the position.

   PURPOSE: This section can be a "marketing" area where you emphasize unique skills you possess.

7. Create a section header for "Certifications and Credentials" and list the active credentials and certifications you have. Include the title of the certification, awarding agency, and the expiration date.

   Note: You may want to consider adding in the date you are taking a credential examination. Employers like to know the status of your credential examination.

   PURPOSE: Employers need to know if you have your medical assistant credential (CMA or RMA). They also might like to know if you have an active cardiopulmonary resuscitation (CPR) card.

8. All information on the resume needs to appear in reverse chronologic order (i.e., newest information is on top). Work experiences should include both the start and end month and year.

   PURPOSE: Employers need to know how long you worked at a specific place. If the position was seasonal or temporary, it is important to note that.

9. The resume needs to look professional and interesting. Use font styles (e.g., bold, underline, italic) to emphasize important words and phrases. Use professional-looking bullets to list job duties and other information. Use the key words from the posting throughout the resume.

   PURPOSE: The more professional and interesting a resume appears, the better the chance that it will be reviewed by the potential employer.

10. Proofread the resume. Correct any spelling, grammar, punctuation, or sentence structure errors you find. If time allows, have another person review the resume and use the feedback to revise your resume.

    PURPOSE: Resumes submitted with errors often are discarded without consideration.

11. Print the resume on resume paper and proofread one final time. Any errors should be corrected, and the document should be reprinted or emailed to the instructor.

PROCEDURE 22.2   Create a Cover Letter

Task: Write an effective cover letter that will accompany the resume.

EQUIPMENT and SUPPLIES

- Computer with word processing software and a printer
- Current job posting
- Resume paper
- Pen

PROCEDURAL STEPS

1. Using the job posting, read through the job description. With a pen, circle the position requirements and the key phrases.
   Your letter should contain the key phrases and position requirements that are found in the job posting.

2. Using the computer with word processing software, create a professional-looking header in the document's header that matches your resume header. Include your name, address, telephone number(s), and email address.
   PURPOSE: To ensure potential employers have a means of contacting you. You can enhance the professional appearance of your documents by having the same header on each document.

3. Type the date in the correct location using the correct format. Have one blank line between the date line and the last line of the letterhead.
   PURPOSE: All letters require a date for legal purposes. The correct format would be month date, year (e.g., May 14, 2023).

4. Type the inside address using the correct spelling, punctuation, and location for the information. Leave 1 to 9 blank lines between the date and the inside address, depending on the location of the body of the letter.
   PURPOSE: The body of the letter needs to be centered vertically from top to bottom of the document. More blank lines can be added to move the body to the correct location.

5. Starting on the second line below the inside address, type the salutation using the correct format. Use a colon after the person's name.
   PURPOSE: A proper greeting helps set the tone of the letter.

6. Type the message in the body of the letter using the proper location and format. There should be a blank line after the salutation and between each paragraph. The message should be clear, concise, and professional. Use proper grammar, punctuation, capitalization, and sentence structure.
   PURPOSE: Proper grammar usage helps convey the message more accurately and professionally.

7. The first paragraph should contain the title and number of the job posting. The middle paragraph(s) should summarize your strengths and include key phrases from the posting. The final paragraph should discuss your availability for an interview. The body should end with an expression of gratitude to the reader.
   PURPOSE: It is important to thank the reader for considering you for the position.

8. Type a proper closing, leaving one blank line between the last line of the body and the closing. Use the correct format and location.
   PURPOSE: The closing helps end the message with a proper tone.

9. Type the signature block using the correct format and location. There should be four blank lines between the closing and the signature block.
   PURPOSE: The four blank lines will provide you with space to sign your name.

10. Spell-check and proofread the document. Check for proper tone, grammar, punctuation, capitalization, and sentence structure. Check for proper spacing between the parts of the letter.
    PURPOSE: The spell-check tool will identify only certain errors; proofreading will help to identify incorrect word usage, improper tone, and errors in formatting. The tone of the letter should be professional, but not aggressive.

11. Make any final corrections. Print the document on resume paper and sign the letter, or email the document to your instructor or employer.
    PURPOSE: It is professional to use resume paper when submitting a resume and cover letter to an employer.

PROCEDURE 22.3   Complete a Job Application

Task: Complete an accurate, detailed job application legibly so as to secure a job offer.

EQUIPMENT and SUPPLIES

- Pen
- Application form
- Information regarding your past education, job experiences, and the skill sets you have developed (e.g., computer skills, keyboarding speed)
- Contact information for former supervisors and references
- Current resume

PROCEDURAL STEPS

1. Read the entire job application before completing any part of the document.
   PURPOSE: Reading through the entire application helps prevent errors when filling out the document.

2. Refer to your information on past jobs, education experiences, and skill sets you have developed as you complete the application. Answers to the questions need to be accurate and honest.

Continued

PROCEDURE 22.3   Complete a Job Application—*continued*

PURPOSE: The application is a legal document, and the answers must be correct and true.

3. Use proper grammar, sentence structure, punctuation, spelling, and capitalization. Handwriting should be legible to the reader.
   PURPOSE: Errors on the application or illegible sections may affect whether you are hired.

4. Do not leave any space blank. Answer each question on the document. If the question does not apply, write "not applicable."
   PURPOSE: Leaving a space blank on the application may suggest that the candidate did not want to answer a certain question or accidentally overlooked it. By writing "not applicable" on such questions, the candidate demonstrates competence and attention to detail.

5. Do not write "See resume" anywhere on the document.
   PURPOSE: Many supervisors view this practice as laziness. Always fill out the job application completely and do not leave blank spaces.

6. Include information on the application that exhibits dependability, punctuality, teamwork, attention to detail, a positive work ethic and initiative, the ability to adapt to change, a responsible attitude, and use of technology.
   PURPOSE: These phrases send an important message to employers. It is important to use words they are looking for.

7. Sign the document and date it.
   PURPOSE: Because this is a legal document, read the fine print before signing the document and dating it.

8. Proofread the document and make sure none of the information conflicts with the resume.
   PURPOSE: Proofreading helps the candidate to catch any errors before submitting the application.

PROCEDURE 22.4   Create a Career Portfolio

Task: Create a custom portfolio that provides potential employers evidence of your skills and knowledge as a medical assistant.

EQUIPMENT and SUPPLIES

- Three-ring binder or folder
- Plastic sleeves for the three-ring binder
- Dividers with tabs for the three-ring binder
- Current resume and cover letter
- Documents providing evidence of your skills and knowledge (e.g., transcripts, job and practicum evaluation forms, practicum skill checklist, projects completed in school, letters of recommendation, copies of certifications [e.g., CPR card])

PROCEDURAL STEPS

1. Group documents in a logical manner, putting similar documents together. Identify the arrangement for the portfolio. An arrangement could include cover letter and resume, education section (e.g., transcript, practicum evaluation form and skills checklist, awards), prior job-related documents (e.g., evaluations), reference letters, and work products (e.g., projects you created in your medical assistant program).
   PURPOSE: Organizing the documents in a logical manner will help the reader identify the important documents. The arrangement will also show the reader your ability to organize content.

2. Insert one document per plastic pocket. Place all documents in plastic pockets.
   PURPOSE: The plastic pockets will keep the documents clean and neat.

3. Neatly write the topic area on the tab of the dividers. Insert the tabbed dividers in the binder or folder.
   PURPOSE: This will help the reader find the content easier.

4. Place all documents in the binder or folder behind the correct divider. Place your cover letter and resume in the front of all the other documents.
   PURPOSE: The reader can review the letter and resume as needed before looking at the other documents in the portfolio.

5. Create a table of contents to identify the tabbed areas.
   PURPOSE: Organizing the documents in a logical manner will help the reader identify the important documents. The arrangement will also show the reader your ability to organize content.

6. After the portfolio is assembled, review the entire portfolio to ensure it looks professional and the documents provide positive support of your skill set and knowledge.
   PURPOSE: Minimize the negative documents in your portfolio. They will not help you obtain a job as much as the positive, supporting documents.

PROCEDURE 22.5   Practice Interview Skills During a Mock Interview

Task: Project a professional appearance during a job medical assistant interview and to be able to express the reasons you are the best candidate for the medical assistant position.

EQUIPMENT and SUPPLIES

- Current job posting
- Resume
- Cover letter
- Interview portfolio (optional)
- Application (optional)
- Interviewer
- Mock interview questions

PROCEDURAL STEPS

1. Wear interview-appropriate attire and be groomed professionally.
   PURPOSE: Your appearance will influence the first impression made on this potential employer. Most medical facilities prefer conservative dress.
2. Portray a professional image by shaking hands firmly prior to the start of the interview. Ensure that each interviewer has a copy of your resume and cover letter. Refrain from nervous behaviors (e.g., saying "um," tapping a pen or your foot) during the interview.
   PURPOSE: Many employers feel a firm handshake is important. Each interviewer may need a copy of your documents to reference during the interview.
3. Answer introductory questions by providing only professional information. This may include information about your education, experience, and career goals.

PURPOSE: Many people are tempted to answer with personal information (e.g., if they are married, have children). Personal information should not be discussed during the interview.

4. Answer interview questions with open, honest, and positive responses. Completely answer questions, provide information or examples, and do not answer in single sentences or with limited responses.
   PURPOSE: The goal of the interview is for the employer to get to know you. Limited responses negatively affect this goal.
5. Use key words from the job posting when answering the interview questions.
   PURPOSE: This helps to prove the interviewee has exactly what the organization is looking for.
6. Ask the interviewer two to three appropriate questions about the facility or the position.
   PURPOSE: This demonstrates an interest in the organization and the position.
7. Express interest in the job and politely complete the interview by shaking hands and thanking the interviewer for the opportunity for the interview.
   PURPOSE: The employer wants to know that you are interested in the job. It is professional to thank the interviewer for the interview opportunity.

PROCEDURE 22.6   Create a Thank-You Note for an Interview

Task: Create a meaningful thank-you note to be sent after the interview process.

EQUIPMENT and SUPPLIES

- Computer with word processing software and a printer
- Job description
- Contact name from interview

PROCEDURAL STEPS

1. Using word processing software, compose a professional letter using the business letter format. Include all of the required elements in the letter. Use correct spacing between the elements.
   PURPOSE: Creating a letter that reflects a professional business letter shows the employer you pay attention to detail.
2. Emphasize the particulars of the interview in the body of the letter.
   PURPOSE: Providing highlights of the interview will assure the employer that you took the time to write an individual thank-you letter.

3. Include positive information you wish you had covered in the interview.
   PURPOSE: This allows you to present any missed skills or details in a professional manner.
4. Create a message that is concise and to the point.
   PURPOSE: Keep the letter short and concise. Employers look for employees who can summarize a message and communicate that message.
5. Proofread the letter and make any revisions as needed. Sign and send the thank-you note.
   PURPOSE: It is important to make sure your note is written correctly. You want to leave a positive perception with the employer.

Abscess Localized collections of pus, which may be under the skin or deep in the body, that cause tissue destruction.

Abstract Collecting important information from the health record.

Abuse An action that purposely harms another person.

Accessory muscles Muscles in the neck, abdomen, and back that assist in breathing.

Accommodation Adjustment of the eye that allows a person to see various sizes of objects at different distances.

Accounts payable Money owed by a company to other companies for services and goods; pertains to paying the facility's bills.

Acute phase The phase during which rapid multiplication of the pathogen takes place. Symptoms are very distinct. A strong response of the immune system takes place during this stage.

Addiction A disease that occurs when a person cannot stop or limit the use of a drug, even after negative consequences have been experienced.

Adherence (ad HEER ehns) The act of sticking to something.

Adhesions (ad HEE zhuns) Bands of scar tissue that can bind anatomic structures together.

Adjudicate (uh JOO di kayt) To settle or determine judicially.

Advance directives Written instructions about healthcare decisions in case a person is unable to make them.

Affect The external emotional expression.

Afferent (AF er uhnt) Pertaining to carrying toward a structure.

Age of majority The age at which the law recognizes a person to be an adult; it varies by state.

Albumin (al BYOO men) Most abundant plasma protein in human blood. It is important in regulating the water balance of blood.

Allopathic (al uh PATH ik) A system of medical practice that treats disease by the use of remedies, such as medications and surgery, to produce effects different from those caused by the disease under treatment; medical doctors (MDs) and osteopaths (DOs) practice allopathic medicine; also called *conventional medicine.*

Alphabetic filing Any system that arranges names or topics according to the sequence of the letters in the alphabet.

Alphanumeric Describes systems made up of combinations of letters and numbers.

Amblyopia (am blee OH pee ah) Dull or dim vision, with no apparent organic defect.

Amenorrhea (ey men uh REE uh) Lack of menstrual flow.

Amino (ah MEE noe) acids Released during the digestion of protein foods in the intestines; carried by the blood to cells, where they are used to make proteins. Used for growth, maintenance, and repair of cells; they also transport nutrients.

Amnesia (am NEE zhah) Memory loss.

Amygdala (ah MIG dah lah) A small mass of gray matter found in each temporal lobe of the cerebrum and involved with memories, emotions, and activating the fight-or-flight response; part of the limbic system.

Analgesic (an ahl JEE zik) A drug that reduces or eliminates pain.

Analyte (AN e lit) The substance or chemical being analyzed or detected in a specimen.

Anaphylaxis (an ah fah LAK sis) A rapidly progressing, life-threatening allergic reaction; characterized by hives, swelling of the mouth and airway, difficulty breathing, wheezing, and loss of consciousness.

Anaplastic (an uh PLAS tic) A rapidly dividing cancer cell that has little to no similarity to normal cells.

Anemia A deficiency of hemoglobin in the blood. Accompanied by a reduced number of red blood cells, pale skin, weakness, and shortness of breath among other symptoms.

Anencephaly (an en SEF uh lee) Congenital absence of part or all of the brain.

Anesthetic (an ehs THET ik) An agent that causes partial or complete loss of sensation.

Aneurysm (AN yeh rizm) An abnormal blood fill sac formed from a localized dilatation of the wall of a vein, artery, or heart.

Anhedonia (an hee DOE nee ah) The inability to feel or experience pleasure during a pleasurable activity.

Anovulation Failure of the ovaries to release an ovum at the time of ovulation.

Answering service A commercial service that answers telephone calls for its clients.

Anthropometric (an thruh PO me trik) The measurement of the size and proportions of the human body.

Antiarrhythmic (an tee ah RITH mik) A drug that prevents or alleviates heart arrhythmias.

Antibiotic (an ti bie OT ik) A drug that destroys or inhibits the growth of bacteria.

Antibody A protein substance produced in the blood or tissues in response to a specific antigen, which destroy or weaken the antigen; part of the immune system.

Anticoagulant (an tee koe AG yuh lunt) A substance (i.e., medication or chemical) that prevents clotting of blood.

Anticonvulsant (an tee kahl VUL sahnt) A drug used to prevent or treat seizures.

Antigen A substance that stimulates the production of an antibody when introduced into the body. Antigens include toxins, bacteria, viruses, and other foreign substances.

Antihistamine (an tee HIS tah meen) A drug that counteracts the effects of histamine.

Antihyperlipidemic (an tie hie per lip i DEE mik) A drug that lowers the lipid levels in the blood.

Antihypertensive A drug that reduces high blood pressure.

Anti-inflammatory (an TEE in FLAM ah tor ee) A medication that prevents or reduces inflammation.

Antimalarial (an TEE mah LAR ee ahl) A drug used to treat or prevent malaria.

Antioxidant (an tee OK si dahnt) Synthetic or natural substance found in food and supplements; may prevent or delay some types of cell damage.

Antipyretic (an tee pie RET ik) A drug that is used to reduce a fever.

Antiseptic (an ti SEP tik) Substances that inhibit the growth of microorganisms on living tissue (e.g., alcohol and povidone-iodine solution [Betadine]); they are used to cleanse the skin, wounds, and so on.

Aphasia (ah FAY zhah) Partial or complete loss of the ability to articulate ideas or understand written or spoken language.

Apnea (AP nee ah) Abnormal, periodic cessation of breathing.

Approximated (uh PROK si may ted) Near, close together.

Arbitration (ahr bi TRAE shuhn) The process in which conflicting parties in a dispute submit their differences to a court-appointed person (arbitrator), who submits a legally binding decision.

Arrhythmia (ah RITH mee ah) An abnormal heart rate or rhythm.

Arterioles (ar TEER ee ohlz) Small arteries.

Arteriosclerosis (ar teer ee oh sklah ROH sis) Thickening, decreased elasticity, and calcification of arterial walls.

Arteriovenous Pertains to the arteries and veins.

Arteriovenous fistula An abnormal joining of an artery and vein.

Arthropod Any animal that lacks a spine, such as insects, crustaceans, arachnids, and others.

Artifact A substance, structure, or event that does not naturally occur in a situation. Examples include interference, or electrical "garbage," on an ECG, or crystals, lint, or contamination of a staining technique.

Artificial insemination The injection of semen into the vagina or uterus using a catheter or syringe. Nonsexual.

Aseptically (ay SEP tick ah lee) Free from living pathogenic organisms.

Asexual Describes reproduction that does not involve the fusion of male and female sex cells.

Aspirate (AS pi rayt) To withdraw fluid using suction. Example: a specimen that has been removed from the body using a needle and syringe.

Aspirating (AS puh rayt ing) To draw off or remove by suction.

Assets All property available for the payment of debts.

Atheroma (ath uh ROH mah) A waxy lesion of cholesterol, fat, calcium, cells, and other substances that builds up on the inner wall of an artery.

ATP (adenosine triphosphate) A high-energy molecule, found in every cell, that supplies large amounts of energy for various biochemical processes.

Attenuated (uh TEN yoo ayt ed) Weakened or changed.

Atypical lymphs In many viral infections stimulated or reactive lymphs are called atypical lymphs. They are commonly seen in infectious mononucleosis.

Audible (AW duh buh l) Capable of being heard.

Audiologist (aw dee OL uh jist) Allied healthcare professional who specializes in evaluation of hearing function, detection of hearing impairment, and determination of the anatomic site of impairment.

Audit A process completed before claims submission in which claims are examined for accuracy and completeness.

Auditory cortex The region of the cerebral cortex that receives auditory data.

Auscultated (AW skuh l teyt d) Listened to with a stethoscope.

Authorized agent A person who has written documentation that he or she can accept a shipment for another individual.

Autoimmune An immune response against a person's own tissues, cells, or cell parts, as in autoimmune disease, leading to the deterioration of tissue.

Automatic call routing A system that distributes incoming calls to a specific group or person based on customer need; for example, the customer presses 1 for appointments, 2 for billing questions, and so on.

Autonomy (aw TON uh mee) The ability to function independently.

Axon (AK son) A long extension of a nerve fiber that conducts the impulse away from the nerve cell body.

Backordered An order placed for an item that is temporarily out of stock and will be sent at a later time.

Bacteria Microorganisms that are single celled, lack a nucleus, reproduce asexually, or can form spores. Some can cause disease. The most abundant life form on earth.

Bartholin (BAR thoh lin) cyst A fluid-filled cyst in one of the vestibular glands located on either side of the vaginal orifice.

Basal Bottom layer.

Belligerent (buh LIG er ent) Hostile and aggressive.

Beneficiary A designated person who receives funds from an insurance policy.

Benign A non-cancerous condition, not malignant, harmless.

Biconvex (bie KON veks) Having two outward curving surfaces, on a lens.

Bilaterally (bie LAT er uhl ee) Pertaining to, involving, or affecting two or both sides.

Bilingual (bie LING gwuhl) Ability to communicate effectively in two languages.

Bilirubin (bil i ROO bin) A reddish pigment that results from the breakdown of red blood cells in the liver.

Billable service Assistance (i.e., service) that is provided by a healthcare provider and can be billed to the insurance company or patient.

Binary fission Asexual reproduction in single-celled organisms during which one cell divides into two daughter cells.

Binocular (buh NOK yuh ler) Involving, relating, or seeing with both eyes.

Binomial A name consisting of a generic and a specific term.

Bioethicists (BYE oh eth i sists) People who study the ethical effect of biomedical advances (e.g., drugs and genetic engineering).

Biomarkers Detectable cellular indicators used as a marker for a substance or disease process.

Biopsy (BIE op see) Process of viewing living tissue that has been removed for the purpose of diagnosis and/or treatment.

Bipolar Having two poles or electrical charges.

Blood agar plate (BAP) A solid agar medium that contains nutrients and 5% washed sheep's blood. The blood is added as an extra nutrient source for bacteria.

Blood culture A microbiological procedure ordered when a provider suspects a bacterial infection is causing a fever of unknown origin (FUO). A blood sample is collected into a nutrient media and held at body temperature. If bacteria are in the blood sample, the culture media should encourage the growth of the infecting bacteria in the laboratory.

Bonded A term describing employees for whom an employer has obtained a fidelity bond from an insurance company, which will cover losses from any dishonest acts (e.g., embezzlement, theft) committed by those employees.

Bookkeeping   The process of recording financial transactions.

Boot   The process of starting or restarting a computer when the operating system is loaded.

Bounding   Describes a pulse that feels full because of the increased power of cardiac contraction or as a result of increased blood volume.

Bradycardia (brad ee KAHR dee uh)   A slow heartbeat; a pulse below 60 beats per minute.

Bradypnea (brad IP nee ah)   Abnormally slow breathing.

Breach   Disclosure of protected health information, without a reason or permission, which compromises the security or privacy of the information.

Bronchiolitis   Occurs when the small airways of the lungs become inflamed because of a viral infection.

Bronchodilator   A drug that relaxes smooth muscle contractions in the bronchioles to improve lung ventilation.

Bruit (broot)   An abnormal sound or murmur heard on auscultation of an organ, vessel (e.g., carotid artery), or gland.

Business associate   A person or business that provides a service to a covered entity that involves access to PHI. Examples include legal, billing, and management services; accreditation agencies; consulting firms; and claims-processing organizations.

Buying cycle   Refers to how often an item is purchased and depends on how frequently the item is used and the storage space available for it.

Calcium   A naturally occurring element that is necessary for many body functions, including strong bones and teeth, proper blood clotting, nerve conduction, and muscle contractions.

Calculi (KAL kyuh lie)   Stones formed in the kidneys, gallbladder, and other parts of the body.

Calibrated (KAL uh bray ted)   Determined by or checked against those of a standard (as in readings).

Calibration (kal uh BRAY shun)   Determining the accuracy of an instrument by comparing its output with that of a known standard or another instrument known to be accurate.

Caliper   A pocket-sized tool used for measuring the height and width of the ECG waves and intervals.

Call forwarding   A telephone feature that allows calls made to one number to be forwarded to another specified number.

Caller ID   A feature that identifies and displays the telephone numbers of incoming calls made to a particular line.

Candidiasis (kan di DIE i sis)   An infection caused by a yeast, *Candida albicans*, that typically affects the vaginal mucosa and skin.

Cannula (KAN yuh la)   A rigid tube that surrounds a blunt trocar or a sharp, pointed trocar, which is inserted into the body; when the trocar is withdrawn, fluid may escape from the body through the cannula, depending on the insertion site.

Capitation (ka pi TAY shun)   A payment arrangement for healthcare providers. The provider is paid a set amount for each enrolled person assigned to him or her, per period of time, whether or not that person has received services.

Caption   A heading, title, or subtitle under which records are filed.

Cardiopulmonary resuscitation (ri sus i TAY shun) (CPR)   The application of manual chest compressions and ventilations (also called rescue breathing) to patients who are not breathing or do not have a pulse; also known as basic life support (BLS).

Cartilage (KAR tih lij)   Flexible connective tissue that covers the ends of many bones at the joint.

Cash on hand   The amount of money the healthcare facility has in the bank that can be withdrawn as cash.

Cataract (KAT ur ackt)   Progressive loss of transparency of the lens of the eye.

Catheter   A hollow, flexible tube that can be inserted into a vessel, organ, or cavity of the body to withdraw or instill fluid, monitor information, and visualize a vessel or cavity.

Caustic (KAW stik)   Capable of burning, corroding, or damaging tissue by chemical action.

Centrifuge (SEN truh fyooj)   A machine that rotates at high speed and separates substances of different densities by centrifugal force. Example: a tube of blood is separated into plasma/serum, white blood cells, platelets, and red blood cells.

Certified Registered Nurse Anesthetist (CRNA)   A nursing healthcare professional who is certified to administer anesthesia.

Cerumen (si ROO muhn)   A waxy secretion in the ear canal; commonly called *ear wax*.

Cessation (se SAY shuhn)   Bringing to an end.

Cheyne-Stokes respiration   Deep, rapid breathing followed by a period of apnea.

Chief complaint   A statement in the patient's own words that describes the reason for the visit.

Choroid plexus (KOR oid PLEK sus)   A network of capillaries found in the lateral ventricles and the third and fourth ventricles that secrete cerebrospinal fluid.

Chromosomes (KROE mah sohms)   Rod-shaped structures found in the cell's nucleus, which contain genetic information.

Chronic   Developing slowly and lasting for a long time, generally 3 or more months.

Chronic obstructive pulmonary disease (COPD)   A progressive, irreversible lung condition that results in diminished lung capacity.

Chronologic (kroon l OJ ick)   Arranged in the order of time.

Cicatrix (SIK uh triks)   Early scar tissue that appears pale, contracted, and firm.

Claim   An itemized statement of services and costs from a healthcare facility submitted to the health (insurance) plan for payment.

Claim scrubbers   Software that finds common billing errors before the claim is sent to the insurance company.

Claims clearinghouse   An organization that accepts the claim data from the provider, reformats the data to meet the specifications outlined by the insurance plan, and submits the claim.

Clarification (KLAR uh fa kay shuh n)   Allows the listener to get additional information.

Clitoris (KLIT uh ris)   Sensitive, erectile tissue.

Clot activators   Substances added to a venipuncture tube to enhance and speed up blood clotting.

Clubbing   Abnormal enlargement of the distal phalanges (fingers and toes) associated with cyanotic heart disease or advanced chronic pulmonary disease.

CMS-1500 Health Insurance Claim Form (CMS-1500)   The standard insurance claim form used for all government and most commercial insurance companies.

Coaching   Providing information in a supportive environment that allows people to grow, change, or improve their situation.

Code   A term used in healthcare settings to indicate an emergency situation and to summon the trained team to the scene.

Coding system   A system designed to use characters (i.e., numbers and letters) to represent something like a medical procedure or a disease.

Cohesive (koh HEE siv)   Sticking together tightly; exhibiting or producing cohesion.

Collaboration (kuh lab uh RAY shun)   The act of working with another or other individuals.

Collagen (KAH lah jen)   The most abundant structural protein found in skin and other connective tissues. It provides strength and cushioning to many parts of the body.

Colonoscopy (kohl uh NOS kuh pee)   A procedure in which a fiber-optic scope is used to examine the large intestine.

Colostomy (koh LOS tuh mee)   A surgical procedure in which the large intestine is brought though the abdominal wall, creating either a temporary or permanent opening (stoma) to allow stool to pass out of the body.

Colposcopy (kol PAW skoh pee)   Using a microscope with a light source, the vagina and cervix are visually examined to locate and evaluate abnormal cells. A biopsy of abnormal cells may be taken during this procedure.

Combining forms   The "subjects" of most terms. They consist of the word root with its respective combining vowel.

Common law   Unwritten laws that come from judicial decisions based on societal traditions and customs.

Communicable diseases (kuh MYOO ni kuh buh l)   Diseases spread from person to person either by direct contact or nondirect contact (i.e., insects).

Compartment syndrome   A serious condition that involves increased pressure, usually in the muscles; which leads to compromised blood flow and muscle and nerve damage.

Compassion   Having a deep awareness of the suffering of another and a wish to ease it.

Complementary and alternative medicine (CAM)   A group of diverse medical and healthcare systems, practices, and products that are not generally considered part of conventional medicine. Complementary medicine is used in combination with conventional medicine (allopathic or osteopathic); alternative medicine is used instead of conventional medicine.

Compliance (kuhm PLIE ahns)   The act of following through on a request or demand. Patient compliance sounds negative, thus patient adherence is now being used.

Compliant (kum PLIE unt)   Obeying, obliging, or yielding.

Computer network   A system that links personal computers and peripheral devices to share information and resources.

Computer on wheels (COW)   A wireless mobile workstation; also called a *workstation on wheels* (WOW).

Computerized provider/provider order entry (CPOE)   The process of entering medication orders or other provider instructions into the EHR.

Concise (kuhn SICE)   Using as few words as possible to express a message.

Concussion (kuhn KUSH uhn)   A traumatic brain injury caused by a blow to the head.

Cone biopsy   An extensive cervical biopsy during which a cone-shaped wedge of tissue is removed from the cervix and examined under a microscope. Abnormal tissue, along with a small amount of normal tissue, is removed.

Conference call   A telephone call in which a caller can speak with several people at the same time.

Congruence (kuh n GROO uh ns)   Agreement; the state that occurs when the verbal expression of the message matches the sender's nonverbal body language.

Conscientious (kon shee EN shuhs)   Meticulous, careful.

Consensus (kun SEN sus)   General agreement.

Constrict   To contract or shrink.

Contamination (kun tam i NAY shun)   The process by which something becomes harmful or unusable through contact with something unclean.

Continuity of care   The smooth continuation of care from one provider to another. This allows the patient to receive the most benefit and no interruption or duplication of care.

Contraindicate (kon truh IN di keyt)   To suggest that it should not be used.

Control materials   Manufacturer-prepared samples that have a known quantity of a specific analyte. Used for quality control purposes. Testing results should fall within a manufacturer defined range of results. Also called *controls* or *quality controls*.

Convalescent stage   The phase during which the host recovers gradually and returns to baseline or normal health.

Copayment (copay)   A set dollar amount that the patient must pay for each office visit. There can be one copayment amount for a primary care provider, a different copayment amount (usually higher) to see a specialist or be seen in the emergency department.

Coping mechanisms   Behavioral and psychological strategies used to deal with or minimize stressful events.

Correlate (KAWR uh leyts)   To establish an orderly relationship or connection.

Corrosive (kuh ROH siv)   Causing or tending to cause the gradual destruction of a substance by chemical action.

Corticosteroids (kor ti koe STER oids)   A group of steroid hormones produced in the body or given as a medication. Some have metabolic functions, and others reduce tissue inflammation. Glucocorticoids and mineralocorticoids are two types.

Counterfeit (KOWN ter fit)   An imitation intended to be passed off fraudulently or deceptively as genuine; forgery.

Counteroffer   Return offer made by one who has rejected an offer or a job.

Covered entity (KUV er ed EN ti tee)   A healthcare facility, healthcare provider, pharmacy, health (insurance) plan, or claims clearinghouse that transmits protected health information electronically.

CPT Assistant   An online CPT coding journal, supported by the AMA, that addresses subjects such as appealing insurance denials, validating coding to auditors, training staff members, and answering day-to-day coding questions.

Crash cart   Emergency medications and equipment (e.g., oxygen, intravenous [IV] and airway supplies) stored in a cart and ready for an emergency.

Creatinine clearance rates   Result from a procedure used to evaluate the glomerular filtration rate of the kidneys.

Credential (kri DEN shus l)   Evidence of authority, status, rights, entitlement to privileges.

Crepitation (krep i TAY shun)   A dry, crackling sound or sensation.

Critical thinking   The constant practice of considering all aspects of a situation when deciding what to believe or what to do.

Cryopreservation (KRIE oh pri zur vae shun)   To preserve by freezing at low temperatures.

Cryosurgery   The technique of exposing tissue to extreme cold to produce a well-defined area of cell destruction.

Crystals   Solid substances with a regular shape that is due to the structure of molecules.

Culture media   A solid, liquid, or semi-solid medium designed to support the growth of microorganisms, especially bacteria and fungus.

Curettage (kyoo rhe TAHZH)   The act of scraping a body cavity with a surgical instrument, such as a curette.

Cystic fibrosis (CF)   A disorder that affects all the exocrine cells, but affects the respiratory system the most. Mucus is abnormally thick and blocks the alveoli, causing dyspnea.

Cytology (sie TOL oh jee)   The study of cells using microscopic methods.

Cytoplasm   The cell substance that fills the area between the nucleus and the cell membrane. It contains the organelles of the cell.

Damages   A monetary settlement the defendant pays the plaintiff in a civil case for loss or injury. Also, one of the 4 Ds of negligence, meaning the patient suffers a legally recognized injury.

Data server   Computer hardware and software that perform data analysis, storage, and archiving; also called a *database server.*

Debridement   The surgical removal of dead, damaged, or infected tissue to improve the function of healthy tissue.

Debris (duh BREE)   The remains of anything broken down or destroyed; ruins, rubble.

Decanting   Pouring a liquid gently so that it does not disturb the remaining sediment.

Declaratory judgment   A court judgment that defines the legal rights of the parties involved.

Decongestant   A drug that is used for nasal congestion.

Decryption (dee KRIP shun)   The computer process of changing encrypted text to readable or plain text after a user enters a secret key or password.

Decubitus ulcers (deh KYOO bi tus)   Sores or ulcers that develop over a bony prominence as the result of ischemia from prolonged pressure; also called *bed sores* or *pressure sores.*

De-escalating   Reducing the level or intensity; bringing down a person's anger or elevated emotions.

Defecation (DEF i kay shun)   The act of voiding waste from the bowels through the anus; the act of having a bowel movement.

Defendant (dih FEN dant)   An individual or business against whom a lawsuit is filed.

Defense (di FENS)   A strategy used by the defendant to avoid liability in a lawsuit.

Defense mechanisms   Unconscious mental processes that protect people from anxiety, loss, conflict, or shame.

Degenerative (dih JEN er uh tiv)   An illness resulting from the deterioration of tissues and organs.

Delegate   To appoint a person as a representative.

Delusion (de LOO zhun)   Unshakable belief in something untrue; may be accompanied by hallucinations and/or paranoia.

Demeanor (dih MEE ner)   Behavior toward others; outward manner.

Dementia (dih MEN shah)   A mental disorder in which the individual experiences a progressive loss of memory, personality alterations, confusion, loss of touch with reality, and stupor (seeming unawareness of, and disconnection with, one's surroundings).

Demographic (dem uh GRAF ik)   Statistical data of a population. In healthcare this includes the patient's name, address, date of birth, employment, and other details.

Density   Describes how compact or concentrated something is.

Deoxygenated   Oxygen deficient; oxygen was removed.

Dependent adults   People between the ages of 18 and 64 who have a mental or physical impairment that prevents them from doing normal activities or from protecting themselves.

Depersonalization   Alternative perception of the self; a person's own reality is lost. People feel they are not in control of their own actions or speech.

Deposition (dep ah ZISH uhn)   A sworn testimony made before a court-appointed officer; it is used in the discovery process and may be used in the trial.

Depreciate   To diminish in value (such as the value of an item) over a period of time; a concept used for tax purposes.

Derealization   Loss of sensation of the reality of one's surroundings.

Dermatome (DUR mah tome)   Skin surface areas supplied by a single afferent spinal nerve.

Detrimental (de truh MEN tl)   Harmful.

Dextrocardia (dek stro KAHR dee ah)   The heart is located on the right side of the chest and the apex is pointing to the right.

Diabetic retinopathy (die ah BET ik reh tin OP ah thee)   Diabetes mellitus damages the blood vessels in the retina leading to loss of vision and eventual blindness.

Diagnosis (die ag NOH sis)   Determining the cause of a condition, illness, disease, injury, or congenital defect.

Diagnostic statement   Information about a patient's diagnosis or diagnoses that has been taken from the medical documentation.

Diaphragm (DIE uh fram)   A broad, dome-shaped muscle used for breathing. It separates the thoracic and abdominopelvic cavities.

Dictation (dik TEY shuh n)   To say something aloud for another person to write down.

Differentiate (dif uh REN shee eyt)   To distinguish one thing from another. To make a distinction between items.

Differentiated (dif uh REN shee ayt)   Describes how malignant tissue looks like the normal tissue it came from; poorly differentiated means it does not look like the normal tissue, and well differentiated means it looks like the normal tissue.

Diffuse   To spread, scatter, disperse, or move.

Dignity (DIG ni tee)   The inherent worth or state of being worthy of respect.

Dilation (die LAY shuhn)   The opening or widening of the circumference of a body orifice with a dilating instrument.

Diluent (die LU ent)   A liquid substance that dilutes or lessens the strength of a solution or mixture.

Dilution   Reducing the concentration of a mixture or solution by adding a known volume of liquid.

Direct filing system   A filing system in which materials can be located without consulting another source of reference.

Discipline   A branch of knowledge, learning, or instruction; for instance medicine, nursing, social work, and physical therapy.

Discrepancy   A lack of similarity between what is stated and what is found; for instance, the computer inventory count is different than the physical count.

Discretionary income   Money in a bank account that is not assigned to pay for any office expenses.

Discrimination (dis krim eh NAE shuhn)   Unfair treatment of another person based on the person's age, gender (sex), ethnicity, sexual orientation, disability, marital status, or other selective factors.

Disinfect   To destroy or render pathogenic organisms inactive; does not include spores, tuberculosis bacilli, and certain viruses.

Disinfectant (dis in FEK tuh nt)   Any chemical agent used on nonliving objects to destroy or inhibit the growth of harmful organisms; not effective against bacterial spores.

Disparaging (di SPAR a jing)   Slighting; having a negative or degrading tone.

Disruption   An unexpected event that throws a plan into disorder; an interruption that prevents a system or process from continuing as usual or as expected.

Dissect   To cut or separate tissue with a cutting instrument or scissors.

Diuretic   A drug that increases the amount of urine produced.

Diurnal (die UR nl) variation   Fluctuations that occur during each day.

Diversity   The differences and similarities in identity, perspective, and points of view among people.

Docking station   Also known as a *universal port replicator*; this hardware device allows laptops to connect with other devices, making it into a desktop computer.

Dosage   May also be referred to as *dose*; the quantity of medication to be administered at one time.

Down syndrome   A genetic disorder in which abnormal cell division results in an extra chromosome 21.

Downtime   The interval of time where something, such as hardware or software, is not functioning.

Drive   A computer device that reads data from and may write data to a storage medium.

Dumb terminal   A personal computer that does not contain a hard drive and allows the user only limited functions, including access to software, the network, or the internet.

Dynamic (die NAM ik) equilibrium   Relating to balance when moving at an angle or rotating.

Dysmenorrhea (dis men uh REE uh)   Painful menstrual flow, cramps.

Dyspareunia (dis ph ROO nee ah)   Painful or difficult intercourse.

Dysphagia   Difficulty swallowing.

Dyspnea (DISP nee uh)   Difficult or painful breathing.

Ecchymosis (ek i MOH sis)   Discoloration of the skin caused by the escape of blood into the tissues from ruptured blood vessels; typically caused by bruising.

Echocardiography (ECHO) (eck oh KAR dee AH gruh fee)   The use of ultrasonic waves directed through the heart to study the structure and motion of the heart. The visual record produced is called an *echocardiogram*.

Ectopic pregnancy (eck TAH pick)   A pregnancy in which the fertilized egg implants outside of the uterus (e.g., fallopian tubes).

Efferent (EF er uhnt)   Pertaining to carrying away from a structure.

Egress (EE gress)   Leaving a place; exit route.

Elastin (ih LAS tin)   A highly elastic protein in connective tissue that allows tissues to resume their shape after stretching or contracting. It is found abundantly in the dermis of the skin.

Electrocardiogram (ECG, EKG)   A record or recording of electrical impulses of the heart produced by an electrocardiograph.

Electrodes   Adhesive patches that conduct electricity from the body to the machine wires (e.g., ECG and transcutaneous electrical nerve stimulation [TENS] unit).

Electrolyte   An inorganic compound, usually a salt. A major factor in controlling fluid balance within the body.

Electronic health record (EHR)   An electronic record conforms to nationally recognized standards and contains health-related information about a specific patient. It can be created, managed, and consulted by authorized clinicians and staff from more than one healthcare organization.

Electronic transaction   The electronic exchange of information between two agencies to accomplish financial or administrative healthcare activities.

Eligibility (el i ji BILL i tee)   Meeting the stipulated requirements to participate in the healthcare plan.

Emancipated minor (i MANS i pa ted MIE nohr)   A minor who has been granted emancipation by the court; the minor can assume the rights and responsibilities of adulthood.

Embezzlement (em BEZ uh l ment)   The misuse of funds for personal gain.

Embolus (EM boh lus)   An air bubble, blood clot, or foreign body that travels through the bloodstream and blocks a blood vessel.

Embryo (EM bree oh)   A developing organism from the moment of conception through the eighth week of development.

Emergency   An unexpected, life-threatening situation that requires immediate action.

Empathy (EM pah thee)   The ability to understand another's perspective, experiences, or motivations.

Emphysema (em fuh ZEE muh)   Thinning and eventual destruction of the alveoli; usually accompanies chronic bronchitis.

Emulsifies (ee MUL sih fyez)   When a substance suspends tiny droplets of one liquid into a second liquid. By creating an emulsion, you can mix two liquids that usually do not mix well, such as oil and water.

EMV chip technology   Global technology that includes imbedded microchips that store and protect cardholder data; also called *chip and PIN* and *chip and signature*.

Encoder   Software that will apply diagnostic or procedure codes to medical conditions or procedures.

Encounter form   A document used to capture the services/procedures and diagnoses for a patient visit. The fees for the services/procedures are usually included on the encounter form.

Endocrine   A glandular secretion that is released into the blood or lymph directly (does not go through a duct).

Endoscopy (en DOS kuh pee)   An examination using a scope with a camera attached to the long, thin tube that can be inserted into the body.

Endoscope   A scope with a camera attached to a long, thin tube that can be inserted into the body.

Endotracheal (EN doe TRAY kee al) (ET) tube   A catheter that is inserted into the trachea through the mouth; provides a patent airway.

Enriched Nutrients are added back into a food, after they were loss during food processing.

Enunciation (ih nuhn see EY shuh n) The use of articulate, clear sounds when speaking.

Enzymes (EN zimes) Special proteins that speed up a chemical reaction in the body.

Epidemiological (ep i dee mee o LOJ i kuh l) The branch of medicine dealing with the incidence, distribution, and control of disease in a population. It also involves the prevalence of disease in large populations, in addition to detection of the source and cause of epidemics of infectious disease.

Epiglottis (ep i GLOT is) Lid-like structure over the glottis that prevents food and liquids from entering the trachea when swallowing occurs.

Epiphyseal plate (eh pi FIZ ee uhl) A thin layer of cartilage located at the ends of a long bone where new bone forms.

Epithelial cells (ep i THEE lee al) Form cellular sheets that cover surfaces, both inside and outside the body. Epithelial cells are closely packed, take on different shapes, and strongly stick to each other.

Eponym (EP uh nim) In medical terms, a medical diagnosis or procedure named for the person who discovered it.

E-prescribing The use of electronic software to communicate with pharmacies and send prescribing information. It takes the place of writing a prescription by hand and giving it to a patient; most new or refill prescriptions can be submitted electronically, cutting down on fraud and errors.

Equilibrium (ee kwuh LIB ree uh m) A state of rest or balance due to the equal action of opposing forces.

Ergonomics (ur guh NOM iks) An applied science concerned with designing and arranging things needed to do your job, in an efficient and safe way.

Erythema (er ee THEE mah) Redness.

Erythropoietin (eh rith roh POY eh tin) A hormone that is produced by the kidney cells and travels to the bone marrow to stimulate red blood cell formation.

Essential hypertension Elevated blood pressure of unknown cause that develops for no apparent reason; sometimes called *primary hypertension.*

Established patient A patient who has been treated previously by the healthcare provider within the past 3 years.

Esterase Any enzyme that breaks down esters (a type of organic molecule) into alcohols and acids.

Ethernet (EE thuhr net) A communication system for connecting several computers so information can be shared.

Ethics (ETH iks) Rules of conduct that differentiate between acceptable and unacceptable behavior.

Ethics committee A group composed of members from a variety of disciplines that analyzes ethical issues.

Etiology (ee tee OL uh jee) The study of the causes or origin of diseases.

Eukaryote (yoo KAR ee oht) Any single-celled or multicellular organism that has genetic material contained in a distinct membrane-bound nucleus.

Euphoria (yoo FOR ee ah) An exaggerated sense of physical and mental well-being.

Evacuated To create a vacuum in a tube, flask, or reaction vessel.

Evert (ih VURT) To turn the eyelid inside out; this typically is done by the provider to inspect the area for foreign bodies.

Evidence-based practice Healthcare practice that incorporates the most current and valid research results, thus providing the best patient care.

Evoked potential test A nerve response test that uses electrodes, which are placed on the scalp to measure brain reaction to a stimulus.

Exclusivity (ik SKLOO siv i tee) The sole right to market an approved medication granted by the FDA; may occur with the patent.

Excoriated (ik SKOHR ee ay ted) To strip off or remove the skin from an area.

Excoriation (ik skawr ee EY shun n) Inflammation and irritation of the skin.

Executor An individual assigned to make financial decisions about the estate of a deceased patient.

Exocrine A glandular secretion released through a duct.

Expediency (ik SPEE dee uh n see) A means of achieving a particular end, as in a situation requiring urgency or caution.

Expert witnesses People who are educated and knowledgeable in the area of concern; they testify in court and provide an expert opinion on the topic of concern.

Expiration Exhaling; movement of waste gases from the alveoli into the atmosphere.

Explanation of benefits (EOB) A document sent by the insurance company to the provider and the patient explaining the allowed charge amount, the amount reimbursed for services, and the patient's financial responsibilities.

Expletive (EK sple tiv) An oath or swear word.

Explicit (ik SPLIS it) Fully and clearly expressed or demonstrated; leaving nothing merely implied.

Exploitation (EKS ploi TAY shuhn) The act of using another person for one's own advantage.

Extension The process of stretching out; increasing the angle of a joint.

Extraction A process by which a specific substance is separated from a group or solution.

Exudates (EKS yoo dayts) Fluids with high concentrations of protein and cellular debris that have escaped from the blood vessels and have been deposited in tissues or on tissue surfaces.

Fact witnesses People who observed the situation and testify in court about the facts of the case.

Familial (fuh MIL yuh l) Occurring in or affecting members of a family more than would be expected by chance.

Fascia (FASH ee ah) A tough fibrous covering of the muscles.

Fatigue (fuh TEEG) Extreme tiredness.

Fatty acids Result when fats are broken down; used by the body for energy and tissue development.

Febrile (FEB ruh l) Pertaining to an elevated body temperature.

Federal Reserve Bank The central bank of the United States. The Federal Reserve system consists of a seven-member Board of Governors with headquarters in Washington, D.C., and 12 Federal Reserve banks in major cities throughout the country.

Fee schedule A list of fixed fees for services.

Filamentous (fil ah MEN tuhs) Composed of or containing filaments or strands of a substance.

File A collection of data or program records stored as a unit with a specific name.

Filtrate Fluid and substances that are filtered out of the blood in the Bowman capsule.

Fire doors Doors made of fire-resistant materials; they close manually or automatically during a fire to prevent it from spreading.

Fissure (fish EHR) A groove that divides an organ into lobes or parts.

Flexion The process of decreasing the angle of a joint.

Fluctuate (FLUHK choo ayt) To shift back and forth.

Follicle-stimulating hormone (FSH) A glycoprotein hormone secreted by the anterior pituitary gland. It stimulates the growth of ovum (eggs) in the ovary and induces the formation of sperm in the testis.

Follow-up appointment An appointment type used when a patient needs to see the provider after a condition should have been resolved or to monitor an ongoing condition, such as hypertension. Also known as a *recheck appointment*.

Fontanel / Fontanelle (fon tah NEL) A soft membranous gap between the incompletely formed cranial bones of an infant; also called a *soft spot*.

Foramen magnum A large opening in the base of the skull. It forms a passageway for the spinal cord.

Forensic (fuh REN sik) Scientific tests or techniques used regarding the detection of crime.

Form Physical characteristics of a medication (e.g., tablet, suspension).

Fornix (FORE niks) A recess in the upper part of the vagina caused by protrusion of the cervix into the vaginal wall.

Fortified Nutrients are added to a food; these nutrients were never originally in the food.

Fungus Any of a diverse group of single-celled organisms, including mushrooms, molds, mildew, smuts, rusts, and yeasts and classified in the kingdom Fungi.

Gait The manner or style of walking.

Gamete (GAM eet) A mature sexual reproductive cell; spermatozoa or ovum.

Gatekeeper The primary care provider, who is in charge of a patient's treatment. Additional treatment, such as referrals to a specialist, must be approved by the gatekeeper.

Germicides (JUR muh sahyds) Agents that destroy pathogenic organisms.

Germline cells Sperm and egg cells.

G-force A force acting on an object because of gravity. Example: A centrifuge spins and exerts g-force.

Girth The measurement around something; when referring to mail, it is the measurement around the middle of the package that is being shipped.

Glasgow coma scale A scale used to measure the level of consciousness and severity of a head injury; ability to open eyes, verbal response, and motor response are evaluated and the score is determined based on the findings.

Glaucoma (glou KOE mah) Increase in the fluid pressure in the eye; can lead to blindness if not treated.

Global services For purposes of CPT coding, medical services and procedures performed for the patient before, during, and after a surgical procedure, that are included with the assigned CPT code.

Glomerulonephritis (gloh mer yuh loh neh FRIE tis) Kidney disease affecting the capillaries of the nephron (glomeruli); characterized by albuminuria, edema, and hypertension.

Glucagon (GLOO kah gon) A hormone produced by the alpha cells in the pancreas; works on the liver to release glycogen and thereby prevent dangerously low blood glucose levels.

Glucose A simple sugar that is absorbed by the intestines and found in the blood. Used by cells for energy and the extra is stored in the liver as glycogen.

Glycolysis (glie KOL uh sis) The chemical breakdown of carbohydrates (glucose) by enzymes, with the release of energy.

Gonads (GOH nad) Organs that produce sex cells in both males and females.

Gonioscopy (goh nee AH skuh pee) Used to diagnose glaucoma and to inspect ocular movement.

Graduated cylinder A narrow, tube-shaped container marked with horizontal lines to represent units of measurement. Used to precisely measure the volume of liquids.

Graft Tissue taken from one area in the body and inserted into another area or person.

Gray matter Nerve tissue that lacks the insulation that causes a white appearance to other nerves; thus, gray matter looks gray.

Gross The amount earned before any tax deductions or adjustments.

Guarantor The person legally responsible for the entire bill. This is usually the patient, but in the case of a minor it would be a parent or legal guardian.

Gyri (JIE rie) Folds or convolutions on the surface of the cerebral hemisphere, which increase the gray matter surface area. **Gyrus** (JIE rus) is the singular form.

Hackers Unauthorized users who attempt to break into computer networks.

Hallucination (hah LOO si nae shun) A sensory experience (e.g., a smell, sound, sight, touch, or taste) involving something that is not present.

Harassment (hah RAS ment) The continued, unwanted, and annoying actions done to another person.

Hardware Physical equipment of the computer system required for communication and data processing functions.

Headset A set of headphones with a microphone attached, used especially in telephone communication.

Health insurance exchange An online marketplace where you can compare and buy individual health insurance plans. State health insurance exchanges were established as part of the Affordable Care Act.

Hematologist (hee mah TOL uh jist) A person trained in the nature, function, and diseases of the blood and blood-forming organs. Can be a physician, trained laboratory personnel, or researcher.

Hematoma (hee mah TOH mah) An abnormal buildup of blood in an organ or tissue of the body, caused by a leak or cut in a blood vessel.

Hematopoiesis (hee mah toh poh EE sis) The formation of the blood cells and platelets.

Hemoconcentration (hee muh kon sun TRAY shun) A condition in which the concentration of blood cells is increased in proportion to the plasma.

Hemoglobin (HEE muh gloh bin)   The oxygen-carrying pigment of red blood cells.

Hemolysis (hee MOL i sis)   The breakdown of red blood cells with the release of hemoglobin.

Hemolytic uremic syndrome   Kidney disorder that can occur after a digestive infection with E. coli, shigella, or salmonella; red blood cells are destroyed and block the kidneys' filtering system causing acute kidney failure.

Hemolyzed (HEE muh liezd)   A blood sample in which the red blood cells have ruptured.

Hemophilia (hee moh FEE lee ah)   A group of inherited blood disorders characterized by a deficiency of one of the factors necessary for the coagulation of blood.

Hemostasis (hee muh STAY sis)   The stoppage of bleeding.

Hereditary (huh RED i ter ee)   Passed from parents to offspring through the genes.

Hertz (hurts)   The unit of measurement used in hearing examinations; a wave frequency equal to one cycle per second.

Hierarchy (HIE er ar kee)   Things arranged in order and rank.

Hippocampus (Hip oh KAM pus)   A ridge in the floor of the lateral ventricle; composed of gray matter. Involved with the limbic system and with creating and filing new memories.

Histology (hi STOL oh jee)   The study of tissues.

History of present illness (HPI)   Describes the signs and symptoms from the time of onset.

Holistic (hoh LIS tik)   A form of healing that considers the whole person (i.e., body, mind, spirit, and emotions) in individual treatment plans.

Homeostasis (hoh mee oh STAY sis)   The internal environment of the body that is compatible with life. A steady state that is created by all the body systems working together to provide a consistent and unvarying internal environment.

Hormone   A chemical substance produced in an endocrine gland and transported in the blood to a specific tissue, where it applies a specific effect.

Hospice (HOS pis)   A concept of care that involves health professionals and volunteers who provide medical, psychological, and spiritual support to terminally ill patients and their loved ones.

Human resources file (HR file)   Contains all documents related to an individual's employment.

Hydrocephalus (HIE droe sef ah luhs)   An abnormal accumulation of cerebrospinal fluid that causes enlargement of the skull and compression of the brain.

Hydronephrosis (hie droh nuh FROH sis)   A backup of urine that causes dilation of the ureters and calyces; can increase pressure on the nephron units.

Hyperlipidemia (hie per lip i DEE mee ah)   An elevated level of lipids in the blood.

Hyperplasia (hahy per PLEY zhee uh)   Enlargement due to an abnormal multiplication of cells.

Hyperpnea (hie PURP nee ah)   Excessively deep breathing.

Hyperventilation (hie pur ven ti LAY shun)   Abnormally increased breathing.

Hypoalbuminemia (hie poh al byoo mi NEE mee ah)   A decreased level of albumin (protein) in the blood.

Hypotension   Blood pressure that is below normal (systolic pressure below 90 mm Hg and diastolic pressure below 50 mm Hg).

Hysterectomy   Surgical removal of the uterus and cervix. The ovaries and fallopian tubes may also be removed.

Idiopathic (id ee uh PATH ik)   Of unknown cause.

Immunoglobulins (im yuh noh GLOB yuh linz)   A group of related proteins that functions as antibodies. Are found in plasma and other body fluids.

Immunosuppressant   A drug used to suppress the immune system.

Impending   A term used in the diagnosis of a condition that can be imminently threatening. For example, a patient showing signs of prediabetes may in the near future develop diabetes; therefore, in this case, diabetes is an impending condition.

Impervious (im PUR vee uhs)   Not permitting penetration.

In vitro   Latin term meaning "in glass" and commonly known as "in the laboratory."

Inanimate   Not animate; lifeless.

Incentive   Things that incite or spur to action; rewards or reasons for performing a task.

Incidence (IN si duh ns)   How often something happens or occurs.

Incompetence (in KOM pi tahns)   The state of being incompetent or lacking the ability to manage personal affairs due to mental deficiency; an appointed guardian or conservator manages the person's affairs.

Incompetent valves   Valves do not close completely and blood leaks backward into the prior chamber; also called "leaky valves."

Inconspicuous (in kuh n SPIK yoo uh s)   Not noticeable or prominent.

Incurred   To come into or acquire.

Indicator (IN di kay ter)   An important point or group of statistical values that, when evaluated, indicates the quality of care provided in a healthcare facility.

Indigent (IN di juh nt)   Poor, needy, impoverished.

Infarction (in FARK shuhn)   Tissue death.

Infection   Invasion of body tissues by microorganisms, which then multiply and damage tissues.

Infectious agents   Living and nonliving pathogens—such as bacteria, viruses, fungi, protozoa, parasite, helminths, and prions—that can cause disease. Also called infectious particles.

Inflammation (in fluh MAY shuhn)   A pathology characterized by redness, swelling, pain, tenderness, heat, and disturbed function of an area of the body. Especially a reaction of tissues to injury.

Ingested   Taken, as food, into the body.

Inhalant (in HAY lunt)   Any substance that can be breathed into the lungs.

Inhalation (in huh LEY shuh n)   The act of breathing in.

Initiative (i NISH eh tive)   The ability to determine what needs to be done and take action on your own.

Injunction (in JUNGK shuhn)   A court order by which an individual or institution is required to perform or restrain from performing a certain act.

INR   INR stands for International Normalized Ratio and is also called a prothrombin time (PT). It is used to test the effectiveness of blood thinning medication.

Insidious (in DID ee uh s)   Proceeding in a gradual, subtle way, but with harmful effects.

Inspiration   Inhaling; movement of O_2 from the atmosphere into the alveoli.

Insufficiency Also called regurgitation or incompetence; the valve does not close completely, and blood leaks backward across the valve into the prior chamber.

Insulin (IN suh lin) A hormone produced by the beta cells in the pancreas; moves glucose into the cells so it can be used for energy.

Intact (in TAKT) Complete or whole. Not altered; unbroken.

Intangible (in TAN juh buhl) Something of value that cannot be touched physically.

Integral (IN ti gruhl) Essential; being an indispensable part of a whole.

Integrity (in TEG ri tee) Adhering to ethical standards or right conduct standards.

Intercellular Located between cells.

Intercom A two-way communication system with a microphone and loudspeaker at each station; often a feature of business telephones.

Intercostal muscles (in tur KOS tul) Muscles located between the ribs that help with quiet respiration.

Interest Money the bank pays the account holder, on the amount in his or her account, for using the money in the account.

Interface An interconnection between systems.

Interferon (in ter FEER on) A protein formed when a cell is exposed to a virus; the protein blocks viral action on the cell and protects against viral invasion.

Intermittent Occurring in intervals.

Intermittent pulse A pulse in which beats occasionally are skipped.

Interoperability (in ter OP er uh bi li tee) The ability to work with other systems.

Interpersonal skills The ability to communicate and interact with others; sometimes referred to as "soft skills."

Interrogatory (IN tah rog ah TOOR ee) Written or oral questions that must be answered under oath.

Interstitial (in ter STISH ul) Between the cells.

Interstitial cells Testosterone-secreting cells of testes that are found in the spaces between the seminiferous tubules.

Interval Space of time between events.

Intracellular pathogens A disease causing organism that is within or inside of a cell.

Intranet (IN trah net) A private computer network that can only be accessed by authorized people (e.g., employees of the facility, that owns the network).

Intraosseous (in tra OS ee us) Within bone; route for delivery of fluids and medications through a needle inserted into the marrow of certain bones (e.g., humerus, tibia, and femur).

Intravenous (IV) Through a vein; fluids and medications can be given through a vein.

Intrinsic factor Secreted by the parietal cells of the stomach; necessary for the absorption of vitamin B_{12} to prevent pernicious anemia.

Inventory A detailed list of equipment and supplies owned and stored; the process of counting the supplies in stock.

Invoices Billing statements that list the amount owed for goods or services purchased.

Ion (AHY ons) An electrically charged atom, or the smallest component of an element.

Jargon (JAHR guhn) The vocabulary of a particular profession as opposed to common, everyday terms.

Jaundice A yellow discoloration of the skin and mucous membranes caused by deposits of bile.

Job boards Websites where employers post jobs, that can be used by job seekers to identify open positions.

Judicious (joo DISH uhs) Using good judgment; being discreet, sensible.

Labia majora (LAY bee ah muh JOR ah) The larger external folds of skin surrounding the opening of the vagina.

Labia minora (LAY bee ah min NOR uh) The smaller inner folds of skin surrounding the opening of the vagina.

Lacrimation (lak ri MAY shun) The secretion or discharge of tears.

Laparoscopy (lap ar AW scoh pee) A procedure used to visually examine the abdomen.

Larynx (LAR inks) The voice box.

Lateral flow immunoassay (im yuh noh AH say) A laboratory or clinical technique that uses the specific binding between an antigen and antibody to identify and quantify a substance in a sample. The sample in this technique moves in a sideways motion, usually on an absorbent paper.

Learning style The way an individual perceives and processes information to learn new material.

Lethargy (LETH er jee) The state of being drowsy and dull, listless and unenergetic.

Leukoderma Lack of skin pigmentation, especially in patches.

Liability (LIE ah bil i tee) The state of being liable or responsible for something.

Liable Legally responsible or obligated.

Libido Sexual drive or instinct.

Licensure (LIE sen shur) A mandatory process established by state law that ensures a person has met the legal standards for practicing an occupation in that state.

Ligaments (LIH gah ments) Supportive connective tissue that connects bones at a joint.

Limbic system Consists of several structures including the amygdala, hippocampus, and hypothalamus; plays an important role with behavior, memories, and emotions.

Litigious (LI ti jehs) Prone to lawsuits.

Local Affecting the area where applied.

***Locum tenens* (LOE kuhm TEE nenz)** Latin for "to substitute for"; physicians or advance practice professionals who temporarily contracted to provide healthcare services when a facility has a vacancy, vacation, or a leave of absence.

Loop electrosurgical excision procedure (LEEP) After an anesthetic has been injected into the cervix, a high-frequency electrical current running through a wire is used to remove abnormal tissue from both the cervix and the endocervical canal.

Lumen The cavity, channel, or open space within a tube or tubular organ.

Lumpectomy (luhm PEK tuh mee) Removal of the breast tumor and a small amount of the surrounding tissue.

Luteinizing hormone (LH) A hormone produced by the anterior pituitary gland. LH stimulates ovulation and the development of the corpus luteum in females and the production of testosterone in males.

Lymph (limf) A clear, yellowish fluid containing white blood cells in a liquid similar to plasma. The fluid comes from the tissues of the body and is moved through the lymphatic vessels and the bloodstream.

Lymphedema (lin fuh DEE mah)   A condition in which extra lymph fluid builds up in tissues and causes swelling. It may occur in an arm or leg if lymph vessels are blocked, damaged, or removed by surgery.

Lymphocyte (LIM fuh site)   A type of white blood cell that has a large, round nucleus that is surrounded by a thin layer of agranular cytoplasm.

Lymphostasis (lim foh STAY sis)   Obstruction or interruption of normal lymph flow.

Macromolecules   Molecules needed for metabolism: carbohydrates, lipids, proteins, amino acids, and nucleic acids.

Macrophages (MACK roh fay jehs)   Large white blood cells that live in the tissues. They engulf foreign particles, microorganisms, and cell debris.

Malaise (ma LAYZ)   A condition of general bodily weakness or discomfort, often marking the onset of a disease.

Malignant   A cell with uncontrolled growth that spreads rapidly, with the potential for serious harm.

Malpractice (mal PRAK tis)   A type of negligence in which a licensed professional fails to provide the standard of care, causing harm to a person.

Malware (MAL wair)   Malicious software designed to damage or disrupt a system (e.g., a virus).

Mania (MAY nee ah)   Abnormally elated mental state; the person may have feelings of euphoria, lack of inhibitions, sleeplessness, talkativeness, risk-taking behaviors, and irritability.

Manipulation   Movement or exercise of a body part by means of an externally applied force.

Mastectomy (ma STEK tuh mee)   Removal of the entire breast.

Matrix (MAY triks)   The environment where something is created or takes shape. A base on which to build.

Mature minor   A person under the age of adulthood who demonstrates the maturity to make a personal healthcare decision and can give informed consent for treatment.

Meatus   A body opening or passage, especially the external opening of a structure.

Media (ME de ah)   Types of communication (e.g., social media sites); with computers, the term refers to data storage devices.

Mediastinum (mee dee AH sti nuhm)   The space in the thoracic cavity that lies between the lungs, containing the heart, trachea, and esophagus.

Mediation (MEE dee ae shuhn)   The process of facilitating conflicting parties to make an agreement, settlement, or compromise.

Medical necessity   Services or supplies (CPT and HCPCS codes) that are used to treat the patient's diagnosis (ICD codes) meet the accepted standard of medical practice.

Medically necessary   Accepted healthcare services that are appropriate for the evaluation and treatment of a disease, condition, illness or injury and are consistent with the applicable standard of care.

Medulla oblongata (muh DUHL uh ob lawng GAH tuh)   The lowest part of the brain, continuous with the top of the spinal cord.

Melanocytes (meh LAN oh sites)   Cells of the stratum germinativum that produce a brownish pigment called melanin. Melanin gives us our skin color.

Ménière's (mayn YAIRZ) disease   Chronic disease of the inner ear causing recurrent episodes of vertigo, progressive sensorineural hearing loss, and tinnitus.

Meninges (meh NIN jeez)   A protective covering around the brain and spinal cord.

Meningocele (meh NING goh seel)   The protrusion of the meninges through an opening in the spinal column or skull.

Menometrorrhagia (men oh meh troh RAH zsa)   Excessive menstrual flow and uterine bleeding other than that caused by menstruation.

Menorrhagia (men or RAH zsa)   Abnormally heavy menstrual flow or prolonged menstrual periods.

Mentor   A steady employee whom a new staff member can approach with questions and concerns.

Metabolic   relating to or resulting from metabolism (the chemical process where cells produce the substances and energy needed to sustain life).

Metabolism (me TAB oh lizm)   The chemical process that occurs within a living organism in order to maintain life.

Metabolites (meh TAB uh lites)   By-products of drug metabolism.

Microbiome (mie kroh BIE ohm)   The total collection of microorganisms, and their genetic material, present on or in the human body or a specific site in the human body.

Microcephaly (mie kroh SEF ul ee)   Abnormally small head associated with incomplete brain development.

Microcuvette (MIE kroh koo vet)   A small plastic or glass tube designed to hold samples for laboratory tests that detect light or color changes.

Microorganism   Any living organism—such as bacterium, protozoan, fungi, parasite, or helminth—of microscopic size. Some definitions include viruses, which are not alive.

Minor   One who has not reached adulthood; usually age 18 or 21, depending on the jurisdiction.

Miotic (my OT ik)   Any substance or medication that causes constriction of the pupil.

Mitosis (mie TOH sis)   A cell division process by which two daughter cells are formed from one parent cell; each daughter has a complete copy of parent's chromosomes.

Mnemonic (ni MON ik)   A learning device (e.g., an image, a rhyme, or a figure of speech) that a person uses to help him or her remember information.

Mock   Simulated; intended for imitation or practice.

Modalities (moe DAL i tees)   A therapeutic treatment for a disorder.

Modem (MOE duhm)   Peripheral computer hardware that connects to the router to provide internet access to the network or computer.

Mold   Growth of tiny fungi forming on a substance. Often looks downy or furry and is associated with dampness or decay.

Molecule   The simplest unit of a chemical compound that can exist, consisting of two or more atoms held together with chemical bonds.

Monocytes (MON uh site)   Agranulocyte that engulfs foreign particles, microorganisms, and cell debris.

Monotone (MON uh tohn)   A succession of syllables, words, or sentences spoken in an unvaried key or pitch.

Morale (muh RAL)   Emotional or mental condition with respect to cheerfulness or confidence.

Morals (MORE ahls)   Internal principles that distinguish between right and wrong.

Morbidity (more BID i tee)   The rate of a disease in a population.

Mortality (more TAL i tee)   The relative frequency of deaths in a specific population.

Mucous membrane   A mucus-producing membrane that lines tracts and structures of the body (e.g., GI tract, respiratory tract); also called *mucosa.*

Multiple-line telephone system   A business telephone system that allows for more than one telephone line.

Murmur   An abnormal sound heard during auscultation of the heart that may or may not have a pathologic origin; it is associated with valve disease or a congenital heart defect.

Myelin sheath (MIE uh lin sheeth)   A protective insulation that covers the axons and help with the transmission of nerve impulses.

Myocardium (mie oh KAR dee um)   The middle layer and the thickest layer of the heart; composed of cardiac muscles.

Myoglobin   Type of hemoglobin found in the muscle.

Myxedema (mick suh DEE mah)   Advanced hypothyroidism in adulthood.

Nasal wash   Also called a nasal aspirate. A syringe is used to gently squirt a small amount of sterile saline into the nose, and the resulting fluid is collected into a cup (for a wash). Or after the saline is squirted into the nose, gentle suction is applied (for the aspirate).

Nasopharyngeal (nae zoe fah RIN jee ahl) airway (NPA)   A soft flexible tube that is inserted in the nose and provides a patent airway; also known as a *nasal trumpet.*

National Provider Identifier (NPI)   An identifier assigned by the Centers for Medicare and Medicaid Services (CMS) that classifies the healthcare provider by license and medical specialties.

Necrosis (neh KROH sis)   Tissue death.

Negative feedback   An output or response that affects the input of a system.

Neglect   Failure to provide proper attention or care to another person.

Negligence (NEG li juhns)   Failure to act as a reasonably prudent person would under similar circumstances; such conduct falls below the standards of behavior established by law for the protection of others against unreasonable risk of harm.

Negotiable (ni GOH shee uh buhl) instrument   A document guaranteeing payment of a specific amount of money to the payer named on the document.

Nephrectomy   Surgical removal of a kidney.

Nephrotoxic   Damaging or destructive to the kidneys.

Net   The amount someone is paid after taxes and other deductions have been subtracted.

Neuralgia (noo RAL jah)   Sharp, spasm-like pain in a nerve or along the course of one or more nerves.

Neuropathy (nu ROP a thee)   A nervous system disorder of the peripheral nerves that causes discomfort, numbness, and weakness, especially in the extremities.

Neurotransmitter   A chemical that helps a nerve cell communicate with another nerve cell or muscle.

Nocturia (nok TOOR ee uh)   Frequent urination at night.

Nodules (NOJ ool)   Small lumps, lesions, or swellings that are felt when the skin is palpated.

Nomenclature (NOH muh n kley cher)   A system of names or terms, used in science and art to categorize items.

Nondecodable terms   Words used in healthcare whose definitions must be memorized without the benefit of word parts.

Noninvasive procedures   Procedures that do not penetrate human tissue.

Nonorganic (nahn or GAN ik)   Not having an organic or physiologic cause; a disorder that does not have a cause that can be found in the body.

Nonverbal communication   A type of communication that occurs through body language and expressive behaviors rather than with verbal or written words.

Normal flora   Microorganisms (mostly bacteria and yeast) that live on or in the body. Normal microscopic residents of the body.

No-show   Failure of a patient to keep an appointment without advance notice.

Nosocomial (nos uh KOH mee uh l)   Also known as Healthcare-Acquired Infections (HAI).

Nosocomial (nos uh KOH mee ul) infections   Infections acquired in a healthcare setting.

Notice of Privacy Practices (NPP)   A written document describing the healthcare facility's privacy practices. The patient must be provided with the NPP and sign an acknowledgment of receipt.

Nucleus   A specialized organelle of a cell that is encased in a membrane and directs growth, metabolism, and reproduction of the cell.

Numeric filing   The filing of records, correspondence, or cards by number.

Objective information   Data obtained through physical examination, laboratory and diagnostic testing, and by measurable information.

Obliteration (uh blit uh REY shun)   To remove or destroy all traces of; do away with; destroy completely.

Obturator (OB tuh rayt oar)   A metal rod with a smooth, rounded tip that is placed in hollow instruments to reduce injury to body tissues during insertion.

Occlude   To close, shut, or stop up.

Occult   Hidden or unseen.

Oncologist   A specially trained doctor who diagnoses and treats cancer.

Online insurance web portal   An online service provided by various insurance companies for providers to look up a patient's insurance benefits, eligibility, claims status, and explanation of benefits.

Oocyte (OO eh site)   An immature ovum (egg).

Oophorectomy (oo for ECK tuh mee)   Surgical removal of the ovaries.

Opaque (oh PAYK)   Not transparent; cloudy or murky.

Operating system   System software; it acts as the computer's software administrator by managing, integrating, and controlling application software and hardware. Windows is an example.

Organelles   Structures inside of a cell that perform specific functions.

Orientation   Awareness of one's environment, with reference to people, place, and time.

Orifice (ORE ih fis)   The vaginal opening.

Orthopnea (or THOP nee ah)   Condition of difficult breathing unless in an upright position.

Orthostatic (postural) hypotension   A temporary fall in blood pressure that occurs when a person rapidly changes from a recumbent position to a standing position.

Ossicles (OS i kahls)   The three small bones of the middle ear (malleus, incus, and stapes) that transmit sound vibrations from the eardrum to the inner ear.

Osteoblasts (OS tee oh blasts)   Bone-forming cells.

Osteoclasts (OS tee oh clasts)   Bone cells that break down bone.

Osteoporosis (os tee oh puh ROH sis)   Abnormal thinning of the bone structure causing bones to become brittle and weak.

Otitis externa   Inflammation or infection of the external auditory canal; commonly called *swimmer's ear.*

Otosclerosis (oh tuh skli ROH sis)   The ossicles of the middle ear (malleolus, incus, and stapes) become fused and act as a single unit instead of individual bones.

Ototoxic (oh tuh TOK sik)   A medicine or substance capable of damaging cranial nerve VIII or the organs of hearing and balance.

Out guides   Sturdy cardboard or plastic file-sized cards used to replace a folder temporarily removed from the filing space.

Output device   Computer hardware that displays the processed data from the computer (e.g., monitors and printers).

Overlearn   To learn or memorize beyond the point of proficiency or immediate recall.

Ovulation (OV yuh ley shun)   The release of the ovum from the ovarian follicle.

Packing slip   A document that accompanies purchased merchandise and shows what is in the box or package.

Palpation (PAL pey shuh n)   The use of touch during the physical examination to assess the size, consistency, and location of certain body parts.

Parameters (puh RAM it ers)   Rules that control how something should be done; guidelines or boundaries.

Paranasal sinuses (pair uh NAY zul SIE nus suhs)   Hollow, air-filled cavities in the skull and facial bones. They lighten the weight of the skull and increase the tone, or resonance, of speech.

Paraphrasing   Rewording a statement to check the meaning and interpretation; also shows you are listening and understanding the speaker.

Parasitic   Pertaining to a parasite (an organism that lives on or in another organism, known as the host). Benefits from the host; the host does not benefit from the parasite.

Parenteral (pa REN ter uh l)   Taken into the body by any route other than the digestive tract (e.g., subcutaneous, intravenous, or intramuscular administration).

Participating provider   A physician or other healthcare provider who enters into a contract with a specific insurance company or program and by doing so agrees to abide by certain rules and regulations set forth by that particular third-party payer.

Patency (PAT en see)   Open condition of a body cavity or canal.

Patent (PAT nt)   A grant from the government that gives a creator (or manufacturer) of an invention the sole right to produce, use, and sell the product for a set period of time.

Patent (PAY tent)   Open.

Pathogen   A disease-causing organism.

Pathogenic   Capable of producing disease.

Pathologic   Caused by or involving disease.

Pathologist (pah THOL uh jist)   A physician specially trained in the nature and cause of disease.

Pathology   Study of disease.

Patient abandonment   A form of medical malpractice, also called *negligent termination*; the provider ends the provider-patient relationship without reasonable or adequate notification.

Patient account   A running balance of all financial transactions for a specific patient.

Patient navigator   A person who identifies patients' needs and barriers; then assists by coordinating care and identifying community and healthcare resources to meet the needs. May also be called *care coordinator*.

Patient portal   A secure online website that gives patients 24-hour access to personal health information using a username and password.

Pegboard system   A manual bookkeeping system that uses a day sheet to record all financial transactions for the date of service and maintains patient account balances by using physical ledger cards.

Perceiving (per SEEV ing)   How an individual looks at information and sees it as real.

Percutaneous   Puncture through the skin.

Performance measurement   The regular collection of data to assess whether the correct processes are being performed and desired results are being achieved.

Perineal (pair ih NEE uhl)   Pertaining to the area between the vaginal opening and the rectum (perineum).

Perineum (pair ih NEE um)   The area between the opening of the vagina and the anus.

Peripheral (puh RIF er uhl)   Refers to an area outside of or away from an organ or structure.

Peripheral neuropathy (puh RIF er uh l noo ROP uh thee)   A problem with the function of the nerves outside the spinal cord; symptoms include weakness, burning pain, and loss of reflexes; a frequent complication of diabetes mellitus.

Peristalsis (payr i STAHL sis)   Wave-like movement from alternating contraction and relaxation of a tubular structure (e.g., intestine), which propels the content forward.

Peritoneum (per i tuh NEE um)   A serous membrane lining of the abdominal cavity, which folds inward to enclose the viscera (internal organs).

Peritubular capillaries (PER i too bu lar)   Blood capillaries surrounding the proximal and distal convoluted tubules in the kidneys.

Permeability (PUR mee ah bil i tee)   A quality or characteristic of a material that allows another substance to pass through it.

Permeable (PUR mee uh buhl)   Allowing for penetration.

Personal ethics   An individual's code of conduct.

Petechiae (pi TEEK kee uh)   Very small, round hemorrhage in the skin or mucous membrane.

Peyer patches (PEYH urh PACH ehs)   Small masses of lymphatic tissue found mostly in the ileum of the small intestine. They are an important part of the immune system, because they monitor intestinal bacteria populations and prevent the growth of pathogenic bacteria in the intestines.

Pharyngitis   Inflammation or infection of the pharynx, usually causing the symptoms of a sore throat.

Phenylalanine   An essential amino acid found in milk, eggs, and other foods.

Phenylketonuria (PKU)   A deficiency in the enzyme phenylalanine hydroxylase, which is responsible for converting phenylalanine into tyrosine.

Photophobia (foh toh FOH bee ah)   Extreme sensitivity to light.

Photosensitivity (FOE toe sen si TIV i tee)   Increase in the reactivity of the skin to sunlight or ultraviolet radiation.

Physiologic   Consistent with the normal function of the body.

Pineal gland   A small organ in the brain that secretes melatonin, a hormone that regulates the sleep/awake cycle.

Pipet (pie PET)   A slender tube attached to or including a bulb, for transferring or measuring small amounts of a liquid, often used in a laboratory.

Pitch   The depth of a tone or sound; a distinctive quality of sound.

Pitting edema   Excessive fluid in the intercellular spaces in the tissue; when external pressure (e.g., socks, finger pressure) is relieved, a depression is seen in the tissue.

Plaintiff (PLAIN tif)   An individual or party who brings a lawsuit to court.

Plaque   Sticky substance made of mucus, food particles, and bacteria that builds up on the exposed part of the tooth.

Plasma (PLAZ muh)   The liquid portion of a whole blood sample that has not clotted due to an anticoagulant. Liquid portion of blood that contains clotting factors. Liquid portion of the blood found in the body.

Plume   Vapor, smoke, and particle debris produced by laser procedures.

Pneumonia   Inflammation of the lungs with congestion of the air sacs (alveoli). Can be caused by a bacterium or virus.

Pocket face mask   A device used to deliver a rescue breath.

Point-of-care   Something designed to be used at or near where the patient is seen; point-of-care tools and apps are resources for the provider to use when working directly with the patient.

Poised (poizd)   Having a composed and self-assured manner.

Policy   A written agreement between two parties, in which one party (the insurance company) agrees to pay another party (the patient) if certain specified circumstances occur.

Polycythemia (pol ee sie THEE mee ah)   A disorder characterized by an abnormal increase in the number of red blood cells in the blood.

Pores   Tiny openings in the surface of the skin that allow gases, liquids, or microscopic particles to pass.

Portrait orientation   The most common layout for a printed page; the height of the paper is greater than its width.

Postherpetic neuralgia (noo RAL juh)   Nerve pain that occurs after a shingles outbreak and may become chronic.

Practice management software   A type of software that allows the user to enter demographic information, schedule appointments, maintain lists of insurance payers, perform billing tasks, and generate reports.

Preauthorization   A process required by some insurance carriers in which the provider obtains permission to perform certain procedures or services.

Precedence (PRES i dehns)   Followed first.

Precedent (PRES i dent)   A prior court decision that serves as a model for similar legal cases in the future.

Precertification   The process of determining if a procedure or service is covered by the insurance plan and what the reimbursement is for that procedure or service.

Precipitate (pri SIP i tate)   Solid particles that settle out of a liquid.

Preeclampsia (pree ih KLAMP see ah)   A form of toxemia during pregnancy, characterized by high blood pressure, fluid retention, and protein in the urine. May progress to eclampsia.

Preexisting condition   A health problem that was present before new health insurance coverage started.

Prefixes   Word parts that appear at the beginning of some terms.

Premium   The amount paid or to be paid by the policyholder for coverage under the contract, usually in periodic installments.

Privacy filters   Devices attached to the monitor that allow visualization of the screen contents only if the user is directly in front of the screen; also called *monitor filters* or *privacy screens*.

Privileged communication   Communication that cannot be disclosed without authorization of the person involved; includes provider-patient and lawyer-client communications.

Processing (prah CES ing)   How an individual internalizes new information and makes it his or her own.

Product   The number obtained by multiplying two or more numbers together.

Productive cough   A cough that produces phlegm or mucus.

Proficiency (pruh FISH uh n see)   Skilled as a result of training or practice.

Prognosis (prog NOH sis)   The likely outcome of a disease, including the chance of recovery.

Progress notes   Documentation in the paper health record that can be used to track the patient's condition and progress.

Prokaryote (proh KAR ee ote)   Any organism that is made up of at least one cell and has genetic material that is not enclosed in a nucleus. Bacteria are prokaryotes, primitive organisms.

Proofread   To read and mark corrections.

Protected health information (PHI)   Individually identifiable health information stored or transmitted by covered entities or business associates. Includes verbal, paper, or electronic information.

Protozoa (pro tuh ZOH ah)   Single-celled organisms that are the most primitive form of animal life. Most are microscopic. Examples are amoebas, ciliates, flagellates, and sporozoans.

Provider network   An approved list of physicians, hospitals, and other providers.

Provider Web portal   A secure online website that gives contracted providers a single point of access to insurance companies. This allows the provider to determine patient eligibility and deductible status, submit preauthorizations/precertifications, and check the status of claims.

Provider   An individual or company that provides medical care and services to a patient or the public.

Provisional diagnosis (dahy uh g NOH sis)   A temporary diagnosis made before all test results have been received.

Pruritus (proo RYE tuss)   Itching.

Psoriasis (sah RIE ah sis)   A usually chronic, recurrent skin disease marked by bright red patches covered with silvery scales.

Psychiatrists   Medical doctors who have been specially trained to diagnose and treat patients with mental, emotional, and behavioral conditions.

Psychotherapy (sie KOE ther ah pee) The treatment of behavioral health disorders through the use of psychological techniques, which encourage communication of conflicts and insights into the person's problems. The goals of this treatment include symptoms relief, changes in behavior leading to improved social and vocational function, and personality growth.

Psychotherapy notes Patient-provider details from private, group or family therapy, including what the patient stated and the provider's analysis of the statements and situation.

Puberty (PYOO bur tee) The stage of life in which males and females become functionally capable of sexual reproduction.

Pulmonary hypertension High blood pressure that affects the pulmonary system (pulmonary arteries and the right side of the heart).

Pulse deficit A condition in which the radial pulse is less than the apical pulse; it may indicate a peripheral vascular abnormality.

Pulse pressure The difference between the systolic and diastolic blood pressures (30 to 50 mm Hg is considered normal).

Purchase order number A unique number assigned by the ordering facility that allows the facility to track or reference the order.

Pure culture The growth of only one microorganism in a culture, or on a nutrient surface.

Purulent (PYOOR yoo lent) Pus like.

Pyemia (pahy EE mee uh) The presence of pus-forming organisms in the blood.

Pyrexia (pahy REK see uh) A febrile condition or fever.

Qualified Medicare Beneficiaries (QMBs) Low-income Medicare patients who qualify for Medicaid for their secondary insurance.

Quality control A process to ensure the reliability of test results, often using manufactured samples with known values.

Quantitative Describes a test result that is expressed as a number, usually with units of measure attached to numeric values.

Rales [rayls] An abnormal lung sound heard on auscultation, characterized by discontinuous bubbling noises.

Rapport (ra PORE) A relationship of harmony and accord between the patient and the healthcare professional.

Reagent (re-AY-jent) A substance for use in a chemical reaction.

Rebound pain Pain felt when the pressure on the abdomen is released.

Receptors Structures or sites on or in a cell that bind with substances such as hormones, antigens, or drugs.

Recommended dietary allowance (RDA) Average daily level of food intake needed to meet the nutrient requirements of most healthy people.

Reconciliation (rek uh n sill ee EY shuh n) To bring into agreement.

Reconciling Comparing a document with another document to ensure that they are consistent.

Reconstituted (ree KON sti toot ed) A dried substance (powder) that has been restored to a fluid form, so it can be injected.

Recovery position A position on the person's side that helps to keep the airway open and clear.

Referral An order from a primary care provider for the patient to see a specialist or to get certain medical services.

Referral laboratory A laboratory that performs testing for another laboratory. Testing varies from high-volume routine testing to low-volume unique or unusual testing. Also called reference,

diagnostic, or commercial testing laboratories. Often privately owned.

Reflecting Putting words to the patient's emotional reaction, which acknowledges the person's feelings.

Reflection (ree FLEK shun) The process of thinking about new information so as to create new ways of learning.

Reflexes Movements or processes caused by a reflex response; reflex is an automatic response that doesn't require thought.

Registered dietitian (die eh TISH an) A credentialed healthcare professional who is trained in nutrition and is able to apply the information to the dietary needs of healthy and ill patients.

Regular diet The food and drink a person typically consumes when there are no dietary limitations.

Reimbursement (ree im BURS ment) To make repayment for an expense or a loss incurred.

Relapse The recurrence of the symptoms of a disease after apparent recovery.

Release of information A form completed by the patient that authorizes the medical office to release medical records to the insurance company for health insurance reimbursement.

Reliable (ree LIE ah bul) Dependable, able to be trusted.

Remission The partial or complete disappearance of the clinical and subjective characteristics of a chronic or malignant disease.

Renal ischemia A blood flow deficiency to the kidney(s).

Renal threshold The blood level of a substance, above which the kidneys fail to reabsorb it, so the substance will appear in the urine.

Replication The production of exact copies of a complex molecule, such as DNA.

Res ipsa loquitur (RASE ipsah low kwah tuhr) Latin term meaning "the thing speaks for itself." A legal concept under which the plaintiff's burden to prove malpractice is minimal, since the jury can clearly understand the details of the injury. For example, a surgical instrument was left in the body during surgery.

Res judicata (RASE JOO di kah tah) Latin for "a thing decided." Once a case has been decided by the court, it cannot be litigated again.

Resection Surgical removal of all or part of an organ.

Resident A physician who has graduated from medical school and is finishing specialized clinical training.

Residual urine Urine that remains in the bladder after micturition or urination.

Resource-based relative value system (RBRVS) A system used to determine how much providers should be paid for services provided. It is used by Medicare and many other health insurance companies.

Respect Showing consideration or appreciation for another person.

Respiratory arrest Stoppage of breathing.

Respondeat superior (re SPON dee at soo PIR ee ahr) Latin for "let the master answer"; a legal doctrine by which the employer/provider is legally responsible for the wrongful actions or lack of actions of employees if done within the scope of employment.

Restock The process of replacing the supplies that were used.

Retaliation (ree tal ee A shuhn) Getting back at others for something they did to you.

Retention A term referring to actions taken by management to keep good employees.

Retention schedule   A method or plan for retaining or keeping health records and for their movement from active to inactive to closed.

Retractions (re TRAK shuns)   The sucking in of tissues between the intercostal spaces and neck due to respiratory distress; classic sign of severe asthma.

Retribution (reh trih BYOU shuhn)   Punishment inflicted on someone as vengeance for a wrong or criminal act; the act of taking revenge.

Revenue (REV eh noo)   Money collected for providing a product or service.

Reverse chronologic order   The most recent item is on top and the oldest item is last.

Review of systems   A list of questions related to each organ system, designed to uncover potential disease processes.

Rhonchi (RON kye)   An abnormal rumbling sound heard on auscultation, caused by airways blocked by secretions or muscle contractions.

Route   The means by which a drug enters the body.

Rugae (ROO gah)   Folds in the wall of the organ; when organ (e.g., stomach, bladder, uterus) fills or needs to expand, the rugae unfold.

Salary   A fixed compensation periodically paid to a person for regular work.

Salpingo-oophorectomy (sal ping goh oh of or EK toh mee)   Surgical removal of the fallopian tube and ovary.

Sanitize   The process of cleaning equipment and instruments with detergent and water in order to remove debris and reduce the number of microorganisms.

Sclera (SKLEER uh)   The white part of the eye that forms the orbit.

Scope of practice   Range of responsibilities and practice guidelines that determine the boundaries within which a healthcare worker practices.

Scored tablet   A tablet with a groove on the surface, used for splitting it in half.

Screen   A system for examining and separating into different groups; in the healthcare facility, it means determining the severity of illness that patients experience and prioritizing appointments based on that severity.

Screening   A system for examining and separating into different groups; in the healthcare facility, it means determining the severity of illness that patients experience, and prioritizing appointments based on that severity.

Seborrhea (seb uh REE ah)   An excessive discharge of sebum from the sebaceous glands, forming greasy scales or crusty areas on the body.

Secondary storage devices   Media (e.g., jump drive, flash drive, hard drive) capable of permanently storing data until they are replaced or deleted by the user.

Security risk analysis   Identification of potential threats of computer network breaches, for which action plans for corrective actions are instituted.

Sediment   An insoluble material that settles to the bottom of a liquid specimen and to the bottom of centrifuged sample.

Senescent (si NES ent) cell   An old or aging cell that can no longer divide and reproduce.

Sensorineural (sen suh ree NOOR uhl)   Involving the sensory nerves, especially as they affect hearing.

Sentinel node biopsy   Removal of a limited number of lymph nodes to determine if the cancer has spread to the lymph nodes.

Septicemia (sep tih SEE mee ah)   A systemic infection involving pathologic microbes in the blood as a result of an infection that has spread from elsewhere in the body.

Sequela (si KWEL uh) (singular), Sequelae (plural)   An abnormal condition resulting from a previous disease.

Serous (SEER uhs)   A thin, watery serum-like drainage.

Serum (SEER um)   The liquid portion of a clotted blood specimen. It no longer contains active clotting agents.

Shaken baby syndrome   Condition resulting from internal head injuries that occur when a baby or young child is violently shook.

Sharps   Medical term for devices with sharp points or edges that can puncture or cut skin. Examples include needles, scalpels, or broken glass.

Sickle cell anemia   An inherited anemia characterized by crescent-shaped red blood cells (RBCs). This causes RBCS to block capillaries, reducing the oxygen supply to the cells.

Side effects   Unpleasant effects of a drug in addition to the desired or therapeutic effect.

Signs   Objective findings determined by a clinician, such as a fever, hypertension, or rash.

Sinus arrhythmia   An irregular heartbeat that originates in the sinoatrial node (pacemaker).

Skill set   A person's abilities, skills, or expertise in an area.

Small claims court   A special court established to handle small claims or debts without the services of lawyers.

Software   A set of electronic instructions to operate and perform different computer tasks.

Solvent   A liquid that is able to dissolve other substances.

Solvent (SOL vuhnt)   Able to pay all debts.

Somatic cells (soe MAT ik)   Nonreproductive cells; they do not include sperm and egg cells.

Speakerphone   A telephone with a loudspeaker and a microphone; it can be used without having to pick up and hold the handset.

Special report   Additional medical documentation required to confirm the need for the use of unlisted, unusual, or newly adopted medical procedures code.

Specificity (spes i FIS i tee)   The quality or state of being specific.

Speed dialing   A telephone function in which a selected stored number can be dialed by pressing only one key.

Spermatozoa (spur mat ah ZOH ah) (singular, spermatozoon)   Mature male reproductive cells.

Sphincter (SFINGK ter)   A circular muscle that either constricts and closes the opening or relaxes and allows substances to pass through the opening.

Spina bifida (SPY nah BIF id dah)   A condition in which the spinal column has an abnormal opening that allows protrusion of the meninges and/or the spinal column.

Spore   A thick-walled, dormant form of bacteria that is very resistant to disinfection measures.

Stains   Reagents or dyes used to prepare specimens for microscopic examination.

Standard of care   The level and type of care an ordinary, prudent healthcare professional with the same training and experience in a similar practice would have provided under a similar situation.

Standard operating procedures (SOP)   A set of step-by-step instructions to help employees carry out routine operations efficiently, with high quality, and uniformity of performance.

Standard Precautions   A set of infection control practices used to prevent the transmission of diseases that can be acquired by contact with blood, body fluids, nonintact skin, and mucous membranes.

STAT   The medical abbreviation for the Latin term *statum*, meaning immediately; at this moment.

Static (STAT ik) equilibrium   Relating to balance when moving in a straight line.

Stem cells   Undifferentiated cells that can become specialized cells in the body.

Stenosis (sten OH sis)   Occurs when the heart valve flaps are stiff or fused together, thus narrowing the valve.

Sterile (STER il)   Free of all microorganisms, pathogenic and nonpathogenic.

Sterilize   The process of removing all microorganisms.

Stertorous (STUR ter uhs)   Heavy, as related to snoring.

Stoma (STOH mah)   A temporary or permanent surgically created opening used for drainage (i.e., urine, stool).

Strata   Naturally or artificially formed layers of material, usually multiple layers.

Stretch receptor   A sensory nerve ending that responds to a stretch stimulus.

Stylus (STI luhs)   A metal probe that is inserted into or passed through a catheter, needle, or tube used for clearing purposes or to facilitate passage into a body orifice.

Stylus (STI luhs)   A pen-shaped device with a variety of tips that is used on touchscreens to write, draw, or input commands.

Subcultured   Occurs when an organism (a bacterium) has been cultivated again on a new nutrient surface.

Subjective information   Data or information obtained from the patient, including the patient's feelings, perceptions, and concerns; obtained through interview or questions.

Subpoena (suh PEE nuh)   A court order requiring a person to appear in court at a specific time to testify in a legal case.

Subpoena duces tecum (suh PEE nuh DOO seez TEE kuhm)   A legal document commanding a person to bring a piece of evidence (such as the plaintiff's health record) to court.

Subsequent (SUHB si kwuhnt)   Occurring later or after.

Suction (SUHK shun)   The production of a partial vacuum by the removal of air in order to force fluid into a vacant space.

Suffixes   Word parts that appear at the end of some terms.

Sulci (SUL sie)   Grooves or depressions on the surface of the brain between the gyri. **Sulcus (SUL kus)** is the singular form.

Summarizing   Allowing the listener to recap and review what was said.

Supernatant   The clear liquid above the sediment in a centrifuged urine specimen.

Suppurative (SUHP yuh ray tiv)   Characterized by the formation and/or discharge of pus.

Surfactant (sur FACK tunt)   A mixture of protein and fats that lines the alveoli and prevents the tissues from sticking together and collapsing during exhalation.

Surrogate (SUR ah git)   A person who acts on behalf of another person or takes the place of another person. Examples include a surrogate mother or a healthcare agent.

Symmetry (SIM ih tree)   Similarity in size, form, and arrangement of parts on opposite sides of the body.

Symptoms   Subjective complaints reported by the patient, such as pain or nausea.

Synapse (SIN aps)   A point of communication between two cells.

Syncope (SING kuh pee)   Fainting; a brief lapse in consciousness.

Synthesis (SIN theh sis)   Formation of a chemical compound from simpler compounds or elements.

Syringe (suh RINJ)   A device with a slender barrel and needle used to withdraw blood from a vein or artery.

Systemic   Affecting the entire body.

Tachycardia (tak i KAHR dee uh)   A rapid but regular heart rate; one that exceeds 100 beats per minute.

Tachypnea (tack ip NEE ah)   Rapid, shallow breathing.

Tactful   The quality of having a sense of what to do or say to maintain good relations with others or to prevent offense.

Target cells   A cell selectively affected by a specific agent, such as a drug, hormone, or virus.

Target tissue   The destination, or intended tissue in the nervous impulse (e.g., a muscle).

Telehealth   Refers to remote clinical services and nonclinical services, such as provider training, meetings, and continuing education.

Telemedicine (TEL i med i sin)   The use of telecommunication technology to provide healthcare services to patients at a distance; it is usually used in rural communities.

Template (TEM plit)   A document or file that has a preset format; used as a starting point when composing something and saves from recreating it each time it is used.

Tendons   (TEN duns) Connective tissue that attaches muscles to bone.

Termination letters   Documents sent to patients explaining that the provider is ending the physician-patient relationship and the patients need to see other providers.

Testis (TES tis) (plural, testes)   The male gonad, also called a **testicle** (TESS tick kul).

Testosterone (tess TOSS tur rohn)   Male sex hormone produced by the interstitial cells in the testes.

Thalamus (THAL uh muh s)   The middle part of the brain through which sensory impulses pass to reach the cerebral cortex.

Therapeutic range   Is reached when the blood concentration of a medication is high enough for the therapeutic effect to occur.

Third-party administrator (TPA)   An organization that processes claims and provides administrative services for another organization. Often used by self-funded plans.

Thoracentesis (thor ah sen TEE sis)   Aspiration of a fluid from the pleural cavity.

Thready   Describes a pulse that is thin and feeble.

Thrombus (THRAHM bus)   A blood clot that blocks the flow of blood.

Tickler file   A chronologic file used as a reminder that something must be dealt with on a certain date.

Tinea (TIN ee uh)   Any fungal skin disease that results in scaling, itching, and inflammation; examples include ringworm and athlete's foot.

Tinnitus (TIN it uh s)   A noise sensation of ringing heard in one or both ears.

Tissue culture   The technique or process of keeping tissue alive and growing in a culture medium.

Tonometer (toh NOM i ter)   An instrument used to measure intraocular pressure.

Tort   A civil wrongdoing that causes harm to a person or property; excludes breach of contract.

Tortfeasor (TORTE fee zahr)   The individual or entity who committed the tort, either intentionally or as a result of negligence.

Toxicity   The harmful and deadly effect of a medication that can develop due to the buildup of medication or by-products in the body.

Toxicology (tok si KOL oh jee)   The study and science dealing with the effects, antidotes, and detection of poisons or drugs.

Toxins   Substances created by microorganisms, plants, or animals and poisonous to humans.

Tract   A system of tissues (e.g., neuronal axons) and/or organs (e.g., intestines) that function together.

Transcription (tran SKRIP shuh n)   To make a written copy of dictated material.

Transient (TRAN zee uhnt)   Not lasting, enduring or permanent; transitory.

Transillumination (trans i LOO muh ney shun)   Inspection of a cavity or organ by passing light through its walls.

Transitional epithelium   A type of cell found in the lining of hollow organs. It has the ability to stretch with the contraction and distention of the organ.

Transmission   The passage or spread disease.

Transport medium   A medium used to keep an organism alive during transport to the laboratory.

Trauma (TRAW muh)   A physical injury or wound caused by external force or violence.

Triage (tree AHZH)   The process of sorting patients to determine medical need and the priority of care.

Triaging flow map   A written flow map to make triage decisions; based on answers to questions, the person moves through the map until a triage decision is made.

Tripod position   The standing position when using crutches; crutch tips are 4 to 6 inches to the side and front of each foot.

Trustee   The coordinator of financial resources assigned by the court during a bankruptcy case.

Turgor (TUR ger)   Referring to normal skin tension; the resistance of the skin to being grasped between the fingers and released. Turgor decreases with dehydration and increases with edema.

Unipolar   Having one pole or electrical charge.

Unit dose packaging   A packaging method for drugs; holds a specified quantity of medication in a single-use container (e.g., syringe, blister pack).

Unsecured debt   Debt that is not guaranteed by something of value; credit card debt is the most common type of unsecured debt.

Urgent   An acute situation that requires immediate attention but is not life-threatening.

Urostomy (yoo ROS te mee)   A surgically created opening on the abdominal wall used to drain urine.

Urticaria (ur ti KAYR ee ah)   Hives.

Utilization management   A decision-making process used by managed care organizations to manage healthcare costs. It involves case-by-case assessments of the appropriateness of care.

Vascular (VAS kyuh ler)   Having vessels that conduct or circulate liquids (blood).

Vascular access   A surgical procedure that creates a vein to remove and return blood during the hemodialysis procedure.

Vasoconstriction (vas oh kuhn STRIK shuhn)   Contraction of muscles, causing the narrowing of the inside tube of the vessel.

Vectors   Animals or insects (e.g., ticks, rodents, mosquitos) that transmit a pathogen.

Vendors   Companies that sell supplies, equipment, or services to other companies or individuals.

Venule (VEN yuhl)   A very small vein.

Verification of eligibility   The process of confirming health insurance coverage for the patient.

Vertebrae (VUR teh bray)   A series of small, irregular-shaped bones that form the spine. Each vertebra has several projections, joint surfaces, areas for muscle attachment, and a hole where the spinal cord passes.

Vertigo (VER ti goe)   Dizziness; an abnormal sensation of movement when there is none.

Vested   Granted or endowed with a particular authority, right, or property; to have a special interest in.

Viability (vie a BIL ih tee)   The ability to live.

Vigilance (VIJ uh lahns)   Keen watchfulness to detect danger.

Viscosity (vi SKOS I tee)   Resistance to flow; the thicker the liquid, the higher the viscosity.

Voice mail   An electronic system that allows messages from telephone callers to be recorded and stored.

Waiting period   The length of time a patient waits for disability insurance to pay after the date of injury.

Water deprivation test   A test to measure the amount and concentration of urine produced when water is withheld from a patient for a period of time.

Wet mount   A glass slide that holds a specimen suspended in a drop of liquid for microscopic examination.

Wheezing (WHEE zeeng)   Whistling sound made during breathing.

Whistleblower   A person (usually an employee) who reports a violation of the law within the organization. The person reports the information to the public or to a person in authority.

Workplace emergencies   Unforeseen situations that threaten employees and visitors; can disrupt services provided.

Yeast   Any various single-celled fungi, which reproduce by budding and are able to ferment sugars.

Zone   A region or geographic area used for shipping.

ABBREVIATIONS

%TBSA percent of total burn surface area
°C Celsius
(D)HHS Department of Health and Human Services
°F Fahrenheit
s̄ without
3D three-dimensional
A
A&Ox3 alert and oriented to person, place, and time
A/P accounts payable
A/R accounts receivable
A1c glycated hemoglobin
aa of each (used in prescriptions)
AAA abdominal aortic aneurysm
AAFP American Academy of Family Physicians
AAMA American Association of Medical Assistants
AAMT American Association for Medical Transcriptions
AAP American Academy of Pediatrics
AAT alpha-1 antitrypsin
ABG arterial blood gas
ABHES Accrediting Bureau of Health Education Schools
ac before meals
ACA The Affordable Care Act
ACE inhibitor angiotensin converting enzyme inhibitor
Ach acetylcholine
ACL anterior cruciate ligament
ACTH adrenocorticotropic hormone
AD Alzheimer's disease
ad lib as desired
ADA Americans with Disabilities Act
ADA American Diabetes Association
ADAAA Americans with Disabilities Act Amendment Act
ADF scanner automatic document feeder
ADH antidiuretic hormone
ADHD attention deficit hyperactivity disorder
ADLs activities of daily living
ADR alternative dispute resolution
AED automated external defibrillator
AFB acid-fast bacilli
AFP alpha-fetoprotein
AgNO₃ silver nitrate
AHA American Heart Association
AHRQ Agency for Healthcare Research and Quality
AIDS acquired immunodeficiency syndrome
AK astigmatic keratotomy
ALL acute lymphocytic leukemia
ALP alkaline phosphatase
ALS amyotrophic lateral sclerosis
ALT alanine aminotransferase
AM, a.m. morning
AMA American Medical Association
AML acute myeloid leukemia

AML acute myelogenous leukemia
AMT American Medical Technologists
ANA antinuclear antibody test
ANLL acute myeloid leukemia
ANS autonomic nervous system
Anti-CCP anti-cyclin citrullinated peptide
AP Anteroposterior
APAP acetaminophen
APRN advanced practice registered nurse
aq water
ARB angiotensin II receptor blocker
ART assistive reproductive technology
ARV antiretroviral
ASA aspirin
ASA The Anesthesia Society of America
ASCP American Society of Clinical Pathologists
ASD atrial septal defect
ASD autism spectrum disorder
AST aspartate aminotransferase
ATP adenosine triphosphate
AUD alcohol use disorder
AV atrioventricular
aV augmented voltage
B
BAP blood agar plate
BBB blood-brain barrier
BBPS bloodborne pathogen standard
BCG bacille Calmette-Guérin
BD Blu-Ray disc
beta-hCG beta human chorionic gonadotropin
bid twice a day
BLS basic life support
BMI body mass index
BMR basal metabolic rate
BOO bladder outlet obstruction
BP blood pressure
BPD bronchopulmonary dysplasia
BPH benign prostatic hyperplasia
BSE breast self-examination
BTL bottle
BUN blood urea nitrogen
BX box
C
c̄ with
C Celsius
c centi
C&S culture and sensitivity
Ca calcium
CAAHEP Commission on Accreditation of Allied Health Education Programs
CABG coronary artery bypass graft

CAD coronary artery disease
CAM complementary and alternative medicine
cap capsule
CAP College of American Pathologists
CAPTA Child Abuse Prevention and Treatment Act
CARD check, assign, reverse, define
CAT computerized axial tomography
CBC complete blood count
CBT cognitive behavioral therapist
CC chief complaint
cc cubic centimeter
CCB calcium channel blocker
CCK cholecystokinin
CCMA certified clinical medical assistant
CCMS clean-catch midstream urine
CD collecting duct
CD compact disc
CD conduct disorder
CDC Centers for Disease Control and Prevention
CEJA Council of Ethical and Judicial Affairs
CEU continuing education unit
CF cystic fibrosis
cfu colony-forming units
CHAMPVA Civilian Health and Medical Program of the Department of Veterans Affairs
CHD coronary heart disease
CHF congestive heart failure
CHIP Children's Health Insurance Program
Chol cholesterol
CIS clinically isolated syndrome
CK creatine kinase
CKD chronic kidney disease
CK-MB creatine kinase-MB
Cl chloride
CLIA Clinical Laboratory Improvement Amendments
CLL chronic lymphocytic leukemia
CLS clinical laboratory scientist
CLSI Clinical and Laboratory Standards Institute
CLT clinical laboratory technician/technologist
cm centimeter
CMA certified medical assistant
CML chronic myeloid leukemia
CMLA certified medical laboratory assistant
CMP comprehensive metabolic profile
CMPs civil monetary penalties
CMS Centers for Medicare and Medicaid Services
CNM certified nurse midwife
CNS central nervous system
CNS clinical nurse specialist
CO₂ carbon dioxide
COPD chronic obstructive pulmonary disease
COW computer on wheels
CoW certificate of waiver
CPAP continuous positive airway pressure
CPK creatinine phosphokinase
CPOE computerized provider/physician order entry
CPR cardiopulmonary resuscitation

CPT current procedural terminology
CPT certified phlebotomy technician
CPU central processing unit
Creat creatinine
CRNA certified registered nurse anesthetist
CRP C-reactive protein
CS case
CSF cerebrospinal fluid
CSMT color, sensation, motion, and temperature
CT computed tomography
CTA computerized tomography angiography
CVA cerebrovascular accident
CVS cyclic vomiting syndrome
CVS chorionic villus sampling
CWP coal workers' pneumoconiosis
CXR chest x-ray
D
d day
DAP test draw-a-person test
DASH Dietary Approaches to Stop Hypertension
DBS deep brain stimulation
DBT dialectical behavioral therapy
DC Doctor of Chiropractic
DCT distal (convoluted) tubule
DDL digital data loggers
DEA Drug Enforcement Agency
DEA Drug Enforcement Administration
DHE dihydroergotamine
DI diabetes insipidus
DJD degenerative joint disease
DKA diabetic ketoacidosis
DM diabetes mellitus
DMARDs disease-modifying antirheumatic drugs
DNA deoxyribonucleic acid
DNR do not resuscitate
DO Doctor of Osteopathy
DOB date of birth
DRE digital rectal exam
DSL modem digital subscriber line modem
DSM Diagnostic and Statistical Manual of Mental Disorders
DTP diphtheria-tetanus-pertussis
DUB dysfunctional uterine bleeding
DV daily value
DVD digital versatile/video disc
DVT deep vein thrombosis
E
E/M evaluation and management
EA each
EAP employee assistance program
EBV Epstein-Barr virus
ECG electrocardiogram
ECHO echocardiography
ED emergency department
ED erectile dysfunction
EDTA ethylenediaminetetraacetic acid
EEG electroencephalography
EFT electronic funds transfers

EGD   esophagogastroduodenoscopy
EHR   electronic health record
EIA   enzyme immunoassay
EIN   employer identification number
EKG   electrocardiogram
ELISA   enzyme-linked immunosorbent assay
EM   erythema migrans (sometimes called erythema chronicum migrans)
EMDR   eye movement desensitization and reprocessing
EMG   electromyography
EMG   emergency
EMG   electromyography
EMR   electronic medical record
EMS   emergency medical services
EMTs   emergency medical technicians
ENT   ear, nose, throat
EOB   explanation of benefits
EOM   extraocular movement
EP   established patient
EPA   Environmental Protection Agency
EPDS   Edinburgh Postnatal Depression Scale
ePHI   electronic protected health information
EPO   exclusive provider organization
EPS   electrophysiology study
EPSDT   early and periodic screening, diagnosis, and treatment
ER   endoplasmic reticulum
ERCP   endoscopic retrograde cholangiopancreatography
ERV   expiratory reserve volume
ESR   erythrocyte sedimentation rate
ESRD   end-stage renal disease
ESU   electrosurgical unit
ESWL   extracorporeal shock wave lithotripsy
ET   endotracheal
F
F   Fahrenheit
FAERS   FDA adverse event reporting system
FBG   fasting blood glucose
FBS   fasting blood sugar
FDA   Food and Drug Administration
Fe   iron
FECA   Federal Employees Compensation Act
FEV₁   forced expiratory volume in 1 second
FH   family history
FIT   fecal Immunochemical test
fl oz   fluid ounce
FOB   fecal occult blood
FOBT   fecal occult blood test
FRC   functional residual capacity
FSH   follicle-stimulating hormone
FTC   Federal Trade Commission
FUO   fever of unknown origin
FVC   forced vital capacity
G
g   gram
G   gauge
GAD   generalized anxiety disorder
GAS   general adaptation syndrome
GAS   group A streptococcus

GB   gigabyte
GER   gastroesophageal reflux
GERD   gastroesophageal reflux disease
gFOBT   guaiac fecal occult blood test
GGT   gamma glutamyl transferase
GH   growth hormone
GHRL   ghrelin
GI   gastrointestinal
GI   glycemic index
GINA   Genetic Information Nondiscrimination Act
GMOs   genetically modified organisms
GNB   Gram negative bacilli
GN-RH   gonadotropin-releasing hormone
GPC   Gram positive cocci
GPOs   group purchasing organizations
gr   grain
GTT   glucose tolerance test
gtt(s)   drop(s)
H
H&H   hemoglobin and hematocrit
H&P   history and physical
h, hr   hour
H⁺   hydrogen
HAV   hepatitis A virus
HAV   hepatitis A virus
HbA1C or A1C   glycosylated hemoglobin
HBV   hepatitis B virus
hCG   human chorionic gonadotropin
HCPCS   Healthcare Common Procedure Coding System
HCS   hazard communication standard
HCT   hematocrit
HCV   hepatitis C virus
HD   hoarding disorder
HD   Huntington's disease
HDD   hard disk drive
HDL   high-density lipoprotein
HDN   hemolytic disease of the newborn
HDV   hepatitis D virus
HEV   hepatitis E virus
Hgb   hemoglobin
HHR   hybrid health record
HHS   Department of Health and Human Services
HIDA scan   hepatobiliary iminodiacetic acid scan
HIE   health information exchange
HIPAA   Health Insurance Portability and Accountability Act
HITECH   Health Information Technology for Economic and Clinical Health Act
HIV   human immunodeficiency virus
HMIS   hazardous materials information system
HMO   health maintenance organization
HPI   health plan identifier
HPI   history of present illness
HPV   human papilloma virus
HRT   hormone replacement therapy
HSV   herpes simplex virus
HSV-1   herpes simplex virus-1
HZV   herpes zoster vaccine

I

I&D incision and drainage

IAPS International Academy of Phlebotomy Sciences

IBD inflammatory bowel disease

IBS irritable bowel syndrome

IC inspiratory capacity

IC interstitial cystitis

ICD implantable cardioverter defibrillator

ICD International Classification of Disease

ICD-10-CM *International Classification of Diseases, 10th revision, Clinical Modification*

ICP intracranial pressure

ICS intercostal space

ID identification

ID intradermal

IDS integrated delivery system

IE infective endocarditis

IFA immunofluorescence assay

iFOBT immunochemical fecal occult blood test

Ig Immunoglobulin

IM intramuscular

INR international normalized ratio

IOL intraocular lens

IPA independent practice associations

IPAA ileal pouch-anal anastomosis

IPT interpersonal psychotherapy

IQ intelligent quotient

IRV inspiratory reserve volume

ISCLT International Society of Clinical Laboratory Technology

ISP internet service provider

IT information technology

ITP idiopathic thrombocytopenic purpura

IUD intrauterine device

IUFD intrauterine fetal death

IUI intrauterine insemination

IV intravenous

IVIg intravenous immunoglobulin

IVP intravenous pyelogram

J

JA juvenile arthritis

JIA juvenile idiopathic arthritis

K

K potassium

k kilo

KB kilobyte

kg kilogram

KOH potassium hydroxide

KS Kaposi sarcoma

L

L liter

LA left arm

LAGB laparoscopic adjustable gastric band

LAN local area network

LASIK laser-assisted in-situ keratomileusis

lb pound

LCD monitor liquid crystal display monitor

LCL lateral collateral ligament

LCSW licensed clinical social worker

LDH lactate dehydrogenase

LDL low-density lipoprotein

LED light-emitting diodes

LEEP loop electrosurgical excision procedure

LES lower esophageal sphincter

LH luteinizing hormone

LICSW license independent clinical social worker

LL left leg

LLQ left lower quadrant

LP lumbar puncture

LPN licensed practical nurse

LSW licensed social worker

LUQ left upper quadrant

M

m meter

m milli

MA medical assistant

MAC Mycobacterium avium complex

MB megabyte

mc micro

mcg microgram

MCH mean cell hemoglobin

MCHC mean cell ratio of hemoglobin and hematocrit

MCL medial collateral ligament

MCO managed care organization

MCV mean cell volume

MD doctor of medicine

MD muscular dystrophy

MDI metered-dose inhaler

med medicine

mg milligram

MGUS monoclonal gammopathy of undetermined significance

mHealth mobile health

MI myocardial infarction

min minute

mL milliliter

mL milliliter

MLA medical laboratory assistant

MLT medical laboratory technician

mm millimeter

MMPI Minnesota Multiphasic Personality Inventory

MMR measles-mumps-rubella

MOM milk of magnesia

Mono infectious mononucleosis

MPM medical practice management

MRA magnetic resonance angiography

MRI magnetic resonance imaging

MS musculoskeletal system

MS multiple sclerosis

MSAFP maternal serum alpha-fetoprotein (test)

MT medical technologist

MT-sDNA multi-targeted stool DNA (test)

MUGA multiple-gated acquisition

MVD coronary microvascular disease

MVV maximum voluntary ventilation

MY myopia

N

Na   sodium

NAFLD   nonalcoholic fatty liver disease

NAS   nasal

NCA   National Certification Agency

NCA   National Certification Agency for Medical Laboratory
Personnel

NCCI   National Corrective Coding Initiative

NCCT   National Center for Competency Testing

NCMA   National Certified Medical Assistant

NCQA   National Committee for Quality Assurance

NCV   nerve conduction velocity

NCVIA   The National Childhood Vaccine Injury Act

NDC   National Drug Code

NH₃   ammonia

NHA   National Healthcareer Association

NHI   National Institutes of Health

NIDA   National Institute on Drug Abuse

NIH   National Institutes of Health

NK   natural killer

NKA   no known allergies

NKDA   no known drug allergies

nm   nanometer

NMJ   neuromuscular junction

noc, noct   night

NOTA   National Organ Transplant Act

NP   new patient

NP   nurse practitioner

NPA   National Phlebotomy Association

NPI   national provider identifier

NPO   nothing by mouth

NPP   notice of privacy practices

NS   normal saline

NSAID   nonsteroidal anti-inflammatory drug

NTM   nontuberculous mycobacteria

NUCC   National Uniform Claim Committee

O

O&P   ova and parasite

O₂   oxygen

OA   osteoarthritis

OAE   otoacoustic emission

OB/GYN   obstetrics and gynecology

OCD   obsessive-compulsive disorder

OCP   oral contraceptive pills

OCR   Office for Civil Rights

OCR   optical character recognition

ODD   oppositional defiant disorder

OGTT   oral glucose tolerance test

OMT   osteopathic manipulative therapy

ONC   The Office of the National Coordinator for Health
Information Technology

OPIM   other potentially infectious materials

OPTN   Organ Procurement and Transplant Network

ORIF   open reduction and internal fixation

OSA   obstructive sleep apnea

OSH Act   Occupational Safety and Health Act

OSHA   Occupational Safety and Health Administration

OT   oxytocin

OTC   over-the-counter (drugs)

OUI   operating under the influence

OWI   operating while intoxicated

oz   ounce

P

p̄   after

P   phosphorus

PA   physician assistant

PA   posteroanterior

PA-C   physician assistant-certified

PACs   premature atrial contractions

PAD   peripheral artery disease

PAP   Papanicolaou

PAR   participating provider

PBGs   physician buying groups

PBS   painful bladder syndrome

PBS   prune belly syndrome

pc   after meals

PC   personal computer

PCL   posterior cruciate ligament

PCMH   patient-centered medical home

PCP   primary care provider

PCT   proximal (convoluted) tubule

PCV13   13-valent pneumococcal conjugate vaccine

PD   Parkinson's disease

PDA   patent ductus arteriosus

PDD   pervasive developmental disorder

PDR   proliferative diabetic retinopathy

PDR   Physician Desk Reference

PDT   photodynamic therapy

PE   pulmonary embolism

PEP   post-exposure prophylaxis

PET   positron emission tomography

PFO   patent foramen ovale

PG   peptidoglycan

PH   pulmonary hypertension

PH   past history

PHI   protected health information

PHQ-2   Patient Health Questionnaire-2

PHQ-9   Patient Health Questionnaire-9

PHR   personal health record

PID   pelvic inflammatory disease

PIN   personal identification number

PKD   polycystic kidney disease

PKG   package

PKU   phenylketonuria

PLMD   periodic limb movement disorder

PM, p.m.   afternoon

PMDD   premenstrual dysphoric disorder

PMH   past medical history

PMN   polymorphonucleocyte

PMS   practice management software

PMS   premenstrual syndrome

PNL   percutaneous nephrolithotripsy

PNS   peripheral nervous system

PO   purchase order

po   oral (route)

po, PO   by mouth

POCT   point-of-care testing

POL   physician office laboratory

POLST   Physician Orders for Life-Sustaining Treatment

POR   problem-oriented record

POS   place of service

POS   point-of-sale

POTS   postural orthostatic tachycardia syndrome

PPD   purified protein derivative (tuberculin skin test)

PPD   prepaid

PPD   purified protein derivative

PPD   postpartum depression

PPE   personal protective equipment

PPI   proton pump inhibitor

PPM(P)   provider-performed microscopy (procedures)

PPMS   primary progressive multiple sclerosis

PPO   preferred provider organizations

PPP   2-hour postprandial urine specimen

PPSA   Physician Payments Sunshine Act

PPSV23 or PPSV   23-valent pneumococcal polysaccharide vaccine

PRL   prolactin

prn   as needed

PSA   prostate-specific antigen

PSDA   Patient Self-Determination Act

PSI   pounds per square inch

PST   plasma separator tubes

PT   prothrombin time

pt   pint

PT   protime

Pt, pt   patient

PTH   parathyroid hormone

PTSD   post-traumatic stress disorder

PTT   partial thromboplastin time

PTT   activated partial thromboplastin time

PTT   partial thromboplastin time

PUVA   psoralen plus ultraviolet A

PVCs   premature ventricular contractions

PYMT   payment

Q

q2h   every 2 hours

q3h   every 3 hours

q4h   every 4 hours

q6h   every 6 hours

q8h   every 8 hours

QA   quality assurance

qam   every morning

QC   quality control

QFT   QuantiFERON-TB

QFT-GIT   QuantiFERON-TB Gold In-Tube

qh   every hour

qid   four times a day

QMBs   qualified Medicare beneficiaries

qs   quantity sufficient

qt   quart

QTY   quantity

R

RA   remittance advice

RA   right arm

RA   rheumatoid arthritis

RAAS   renin-angiotensin aldosterone system

RAIU   radioactive iodine uptake

RAM   random access memory

RBC   red blood cell

RBRVS   resource-based relative value system

RCC   renal cell carcinoma

RDS   respiratory distress syndrome

REM   rapid eye movement

RF   rheumatoid factor

RICE   rest, ice, compression, and elevation

RL   right leg

RLQ   right lower quadrant

RLS   restless leg syndrome

RLS/WED   restless legs syndrome/Willis-Ekborn disease

RMA   registered medical assistant

RMT   registered medical technician

RN   registered Nurse

RNA   ribonucleic acid

ROM   range of motion

ROM   read-only memory

ROS   review of systems

RPM   remote patient monitoring

RPM   revolutions per minute

RRMS   relapsing-remitting multiple sclerosis

RSV   respiratory syncytial virus

RUQ   Right upper quadrant

RV   residual volume

RVG   relative value guide

RW   read/write

Rx   take

S

SA node   sinoatrial node

SA   sinoatrial

SAFER   Safety Assurance Factors for EHR Resilience

SAMHSA   Substance Abuse and Mental Health Services Administration

SBS   shaken baby syndrome

SDS   safety data sheet

SH   social history

SI   Système International

SIBO   small intestinal bacterial overgrowth

SIDS   sudden infant death syndrome

Sig   give the following directions

SL   semilunar

SL   sublingual

SLADH   syndrome of inappropriate antidiuretic hormone

SLE   systemic lupus erythematosus

SNRI   serotonin and norepinephrine reuptake inhibitor

SOB   shortness of breath

sol, soln   solution

SOP   standard operating procedure

SOR   source-oriented record

SPECT   single-photon emission computerized tomography

SPMS   secondary progressive multiple sclerosis
SpO₂   pulse oximetry
SR   systems review
SS   symptom severity (score)
SSD   solid-state disk or drive
SSN   Social Security number
SSRI   selective serotonin reuptake inhibitors
SST   serum separator tubes
STAT   immediately
STI   sexually transmitted infection
subcut   subcutaneous
T
T₃   triiodothyronine
T₄   thyroxine
tab(s)   tablet(s)
TAT   thematic apperception test
TB   terabyte
TB   tuberculosis
TB   total bilirubin
TBI   traumatic brain injury
Tbs, tbsp   tablespoon
TC   total cholesterol
Td   tetanus and diphtheria
Tdap   tetanus-diphtheria-pertussis (vaccine)
TEE   transesophageal echocardiogram
TENS   transcutaneous electrical nerve stimulation
TFT   thyroid function test
TIA   transient ischemic attack
TIBC   total iron-binding capacity
tid   three times a day
TILA   Truth in Lending Act
TIM   topical immunomodulators
tinct   tincture
TLC   total lung capacity
TM   tympanic membrane
TNF   tumor-necrosis factor
TNM   tumor, number of lymph nodes, metastasized
TOF   tetralogy of Fallot
TP   total protein
TPA   third-party administrator
TPR   temperature, pulse, respirations
TRH   thyrotropin-releasing hormone
Trig   triglyceride
TSE   testicular self-exam
TSE   testicular self-examination
TSH   thyroid-stimulating hormone
tsp   teaspoon
T-Spot   T-SPOT *TB* (test)

TST   tuberculin skin test
TTE   transthoracic echocardiogram
TTM   transtelephonic monitor
TURP   transurethral resection of the prostate
TV   tidal volume
U
UA   urinalysis or uric acid
UAGA   Uniform Anatomical Gift Act
UCD or UCHD   usual childhood diseases
UCR   usual, customary, and reasonable
UDDA   Uniform Determination of Death Act
UES   upper esophageal sphincter
UGI   upper gastrointestinal
ung   ointment
UNHS   universal newborn hearing screening test
UPJ   ureteropelvic junction
US   ultrasound
USAN   U.S. adopted name (council)
USB   universal serial bus
USDA   U.S. Department of Agriculture
USMLE   U.S. Medical Licensing Examination
USP-NP   U.S. Pharmacopeia and the National Formulary
USPS   U.S. Postal Service
UTI   urinary tract infection
UV   ultraviolet
V
VA   visual acuity
VAERS   vaccine adverse event reporting system
VC   vital capacity
V-fib   ventricular fibrillation
VICP   Vaccine Injury Compensation Program
VIS   vaccine information statement
VLDL   very low-density lipids
VO   verbal order
VQ scan   lung ventilation/perfusion scan
VS   vital signs
VSD   ventricular septal defect
V-tach   ventricular tachycardia
VUR   vesicoureteral reflux
W
WAIS   Wechsler Adult Intelligent Scale
WAN   wide area network
WBC   white blood cell
WHO   World Health Organization
WOW   workstation on wheels
WPI   widespread pain index (score)
X
x   times

INDEX

Page numbers followed by "*f*" indicate figures, "*t*" indicate tables, and "*b*" indicate boxes.